Tissue Integration in Oral, Orthopedic, and Maxillofacial Reconstruction

Tissue Integration in Oral, Orthopedic, and Maxillofacial Reconstruction

Edited by

William R. Laney, DMD, MS
Professor
Department of Dentistry
Mayo Clinic—Mayo Medical Center
Rochester, Minnesota

Dan E. Tolman, DDS, MSD
Associate Professor
Department of Dentistry
Mayo Clinic—Mayo Medical Center
Rochester, Minnesota

Proceedings of the Second International Congress on Tissue Integration in Oral, Orthopedic, and Maxillofacial Reconstruction

Mayo Medical Center
Rochester, Minnesota
September 23–27, 1990

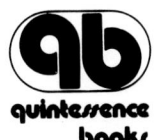
quintessence
books

Quintessence Publishing Co, Inc
Chicago, London, Berlin, São Paulo, Hong Kong, and Tokyo

Library of Congress Cataloging-in-Publication Data

International Congress on Tissue Integration in Oral, Orthopedic, and Maxillofacial Reconstruction
   (2nd : 1990 : Mayo Medical Center)
     Tissue integration in oral, orthopedic, and maxillofacial reconstruction : proceedings of the Second International Congress on Tissue Integration in Oral, Orthopedic, and Maxillofacial Reconstruction, Mayo Medical Center, Rochester, Minnesota, September 23–27, 1990 / edited by William R. Laney, Dan E. Tolman.
       p.   cm.
    Includes bibliographical references.
    ISBN 0-86715-251-6
    1. Tissue-integrated prostheses—Congresses.   2. Osseointegrated dental implants —
Congresses.   3. Implant dentures—congresses.   I. Laney, William R. 1928-
II. Tolman, Dan E.   III. Title.
    [DNLM: 1. Dental Implantion, Endosseous—congresses.   2. Dental Implants—Congresses.
3. Maxillofacial Prosthesis—congresses.   4. Osseointegration—congresses.   WU 600 I612t 1990]
RK667.T57I58   1990
617.6'9—dc 20
DNLM/DLC
for Library of Congress   91-45702
                                                              CIP

quintessence
books

Composition: Midwest Technical Publications, St Louis, MO
Printing and binding: Edwards Brothers Inc, Ann Arbor, MI
Printed in USA

Proceedings of the Second International Congress on Tissue Integration in Oral, Orthopedic, and Maxillofacial Reconstruction

Mayo Medical Center, Rochester, Minnesota
September 23–27, 1990

Organizing Committee

Tomas Albrektsson
Department of Handicap Research
Biomaterials Group
University of Göteborg
Brunnsgatan 2
S-413 12 Göteborg, Sweden

Per-Ingvar Brånemark
The Institute for Applied Biotechnology
Box 33053
S-400 33 Göteborg, Sweden

Patrick J. Henry
The Brånemark Center
64 Havelock Street
West Perth, Western Australia 6005

Kenji W. Higuchi
East 12509 Mission
Spokane, Washington 99216 USA

G. Richard Holt
Division of Otorhinolaryngology
University of Texas Health Science Center
7703 Floyd Curl Drive
San Antonio, Texas 78284 USA

Richard Skalak
Department of Applied Mechanics
and Engineering Science
University of California at San Diego
Bioengineering R 012
La Jolla, California 92093–0412 USA

Daniel van Steenberghe
Department of Periodontology
Faculty of Medicine
Catholic University Leuven
Capucijnenvoer 7
3000 Leuven, Belgium

Philip Worthington
Department of Oral and
Maxillofacial Surgery
Warren G. Magnuson Health Sciences
Center
University of Washington
Room B 241, 5B–24
Seattle, Washington 98195 USA

William R. Laney, Co-Chairman
Department of Dentistry
Mayo Clinic and Mayo Foundation
Mayo Medical Center
Rochester, Minnesota 55905 USA

Dan E. Tolman, Co-Chairman
Department of Dentistry
Mayo Clinic and Mayo Foundation
Mayo Medical Center
Rochester, Minnesota 55905 USA

**Ned B. Van Roekel, Chairman,
Local Arrangements**
Department of Dentistry
Mayo Clinic and Mayo Foundation
Mayo Medical Center
Rochester, Minnesota 55905 USA

Contents

Session III   Moderator, R.P. Desjardins

Contents

Session VI   Moderator, D.E. Tolman

Contributors

J.C. Abarno*
Montevideo, Uruguay

T. Albrektsson
Department of Handicap Research
Biomaterials Group
University of Göteborg
Göteborg, Sweden

C. Aparicio
Barcelona, Spain

J. Awerbuch
Department of Mechanical Engineering Mechanics
Drexel University
Philadelphia, Pennsylvania

C.A. Babbush*
Section of Implant Reconstructive Surgery
Mt. Sinai Medical Center
Cleveland, Ohio

R.E. Baier*
Department of Biomaterials
School of Dental Medicine
State University of New York
Buffalo, New York

T.J. Balshi*
Institute for Facial Esthetics
Fort Washington, Pennsylvania

E. Barth*
Lunceford-Moore Orthopaedic Research
   Laboratory
School of Medicine
University of South Carolina
Columbia, South Carolina

B.E. Becker*
Tucson, Arizona

W. Becker
Department of Periodontics
School of Dentistry
University of Southern California
Los Angeles, California

U. Benzing
Department of Prosthodontic Dentistry
Dental School
University of Tübingen
Tübingen, Germany

L.L. Berge
Department of Orthopedics
Biomechanics Laboratory
Mayo Clinic/Mayo Foundation
Rochester, Minnesota

P. Binon*
Roseville, California

A.T. Bishop
Department of Orthopedics
Biomechanics Laboratory
Mayo Clinic/Mayo Foundation
Rochester, Minnesota

P.-I. Brånemark*
Institute for Applied Biotechnology
Göteborg, Sweden

A.M.S. Brown*
Department of Maxillofacial Surgery
Selly Oak Hospital
Birmingham, England

C.L. Brownd*
Denver, Colorado

D.M. Brunette*
Department of Oral Biology
Faculty of Dentistry
University of British Columbia
Vancouver, Canada

J.B. Brunski*
Department of Biomedical Engineering
Rensselaer Polytechnic Institute
Troy, New York

A. Buchs
Orlando, Florida

D. Buser*
Department of Oral & Maxillofacial Surgery
School of Dental Medicine
University of Berne
Berne, Switzerland

A. Callens
Department of Periodontology
Faculty of Medicine
Catholic University–Leuven
Leuven, Belgium

R. Cellete
Rome, Italy

N. Chafetz
Torrance, California

E.Y.S. Chao*
Department of Orthopedics
Biomechanics Laboratory
Mayo Clinic/Mayo Foundation
Rochester, Minnesota

B. Chehroudi
Department of Oral Biology
Faculty of Dentistry
University of British Columbia
Vancouver, Canada

M. Chipman
Department of Preventative Medicine
Faculty of Dentistry
University of Toronto
Toronto, Canada

G.V.B. Cochran
Orthopedic Engineering & Research Center
Helen Hayes Hospital
West Haverstraw, New York

T.A. Collins*
Springfield, Missouri

P.W. Cowan*
Dublin, Ireland

P. Darius
Laboratory for Statistics & Experimental Design
Faculty of Agricultural Sciences
Catholic University of Leuven
Heverlee, Belgium

M. Deadman*
Department of Maxillofacial Surgery
Queen Elizabeth Hospital
Birmingham, England

D.A. Deporter*
Department of Periodontics
Faculty of Dentistry
University of Toronto
Toronto, Canada

P. Doms
Department of Maxillofacial Surgery
Schaerbeck Hospital
Brussels, Belgium

W.B. Donohue*
Department of Stomatology
Faculty of Dental Medicine
University of Montreal
Montreal, Canada

J. Dootson
Department of Oral & Maxillofacial Surgery
Moncrief Army Hospital
Fort Jackson, South Carolina

L. Duchateau
Department of Periodontics
Faculty of Medicine
Catholic University–Leuven
Leuven, Belgium

P. Ducheyne
Department of Bioengineering
School of Dental Medicine
University of Pennsylvania
Philadelphia, Pennsylvania

R.W. Dykema
Department of Prosthodontics
School of Dentistry
Indiana University
Indianapolis, Indiana

L.E. Ericson
Department of Anatomy
University of Göteborg
Göteborg, Sweden

I. Ericsson*
Department of Periodontology
Faculty of Odontology
University of Göteborg
Göteborg, Sweden

M. Filiaggi
Department of Metallurgy & Materials Science
Center for Biomaterials
University of Toronto
Toronto, Canada

W.D. Gates*
Department of Prosthodontics

College of Dentistry
University of Iowa
Iowa City, Iowa

P.-O. Glantz
Department of Prosthetic Dentistry
Faculty of Odontology
University of Lund
Malmö, Sweden

K. Gotfredsen*
Department of Prosthetic Dentistry
Royal Dental College
Copenhagen, Denmark

T.R.L. Gould
Department of Clinical Dental Sciences
Faculty of Dentistry
University of British Columbia
Vancouver, Canada

R. Greer
Department of Oral Pathology
School of Dentistry
University of Colorado
Denver, Colorado

J. Gunne
Department of Prosthetic Dentistry
University of Umeå
Umeå, Sweden

M. Handelsman
Los Angeles, California

Å. Hansson
Department of Handicap Research
Biomaterials Group
University of Göteborg
Göteborg, Sweden

D. Harris*
Blackrock Clinic and Trinity College
Dublin, Ireland

R.M. Heballi*
Department of Oral Surgery
Government Dental College
Bangalore, India

K.W. Higuchi*
Spokane, Washington

E. Hjörting-Hansen
Department of Oral & Maxillofacial Surgery
Royal Dental College
Copenhagen, Denmark

G. Holt
San Antonio, Texas

S.J. Hoshaw*
Department of Biomedical Engineering
Rensselaer Polytechnic Institute
Troy, New York

S.A. Hum*
Winston-Salem, South Carolina

S.C. Jacks
College of Dentistry
Ohio State University
Columbus, Ohio

M. Jacobsson*
Department of Handicap Research
Biomaterials Group
University of Göteborg
Göteborg, Sweden

O.T. Jensen*
Department of Oral Pathology
School of Dentistry
University of Colorado
Denver, Colorado

C.B. Johansson*
Department of Handicap Research
Biomaterials Group
University of Göteborg
Göteborg, Sweden

K. Johnsson
Department of Handicap Research
Biomaterials Group
University of Göteborg
Göteborg, Sweden

S.A. Jovanovic*
Department of Prosthodontics
University of Aachen
Aachen, Germany

A.H. Kafrawy
Department of Dental Diagnostic Sciences
School of Dentistry
Indiana University
Indianapolis, Indiana

D.H. Kohn*
Department of Biologic & Materials Sciences
School of Dentistry
University of Michigan
Ann Arbor, Michigan

M. Kohri*
Department of Removable Prosthetics
School of Dentistry
Hokkaido University
Kita-ku Sapporo, Japan

M. Koseoglu
Department of Prosthodontics
University of Aachen
Aachen, Germany

J. Krauser*
Palm Beach, Florida

R.A. Kraut*
Montefiore Medical Center
Albert Einstein College of Medicine
Bronx, New York

N.P. Lang
Department of Prosthodontics
School of Dental Medicine
University of Berne
Berne, Switzerland

P.E. Larsen
Department of Oral & Maxillofacial Surgery
College of Dentistry
Ohio State University
Columbus, Ohio

L. Laurell*
Department of Periodontics
Institute for Postgraduate Dental Education
S-Jönköping, Sweden

R.J. Lazzara*
West Palm Beach, Florida

U. Lekholm*
Faculty of Odontology
Brånemark Clinic
University of Göteborg
Göteborg, Sweden

Y.N. Li*
Department of Orthopedics
Biomechanics Laboratory
Mayo Clinic/Mayo Foundation
Rochester, Minnesota

R. Lubar
Northbrook, Illinois

G. Lundborg*
Department of Hand Surgery
Malmö General Hospital
University of Lund
Malmö, Sweden

D. Lundgren*
Department of Periodontics
Institute for Postgraduate Dental Education
S-Jönköping, Sweden

A. McCullen
Veterinary Services
Tripler Army Medical Center
Tripler AMC, Hawaii

E.A. McGlumphy*
Department of Restorative Dentistry
College of Dentistry
Ohio State University
Columbus, Ohio

D.A. Mendel
Department of Restorative Dentistry
College of Dentistry
Ohio State University
Columbus, Ohio

A.E. Meyer
Department of Biomaterials
School of Dental Medicine
State University of New York
Buffalo, New York

P. Meyer
Department of Oral Surgery
School of Dentistry
University of Marseilles
Marseilles, France

I. Naert*
Department of Prosthetic Dentistry
Catholic University–Leuven
Leuven, Belgium

J.R. Natiella
Department of Biomaterials
School of Dental Medicine
State University of New York
Buffalo, New York

G.A. Niznick*
Core-Vent Corporation, Inc
Encino, California

C. Ochsenbein
Dallas, Texas

T.J. O'Leary*
Department of Periodontics
School of Dentistry
Indiana University
Indianapolis, Indiana

J. Olivé*
Barcelona, Spain

D. Patrick*
Dentsply/Core-Vent Implant Division
Encino, California

M. Pharoah
Department of Radiology
Faculty of Dentistry
University of Toronto
Toronto, Canada

R.M. Pilliar*
Center for Biomaterials
Faculty of Dentistry
University of Toronto
Toronto, Canada

D.W. Proops
Departments of Maxillofacial & ENT Surgery
Queen Elizabeth Medical Center
Birmingham, England

M. Quirynen*
Department of Periodontology
Faculty of Medicine
Catholic University–Leuven
Leuven, Belgium

B. Rangert*
Nobelpharma AB
Göteborg, Sweden

E.-J. Richter*
Department of Prosthodontics
University of Aachen
Aachen, Germany

S.L.G. Rothman
Torrance, California

G. Sales*
Montevideo, Uruguay

H.-J. Schmitz*
Department of Maxillofacial & Facial Plastic Surgery
University of Aachen
Aachen, Germany

F.M. Schultz
Department of Orthopedics
Biomechanics Laboratory
Mayo Clinic/Mayo Foundation
Rochester, Minnesota

M.S. Schwarz*
Torrance, California

G. Scortecci*
Department of Oral Surgery
School of Dentistry
University of Marseilles
Marseilles, France

L. Sennerby*
Departments of Anatomy & Handicap Research

University of Göteborg
Göteborg, Sweden

J.M. Slack*
Spokane, Washington

D.C. Smith
Center for Biomaterials
Faculty of Dentistry
University of Toronto
Toronto, Canada

C. Sollerman
Department of Hand Surgery
Malmö General Hospital
University of Lund
Malmö, Sweden

H. Spiekermann*
Department of Prosthodontics
University of Aachen
Aachen, Germany

B. Stauts
Torrance, California

E.A. Stuebner
Department of Oral & Maxillofacial Surgery
School of Dentistry
University of Illinois
Chicago, Illinois

D.Y. Sullivan
Washington, DC

T. Sullivan
Department of Pathology
School of Medicine
University of South Carolina
Columbia, South Carolina

J.L. Taylor*
Department of Biomedical Engineering
Rensselaer Polytechnic Institute
Troy, New York

P. Thomsen*
Department of Anatomy
University of Göteborg
Göteborg, Sweden

I. Turesson
Department of Handicap Research
Biomaterials Group
University of Göteborg
Göteborg, Sweden

D. van Steenberghe*
Department of Periodontology

Faculty of Medicine
Catholic University–Leuven
Leuven, Belgium

M.J.C. Wake
Departments of Maxillofacial & ENT Surgery
Queen Elizabeth Medical Center
Birmingham, England

L. Walker
Department of Prosthodontics
Veterans Affairs Medical Center
San Francisco, California

L. Watanabe
Department of Restorative Dentistry
School of Dentistry
University of California
San Francisco, California

P.A. Watson
Center for Biomaterials
Faculty of Dentistry
University of Toronto
Toronto, Canada

H. Weber*
Department of Prosthodontics
School of Dentistry

University of Tübingen
Tübingen, Germany

D. Weir
Department of Restorative Dentistry
School of Dentistry
University of California
San Francisco, California

T.L. West*
Department of Periodontics
School of Dental and Oral Surgery
Columbia University
New York, New York

G.A. Zarb*
Department of Prosthodontics
Faculty of Dentistry
University of Toronto
Toronto, Canada

H. Zattara
Department of Oral Surgery
School of Dentistry
University of Marseilles
Marseilles, France

J. Zosky
Orthopedic & Arthritic Hospital
Toronto, Canada

Introduction

On May 22–24, 1985, the First International Congress on Tissue Integration in Oral and Maxillofacial Reconstruction was held in Brussels, Belgium. More than 250 participants from 22 countries participated in an exchange of ideas on tissue integration in the craniofacial area during the three-day conference. The Organizing Committee for the First Congress consisted of: Maxwell Abramson (New York), Per-Ingvar Brånemark (Gothenburg, Sweden), Gunnar Carlsson (Gothenburg, Sweden), Leo Coppes (Amsterdam), Gunnar Lidén (Minneapolis), Valle Oikarinen (Helsinki), Richard Skalak (New York), and Daniel van Steenberghe, Chairman (Leuven). The proceedings of the First Congress were edited by Daniel van Steenberghe and published by Excerpta Medica, Amsterdam, in 1986.

The primary aim of the organizers of the First Congress was to consider both the basic scientific and clinical aspects of extraoral and intraoral tissue-integrated implants. The targeted participants were general dentists, oral surgeons, periodontists, prosthodontists, maxillofacial surgeons, ENT surgeons, ophthalmologists, plastic surgeons, and basic scientists. It was envisioned that meetings of this nature could be held periodically to improve international communication and cooperative efforts in treating oral and paraoral defects with tissue-integrated prostheses.

The Second International Congress was scheduled for presentation in the United States 5 years later. The Mayo Medical Center, Rochester, Minnesota, was selected as the host site and meeting dates of September 23–27, 1990, were established. The objectives of the Second Congress remained twofold: (1) to evaluate through scholarly presentations both the scientific and clinical aspects of intraoral and extraoral as well as orthopedic tissue-integrated implants, and (2) to hold concurrent group discussions on the state of the art in the related basic and applicable clinical sciences. The latter portion of the Congress was expanded by the organization of four invited consensus panels of approximately 15 participants each. These groups considered pertinent topics and questions assigned by the Organizing Committee regarding the broad areas of basic science, intraoral, craniofacial, and orthopedic applications of tissue integration. Their deliberations were formalized in panel reports that were presented to the Congress assembly on the last day of the meeting.

A Third International Congress has tentatively been scheduled for 1995. While the general goals and objectives will remain the same, specific topics and subject areas for emphasis have yet to be identified.

Whereas the First Congress emphasized primarily craniofacial reconstruction utilizing bone-anchored implant support, the Second Congress included pertinent related aspects of basic science as well as the application of tissue-integrated prostheses to oral, craniofacial, and, for the first time, orthopedic reconstruction. Some 50 oral scientific presentations were made on such topics as the physical and chemical aspects of implant materials, characterization of the interface between living tissue and alloplastic surfaces, cell biology and biomechanics, load transfer, orthopedic fixation, preparation of tissues, patient selection, and long-term clinical results. Sixteen poster clinics were also presented. All of the speakers and poster clinicians were invited by the Congress Organizing Committee by virtue of their selection based on presubmitted abstracts. Nine keynote speakers with internationally recognized expertise addressed assigned topics in pertinent areas of interest. The presentations by the four consensus panels were also an integral part of this Congress.

Participants, representing 24 countries, were officially welcomed to the Mayo Medical Center by Dr Robert Waller, chairman of the Mayo Board of Governors, chief executive officer of the Mayo Medical Center, and an internationally known ophthalmologist. His introductory remarks included a brief review of the Mayo institutions and the historical evolution of one of the world's largest integrated group practices of medicine. He cited the medical center's mission and objectives in light of its three main areas of activity: clinical practice, education, and research.

The opening keynote speaker, Per-Ingvar Brånemark, Gothenburg, Sweden, set the stage for the Congress by retracing the evolution of the osseointegration concept and its relationship to tissue-integrated prostheses. Whereas the application of tissue-integrated prostheses in the past has been primarily for the replacement of missing teeth, more recently interests have been centered on craniofacial and orthopedic restorations.

Professor Brånemark noted that clinical documentation has established the tissue-anchored prosthesis as a safe and beneficial treatment modality for the rehabilitation of the edentulous patient. This has initiated rapidly growing interest in the understanding of basic mechanisms related to response and behavior of materials and living tissues. It has also identified diagnostic criteria and factors affecting prognostic predictability.

Encouraging long-term intraoral results has prompted the application of similar procedures to extraoral rehabilitation — and more recently, outside the craniomaxillofacial region, to hand surgery and orthopedics. Professor Brånemark suggested that in the development and modification of rational clinical procedures, it is necessary to respect the limitations that are related to our incomplete understanding of the dynamic interface between biologic and nonbiologic components, their composition, reaction, and long-term interaction.

The scientific papers that were presented are provided herein in the order of speaker appearance. Papers that are not printed in their entirety have been included by way of abstract, as some have been submitted for publication or are in press elsewhere. Open discussions that followed the oral presentations are provided to demonstrate the participants' interaction with speakers as well as that between speakers. The abstracts of poster presentations are also printed herein to provide a complete rendering of scientific program content.

The reports of the four consensus panels are appended to the scientific program. These documents represent the state-of-the-art knowledge and clinical procedure as determined by the panels of invited experts who participated.

Acknowledgments

The Organizing Committee of the Second International Congress on Tissue Integration in Oral, Orthopedic, and Maxillofacial Reconstruction is most grateful for and indebted to the following who provided generous educational grants for the conduct of the Congress.

Institute for Applied Biotechnology, Gothenburg, Sweden;
Nobelpharma USA, Inc, Chicago, Illinois;
Quintessence Publishing Co, Inc, Carol Stream, Illinois;
W.L. Gore and Associates, Flagstaff, Arizona;
Core-Vent Corporation, Encino, California

Electron Microscopic Observations on the Effects of Surface Topography on the Behavior of Cells Attached to Percutaneous and Subcutaneous Implants

D.M. Brunette, B. Chehroudi, and T.R.L. Gould

Dental implants, percutaneous devices (PD), and natural teeth encounter particular difficulties occasioned by their anatomical location, for they penetrate a stratified epithelium and extend into a microbe-rich environment. Factors associated with the success of artificial implants include mechanical stability and the achievement of an epithelial seal.[1] For dental implants, it is generally accepted that osseointegration provides a stable means of anchoring the implant, and osseointegrated implants have functioned in some instances for decades. Percutaneous devices on the other hand are generally placed in soft tissues and have more limited lifetimes.[2] As noted by von Recum et al,[3] the skin/implant interface generally fails to heal and the device needs to be removed because of extrusion and infection. Such considerations lead to the hypothesis that percutaneous devices would be more successful if means were adopted so that the device could be embedded in bone. Jansen et al[4] observed that direct and indirect bone anchoring favors the longevity of percutaneous implants.

A second approach is to alter the surface topography of the device to stabilize the cell-device interactions. The inherent problem with this approach, however, is that two populations of cells, fibroblasts and epithelium, are involved, and these cell populations differ markedly in their locomotory and proliferative behavior. For example, velours have been used on the surface of PD to facilitate soft connective tissue ingrowth, but the connective tissue could not resist the processes of epithelial permigration and marsupialization of the surface, and the devices consequently failed.[3]

Another approach has been to employ micromachining to tailor grooved surfaces specifically for epithelial cells and fibroblasts so that their behavior is controlled appropriately, but micromachined surfaces have been tested only in brief experiments less than 3 weeks in duration.[5–7] In this paper we report light and electron microscopic observations on the response of epithelium and soft connective tissue to micromachined grooved surfaces implanted in the rat percutaneously for 1 week and subcutaneously for as long as 10 weeks. It was found that 19-μm-deep grooved surfaces oriented connective tissue cells but that the time course for producing this orientation differed between the subcutaneous and percutaneous locations. An unexpected observation was that the grooved, but not control smooth, surfaces produced in some instances a bonelike tissue adjacent to the implant.

Materials and methods

Fabrication of implants

Grooves were etched on silicon substrata by micromachining, a method that was developed originally for fabrication of high-quality photomasks for solar cells.[8] The depth and spacing of an anisotropically etched groove or pit can be regulated by the time of etching and the crystalline orientation of the silicon wafer. This study employed 19-μm-deep, V-shaped grooves whose walls formed a 55° angle with the surface. The grooves were 15-μm wide across the top and separated by 15-μm flat ridges.

Impressions of the micromachined surfaces were made in a vinyl silicone impression material (Exaflex, G-C Dental, Tokyo, Japan), and the impressions were used to cast replicas of the original patterns in epoxy resin (Epotek 3 oz-3, Epoxy Technology, Billerica, Mass). Replicas were then used to make implants as described previously.[5,6] The subcutaneous implants (SCI) were U-shaped and had two protruding parts connected to each other by a flat pedestal. Each protruding part was 2 mm tall and had an outer surface that faced laterally and an inner surface that faced medially. The percutaneous implants (PI) were similar to the subcutaneous implants; however, they were made taller ($\approx$ 5 mm) to penetrate the skin. Grooves were cast on the four test surfaces so that the long axis of the grooves would parallel the surface of the skin when placed in situ. The SCI and PI were baked at 60°C for 3 days, and then coated with $\approx$ 50 nm titanium using a sputter coater (Randex, Palo Alto, Calif).

Preparation and characterization of surfaces

The titanium-coated implants were cleaned ultrasonically for 20 minutes in a detergent specifically formulated for tissue culture (7X Flow Labs, McLean, Va). After being rinsed 20 times with deionized, sterile distilled water, they were dried overnight in a tissue culture laminar-flow hood, treated for 3 minutes in an argon gas glow-discharge chamber, and immediately stored in deionized, degassed, sterile distilled water in exhaustively cleaned, watertight Teflon vials. Three components of each implant were numbered and packed individually. At least one randomly chosen sample from each batch of titanium-coated implants was inspected by

scanning electron microscopy (SEM) for the quality of groove shape as well as the smoothness and continuity of the titanium coating. In addition, the titanium surfaces resulting from the cleaning procedure were analyzed by x-ray photoelectron spectroscopy (XPS) at the National ESCA and Surface Analysis Center for Biomedical Problems, University of Washington, Seattle, Washington.

Implantation procedure

The implantation procedure has been described in detail previously.[5] In brief, inbred Sprague-Dawley rats, weighing from 400 to 450 g, were intubated and anesthetized using halothane. Then the fur above the parietal area was shaved and treated with depilatory, and the underlying skin scrubbed with Betadine (Purdue Frederich Inc, Toronto, Canada) for 1 minute followed by 70% ethanol for 1 minute. For percutaneous implantation, an access incision was made distally from the base of one ear to the other, then two parallel incisions were made at right angles to the access incision and approximately 5 mm medial to it, so that they were just sufficient in size to accommodate the two protruding skin-penetrating components with a tight fit. The epidermal and dermal layers over the periosteum were reflected from the access incision toward the two parallel incisions. The implant was then placed through the access incision so that after manipulation, the two skin-penetrating components were threaded through the two parallel incisions. Finally, the access incision was sutured using 4-0 silk sutures and the animals received a prophylactic intramuscular injection of antibiotics (Pen-Di-Stred, Roger STP, London, Canada). All surgery was performed under full sterile conditions, and animals were kept in 60-cm-tall cages to reduce the chances of the implant rubbing against the ceiling of the cage. In addition, the animals with percutaneous devices were fitted with Elizabethan collars to reduce their ability to disturb the implant by rubbing it with their paws.

For subcutaneous implantation, an access incision in the parietal area was made distally from one ear to the other. The epidermal and dermal layers as well as the periosteum were removed by a combination of blunt and sharp dissection to form a pouch sufficient for the implant. In addition, the discontinuity of the bone under the implant was smoothed by means of a bone file. Implants were then placed on the parietal bone and the access incision was sutured using 4-0 silk. Animals received a prophylactic intramuscular injection of antibiotics.

Specimen collection and preparation

For subcutaneous implants, two animals were sacrificed every week up to the 11th week after placement. Animals with percutaneous implants were terminated by an overdose of sodium pentobarbital 1 week after surgery and the implants removed. Prior to complete collapse of the heart, perfusion was carried out through the left ventricle with a solution of 2.5% glutaraldehyde in 0.1 M sodium phosphate buffer, preceded by a 5-minute flush of warm, heparinized normal saline into the blood circulation. The implant and the tissue around it were gently removed using a no. 15 scalpel blade and placed in Karnowsky's fixative for 24 hours at 4° C. Secondary fixation was with 2% buffered OsO_4 on a rotator for 3 hours. At this stage the SCI and the PI were cut in two, and fixation was allowed to continue for an additional 2 hours. Because the standard dehydrating agent, alcohol, had been previously found to damage the grooves and undermine the titanium coating, Aquembed (Ladd, Burlington, Vt), a water-miscible resin, was used. Specimens were dehydrated in graded Aquembed (50% to 100%, 1 hour in each change), then infiltrated with graded Aquembed/Epon (J.B. EM Dorval, Canada) (50% to 100%, 1 hour in each change) on the rotator. The specimens stayed on the rotator overnight in fresh Epon. The next day, infiltration was carried out with three changes of fresh Epon without accelerator (2 hours in each change), followed by three changes of Epon with accelerator (2 hours in each change).

Specimens were then placed under vacuum at 4°C overnight and finally embedded in Epon.

Histology

Sections were taken throughout the length of the implant using a Sorvall MT2 microtome. For light microscopy, two μm-thick sections were cut in an orientation such that the horizontal grooves were cross sectioned. Sections were stained with toluidine blue and examined under the microscope at ×500 magnification. For transmission electron microscopy (TEM), 50- to 60-nm-thick sections of the implants were cut with a diamond knife from various regions of the epithelial and connective tissue attachment. The sections were then stained with alcoholic uranyl acetate and aqueous lead citrate and viewed under an electron microscope.

Results

Implant surface preparation

Scanning electron microscopic observations of the test surfaces indicated that grooves were replicated identically to the master pattern on the silicon wafers, and the titanium coating was smooth and continuous. X-ray photoelectron spectroscopy analysis, which characterizes the outer 50 to 100 Å of the test surfaces, disclosed that the major titanium class was Ti^{+4} (binding energy = 459 eV). As another major element present was oxygen, it was probable that the surface consisted largely of TiO_2. Other elements found on the implant surface included carbon and traces of nitrogen.

Clinical observations

Clinical signs of inflammation, such as swelling and redness, were apparent after placement of the SCI. The swelling gradually resolved after

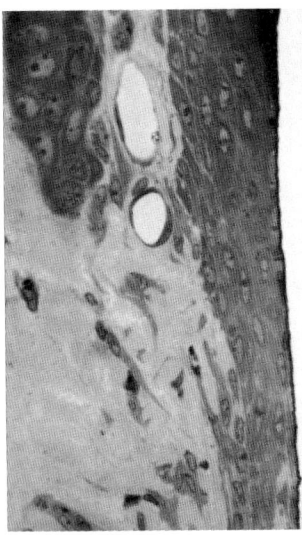

Fig 1 Light micrograph of a toluidine-blue-stained section of a titanium-coated, percutaneous, smooth-surfaced implant in the region of epithelial attachment to the implant. The implant had been in place 1 week (original magnification $\times 700$).

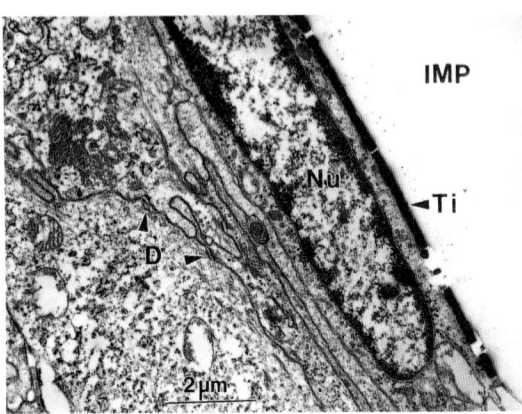

Fig 2 Electron micrograph of a titanium-coated, percutaneous, smooth-surfaced implant in the region of epithelial attachment to the implant. The implant had been in place 1 week. Note close adaptation of epithelium to the surface. The labels *D, Ti, IMP,* and *Nu* indicate desmosomes, titanium coating, implant, and nucleus, respectively.

the first week of implantation. Percutaneous implants also demonstrated some evidence of inflammation, which resolved itself within 2 days of surgery. In this series of experiments, 20

implants were placed percutaneously, of which 18 were recovered and processed for light and for electron microscopy. All 22 of the subcutaneous implants were recovered and processed for light and electron microscopy.

Light and electron microscopy observations

Percutaneous implants

Both connective tissue and epithelium were closely attached to at least part of the test surfaces of implants, and at $\times 400$ magnification, a clear outline of the cell nucleus and often the entire cell boundary could be identified. Differences were found between epithelial and connective tissue cells' location, orientation, and extent of attachment on grooved and smooth surfaces, as will be described shortly.

As observed previously,[7] 1 week after implantation a close epithelial attachment was observed on the smooth surface (Figs 1 and 2). However, on the 19-μm-deep grooved surface the epithelial cells were found to attach closely only to the ridges, and the cells did not enter the grooves (Figs 3 and 4).

One week after placement, the connective tissue could be categorized as young granulation tissue. However, this tissue was more organized and contained more fibroblasts and fewer inflammatory cells and contacted the implant surface more intimately than the subcutaneous implants at 1 week (Fig 5). In some instances, the fibroblasts had adopted a perpendicular or oblique orientation to the 19-μm-deep grooved surface (Fig 6). Examination of the fibroblasts attached to grooved surfaces in the electron microscope demonstrated that cell processes extended deeply into the grooves (Fig 7).

Subcutaneous implants

One week after implantation, an immature granulation tissue comprising remnants of red blood cells, fibrin meshwork, neutrophils, macrophages, and occasional large fibroblasts was found. Fibroblasts could be located within

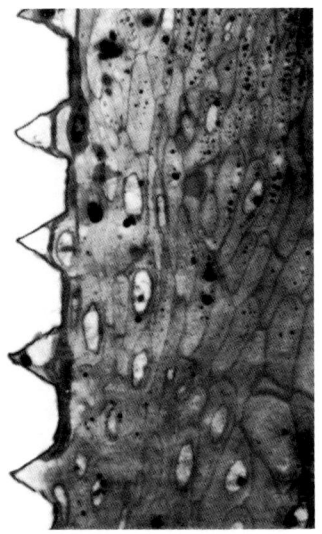

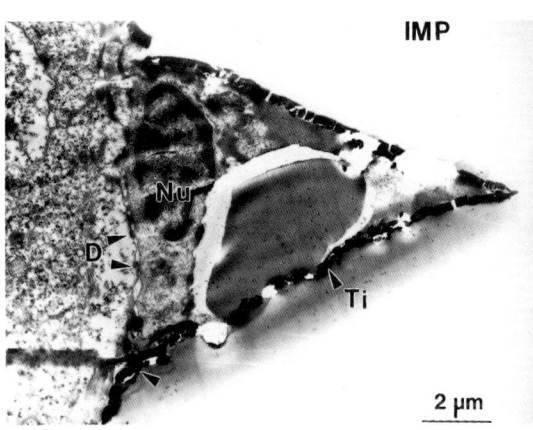

Fig 4 Electron micrograph of a section of a titanium-coated, percutaneous implant with 19-μm-deep grooves in the region of epithelial attachment to the implant. The implant had been in place 1 week. Note that the epithelial cell body is not found in the deeper regions of the groove. The labels *D, Ti, IMP,* and *Nu* indicate desmosomes, titanium coating, implant, and nucleus, respectively.

Fig 3 Light micrograph of a toluidine-blue-stained section of a titanium-coated, percutaneous implant with 19-μm-deep grooves in the region of epithelial attachment to the implant. The implant had been in place 1 week. Note that the epithelium bridged over the grooves and was tightly attached at the ridges (original magnification × 700).

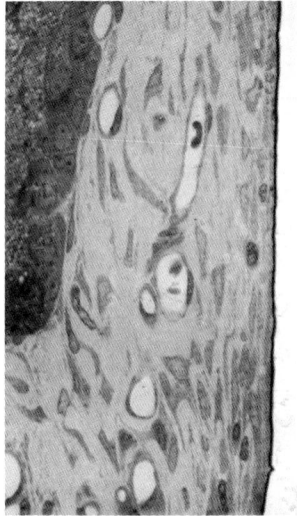

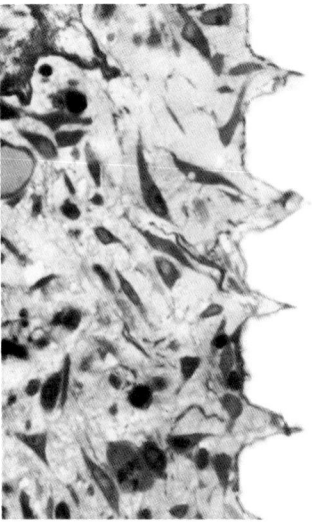

Fig 5 Light micrograph of a toluidine-blue-stained section of a titanium-coated, percutaneous, smooth-surfaced implant in the region of connective tissue attachment to the implant. The implant had been in place 1 week. Note that the fibroblasts are oriented parallel to the long axis of the implant (original magnification × 700).

Fig 6 Light micrograph of a toluidine-blue-stained section of a titanium-coated, percutaneous implant with 19-μm-deep grooves in the region of connective tissue attachment to the implant. The implant had been in place 1 week. Note the oblique orientation of the fibroblasts relative to the grooved implant surface (original magnification × 700).

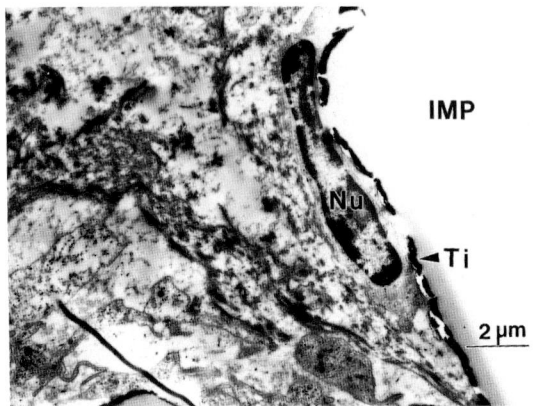

Fig 7 Electron micrograph of a section of a titanium-coated, percutaneous implant with 19-μm-deep grooves in the region of connective tissue attachment to the implant. The implant had been in place 1 week. Note that the fibroblast processes penetrate deeply into the groove. The labels *Ti, IMP,* and *Nu* indicate titanium coating, implant, and nucleus, respectively.

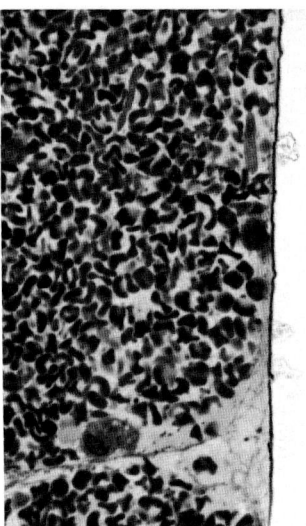

Fig 8 Light micrograph of a toluidine-blue-stained section of a titanium-coated, subcutaneous, smooth-surfaced implant. The implant had been in place 1 week. The tissue in the vicinity of the implant could be described as immature granulation tissue (original magnification ×700).

grooves as well as in the vicinity of the smooth surfaces (Fig 8). After 2 weeks, the dominant cells were large fibroblasts, macrophages, and a few neutrophils. On the smooth surface, several cells were aligned in such a manner as to suggest that a capsule was being formed. On the grooved surface, fibroblasts were located within the grooves and in close contact with the ridges, but there was no evidence of capsule formation. Some fibroblasts were oriented at an oblique or near perpendicular angle to the long axis of the implant. After 3 weeks, the capsule had become thicker on the smooth surface (Fig 9) and a thin capsule comprising ≈ two layers of fibroblasts had formed on the grooved surfaces (Fig 10). Fibroblasts within the grooves appeared either rounded or elongated in the direction of the grooves.

Although the thickness of the capsule continued to increase on the smooth surfaces, no apparent changes were noted in the thickness of the capsule near the grooved surfaces in the fourth or fifth week. However, the cytoplasm of cells located inside the grooves became con-

densed and the cell boundary became indistinct. These cells stained distinctively darker than other cells located farther from the implant surface. Five weeks postimplantation, an increase in the number of mast cells with distinct cytoplasmic granules was noted in the vicinity of both the smooth and grooved implants (Fig 11).

Mineralization

Ten weeks after implantation, densely staining foci were observed on some of the 19-μm-deep grooved surfaces, and some cells in the vicinity of the implant had the appearance of osteoblasts (Fig 12). In some instances, portions of blocks had to be demineralized in ethylenediamine tetraacetic acid (EDTA) and embedded again in Epon before they could be sectioned. Cells within the foci had an osteocytelike appearance, as they resided in distinct lacunae and had several extended cell processes (Fig 13). Thus, as these foci contained osteoblast-like and osteocytelike cells and mineralized extracellular matrix, they are referred to as bone-

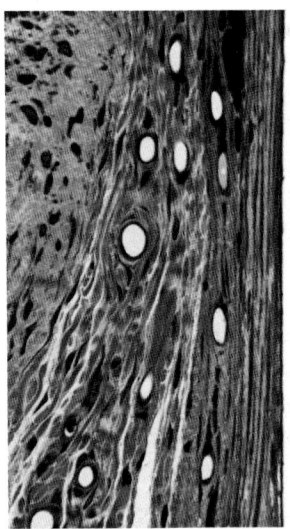

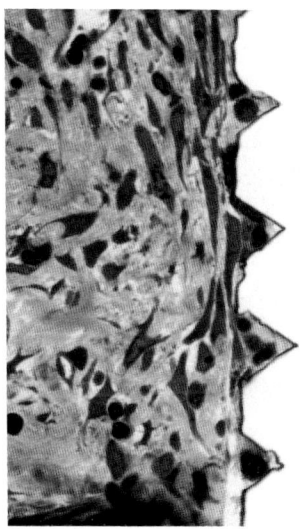

Fig 9 Light micrograph of a toluidine-blue-stained section of a titanium-coated, subcutaneous, smooth-surfaced implant. The implant had been in place 3 weeks and a connective tissue capsule had formed (original magnification ×700).

Fig 10 Light micrograph of a toluidine-blue-stained section of a titanium-coated, subcutaneous implant with 19-μm-deep grooves. The implant had been in place 3 weeks. A thin capsule comprising about two cell layers had formed and cells within the grooves were either round or oriented with their long axis running in the direction of the grooves (original magnification ×700).

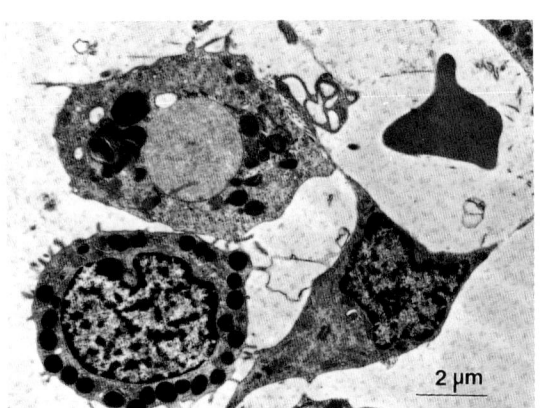

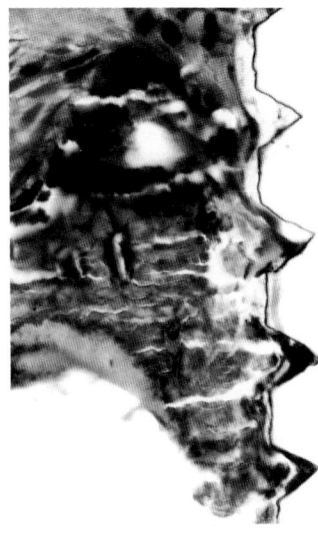

Fig 11 An electron micrograph of a mast cell observed in the vicinity of a subcutaneous implant that had been in place 11 weeks.

Fig 12 Light micrograph of a toluidine-blue-stained section of a titanium-coated, subcutaneous implant with 19-μm-deep grooves. The implant had been in place 11 weeks. A nodule of mineralized tissue had formed adjacent to the grooves. Arrows indicate osteocytelike cells within the nodule (original magnification ×700).

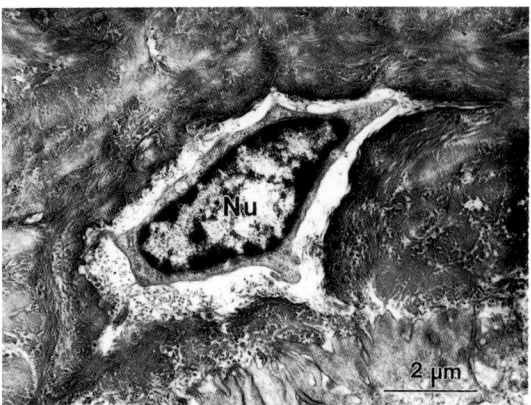

Fig 13 An osteocytelike cell from one of the minera-lized nodules formed adjacent to the grooved surface of a subcutaneous implant in place 11 weeks. *Nu* indicates nucleus.

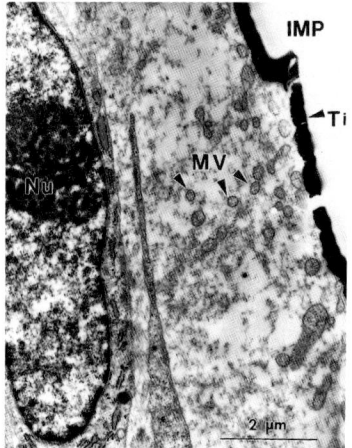

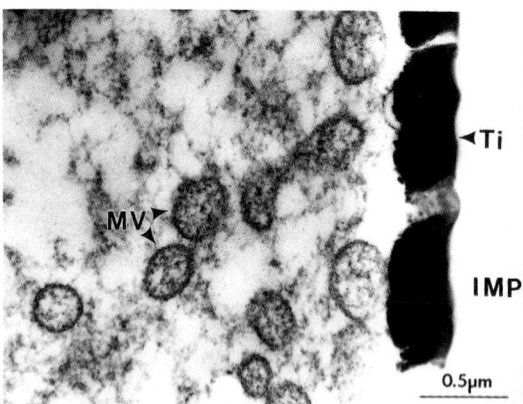

Figs 14a and b Matrix vesicles (*MV*) formed on an implant in the vicinity of a grooved substratum. *Nu, Ti,* and *IMP* indicate nucleus, titanium coating, and implant, respectively.

like tissue in this paper. Further evidence that the 19-μm-deep grooved surface produced mineralization was that matrix vesicles were observed subjacent to some connective tissue cells on this surface (Fig 14a). Some of the vesicles appeared to be in intimate contact with the titanium surface (Fig 14b). No foci of minera-lized tissue were observed adjacent to smooth surfaces in any sections.

Discussion

The importance of connective tissue organiza-tion in the behavior of epithelium attached to a percutaneous device has long been noted in the biomaterials literature, where Winter catalogued several examples of the inhibition of epithelial movement by collagen fibers.[9] Lundgren et al[10] implanted monofilament polyester fabrics with and without titanium coating with four different mesh sizes into the back skin of rats and con-cluded that successful healing was associated with ingrowth into the mesh apertures of a cell-rich collagenous tissue that seemed to block-ade epithelial downgrowth. Similarly, Squier and Collins[11] demonstrated the inhibitory influence of the connective tissue on the epithelial down-growth at the tissue/implant interface when Milli-pore filters were implanted percutaneously. Epithelial downgrowth was inhibited only in filters in which fibroblasts and fibers infiltrated the pores and were oriented perpendicular to the filter. In our study, both light and electron microscopic observations indicated that the 19-μm-deep grooved surfaces induced oblique or nearly perpendicular orientation of fibroblasts. Previous morphometric measurements of cell migration,[7] which are summarized in Fig 15, demonstrated that epithelial downgrowth was inhibited on 19-μm-deep micromachined grooved surfaces.

In summary, 1 week after placement, recession and epithelial attachment were greater, while connective tissue attachment was less on the smooth surfaces than on the grooved surfaces. Because the epithelium does not enter the 19-μm-deep grooves, the effect on these parameters must be related to the behavior of the connective tissue. Moreover, as significant attachment and organization of the connective tissue does not occur until several days after placement, the inhibitory effect on epithelial downgrowth probably happened during the last 3 days the implant was in place. Thus these data suggest that over longer periods of time the difference in epithelial downgrowth between grooved and smooth surfaces could be even greater. Preliminary data from experiments currently in progress in this laboratory suggest that epithelial downgrowth can be slowed or possibly stopped on percutaneous devices that interface with some grooved surfaces so that no significant difference in recession can be discerned between 2 to 3 weeks.

A striking difference between fibroblast interaction with SCI and PI was that the cells took much longer to form a tight attachment to the SCI. This delay in colonization was probably related to the surgical technique employed. The SCI was located in a pouch formed by surgical dissection, and healing in this area could perhaps be considered as healing by secondary intention. In contrast, tissues were tightly adapted to the PI at placement, and fibroblasts attached to the surfaces much sooner.

Pathologic calcification, defined as the deposition of crystalline calcium phosphate material, consisting primarily of hydroxyapatite in an ectopic site (ie, a site other than in normally mineralized tissue such as bone),[12] has been observed to occur not only in diseases such as atherosclerosis and crystal-deposition arthritis, but also in response to a wide variety of artificial implants, including percutaneous devices,[9] subcutaneous implants,[13] mammary prostheses,[14] and cardiovascular biomaterials.[15] Schoen[15] has advocated the use of rat subcutaneous implantation as a rapid, convenient, and economical means of investigating host and implant deter-

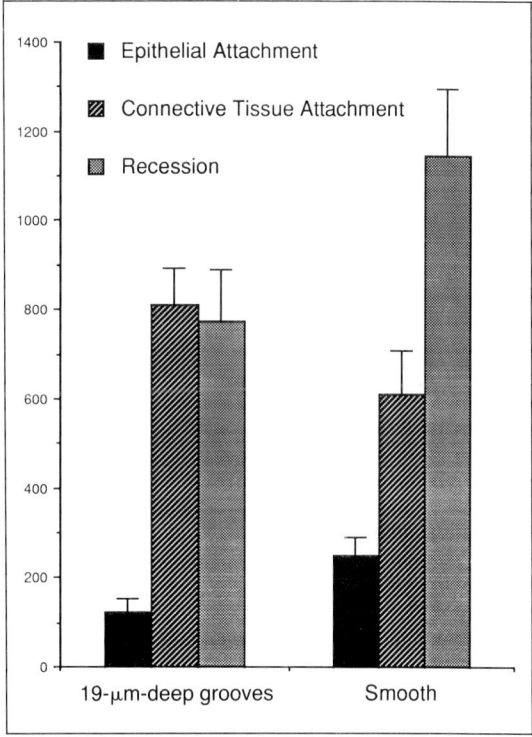

Fig 15 Comparison of length of epithelial attachment, length of connective tissue attachment, and recession between smooth and grooved surfaces. Vertical axis is in micrometers.

minants of mineralization. However, unlike many instances of mineralization, the response to the grooved implants was not limited to the development of crystalline material, but rather resulted in the production of bonelike tissue. At present we have not characterized these foci of mineralization; and chemical as well as morphological analysis is clearly required. Moreover it should be emphasized that bonelike tissue is not produced on all the subcutaneously implanted grooved substrata, a situation that indicates that we have not yet achieved full experimental control of the phenomenon. Nevertheless, our data on the 19-μm-deep grooved surfaces, as well as other micromachined surfaces, indicate that mineralization occurred on a statistically significantly greater proportion of grooved (and other micromachined substrata) surfaces than on smooth surfaces. In fact, mineralization of a smooth-surfaced SCI has not been observed in these experiments.

The observation that surface topography can affect mineralization is not novel and has been observed in a number of systems. Perhaps the earliest example of the possible effects of an implant forming a bone-inductive microenvironment in vivo is the work of Selye et al,[16] who implanted glass cylinders of various shapes into rats so as to direct tissue ingrowth in desired directions. A striking observation was that bone and cartilage formation occurred, but only in some sizes and shapes of cylinders. Bone formation has been observed in conjunction with a variety of porous and textured surfaces, as well as machined surfaces having microscopic grooves, on a number of dental implant systems.[17] Such textured substrata could act through several mechanisms. Two possibilities are of particular interest on a theoretical basis for grooved micromachined surfaces: the ability of the surface to produce a bone-inductive microenvironment and/or induce cell polarity.

1. Bone-inductive microenvironment (BIM). Grooved or pitted surfaces could act by allowing cells in a restricted location to alter their microenvironment so that it favors calcified tissue production. In vitro evidence for this possibility is afforded by the experiments by Nijweide,[18] as well as Tenenbaum and Heersche,[19] who demonstrated that periosteal sheets have to be folded before they will form osteoid. This mechanism predicts that grooves or other types of texture might have an optimum size that would determine the amount of bone formation.
2. Cell polarity. Another possibility is that bone formation will be enhanced by producing cell orientation that will aid in the development of functional cell polarity. In vivo osteogenic cells polarize to become osteoblasts. Thus if cell orientation itself is sufficient to promote bone formation, shallow grooves would be predicted as being as effective as deeper grooves, because both types of grooves orient cells.

It may be possible to distinguish between those possibilities, and other mechanisms as well, by implanting surfaces with systematically varying surface topographies. Because micromachining can produce surfaces with precisely controlled topography that can be varied in shape, depth, and spacing, the implantation of micromachined surfaces could be a valuable method of investigating the topographical control of bone formation on artificial implants.

References

1. von Recum AF. Permanent percutaneous devices. *CRC Crit Rev Bioeng* 1981;5:37–77.
2. von Recum AF. Applications and failure modes of percutaneous devices: A review. *J Biomed Mater Res* 1984;18:323–336.
3. von Recum AF, Yan J, Schreuders PD, Powers DL. Basic healing phenomena around permanent percutaneous implants. pp 159–169 In *Tissue Integration in Oral and Maxillofacial Reconstruction*. Amsterdam: Excerpta Medica, 1986.
4. Jansen JA, van der Waerden PCM, van der Lubbe HBM, de Groot K. Tissue response to percutaneous implants in rabbits. *J Biomed Mater Res* 1990;24: 295–307.
5. Chehroudi B, Gould TRL, Brunette DM. Effects of a grooved epoxy substratum on epithelial cell behaviour in vitro and in vivo. *J Biomed Mater Res* 1988;22: 459–473.
6. Chehroudi B, Gould TRL, Brunette DM. Effects of a grooved titanium-coated implant surface on epithelial cell behavior in vitro and in vivo. *J Biomed Mater Res* 1989;23:1067–1085.
7. Chehroudi B, Gould TRL, Brunette DM. Titanium-coated micromachined grooves of different dimensions affect epithelial and connective-tissue cells differently in vivo. *J Biomed Mater Res* 1990;24: 1202–1219.
8. Camporese DS, Lester TP, Pulfrey DL. A fine line silicon shadow mask for inversion layer solar cells. *IEEE Electron Device Letters* 1981;EDL-2:61–63.
9. Winter GD. Transcutaneous implants: Reactions of the skin-implant interface. *J Biomed Mater Res Symposium* 1974;5(pt1):99–113.
10. Lundgren D, Hakansson JP, Bodo P. Morphometric analysis of tissue components adjacent to percutaneous implants. pp 173–180 In *Tissue Integration in Oral and Maxillofacial Reconstruction*. Amsterdam: Excerpta Medica, 1986.
11. Squier CA, Collins P. The relationship between soft tissue attachment, epithelial downgrowth and surface porosity. *J Periodont Res* 1981;16:434–440.
12. Anderson HC. Calcific diseases. *Arch Pathol Lab Med* 1983;107:341–348.

13. Holund B, Junker P, Garbarsch C, Christoffersen P, Lorenzen I. Formation of granulation tissue in subcutaneous implanted sponges in rats. *Acta Pathol Microbiol Immunol Scand* 1979;87(sec A):367–374.

14. Rolland C, Guidoin R, Marceau D, Ledoux R. Nondestructive investigations on ninety-seven surgically excised mammary prostheses. *J Biomed Mater Res* 1989;23(A3):285–298.

15. Schoen FJ. Special considerations for pathological evaluation of explanted cardiovascular prostheses. pp 412–435 In A.F. von Recum (ed) *Handbook of Biomaterials Evaluation*. New York, NY: Macmillan Publ Co, 1986.

16. Selye H, Lemire Y, Bajusz E. Induction of bone, cartilage and hemopoietic tissue by subcutaneously implanted tissue diaphragms. *Roux' Archiv für Entwicklungsmechanik* 1960;151:572–585.

17. Brunette DL. The effects of implant surface topography on the behavior of cells. *Int J Oral Maxillofac Implants* 1988;3:231–246.

18. Nijweide PJ. Calcium and strontium metabolism of bone in vitro. *Proc Kon Ned Akad Wet* 1975;C78: 416–417.

19. Tenenbaum HC, Heersche JNM. Differentiation of osteoblasts and formation of mineralized bone in vitro. *Calcif Tissue Int* 1982;34:76–79.

Transmission Electron Microscopy of the Bone/Titanium Interface

L. Sennerby, P. Thomsen, and L.E. Ericson

Two different techniques were used to prepare sections for transmission electron microscopy (TEM) of the undecalcified bone/titanium interface of threaded titanium implants inserted in a rabbit tibia for 12 months and clinical dental implants that were retrieved 1 to 16 years after insertion. All implants were removed en bloc with surrounding tissue, fixated, dehydrated, and embedded in plastic resin. No specimens were decalcified. One technique involved electrochemical dissolution (electropolishing) of the bulk part of the embedded implant, leaving the implant surface oxide layer in the embedded tissue. With the other technique, the fracture technique, the implant was separated from the embedded tissue before sectioning. The electropolishing procedure was found to induce serious artifacts including demineralization of the interface tissue. In these specimens, the implant surface was indicated by an electron-dense material in the sections. An unmineralized zone, 2- to 10-μm wide, with the characteristic of osteoid was detected between the implant surface and the mineralized bone. Using the fracture technique, sometimes a space was seen between the mineralized bone and the presumed implant surface. This space did not correspond to the unmineralized interface zone detected with the electropolishing technique, but was most certainly an artifact due to shrinkage during the processing of the tissue and/or manipulation of the implants at the time of retrieval. With the fracture technique, mineralized bone reached close to the presumed implant surface and formed a dense osmiophilic line, a lamina limitans. The lamina limitans was about 100-nm wide and was often in continuity with the lamina limitans lining osteocyte lacunae and canaliculi. Most often, an amorphous layer separated the mineralized bone from the implant. This layer was about 150- to 400-nm wide and was often missing or detached from the mineralized bone. It is concluded that the interface zone previously reported by the authors is an artifact induced by the electropolishing technique.

Complement Fixation by Polymethyl Methacrylate and Titanium, and the Impact on Macrophage Migration

E. Barth and T. Sullivan

A small but significant number of total joint replacements are subject to severe foreign body reactions with subsequent implant loosening.[1,2] These foreign body reactions, which presumably are wear debris related, have evoked an interest in immunological aspects of biomaterial usage.[3] Complement activation induced by biomaterials could underlie the foreign body reaction to some materials since C5a generated during activation is strongly chemotactic for neutrophils and monocytes.[4] Complement activation has been found to be proportional to critical surface tension for a series of biomedical polymers intended for vascular surgery.[5] Moreover, polymethyl methacrylate (PMMA) kidney dialyzers can activate complement.[6] Whether wear debris or in vitro *N* manufactured particles from orthopedic biomaterials can activate complement is not known.

In this study, the complement binding and activation induced by various concentrations of unopsonized or opsonized particles of titanium or PMMA were tested using fresh serum as substrate. The extent of complement *binding* was demonstrated in a sheep erythrocyte hemolysis assay. Complement *activation* was documented by a standard macrophage migration assay.

Materials and methods

Biomaterials

A prepared powder of titanium (Nuclear Metals Inc, Concord, Mass) was screened down through a Fisher Precision sieve mesh no. 5, yielding particles of diameter 5 μm or less. Polymethyl methacrylate powder (diameter 1 to 10 μm) (Howmedica, Rutherford, NJ) was also sifted to obtain particles of diameter 5 μm or less. The particles were suspended in saline with 10% (vol/vol) bovine serum albumin (BSA) to avoid clumping. Particles of diameter 2 to 5 μm were sorted out in a 753 Dual Epic (Coulter Electronics, Hialeah, Fla) flow cytometer. Polystyrene beads (diameter 1 to 2 μm; Polysciences Inc, Warrington, Pa) served as presumably inert control material.

Opsonization

Half the quantity of each particulate biomaterial was opsonized by incubation with excess fresh serum on a clinical rotator for 1 hour at 37°C, washed three times in saline, and resuspended.

Preparation of serum samples for the sheep erythrocyte hemolysis and macrophage migration assays

The suspensions of either unopsonized or opsonized particles were adjusted to a concentration of 10^7 particles per mL saline. The suspensions were spun down, the saline supernate removed, and the particles resuspended in an equal volume of serum. Dilutions of 1:1 and 1:10 were also prepared for subsequent dose-response studies. After incubation at 37°C for 1 hour under constant shaking, the particle suspensions were filtered through Acrodisc (Gelman Sciences, Ann Arbor, Mich) filters (pore size 0.2 μm). The harvested filtrates of serum were then analyzed for remaining complement activity using the sheep erythrocyte hemolysis assay.[7] An end product of the activation of the complement cascade is a macrophage migration inhibition factor (Bb). The presence of this factor in the serum filtrates could be demonstrated in a standard macrophage migration assay.[8] Fresh normal serum served as control samples in the two assays.

Sheep erythrocyte hemolysis assay

Sheep erythrocytes were obtained as 20% red blood cells (RBC) (vol/vol) in citrate (Flow Laboratories, Dublin, Va) and lyophilized rabbit Anti-Sheep Red Blood Cell Stroma (hemolysin) antiserum from Sigma Chemical Company (St Louis, Mo). A 1% (vol/vol) suspension of RBC with 3% (vol/vol) BSA to minimize nonspecific hemolysis was sensitized with a 1:150 dilution of antiserum for 15 minutes at 37°C and then washed twice in ice-cold phosphate-buffered saline (PBS) with BSA. Thereafter the volume of normal serum that would give 50% hemolysis was determined in a spectrophotometric microtiter assay at a wavelength of 620 nm.[7] The volume of normal serum that gave 50% hemolysis was 45 μL. As the parameter for biomaterial complement fixation, the percent of hemolysis caused by 45 μL of each of the biomaterial-exposed serum filtrates was determined.

Macrophage migration assay

Pulmonary macrophages were harvested from pathogen-free male, white New Zealand rabbits as described by Myrvik et al.[9] Lavages consistently contained >90% macrophages in Jenner-Giemsa-stained smears. The viability counts using the trypan blue dye exclusion test were >95%. The cells were resuspended in cell culture medium (ie, 1640 RPMI; Automod Sigma R7755, Sigma Chemical Co, St Louis, Mo) with 2 mM glutamine, 5% fetal bovine serum (FBS), and 100 U/mL penicillin and 100 μg/mL streptomycin at pH 7.4; loaded in capillary tubes with one end sealed with soft paraffin; and centrifuged for 10 minutes at 30 g. Thereafter the tubes were broken off at the transition between the packed cells and the supernate, and the macrophage-rich tubes each were placed in a migration chamber filled with cell culture medium and 20% (vol/vol) of either biomaterial-exposed serum filtrate or normal (control) serum. The chambers were incubated for 24 hours at 37°C under conditions of 5% CO_2 in air. The diameter of the projected macrophage migrations was measured with a planimeter and expressed in percentage of the migration of controls.

Statistics

Each assay was run in six replicates for each biomaterial preparation and particle concentration. The values were expressed as the arithmetic means ± 1 standard deviation (SD). The values of the arithmetic means from each group in either assay were contrasted using a one-way ANOVA at a significance level of $P < .05$. Linear regression analysis was conducted using particle concentration as the predictor and either percent hemolysis or macrophage migration inhibition as the dependent variables.

Results

The results are given in Tables 1 to 3. Polymethyl methacrylate was a more potent complement binder and activator than titanium for all particle concentrations tested (Table 1). These differences between PMMA and titanium particles were consistent regardless of whether unopsonized or opsonized particles were employed. The effect of polystyrene-treated serum did not differ from that of normal serum in any of

Table 1 Arithmetic means ± 1 SD of the sheep RBC hemolysis and macrophage migration inhibition assay data for the various particle concentrations tested*

Particle concentration	10^6/mL	5×10^6/mL	10^7/mL
Titanium (A,H)	98 ± 2	90 ± 5	80 ± 3
PMMA (A,H)	94 ± 3	78 ± 4	58 ± 5
Titanium (B,H)	95 ± 1	86 ± 3	75 ± 4
PMMA (B,H)	92 ± 1	78 ± 2	56 ± 6
Titanium (A,I)	5 ± 1	10 ± 3	15 ± 4
PMMA (A,I)	9 ± 2	24 ± 5	47 ± 9
Titanium (B,I)	5 ± 1	12 ± 2	16 ± 5
PMMA (B,I)	8 ± 1	27 ± 3	54 ± 13

*H = sheep RBC hemolysis, I = macrophage migration inhibition. A = unopsonized and B = opsonized particles. One-way ANOVA analysis at a significance level of $P<.05$ showed that PMMA was a significantly more potent complement binder and activator than titanium and that opsonization of the biomaterials did not affect complement binding or activation.

Table 2 Complement fixation assay. Results of linear regression analysis of accumulated data from dose-response studies*

Biomaterial	α	β	R^2
Titanium (A)	-2.1×10^{-6}	100	0.843
PMMA (A)	-4.1×10^{-6}	98	0.783
Titanium (B)	-2.2×10^{-6}	97	0.821
PMMA (B)	-4.3×10^{-6}	99	0.764

*Particle concentrations served as the predictor (x) and percent hemolysis as the dependent variable (y). α = slope of the line and β is the intercept at the y-axis. A = unopsonized and B = opsonized material.

Table 3 Migration inhibition assay. Results of linear regression analysis of accumulated data from dose-response studies*

Biomaterial	α	β	R^2
PMMA (A)	1.5×10^{-6}	3	0.792
Titanium (A)	4.7×10^{-6}	2	0.658
PMMA (B)	1.6×10^{-6}	5	0.806
Titanium (B)	5.6×10^{-6}	4	0.689

*Particle concentrations served as the predictor (x) and percent hemolysis as the dependent variable (y). α = slope of the line and β = intercept at the y-axis. R^2 is the coefficient of determination. A = unopsonized and B = opsonized material.

the assays. In the range of the particle concentrations tested, the complement depletion as demonstrated by percent hemolysis of sheep erythrocytes was a linear function of increasing particle concentration (Table 2). The slope (β) for PMMA had a higher numerical value than for titanium, corroborating that PMMA was a more potent complement fixer than titanium. Complement activation as documented by percent macrophage migration inhibition also was a linear function of biomaterial particle concentration (Table 3) with a higher numerical value of β for PMMA than for titanium.

Discussion

This study showed that particulate PMMA is a more potent complement fixer and activator than particulate titanium. Moreover, complement fixation and activation are also functions of surface area (ie, number of particles) available. The adsorption of serum proteins (ie, opsonization) does not alter the inherent ability of either biomaterial surface to bind or activate complement.

The biocompatibility of an implanted biomaterial is partly determined by the responses of the body's defense system to the material. The role of the foreign body system in determining the acceptability of an implant is recognized, but much less attention has been paid to the possible role of the immune system in response to biomaterials. However, the discovery of transient leukopenia and associated activation of the complement system in patients undergoing dialysis have heightened interest in immunological aspects of biomaterials usage.[10] Whether or not orthopedic implant materials can activate complement is an issue that has not been previously addressed.

Complement activation induced by biomaterials could underlie the foreign body reaction to some materials since C5a generated during activation is strongly chemotactic for neutrophils and monocytes.[11] Moreover, the generated Bb is a potent inhibitor of macrophage migration.

Once monocytes have arrived at the site of tissue repair around an implant, they will mature into macrophages.[12] Their efficacy as scavengers that clean up dead tissue so that normal tissue repair can proceed depends in part on a normal migratory function.[13] The latter can be severely impaired if the adjacent biomaterial surface is a potent complement activator. Our results indicate that orthopedic implant materials (ie, PMMA) can be potent activators of complement. This observation may in part explain the extreme foreign body reactions evoked by cemented artificial joints.[14] By contrast, the biocompatibility of titanium may in part be the result of its lesser capability to activate complement.

Most foreign body reactions to orthopedic implant materials have been attributed to the presence of wear debris particles.[15] These particles offer a comparatively large surface area for host tissue interaction, and our results indicate a proportionality between available surface area and extent of complement activation.

It is also noteworthy that complement activation was unaffected by pretreatment of the biomaterial particles with serum. In vivo, an implant surface will be covered with adsorbed proteinaceous moieties within a matter of seconds after implantation. However, our in vitro results may indicate that a protein-covered biomaterial surface still retains its inherent capability of complement activation. It is therefore possible that a permanently implanted biomaterial that is a potent complement activator will perpetually activate complement and jeopardize the normal repair process and tissue integration of the implant.

Conclusion

Complement activation by orthopedic implant materials may be a causative factor in implant loosening associated with foreign body reactions. The various immunological aspects of biomaterial usage in orthopedic implantology need further elucidation and consideration in preclinical biocompatibility testing.

References

1. Santavirta S, Konttinen YT, Bergeroth V. Aggressive granulomatous lesions associated with hip arthroplasty. J Bone Joint Surg 1990;72A:252–258.
2. Howie DW, Vernon-Roberts B. The synovial response to intraarticular cobalt-chrome wear particles. Clin Orthop Rel Res 1988;232:244–254.
3. Dorson WJ. White cell and complement problems in artificial organs. ASAIO J 1984;7:50–56.
4. Chenoweth DE, Cooper SW, Hugli TE, Stewart RW, Blackstone EH, Kirklin JW. Complement activation during cardiopulmonary bypass; evidence for generation of C3a and C5a anaphylatoxins. N Engl J Med 1981;304:497–503.
5. Ward CA, Koheil A, Johnson WR, Madras PN. Reduction in complement activation from biomaterials by removal of air nuclei from the surface roughness. J Biomed Mater Res 1980;18:255–269.
6. Hoerl WH, Riegel W, Schollmeyer P, Rautenberg W, Neumann SC. Different complement and granulocyte activation in patients dialyzed with PMMA dialyzers. Clin Nephrol 1986;25:304–307.
7. Kankclerski K, Mollby R. A simple and exact two-point interpolation method for determination of hemolytic activity in microtiter plates. Acta Path Immunobiol Scand 1987;95B:175–179.
8. Gordon MR, Chida K, Takata I, Myrvik QN. Macrophage migration inhibition induced by MDP, LPS, PMA, and MIF/MAF: Reversal by macrophage migration enhancement factor (MEF), L-fucose, L-Fucosyl BSA, D-Mannoose, and D-Mannosyl BSA. J Leukocyte Biol 1987;42:197–203.
9. Myrvik QN. Studies on pulmonary macrophages from normal rabbit: A technique to procure them in a high state of purity. J Immunol 1961;126–132.
10. Chenoweth DE. Biocompatibility of hemodialysis membranes. Evaluation with C3a anaphylatoxin radioimmunoassays. ASAIO J 1984;7:44–49.
11. Hugli TE, Muller-Eberhard HJ. Anaphylatoxins C3a and C5a. Adv Immunol 1978;26:1–53.
12. Wesley CV, Witmer MD, Steinmann RM. The phenotype of dendritic cells and macrophages. Symp FASEB 67th Ann Mtg 1983;67:3114–3118.
13. Fukasawa M, Campeau JD, Yassigihara DL, Rodgers KE, Dizerega GS. Mitogenic and protein synthetic activity of tissue repair cells. Control by the post-surgical macrophage. J Invest Surg 1989;2:160–180.
14. Agins HJ, Alcock NW, Bansai M, Salvati E, Wilson PD, Pellici PM, et al. Metallic wear in failed titanium-alloy total hip replacements. J Bone Joint Surg 1988;70A:347–356.
15. Willert HG, Semlitsch M. Tissue reaction to plastic and metallic wear products of joint endoprostheses. pp 205–239 In Total Hip Prosthesis. Stuttgart: Huber Verlag, 1976.

Histologic and Histomorphometric Evaluation of Submerged and Nonsubmerged Titanium Implants

K. Gotfredsen and E. Hjörting-Hansen

The concept of osseointegration was originally introduced by Brånemark[1,2] to describe a direct contact between bone and implant on the light microscopic level.[3] However, the meaning of osseointegration is complex and the interface between bone and biomaterial should be evaluated qualitatively as well as quantitatively. Some endosteal implants are placed in a two-stage procedure, in which the implant is buried in the bone during an initial healing period (submerged implants). Other endosteal implant systems are placed in a one-stage procedure, in which the implants immediately protrude into the mouth (nonsubmerged implants). The aim of the present study was, firstly, to make a quantitative and qualitative comparison between submerged and nonsubmerged implants and, secondly, to compare the initial healing response around nonsubmerged implants with and without oral hygiene performance in the initial healing phase.

Materials and methods

Six 3.5 to 5.5 kg green vervet monkeys had their mandibular first and second molars extracted bilaterally 10 months before implantation. Twenty-four titanium implants with titanium plasma-sprayed surfaces (ITI hollow-cylinder implants, Institut Straumann AG, Waldenburg, Switzerland) were placed in the toothless regions under anesthesia with intramuscularly injected Ketalar (15 mg/kg body weight; Parke-Davis Co) and Rompun (1 mg/kg body weight; Parke-Davis Co).

In the first experiment, three monkeys had two submerged implants tested against two nonsubmerged implants placed contralaterally. Calcein Green (Sigma) was given intravenously after 3 and 4 weeks in a dose of 15 mg/kg of body weight, and Xylenol Orange (Sigma) was given intravenously after 10 and 11 weeks in a dose of 50 mg/kg of body weight. In the next experiment, three monkeys each had two nonsubmerged implants placed bilaterally. Oral hygiene procedures and the administration of 1% Hibitane (ICI, Maccesfield, United Kingdom) were only performed on one side during the test period.

After 22 weeks, the animals were sacrificed under anesthesia with Ketalar and Rompun by vital perfusion with Karnowsky's fixative through the left ventricle of the heart. After immersion in the same fixative for 1 week, 12 undecalcified blocks measuring 20×25 mm, each with two implants, were dehydrated in ascending series of ethanol concentrations with 0.3% basic fuchsin. The tissue blocks were cleared in 100% acetone for 12 days, embedded in methacrylate resin, and prepared for histological examination. A sectioning technique was designed to provide two buccolingual sections of each implant. After re-embedding in methacrylate, the half implant was turned 90° and two approximal sections were obtained.

For light microscopy, an Olympus BH-2 (Olympus, Tokyo, Japan) microscope was used, and for polarization microscopy, a Zeiss (Zeiss,

Oberkochen, Germany) microscope was used. Microradiographs were taken on 0.08-mm approximal sections with an emulsive film (Emulsion 649-0, Kodak, Rochester, NY), 14kV, 12mA, and exposure in 50 minutes. Fluorescence microscopy was done with an epifluorescence (Zeiss) microscope and scanning electron microscopy was done with a Philips SEM 50 microscope after sputtering with 10 nm gold-palladium. The bone-to-implant direct contact lengths were calculated using a semiautomatic computer program made on the IBAS interactive image analysis system (Kontron Bildanalyse GmbH, Eching, Germany). The undecalcified sections were placed under a light microscope (Zeiss IM, West Germany) at 200 × magnification. A television camera was used to transform the transillumination image into a video signal. The signal was digitally converted with a graphic resolution of 512 × 768 pixels, and gray values between 0 and 255. The black-and-white picture on the screen was analyzed using a digitizing tablet. Interfaces between mineralized bone tissue and the implant were outlined and calculated as a percentage of the total interface length.

Results

The histomorphometric evaluation of direct contacts between mineralized bone and implant surface on the light microscopic level is shown in Figs 1 and 2. No significant difference in bone-to-implant contact length fraction was found between submerged and nonsubmerged implants (Fig 1) when tested as paired observations that eliminate the interanimal difference. The bone-to-implant contact length from experiment 2 (Fig 2), showed generally more bone-to-implant contact along the nonsubmerged implants with oral hygiene during healing, than for the nonsubmerged implants without oral hygiene during healing. A higher percentage of bone-to-implant contact length fractions was found in experiment 2 than in experiment 1.

The light microscopic evaluation showed direct bone-to-implant contact to the submerged as well as to the nonsubmerged implants. The interfaces consisted of areas with mineralized bone and areas with a highly cellular connective tissue, the bone marrow. No fibrous tissue was seen around any of the implants. Infrabony defects were detected around 18 of the 24 implants. When no oral hygiene was performed around the nonsubmerged implants, inflammation in the gingival connective tissue around the implant was often detected, and frequently a long junctional epithelium was found migrating down into the infrabony defect.

Polarized light microscopy made it possible to distinguish the area of bone necrosis resulting from surgical intervention, as demarcation lines clearly separated newly generated bone from the original bone. A large number of osteocytes was seen at the demarcation line.

The microradiographs showed a lower density of the bone adjacent to the implants than the surrounding bone, and it was also possible to distinguish newly generated bone from mature, "old" bone (Fig 3). Fluorescence microscopy showed that the primary mineralization of bone around the implants was a direct apposition of bone, and that the mineralization front had reached the implant surface at some places 4 weeks after implantation (Fig 4).

Scanning electron microscopy showed an intimate contact between bone and the plasma-sprayed surface. The bone was growing into surface irregularities and was rich in cells adjacent to the implant surface.

Discussion

Quantitatively this limited study showed bone-to-implant contacts to the same degree around submerged implants as around nonsubmerged implants without "functional load" and with oral hygiene during healing. Also, nonsubmerged implants without oral hygiene and without "functional load" showed a direct bone-to-implant contact in this study.

Other studies[4] have shown fibrous tissue

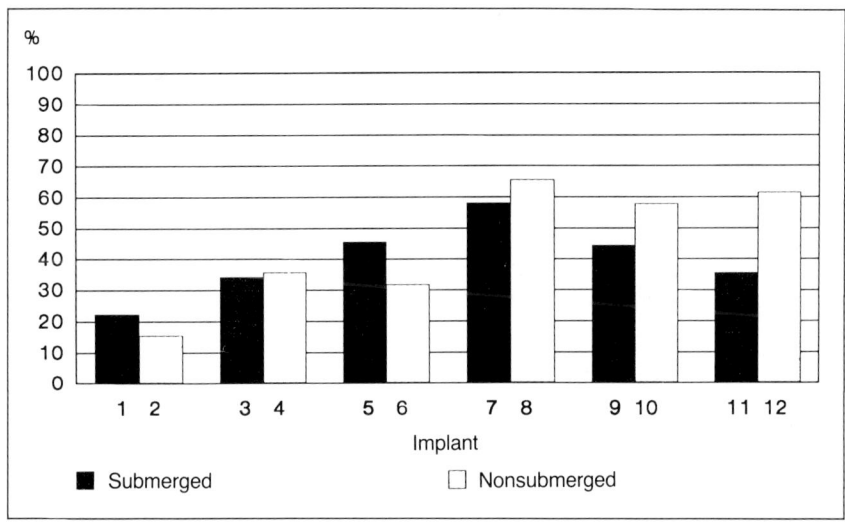

Fig 1 The bone-to-implant contact length fractions on the approximal surfaces in experiment 1. Submerged implants compared with nonsubmerged implants placed contralaterally within the same animal.

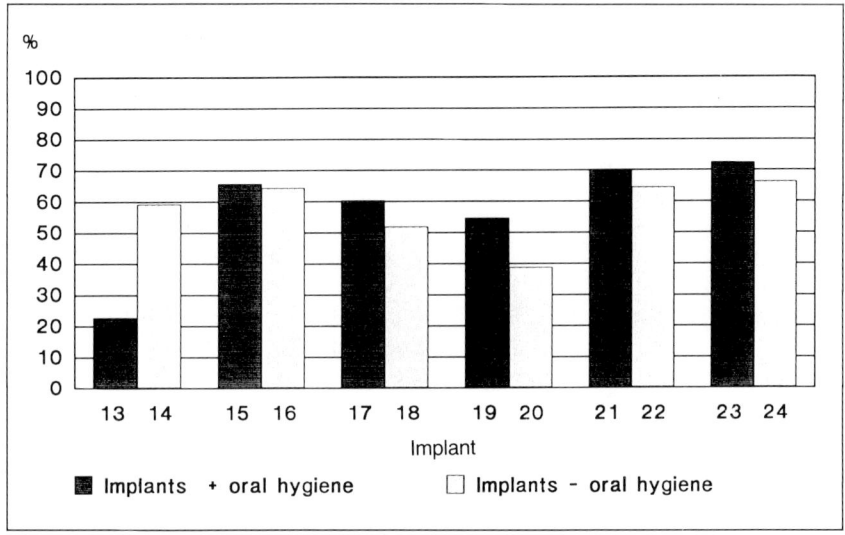

Fig 2 The bone-to-implant contact length fractions on the approximal surfaces in experiment 2. Nonsubmerged implants with oral hygiene compared with nonsubmerged implants placed contralaterally within the same animal.

around nonsubmerged implants with occlusal contact during healing. This confirms the hazard of "functional load" during healing. Micromovements, caused by a "functional load," will probably disturb cell differentiation around the implant.

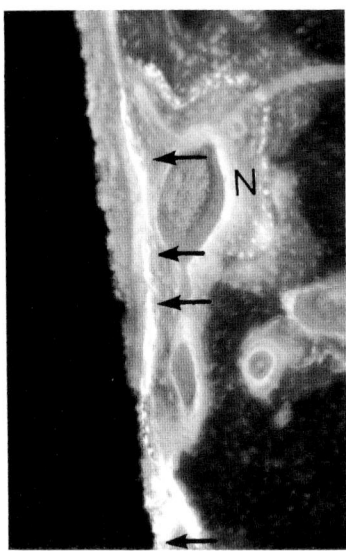

Fig 3 Microradiograph showing lower density of newly generated bone *(N)* than of mature bone. A demarcation line *(arrows)* sharply distinguishes new bone from "old" bone.

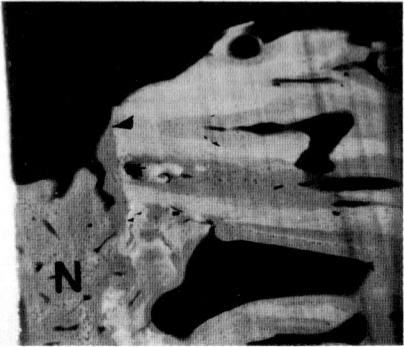

Fig 4 Fluorescence microscopy showing the mineralization front after 3 and 4 weeks. Newly regenerated bone *(N)* was formed as direct apposition of bone.

The study also showed pronounced interanimal and interimplant variations in direct bone-to-implant contacts. These variations are mainly explained by differences in the bony structure between the animals and in the surgical preparation.

Oral hygiene has been emphasized as important for the long-term prognosis of oral implants.[2] In the present study, oral hygiene was not decisive for the achievement of osseointegration but seemed to aggravate infrabony defects around nonsubmerged implants. This would certainly compromise the maintenance of osseointegration around nonsubmerged implants.

Conclusion

It is possible to achieve direct bone-to-implant contact on a light microscopic level around submerged as well as nonsubmerged implants. When nonsubmerged implants are used, "functional load" should be avoided and a strict oral hygiene program followed during the healing phase.

References

1. Brånemark P-I, Hansson BO, Adell R, Breine U, Lindström J, Hallén O, et al. Osseointegrated implants in the treatment of the edentulous jaw. Experience from a 10-year period. *Scand J Plast Reconstr Surg* 1977;11(suppl 16):1–132.
2. Brånemark P-I, Zarb GA, Albrektsson T. pp 11–345 In *Tissue-Integrated Prostheses. Osseointegration in Clinical Dentistry.* Chicago: Quintessence Publ Co, 1985.
3. Albrektsson T, Brånemark P-I, Hansson H-A, Lindström J. Osseointegrated titanium implants. Requirements for ensuring a long-lasting, direct bone-to-implant anchorage in man. *Acta Orthop Scand* 1981;52:155–170.
4. Akagawa Y, Hashimoto M, Kondo N, Satomi K, Takata T, Tsuru H. Initial bone-implant interfaces of submergible and supramergible endosseous single-crystal sapphire endosseous implants. *J Oral Rehabil* 1989;16:581–587.

The Reactions of Periodontal Tissues to Implants and Teeth*

D. van Steenberghe, M. Quirynen, and A. Callens

Incidence of periodontal breakdown in conjunction with teeth

The periodontium consists of epidermal (gingiva and alveolar mucosa) and connective tissues, both mineralized and nonmineralized (the underlying connective tissues of both the gingiva and alveolar mucosa, the root cementum, the periodontal ligament, and the jawbone). The presence of teeth determines the increased height of the jaw process during eruption, while tooth removal leads to jawbone resorption. The latter phenomenon is caused by the absence of intraosseous force transfer. Small positive bone remodeling can also be achieved by endosseous implants providing intimate bone contact.

When teeth erupt, they provoke an epidermal discontinuity that is unique in mammals except for the deer antler. In the latter, an annual shedding occurs, whereas the natural dentition is supposed to maintain itself for a lifetime. In many instances, this does not occur because of periodontal disease such as the disruption of the periodontal ligament caused by tooth trauma. More often a chronic bacterial infection that provokes an inflammatory reaction in the gingival connective tissue can lead to destruction of the connective fibers embedded in the tooth root and allow apical migration of the epithelium. This kind of destructive process depends on the imbalance between bacterial plaque pathogenicity and the local and generalized immune response. Thus few locations in a minority of people will demonstrate important periodontal breakdown,[1] which furthermore appears to be discontinuous in time.[2] An observation based on short-term follow-up examinations or the means of changes in attachment level or marginal bone loss would lead to the false assumption that natural teeth are relatively resistant to periodontal breakdown under the influence of plaque-related inflammatory reactions. Nevertheless, a number of patients still become edentulous and periodontitis plays a prominent role in this regard. Prognostic indicators for periodontal breakdown around natural teeth are lacking.[3] Thus every tooth is at risk when bacterial plaque accumulates on its surface, and especially when an anaerobic environment favors the overgrowth by periodontal pathogens.

In this perspective, an essential question arises when endosseous permucosal implants are concerned. The osseointegration concept has resulted in fewer fibrously encapsulated implants, and more achieve intimate bone apposition. How these different interfaces relate to an eventual breakdown of the surrounding tissues will be the main focus of this paper. A related question is whether the classical periodontal indices also apply to the peri-implant tissues.

The implant/tissue interfaces

When a foreign body penetrates the epidermis, either skin or mucosa, an intimate relationship results between the foreign body surface and

*Keynote presentation.

the epithelial cells. A true connective tissue attachment in which collagen fibers are embedded in the implant surface cannot be expected unless a root cementum was deposited on the implant surface. The latter has been observed when an implant is in contact with the periodontal ligament of a neighboring tooth.[4] However, this phenomenon remains quite removed from regular clinical practice, if indeed it would ever be desirable. This close relationship reveals itself through the presence of hemidesmosomes on the electron microscopic (EM) level, just as is observed in vitro when epithelial cells adhere to the Petri dish on which they are grown.[5,6] Epithelial cells have a tendency to creep along the irregularities of the implant surface by a process known as contact guidance.[7] When adhering to a tooth surface, epithelial cells have a tendency to grow apically unless stopped by the connective tissue attachment.

It is of utmost importance to know by which mechanism epithelial downgrowth is prevented along permucosal implants that achieve an intimate bone apposition. The resistance of epithelial downgrowth can be associated with the underlying bone apposition; but when fibrous scar tissue surrounds the implant, marsupialization usually occurs.[6,8,9] From studies of beagle dogs[9] and man,[10,11] it appears that the subepithelial connective tissue seal, which in man is approximately 1 mm,[12] stops the epithelial downgrowth along the implant surface. What factors play a role in this barrier remains unknown. It is surprising that thus far, no biochemical analysis of the connective tissue layer at the abutment interface around Brånemark implants (Nobelpharma AB, Göteberg, Sweden) has been performed, although this implant type is known to offer a long-term attachment level stability.[13]

From histological and clinical data on some oral implant systems that involve a one-stage placement procedure, it has been shown that apical downgrowth is not necessarily the result of the one-stage technique if underlying intimate bone apposition is achieved. It seems that the implant-bone interface determines the characteristics of the overlying connective tissue interface, which does or does not allow epithe-lial cell ingrowth. Interesting data could be obtained from ankylosed teeth in which some sites demonstrated bone joining the root without the interposition of periodontal ligament. Inflammatory reactions that are associated with bacterial plaque accumulations occur regularly in this supraosseous connective tissue layer and are indistinguishable at the light microscopic level from those occurring around natural teeth.[9,11] This does not mean that permanent anchorage has been obtained because of intimate bone apposition.

Depending upon the surface and configuration properties, either a more or less constant bone level can be maintained over many years,[11] or progressive bone loss occurs.[14] Bone apposition, whether at the light or electron microscopic level, should not be considered synonymous with osseointegration. The latter implies long-term (10 years and more) service under load-bearing circumstances and exposure to bacterial plaque accumulations, while maintaining a constant bone level. This could explain the observed differences in the clinical fate of different implant systems that do achieve bone apposition. d'Hoedt and Schulte[15] reported a more frequent incidence of bone loss and deepening of the probing pocket depth around ITI implants (Institute Straumann AG, Waldenburg, Switzerland) when compared with TPS (Straumann, Ltd, Freiburg, Germany) and IMZ (Implant Support Systems, Inc, Irvine, Calif) while Quirynen et al[14] report a significantly more rapid loss of bone and increased probing pocket depth around IMZ implants than around Brånemark fixtures. In a detailed 3-year study on Brånemark implants, Bower et al[16] revealed that few sites lost considerable bone, while the mean bone loss was minimal. This loss of bone also appeared to be discontinuous, indicating that random bursts of bone loss seem to occur around osseointegrated fixtures as around natural teeth. Thus even if there are clear-cut differences in the anatomy and physiology of the periodontal tissues around teeth and around permucosal implants, more and more similarities seem to emerge.

There is a need to evaluate through worldwide longitudinal studies the fate of the marginal bone level around endosseous implants by means of intraoral long-cone radiographs. The focus should be on the ongoing bone loss or eventual leveling off of this phenomenon, which might otherwise jeopardize implant survival in the long-term perspective. A major clinical problem is the reduced discrimination power of intraoral radiographs. The presence of a radiolucency around the implant definitely indicates that bone apposition was not achieved. However, the absence of it cannot be taken as an indication of an intimate relationship. Another shortcoming of the radiological investigation is that it does not allow for discrimination between the two most frequent causes of nonintegration: occlusal overload or bacterial infection. A narrow radiolucency along the implant surface and parallel to it is indicative of overload. Bone loss caused by marginal inflammation associated with bacterial accumulation on the transgingival implant surface leads to angular bony defects that often have a craterlike morphology. However, clinical observations indicate that overload can lead to similar bony defects caused by lateral components. A longitudinal evaluation could be used to determine whether bone defect morphology might be used to differentiate between overload and infection. Recent introduction of an electronic device, called the Periotest (Siemens AG, Bensheim, Germany), to assess the attachment mode needs to be further assessed.[17]

Bacterial colonization around oral implants

To achieve predictable intimate bone apposition to an implant surface, an atraumatic surgical technique is mandatory. Such a procedure implies no rise in temperature, no mechanical damage, no bacterial contamination, and relative immobility at the implant/bone interface.

Heating and/or mechanical trauma leads to cell necrosis and disruption of the bone microcirculation. The bone is replaced by an ill-defined scar tissue that allows a rapid downgrowth of the epithelium along the interface until the implant is marsupialized. The resulting pocket is invaded by microorganisms that are present even in the edentulous mouth, especially where several microbial habitats are available such as the tonsils and the dorsum of the tongue. The placement of titanium abutments in an edentulous oral cavity favors the appearance of *Neisseria,* a species associated with early plaque formation. In the same study,[18] *Pseudomonas* and enterobacteria were observed for a short period after abutment placement.

Thus the introduction of a nonshedding surface in a completely edentulous oral cavity results in a microbial shift (Fig 1). When teeth or prosthetic surfaces are present, they also offer a retention place. Deep pockets along implants, just as around teeth, offer an anaerobic environment that favors a shift in the microbial flora to gram-negative anaerobic bacteria that are pathogenic to the periodontal tissues. Deep pockets around implants often result from the original thickness of the mucoperiosteum and not from a loss of attachment, as around natural teeth. However, around both teeth and implants, an increasing pocket depth or preferably a decreasing attachment level is indicative of a pathologic process in which marginal bone loss occurs. To avoid deep pockets from the start, it has been advocated that the thickness of the mucoperiosteum be reduced at the abutment connection stage operation.[8]

The microbial ecology around fibrously encapsulated implants with deepening pockets has been described and was associated with clinical symptoms such as pus formation, bleeding tendency, and gingival swelling.[19]

Around implants achieving bone apposition and when the clinical situation is "stable," the subgingival microbial flora is dominated by coccoid cells and gram-positive organisms. Hardly any spirochetes are observed.[20–22] When deepening of the pocket occurred or when radiological signs of fibrous encapsulation appeared, gram-negative anaerobic bacteria classically associated with active periodontitis were detected in a higher proportion.[21] This situation is similarly

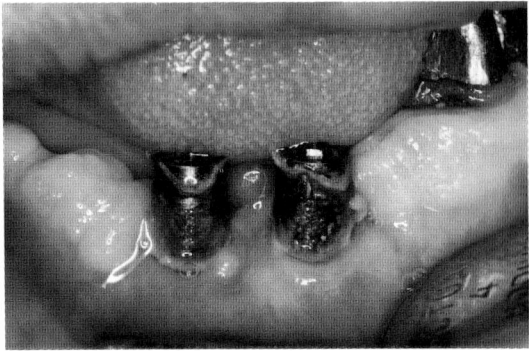

Fig 1 Plaque growth on titanium abutments is more rapid than on natural teeth. If regular monitoring is not organized, this kind of plaque and calculus buildup can occur.

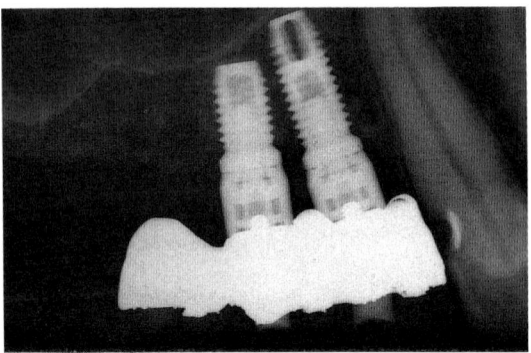

Fig 2 Intraoral radiographs, using a strict paralleling technique, is the only reliable objective method to evaluate progressive bone loss. The threads allow a discriminating power of 0.3 mm.

observed around teeth in the active phase of rapidly advancing periodontitis. Whatever the implant type or surface, there seems to be a constant observation that failing implants are surrounded by subgingival microflora with high proportions of *Bacteroides intermedius, Fusobacterium nucleatum,* and spirochetes.[19,21,23]

This observation should not result in the conclusion that there is a causal relationship. One report indicates some difference between the subgingival flora around Brånemark implants and around natural teeth.[16] Subgingival microbial colonization seems to differ according to

implant surface characteristics. Around some nonfailing titanium implants (TPS) in patients with low to moderate gingivitis, a majority of gram-negative rods was reported, especially in the deeper pockets.[24]

Also of importance is whether patients are completely or partially edentulous. The pockets around natural teeth seem to act as reservoirs for the bacterial colonization of pockets around implants.[22,25] It is essential that microbial oral flora be reduced before placing endosseous implants. A high plaque index and aggressive forms of periodontal infections have been associated with a higher failure rate during the healing phase.[26,27]

After the healing phase, it seems even more logical to assume that gingivitis around implants might influence their survival. In a long-term experimental gingivitis model around Brånemark implants in the dog, no bone loss could be observed at a clinical level,[28] whereas for another titanium implant type, bone loss did occur even if it was slower than around natural teeth in the same dog.[29] The link between different implant surfaces does influence early bacterial colonization and especially the resistance to bone loss, which has clinical implications.

The applicability of periodontal indices

Currently, patient monitoring is dependent upon unsophisticated diagnostic tests such as attachment level determination by means of a pocket probe, intraoral radiographs with a strict paralleling technique, and mobility assessment (Fig 2). Prognostic indicators have not been identified as yet.

Since it is not recommended that fixed prostheses be removed on a regular basis to evaluate the immobility of individual implants, and since radiographs should not be repeated too frequently to avoid undue radiation exposure, the only means for regular control is pocket probing (Fig 3). As with natural teeth, the prognostic value of bleeding upon probing or probing pocket depth is still a matter of debate. Some clinicians claim that these periodontal parameters are thus irrelevant for oral implants,[30] while those involved in periodontology know that even if some aspects remain to be elucidated, their clinical importance cannot be questioned. Otherwise one will have to rely on a clinical perception or infrequent radiological examinations to monitor oral implants and thus may possibly overlook pathologies.

The absence of a ligament interposed between an implant surface and bone means not only clinical immobility, but also that underloading bone resorption can only take place through activation of osteoclasts in bone lacunae near the interface, a so-called undermining resorption. From animal and human experiments, it is known that a whole series of teeth can be moved by anchoring a spring device to osseointegrated fixtures.[31] Thus far this therapeutic approach has been confined to a few centers that have the necessary expertise and ability to document all parameters.

The question has been raised whether a keratinized epithelium should routinely surround permucosal implants or whether the alveolar mucosa would function as well. The same discussion has occurred the past two decades concerning the need for gingiva around teeth. Even if some exceptions can always be found, it has been shown that grafting procedures are obsolete since alveolar mucosa is not more prone to develop inflammation or recessions than gingiva (Fig 4).[32,33] The same seems to apply around oral implants.[34] When a titanium-sprayed surface is used, it has been suggested that gingival penetration was preferable.[35] There is a need for well-documented studies to confirm the clinical observation that the presence or absence of gingiva around osseointegrated implants does not seem to influence the soft tissue reaction, subsequent bone loss, or survival rate. There is the possibility that chronic mechanical trauma resulting from muscle traction in very resorbed jaws can cause marginal irritation when the alveolar mucosa directly adheres to the abutments.[8]

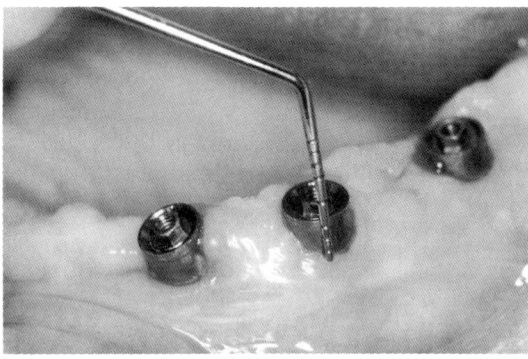

Fig 3 Since radiographs cannot be taken too often, and since there is a good correlation between attachment level measurement by means of a periodontal pocket probe and the bone level, probing should systematically be done at each control visit.

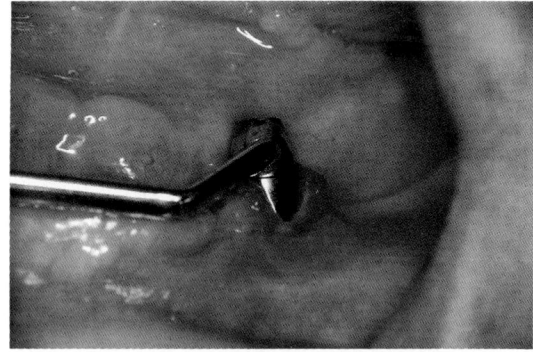

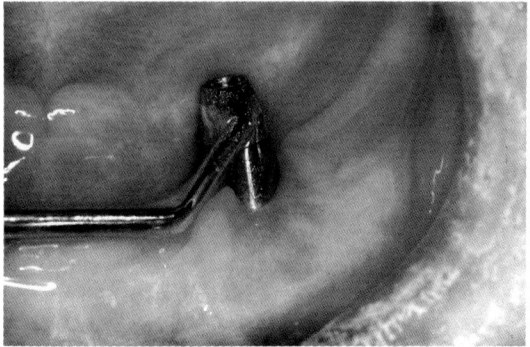

Figs 4a and b Gingival overgrowth should be dealt with by optimal plaque control and prosthetic relining, not by grafting. In this patient, upgrading of oral hygiene resulted in a disappearance of the inflammatory reaction even when no gingiva was present.

Conclusion

Although anatomical differences are evident between the periodontium around teeth and oral permucosal implants, recent investigations indicate numerous similarities. Until more knowledge is gathered, the clinician must rely on classical periodontal parameters such as the use of the periodontal pocket probe to objectively assess gingival inflammation or changes in the attachment level, clinical immobility of individual implants, and the absence of ongoing marginal bone loss. Likewise for natural teeth, prognostic indicators are still lacking. Considering the very few available microbiological reports related to different implant surface characteristics, the knowledge in this field is too limited to draw any conclusions. Available data indicate that, as around natural teeth, deep pockets harbor more organisms associated with periodontal inflammatory reactions.

Generally, patients subject to regular oral hygiene harbor less periodontal pathogens around permucosal titanium implants than around natural teeth. In partially edentulous mouths, where pockets around teeth act as a reservoir, implant surfaces are more rapidly colonized by these pathogens. For some implant systems, an increased resistance to induced periodontitis was documented. This cannot be interpreted as an absolute resistance. Intense gingivitis has been associated with increased marginal bone loss. Thus at the clinical level, there is a need to carefully monitor plaque control and periodontal tissue reactions around permucosal oral implants to avoid problems and eventual failures in the long-term perspective.

References

1. Miller AJ, Brunelle JA, Carlos JP, Löe H. US Department of Health and Human Services: Oral Health of United States Adults. The National Survey of Oral Health in US Employed Adults and Seniors: 1985–1986, National Findings. Washington, DC: US Department of Health and Human Services, Public Health Service, National Institutes of Health, NIH Publication no. 87-2868, 1987.

2. Socransky SS, Haffajee AD, Goodson JM, Lindhe J. New concepts of destructive periodontal disease. *J Clin Periodontol* 1984;11:21–32.

3. Caton J. Periodontal diagnosis and diagnostic aids. pp 1–22 In M. Nevins, W. Becker, K. Kornman (eds) *Proceedings of the World Workshop in Clinical Periodontics.* Chicago: American Academy of Periodontics, 1989.

4. Buser D, Warrer K, Karring T, Stick H. Titanium implants with a true periodontal ligament. An alternative to osseointegrated implants? *Int J Oral Maxillofac Implants* 1990;5:113–116.

5. Gould TRL, Brunette DM, Westbury L. The attachment mechanism of epithelial cells to titanium in vitro. *J Periodont Res* 1981;16:611–616.

6. Hansson H-A, Albrektsson T, Brånemark P-I. Structural aspects of the interface between tissue and titanium implants. *J Prosthet Dent* 1983;50:108–113.

7. Gould TRL. Clinical implications of the attachment of oral tissue to permucosal implants. pp 253–270 In D. van Steenberghe, T. Albrektsson, P-I. Brånemark, P.J. Henry, R. Holt, G. Liden (eds) *Proc Int Congress on Tissue Integration in Oral and Maxillofacial Reconstruction.* Amsterdam: Excerpta Medica, 1985.

8. van Steenberghe D. Periodontal aspects of osseointegrated oral implants. ad modum Brånemark pp 355–370 In M. Bral (ed) *The Dental Clinics of North America,* vol 32. Philadelphia: WB Saunders Co, 1988.

9. Van Drie HJY, Beertsen W, Grevers A. Healing of the gingiva following installment of Biotes implants in beagle dogs. Implant materials in biofunction. *Adv Biomater* 1988;8:485–490.

10. Adell R, Lekholm U, Rockler B, Brånemark P-I, Lindhe J, Eriksson B, et al. Marginal tissue reactions at osseointegrated titanium fixtures. A 3-year longitudinal prospective study. *Int J Oral Maxillofac Surg* 1986; 15:39–52.

11. Lekholm U, Adell R, Lindhe J, Brånemark P-I, Eriksson B, Rockler B, et al. Marginal tissue reactions at osseointegrated titanium fixtures. A cross-sectional retrospective study. *Int J Oral Maxillofac Surg* 1986; 15:53–61.

12. Quirynen M, Naert I, Teerlinck J, Theuniers G, De Clercq M, van Steenberghe D. Periodontal indices around osseointegrated oral implants supporting overdentures. pp 97–112 In E. Schepers, I. Naert, G. Theuniers (eds) *Overdentures on Oral Implants.* Leuven: Leuven University Press, 1990.

13. Adell R, Lekholm U, Rockler B, Brånemark P-I. A 15-year study of osseointegrated implants in the treatment of the edentulous jaw. *Int J Oral Surg* 1981; 10:387–416.

14. Quirynen M, Naert I, van Steenberghe D, Duchateau L, Darius P. Periodontal aspects of Brånemark and IMZ implants supporting overdentures: A comparative study. pp 81–94 In W.R. Laney, D.E. Tolman (eds) *Proceedings of the 2nd International Congress on Tissue Integration.* Chicago: Quintessence Publ Co, 1992.

15. d'Hoedt B, Schulte W. A comparative study of results with various endosseous implant systems. *Int J Oral Maxillofac Implants* 1989;4:95–105.

16. Bower RC, Radny NR, Wall CD, Henry PJ. Clinical and microscopic findings in edentulous patients 3 years after incorporation of osseointegrated implant-

supported bridgework. *J Clin Periodontol* 1989; 16:580–587.

17. Teerlinck J, Quirynen M, Darius P, van Steenberghe D. Periotest®: An objective clinical diagnosis of bone apposition toward implants. *Int J Oral Maxillofac Implants* 1991;6:55–61.

18. Heimdahl A, Köndell PA, Nord CE, Nordenram A. Effects of insertion of osseointegrated prosthesis on the oral microflora. *Swed Dent J* 1983;7:199–204.

19. Rams TE, Roberts TW, Tatun H Jr, Keyes PH. The subgingival micro-flora associated with human dental implants. *J Prosthet Dent* 1984;51:529–534.

20. Lekholm U, Ericsson I, Adell R, Slots J. The condition of the soft tissues at tooth and fixture abutments supporting fixed bridges. A microbiological and histological study. *J Clin Periodontol* 1986;13:558–562.

21. Mombelli A, Van Oosten MAC, Schürch E, Lang NP. The microbiota associated with successful or failing osseointegrated titanium implants. *Oral Microbiol Immunol* 1987;2:145–151.

22. Quirynen M, Listgarten MA. The distribution of bacterial morphotypes around natural teeth and titanium implants ad modum Brånemark. *Clin Oral Implants Res* 1990;1:8–12.

23. Sanz M, Newman MG, Nachnani S, Holt R, Stewart R, Flemmig T. Characterization of the subgingival microbial flora around endosteal sapphire dental implants in partially edentulous patients. *Int J Oral Maxillofac Implants* 1990;5:247–253.

24. Krekeler G, Pelz K, Nelissen R. Mikrobielle Besiedlung der Zahnfleisch taschen am künstlichen Titanpfeiler. *Dtsch Zahnärzt Z* 1986;41:569–572.

25. Apse P, Ellen RP, Overall CM, Zarb GA. Microbiota and crevicular fluid collagenase activity in the osseointegrated dental implants sulcus: A comparison of sites in edentulous and partially edentulous patients. *J Periodont Res* 1989;24:96–105.

26. van Steenberghe D, Lekholm U, Bolender C, Folmer T, Henry P, Herrmann I, et al. The applicability of osseointegrated oral implants in the rehabilitation of partial edentulism: A prospective multicenter study on 558 fixtures. *Int J Oral Maxillofac Implants* 1990;5:272–281.

27. Malmstrom HS, Fritz ME, Timmis DP, Van Dijke TE. Osseo-integrated implant treatment of a patient with rapidly progressive periodontitis. A case report. *J Periodontol* 1990;61:300–304.

28. Brånemark P-I, Breine U, Lindström J, Adell R, Hansson BO, Ohlsson A. Intra-osseous anchorage of dental prostheses. I. Experimental studies. *Scand J Plast Reconstr Surg* 1969;3:81–100.

29. Brandes R, Beamer B, Holt SC, Kornman K, Lang NP. Clinical microscopic observation of ligature induced "periimplantitis" around osseointegrated implants. *J Dent Res* 1988;67:287 (abstract 1397).

30. Cox JF, Zarb GA. The longitudinal clinical efficacy of osseointegrated dental implants: A 3-year report. *Int J Oral Maxillofac Implants* 1987;2:91–100.

31. Roberts WE, Smith RK, Zilberman Y, Mozsary PG, Smith RS. Osseous adaptation to continuous loading of rigid endosseous implants. *Am J Orthod* 1984; 86:95–111.

32. Schoo WH, Van der Velden U. Marginal soft tissue recessions with and without attached gingiva. A five-year longitudinal study. *J Periodont Res* 1985;20: 209–211.

33. van Steenberghe D. La greffe gingivale: abus thérapeutiques et indications. *Parodontol* 1984;3:365–375.

34. Krekeler G, Schilli W, Diemer J. Should the exit of the artificial abutment tooth be positioned in the region of the attached gingiva? *Int J Oral Surg* 1985;14:504–508.

35. Schroeder A, Van der Zypen E, Stich H, Sutter F. The reactions of bone, connective tissue and epithelium to endosteal implants with titanium sprayed surfaces. *J Maxillofac Surg* 1981;9:15–25.

Splinting Osseointegrated Fixtures to Teeth With Normal Periodontiums

T.J. O'Leary, R.W. Dykema, and A.H. Kafrawy

There is substantial evidence attesting to the successful long-term results of titanium fixtures serving as abutments for fixed prostheses in edentulous patients.[1-3] However, little information is available on the use of a combination of implanted fixtures and natural teeth as abutments for partial dentures. In one 10-patient clinical study of 6 to 30 months' duration, a varying number of implanted fixtures were used in combination with remaining natural teeth as supports for fixed prostheses.[4] In six patients, a rigid connector was employed between implant and natural tooth, while in four other patients, nonrigid attachments were used. The investigators reported a high level of oral hygiene around both implants and natural teeth, and a low frequency of bleeding upon probing for the two types of abutments. Mean probing depth and the range of depths were greater around the implanted fixtures than around natural teeth. There was no loss of alveolar bone around natural abutments, whereas a loss of 3 mm was found around two fixtures. In one patient in whom a nonrigid connector was used, the natural tooth was intruded at the 3-month evaluation. Although the report is interesting, it does not provide histologic information on the results of rigidly connecting a single implant to a single natural tooth with a fixed prosthesis, or on the interface between bone and fixture or between the natural root surface, the periodontal ligament, and bone.

A second report stated that the bacterial morphotypes in supra- and subgingival plaque were similar at tooth and fixture sites, with non-motile rods dominating the flora, and that few, if any, spirochetes were present.[5] Histologic analysis of marginal soft tissue biopsies from both fixture and tooth sites revealed only small numbers of inflammatory cells.

In a recent clinical study, 20 jaws were fitted with prostheses; both fixtures and natural teeth were utilized.[6] The authors reported that for most patients, sufficient fixtures were used to support the prosthesis without the natural teeth. They stated that the approach was used for research purposes and did not result in significant findings.

The present study investigated the short- (6 weeks), medium- (6 months), and long-term (1 year) histologic responses of the periodontium when an osseointegrated implant with no mobility was rigidly attached to a natural tooth with normal mobility.

Materials and methods

Six young male beagle dogs with permanent teeth erupted and with healthy periodontiums were used. After a 14-day acclimatization period, the animals' teeth were thoroughly cleaned under general anesthesia. Then the left side of the mandible of three animals was designated as the experimental side; the right side was the control side. In the other three animals, the right side was the experimental side and the left side the control. The mandibular third and fourth premolars (P3 and P4, respectively) on the designated experimental sides were then extracted under general anesthesia, as were the fourth premolars on the control sides. Throughout the study the animals were examined and received a prophylaxis every week. The teeth of each animal were brushed daily with Peridex (Procter & Gamble, Cincinnati, Ohio).

Seven weeks later, the extraction sites (P3 and P4) appeared completely healed. Radiographs confirmed that the sites had filled with new bone. Under intravenous anesthesia, mucoperiosteal flaps were raised from the buccal aspect of the P3, P4 area and extended over the crest of the ridge to the lingual surface. A 7-mm fixture site was then prepared in the P3 area. During preparation of all six experimental sites, the guide drill penetrated 1 to 2 mm into the coronal aspect of the mandibular canal. Implant fixtures measuring 7 by 3.75 mm (Nobelpharma USA, Inc, Chicago, Ill) were placed into the prepared sites and cover screws were affixed. The flaps were returned to their original position and secured with five 4-0 monofilament sutures. Each animal received 1 mL of benzathine penicillin (Flocillin) intramuscularly one time daily for 3 days following implantation of the titanium fixtures. The animals were maintained on a soft diet for 14 days after the fixtures were placed. They also received Liquid Tylenol 300 mg bid orally for 3 days after each surgical procedure. Nine days later, the surgical sites were debrided, irrigated, and the sutures removed.

A minimum of 10 weeks was allowed for healing and osseointegration of the fixtures. The fixtures were then uncovered under general anesthesia, tested for integration, and abutment connectors were placed.

Following a 4-week healing period, the animals were anesthetized and the third premolar and first molar (M1) on the control side and the first molar on the experimental side were prepared and impressions made for gold castings.

Three weeks later, under anesthesia, fixed partial dentures were placed and the occlusion adjusted. On the experimental side, the titanium fixture served as the anterior abutment and the first molar served as the distal abutment for the prosthesis. On the control side, the mandibular third premolar and first molar served as abutments. Radiographs of the experimental and control sides were obtained.

Two dogs were terminated 6 weeks after placement of the fixed partial dentures, two more were sacrificed 6 months after insertion, and the last two dogs were terminated at 1 year. For bone labeling, 10 days before termination each animal received a dose of Procion Brilliant Red H8BS, 100 mg/kg body weight, intraperitoneally.[7] The animals were sacrificed with an overdose of sodium pentobarbital (300 mg/lb body weight) administered intravenously. Death was assured by induction of bilateral pneumothorax.

Jaw segments containing the fixtures, abutments, and adjacent teeth were excised and fixed in 10% formalin and decalcified with 5% formic acid. After decalcification, the fixtures were carefully removed for examination with scanning electron microscopy. The decalcified specimens were then processed for routine paraffin embedding. Semiserial sections 7-μm thick were cut in the mesiodistal plane and stained with hematoxylin and eosin. Unstained sections were examined with fluorescence microscopy for Procion labeling.

Results

Clinical findings: 6 weeks

An interesting find was the rapid acceptance of the fixed partial dentures by the animals. Within 24 hours of placement, the animals were chewing vigorously on both sides of their mouths. The gingiva of both animals was in a high state of health. Probing depths were 2 to 3+ mm around both the control and experimental abutment teeth; areas of isolated bleeding were seen only rarely. Neither the experimental nor the control fixed prostheses exhibited any evidence of mobility or loosening of the castings.

Table 1 Histologic findings: 6-week animals

	Gingival inflammation	Periodontal ligament	Periosteum contiguous to implant	Root surface resorption	Repair of root surface resorption	Alveolar bone
Control sides						
Animal 1: P3	Mild	Normal	NA	No	NA	Physiologic remodeling
Animal 1: M1	Mild to moderate	Normal	NA	No	NA	Quiescent
Animal 2: P3	Minimal to mild	Normal	NA	Yes	Complete	Physiologic remodeling
Animal 2: M1	Minimal	Normal	NA	Yes	Ongoing	Physiologic remodeling
Experimental sides						
Animal 1: implant	Mild to moderate	NA	Yes	NA	NA	Physiologic remodeling
Animal 1: M1	Mild to moderate	Normal	NA	Yes	Ongoing	Quiescent
Animal 2: implant	Mild	NA	Yes	NA	NA	Physiologic remodeling
Animal 2: M1	Minimal	Normal	NA	Yes	Ongoing	Physiologic remodeling

P3 = third premolar; M1 = first molar.

Histologic findings: 6 weeks

Table 1 contains many of the histologic findings. The periodontal ligaments around the roots of the 6-week control and experimental teeth were of normal width (Figs 1 to 4). Strands of a thin layer of connective tissue were evident in some areas at the interface with the implants. These strands possessed the characteristics of a periosteum. When root surface resorption was present, it was superficial and had either been completely repaired or repair was well advanced.

The implants were surrounded with bone, with bony ridges corresponding to the grooves of the implants' surfaces (Fig 5). The bone was in part woven and in part lamellar, with occasional osteons being present. The bone exhibited remodeling with reversal and resting lines. Some endosteal spaces appeared large and lined with active osteoblasts; in some areas, endosteal spaces appeared to be communicating with bone surface.

The inferior alveolar nerves appeared intact and were covered at different levels with fibrous connective tissue alone, with a combination of bone and fibrous connective tissue, or with bone alone.

Clinical findings: 6 months

The two 6-month animals differed in gingival health status. One animal exhibited a high level of gingival health throughout the period. In the fourth month, the second animal began to show signs of gingival inflammation. Despite repeated thorough debridement of the implant sulcus, the inflammation did not subside until the animal was given a long-lasting antibiotic in conjunction with further debridement of the sulcus. The inflammation subsided, but bleeding upon probing was still present just prior to termination of the animal. Mobility could not be detected on the experimental or control fixed partial dentures. Loosening of castings was not seen.

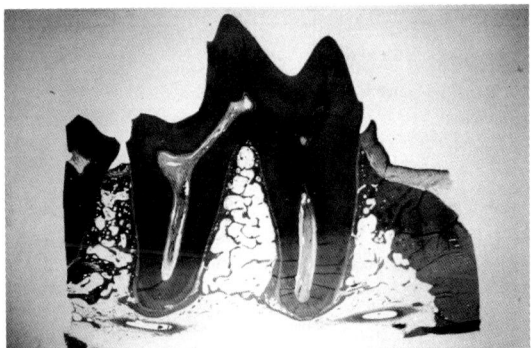

Fig 1 First molar, which served as a posterior abutment on an implant side at 6 weeks (hematoxylin-eosin, original magnification × 15).

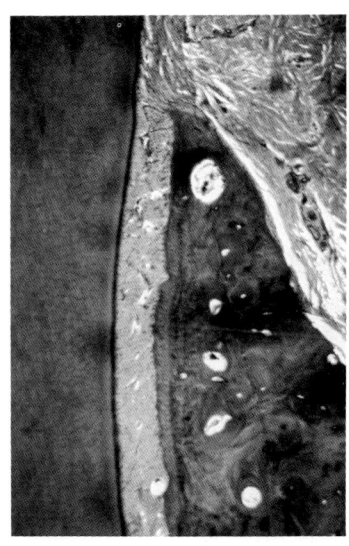

Fig 2 Higher magnification of the cervical region of the mesial surface of the mesial root of the molar of the 6-week experimental specimen. Cementum and periodontal ligament are intact. Alveolar bone surface is quiescent (hematoxylin-eosin, original magnification × 40).

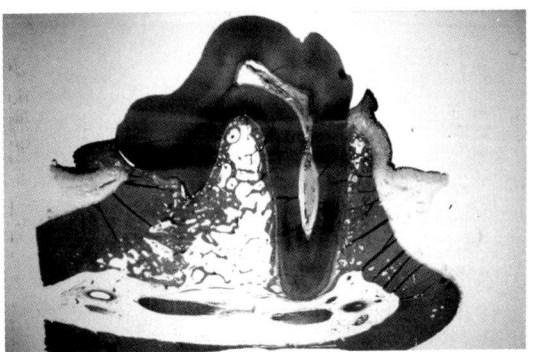

Fig 3 First molar, which served as a posterior abutment on a control side at 6 weeks (hematoxylin-eosin, original magnification × 15).

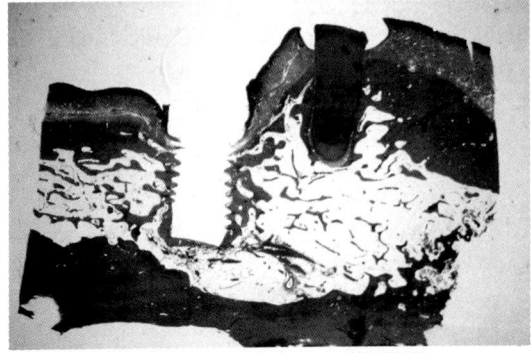

Fig 5 An implant site at 6 weeks. Gingiva surrounds the cervical portion of the fixture. More apically, ridges of bone interdigitate with grooves in the surface of the implant (hematoxylin-eosin, original magnification × 15).

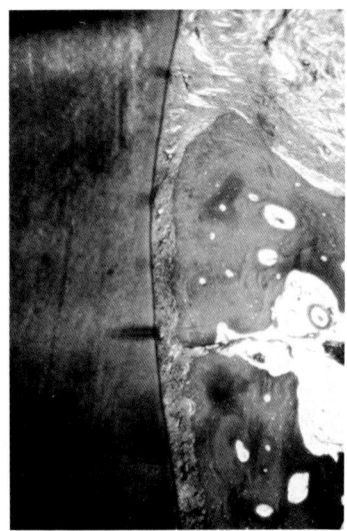

Fig 4 Higher magnification of the cervical region of the mesial surface of the mesial root of the 6-week control specimen. Cementum and periodontal ligament are intact. Alveolar bone surface is essentially quiescent (hematoxylin-eosin, original magnification × 40).

Table 2 Histologic findings: 6-month animals

	Gingival inflammation	Periodontal ligament	Periosteum contiguous to implant	Root surface resorption	Repair of root surface resorption	Alveolar bone
Control sides						
Animal 1: P3	Mild to moderate	Normal	NA	No	NA	Quiescent
Animal 1: M1	Minimal	Normal	NA	No	NA	Quiescent
Animal 2: P3	Mild to moderate	Normal	NA	No	NA	Quiescent
Animal 2: M1	Mild to moderate	Normal	NA	No	NA	Quiescent
Experimental sides						
Animal 1: implant	Moderate to severe	NA	Yes	NA	NA	Physiologic remodeling
Animal 1: M1	Mild	Normal	NA	Yes	Complete	Quiescent
Animal 2: implant	Moderate	NA	Yes	NA	NA	Physiologic remodeling
Animal 2: M1	Mild to severe	Normal	NA	No	NA	Quiescent

P3 = third premolar; M1 = first molar.

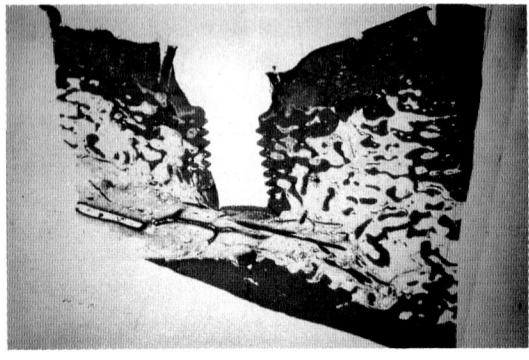

Fig 6 An implant site at 6 months. Gingiva surrounds the cervical portion of the fixture. Bony ridges interdigitate with grooves in the implant surface (hematoxylin-eosin, original magnification × 15).

Histologic findings: 6 months

Table 2 summarizes many of the histologic findings. As with the 6-week animals, there was no periodontal ligament widening around the roots of the control or experimental teeth. A thin layer of connective tissue having the characteristics of periosteum was seen in many areas at the interface with the implants. An isolated area of repaired root resorption was seen on the root of an experimental molar. Both implants were surrounded by lamellar bone with osteons (Fig 6). Physiologic remodeling was evident around both implants, while the bone was quiescent around the experimental and control teeth.

The inferior alveolar nerves appeared intact. The superior aspects of the mandibular canals were covered in part by bone and in part by fibrous connective tissue.

Clinical findings: 1 year

The two 1-year animals displayed a high level of gingival health throughout the study (Figs 7 to 10). Probing depths ranged from 2 to 3½ mm around the abutment teeth and implants. Bleeding upon probing was rare and was found only in isolated areas. As in the other two time groups, mobility of the fixed partial dentures was not found during any weekly examination and there was no evidence of loosening of a casting.

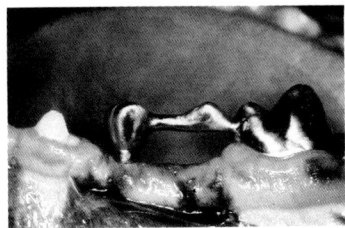

Fig 7 Experimental site at 1 year.

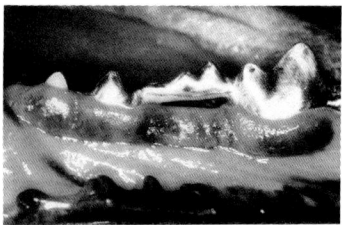

Fig 8 Control site at 1 year.

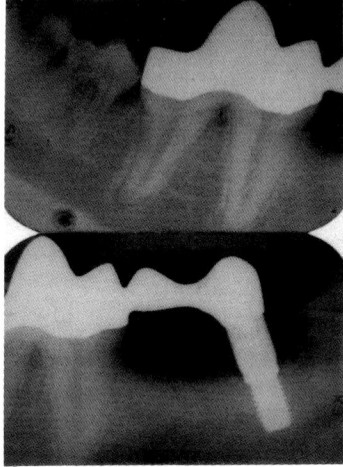

Fig 9 Radiograph of an experimental site at 1 year.

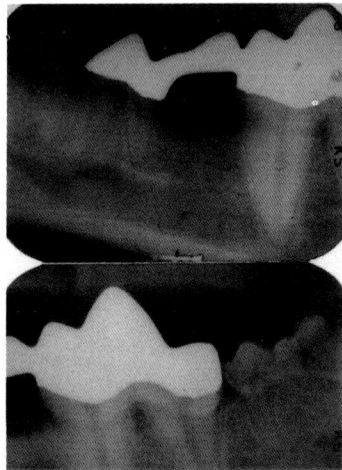

Fig 10 Radiograph of a control site at 1 year.

Histologic findings: 1 year

The major histologic findings at 1 year are presented in Table 3. As in 6-week and 6-month animals, there was no periodontal ligament widening around the roots of any experimental or control teeth. Three roots showed no evidence of resorption, whereas three others exhibited evidence of earlier resorption that had completely repaired itself. The implants were surrounded by lamellar bone, with bony ridges interdigitating with the implants' grooves (Figs 11 to 15). Several bony ridges adjacent to both implants showed a continuous periosteal lining. As in the 6-month findings, physiologic remodeling of the alveolar bone was seen only around the implants. Some of the endosteal spaces communicated with the bone surface. The mandibular canals were covered with bone and showed areas of prominent endosteal osteoblastic activity.

Procion labeling

Unstained sections were examined with fluorescence microscopy for Procion labeling. The implant sites at all study periods showed areas of periosteal (facing the implant) and endosteal bone labeling. Labeling was most intense at the 6-week study period; it declined at 6 months but was still evident at 1 year, indicating physiologic bone remodeling. The natural teeth that served as abutments on both the experimental and control sides showed occasional areas of

Table 3 Histologic findings: 1-year animals

	Gingival inflammation	Periodontal ligament	Periosteum contiguous to implant	Root surface resorption	Repair of root surface resorption	Alveolar bone
Control sides						
Animal 1: P3	Mild to moderate	Normal	NA	No	NA	Quiescent
Animal 1: M1	Mild to moderate	Normal	NA	No	NA	Quiescent
Animal 2: P3	Moderate	Normal	NA	Yes	Complete	Quiescent
Animal 2: M1	Mild	Normal	NA	Yes	Complete	Quiescent
Experimental sides						
Animal 1: implant	Mild	NA	Yes	NA	NA	Physiologic remodeling
Animal 1: M1	Mild to moderate	Normal	NA	Yes	Complete	Quiescent
Animal 2: implant	Mild	NA	Yes	NA	NA	Physiologic remodeling
Animal 2: M1	Moderate	Normal	NA	No	NA	Quiescent

P3 = third premolar; M1 = first molar.

labeling of alveolar bone facing the periodontal ligament (PDL) as well as endosteal labeling and occasional areas of cementum labeling.

Scanning electron microscopy

Scanning electron microscopic examination of the implant surfaces at all study periods exhibited areas of adherent connective tissue composed of fibroblasts and collagen fibers (Figs 16 and 17).

Discussion

Two findings deserve additional comment. None of the first molars that served as distal abutments for the implant-natural tooth fixed prostheses displayed widening of the periodontal ligament space when examined under the light microscope.

Further, microscopic examination did not detect any change in the periodontal ligament spaces of the control abutment teeth. These findings in canines cannot be extrapolated directly to humans because of differences in species and the shearing occlusion in dogs that can place considerable lateral force on the teeth during mastication and other occlusal contacts. The findings do, however, indicate that even in the presence of a less than ideal occlusion, a natural tooth with normal mobility can function satisfactorily as one abutment for a fixed partial denture when used in combination with a screw-type implant.

The routine finding under light microscopy of remnants of periosteum on the bone bordering the implants and on the surface of the metal fixtures was unexpected. Previous reports have stated that when pure titanium fixtures were placed atraumatically and left unloaded until osseointegration had occurred, either they abutted directly against bone or else only a thin proteoglycan layer was interposed between bone and implant.[8,9] Formation of a connective tissue capsule around an implant has been reported when undue trauma was intentionally induced during insertion[10] or when the fixture was immediately loaded.[11]

In the present study, great care was taken to

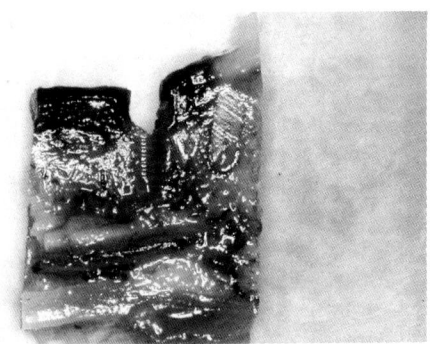

Fig 11 A decalcified, bisected, 1 year specimen after fixture removal.

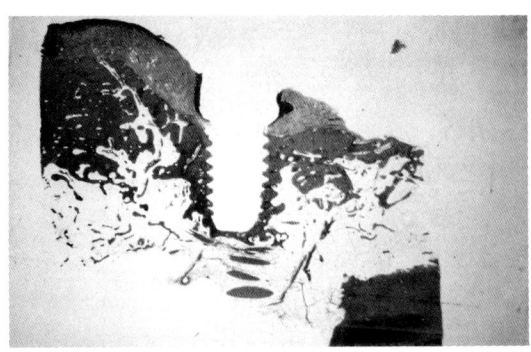

Fig 12 An implant site at 1 year. Gingiva surrounds the cervical part of the fixture. Bony ridges inter-digitate with grooves of the implant surface (hematoxylin-eosin, original magnification ×15).

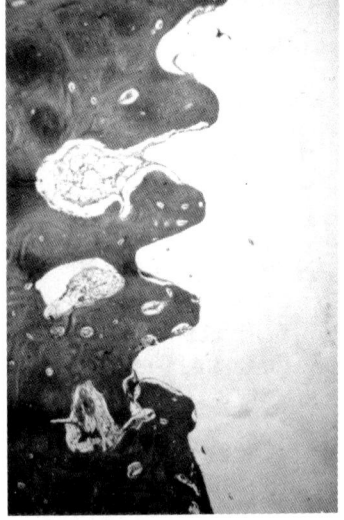

Fig 13 Implant bone interface at 1 year. Endosteal spaces have communicated in some areas with the bone surface (hematoxylin-eosin, original magnification ×40).

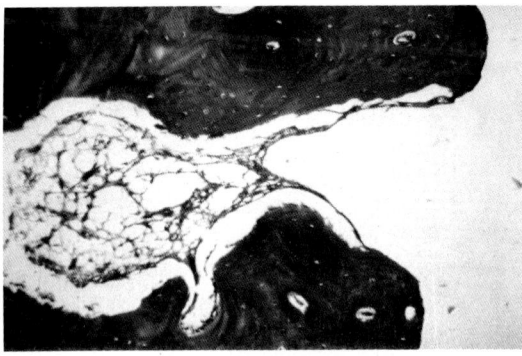

Fig 14 Higher magnification of an area of communication between endosteal space and implant surface (hematoxylin-eosin, original magnification ×100).

Fig 15 Higher magnification of another area of the 1-year specimen. A thin layer of connective tissue is evident over the bone surface. The space between the periosteal covering and the bone surface is arti-factual (hematoxylin-eosin, original magnification ×100).

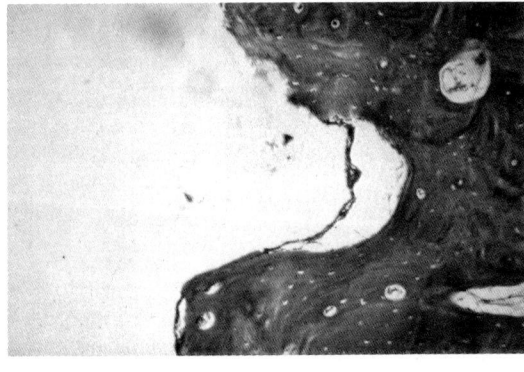

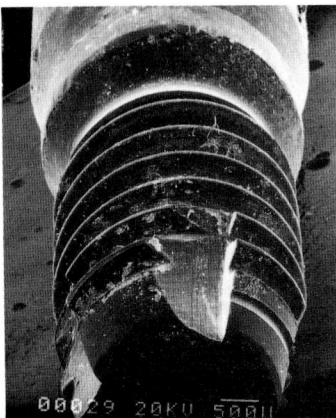

Fig 16 Scanning electron micrograph of an implant at 6 weeks. Fragments of connective tissue are adhering to the implant surface (original magnification ×20).

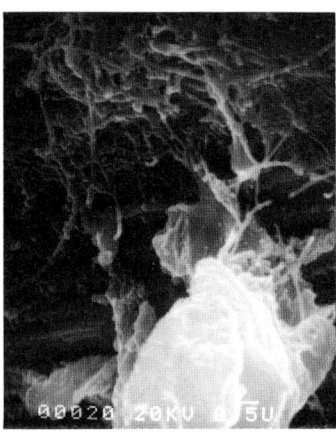

Fig 17 Higher magnification of a fragment of connective tissue that adhered to the implant surface. Fibroblasts and collagen fibers are evident over the implant surface (original magnification ×10,000).

avoid trauma when placing the fixtures and to allow sufficient time, a minimum of 10 weeks, for osseointegration to occur before connecting the abutments. One possible reason for previous reports that titanium fixtures abutted directly against bone could be that, in many instances, ground sections were prepared and the grinding process may have obliterated fine detail.

Finding a periosteum covering bone should have been expected. Except over articular surfaces that are covered either with cartilage or fibrous connective tissue, all external surfaces of bone are covered with periosteum and there is no reason for mandibular bone facing metallic implants to differ.[12,13]

type implant fixture. The surface of bone contiguous to screw-type implants is covered with a thin periosteal lining.

Acknowledgment

This study was supported in part by a grant from the American Academy of Implant Dentistry Research Foundation.

References

1. Brånemark P-I, Hansson BO, Adell R, Breine U, Lindström J, Hallén O, et al. Osseointegrated implants in the treatment of the edentulous jaw. Experience from a 10-year period. *Scand J Plast Reconstr Surg* 1977;11 (suppl 16):1–132.
2. Adell R, Lekholm U, Rockler B, Brånemark P-I. A 15-year study of osseointegrated implants in the treatment of the edentulous jaw. *Int J Oral Surg* 1981; 10:387–416.

Conclusions

A natural tooth with normal mobility can function satisfactorily as one abutment for a fixed partial denture when used in combination with a screw-

3. Adell R. Long-term treatment results. pp 175–186 In P.-I. Brånemark, G.A. Zarb, T. Albrektsson (eds) *Tissue-Integrated Prostheses. Osseointegration in Clinical Dentistry.* Chicago: Quintessence Publ Co, 1985.

4. Ericsson I, Lekholm U, Brånemark P-I, Lindhe J, Glantz P-O, Nyman S. A clinical evaluation of fixed bridge restorations supported by the combination of teeth and osseointegrated titanium implants. *J Clin Periodontol* 1986;13:307–312.

5. Lekholm U, Ericsson I, Adell R, Slots J. The condition of soft tissues at tooth and fixture abutments supporting fixed bridges. A microbiological and histological study. *J Clin Periodontol* 1986;13:558–562.

6. Jemt T, Lekholm U, Adell R. Osseointegrated implants in the treatment of partially edentulous patients: A preliminary study of 876 consecutively placed fixtures. *Int J Oral Maxillofac Implants* 1989;4:211–217.

7. Tomich CE. An evaluation of Procion brilliant red H-8BS as an in vivo hard tissue marking agent. Master's thesis. Indiana University School of Dentistry, Indianapolis, Ind, 1968.

8. Albrektsson T, Brånemark P-I, Hansson H-A, Lindström J. Osseointegrated titanium implants. Requirements for ensuring a long-lasting, direct bone-to-implant anchorage in man. *Acta Orthop Scand* 1981; 52:155–170.

9. Albrektsson T, Brånemark P-I, Hansson H-A, Kasemo B, Larsson K, Lindström I, et al. The interface zone of inorganic implants in vivo. *Ann Biomed Eng* 1983; 11:1–27.

10. Brånemark P-I, Breine U, Adell R, Hansson BO, Lindström J, Ohlsson A. Intra-osseous anchorage of dental prostheses. I. Experimental studies. *Scand J Plast Reconstr Surg* 1969;3:81–100.

11. Armitage J, Natiella J, Green G Jr, Meenaghan M. An evaluation of early bone changes after insertion of metal endosseous implants into the jaws of rhesus monkeys. *Oral Surg* 1971;32:558–567.

12. Leeson CR, Leeson TS. pp 140, 156 In *Histology.* 3rd ed. Philadelphia: WB Saunders Co, 1976.

13. Copenhaver WM, Kelly DE, Wood RL. pp 198, 201–203 In *Bailey's Textbook of Histology.* 17th ed. Baltimore: Williams & Wilkins, 1978.

Mechanical Aspects of a Brånemark Implant Connected to a Natural Tooth

B. Rangert, J. Gunne, and D.Y. Sullivan

In dental implant therapy there sometimes is a need for splinting natural teeth and implants. From a mechanical point of view, the reason for this is either to support teeth by implants or to support implants by teeth. However, the initial vertical flexibility of the implant integrated in bone is considerably less than that of the natural tooth, which is suspended in the periodontal ligament.[1] This difference in flexibility influences the distribution of occlusal forces between implants and teeth when splinted.

One special case of interest is the situation with one implant splinted to one natural tooth so as to allow the implant prosthesis to be extended (Fig 1). If the implant does not get support in this situation, it will be overloaded.[2] Thus the natural tooth connected is expected to share the prosthesis load with the implant.

To investigate this particular situation utilizing the Brånemark implant (Nobelpharma AB, Göteborg, Sweden), an in vitro study was performed.[3] This article summarizes the basic findings of this study.

Flexibility of the Brånemark implant

The gold cylinder and abutment of the Brånemark implant are fastened to the fixture by gold screws and abutment screws. When this screw joint is subjected to a bending moment, the pressure on the cantilever side of the abutment will increase and the pressure on the opposite side will decrease (Fig 2). These changes in surface pressure and gold-screw tension give rise to deformation of the materials involved, and the gold cylinder starts to tilt relative to the abutment. The abutment in turn tilts relative to the fixture. This tilt will be registered as a deflection at the end of the cantilever (Fig 1). As the tilt increases, the surface contacts move to the cantilever side of the abutment and the screw joint eventually opens (Fig 3).

According to the manufacturer (Nobelpharma AB, Göteborg, Sweden) the gold screw should be tightened to about 10 Ncm. Laboratory tests have shown this to correspond to a screw tension force (preload) of about 250 to 300 N (Nobelpharma). With this preload, the combined screw stress from tension and shear is just below the yield strength of the material. When this level (250 to 300 N) is reached because of external load on the gold cylinder, the screw joint will start to open. This means that with a lever arm of about 2 mm, the moment needed to open the screw joint is about 50 to 60 Ncm. Any bending moment below this value will be counteracted by the change in stress distribution within the joint (Fig 2) and will influence screw tension only to a minor extent.[2] Loads below 50 Ncm will therefore have a negligible influence on the screw and neither fatigue problems nor screw loosening need be anticipated at this load level.

Materials and methods

To investigate the mechanical phenomenon of

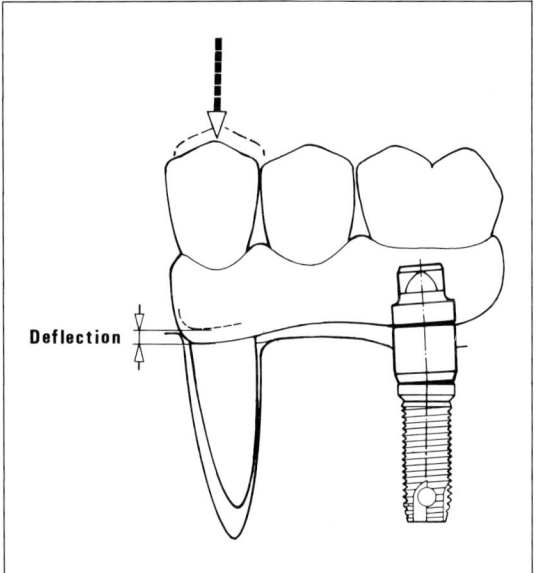

Fig 1 Bridge deflection with one implant and one tooth.

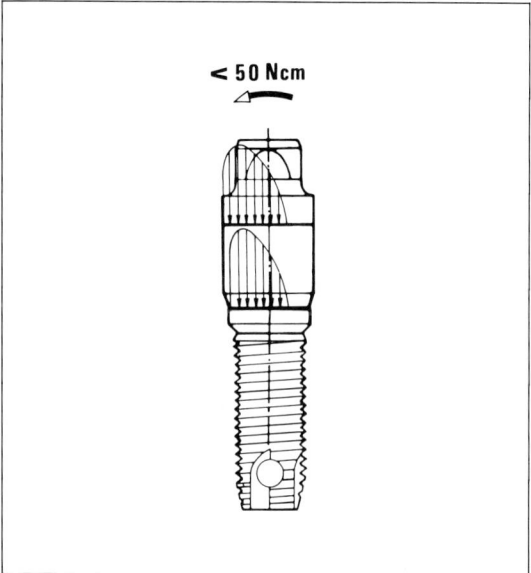

Fig 2 Internal stress distribution in the screw joint compensates for the external load before the screw joint opens. The internal screws are virtually unaffected by the external load.

screw joint flexion described earlier, a bench test was organized (Fig 4), consisting of one implant pillar with the fixture rigidly attached to a steel plate and a Class III gold bar as a 16-mm extension (cross section = 4 mm × 4 mm). This system is assumed to represent the flexibility and mechanical characteristics of the abutment/gold cylinder and extension unit for the clinical situation in which a three-unit fixed prosthesis is supported by one implant and one natural tooth.

The cantilever was loaded at 8 and 16 mm from the center of the implant, and the corresponding deflection at the positions of force was registered. In all tests the abutment screw was tightened to 20 Ncm and the gold screw to 10 Ncm. The tests were carried out with different cantilever lengths to check the results under varying test conditions. Four- and 7-mm abutments were used for both lengths of cantilever and two different abutment configurations were utilized. The implant and extension were also tested against repeated transverse motions in

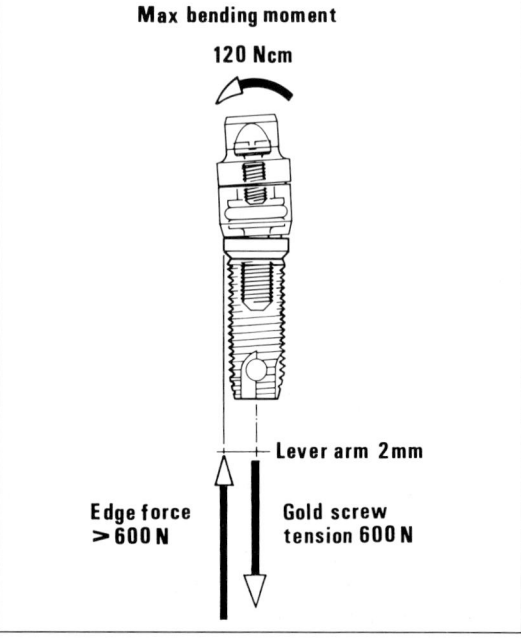

Fig 3 The internal screws are subjected to all the external load when the screw joint has opened.

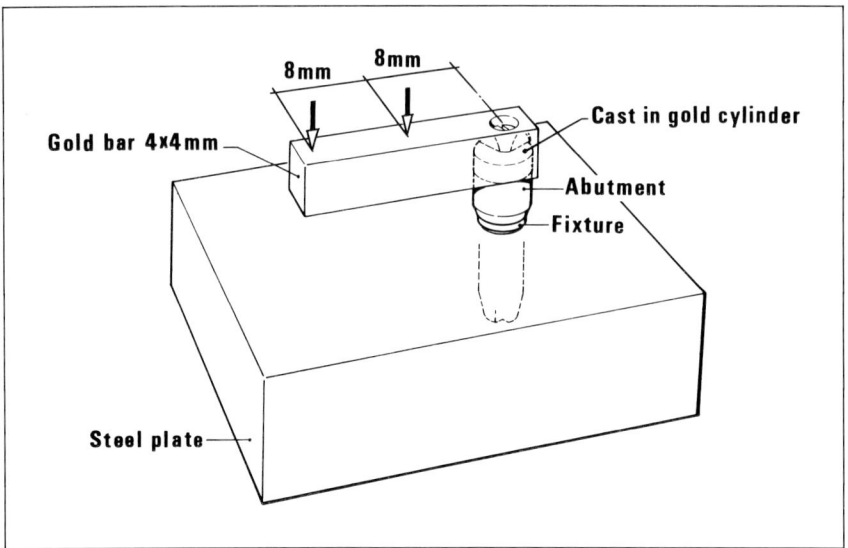

Fig 4 Test configuration.

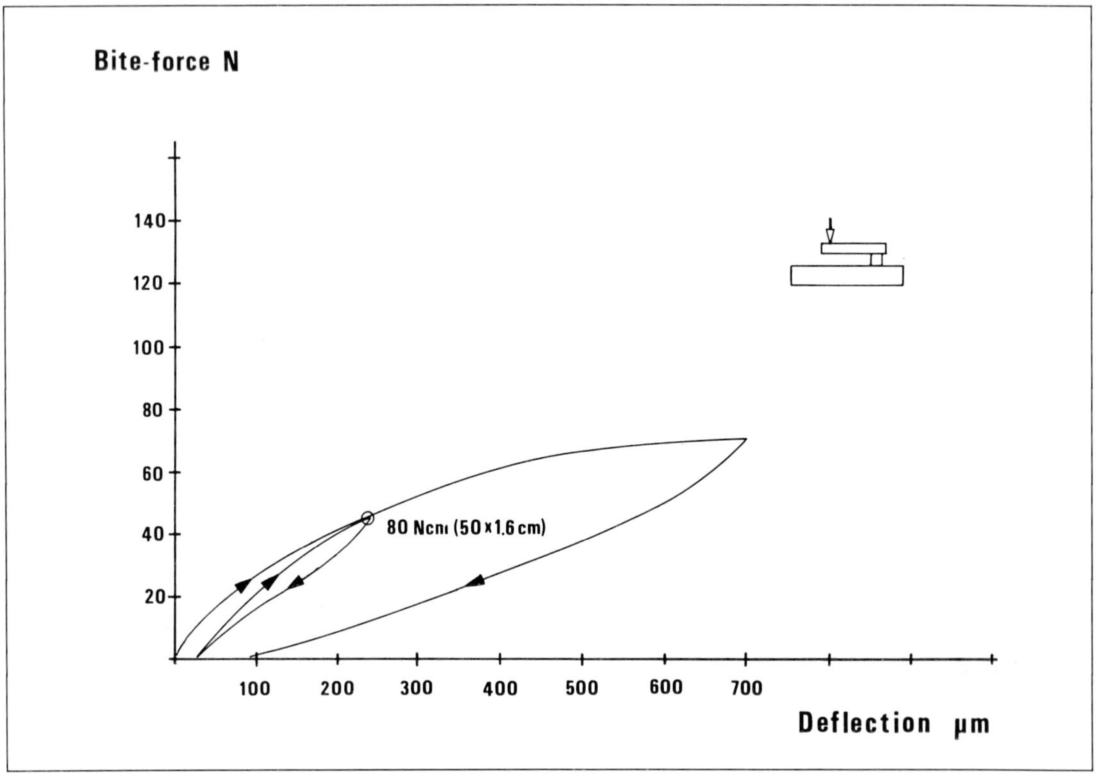

Fig 5 Recorded values for 16-mm extension.

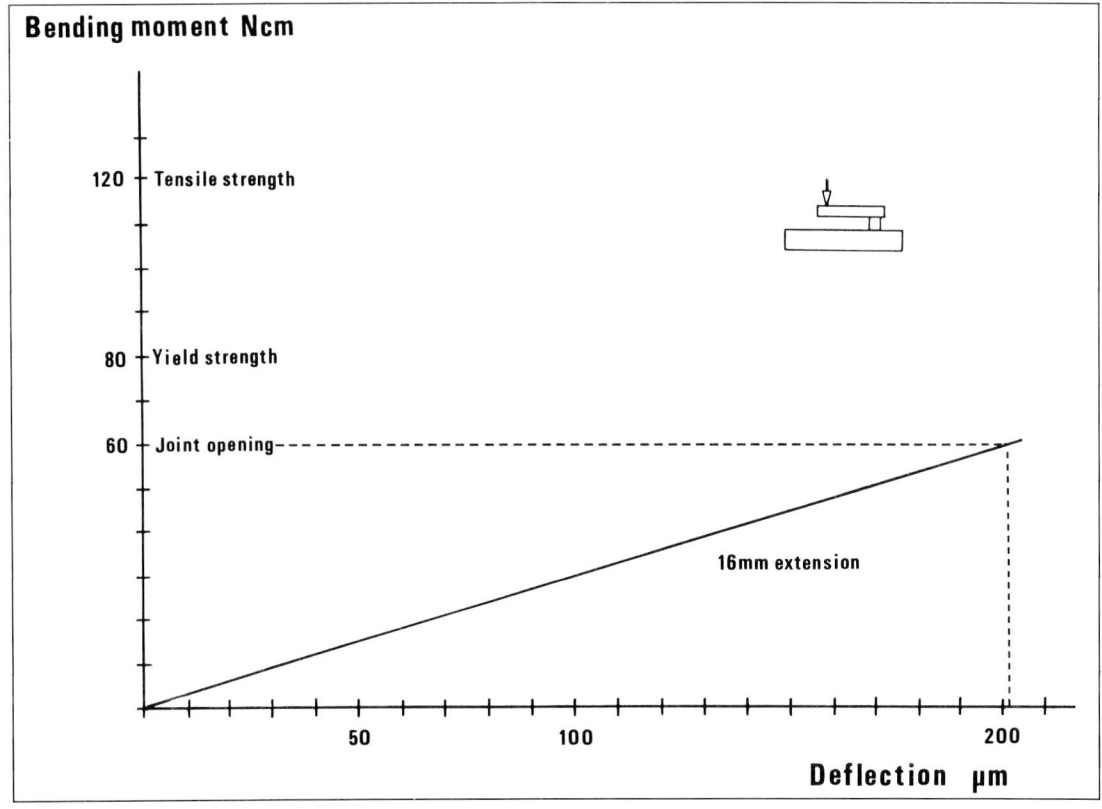

Fig 6 Moment versus deflection of the screw joint with 16-mm extension.

the magnitude of ±50 to 100 μm at the 16-mm position. Vertical load fatigue tests were carried out at load levels of 25 and 50 N at the 16-mm position (40 and 80 Ncm).

Results

A representative recorded diagram for the 16-mm extension is shown in Fig 5. The maximum deviations between different recordings were within 10%. No statistical analysis was performed, however.

Diagrams of recorded force versus deflection show an approximate linearity up to a bending moment of about 80 Ncm (100 and 50 N, respectively), at which point the screw joint starts to yield. This moment (80 Ncm) gives an axial screw force of about 400 N, which corresponds to the yield strength of the gold screw in pure axial loading according to laboratory tests (Nobelpharma). Flexibility increases continuously from this point and the curves flatten out at about 120 Ncm (150 and 75 N, respectively). This moment corresponds to the aforementioned tensile strength of the gold screw, which represents the load capacity of the joint. No significant difference in recorded values was found between the 4- and 7-mm abutments. The relationship was calculated between the applied bending moment on the screw joint and the corresponding angular deflection. The bending stiffness of the screw joint in the elastic range was found to be approximately 5,000 Ncm/rad (90 Ncm/degree).

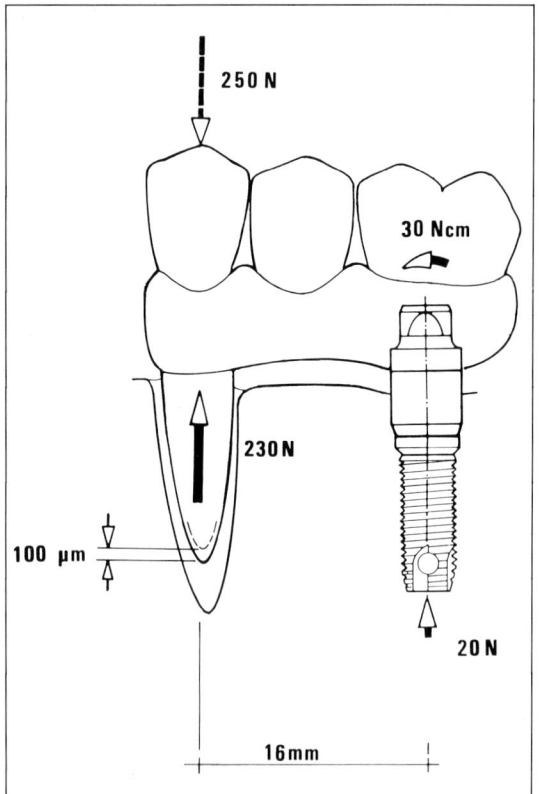

Fig 7 Load distribution with a bite force exerted on the supporting tooth.

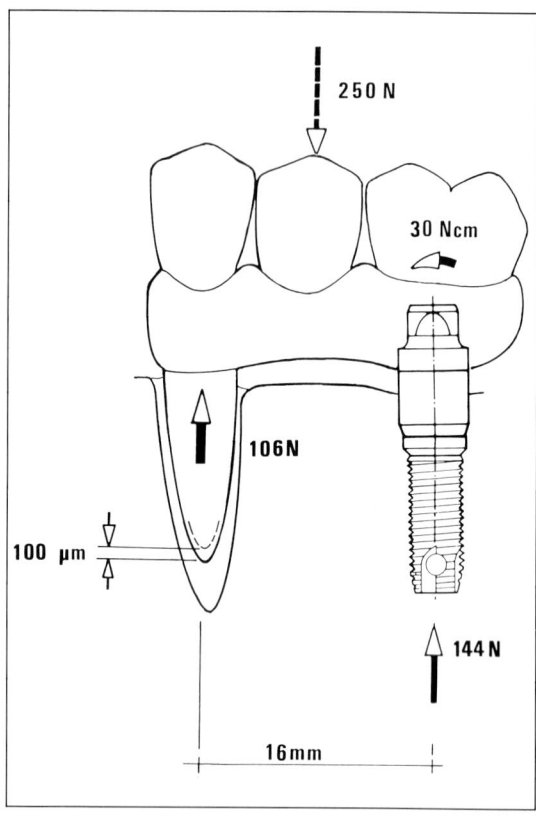

Fig 8 Load distribution with the force exerted between the tooth and the implant.

Repeated vertical loading at the extension, up to the yield strength of the screw joint (80 Ncm), resulted in abutment screw fracture after about 1,000 cycles. With loading below the opening point of the screw joint (40 Ncm), neither screw breakage nor loosening occurred, even at 1,000,000 cycles. This test demonstrates the importance of restricting the loading of the system to below the opening point of the screw joint.

Repeated transverse motion of the cantilever (1,000 cycles) at the 16-mm position at magnitudes of ±50 μm gave screw preload reduction, while magnitudes exceeding about ±100 μm gave rise to screw loosening. This test demonstrates the importance of limiting the transverse mobility of the supporting tooth.

Discussion

Magnitude of flexibility

The theoretical deflection of the cantilever beam can be calculated using the formulae for elastic beams. With a load of 50 N (16-mm extension), the calculated deflection is about 25 μm. Measured values of the axial stiffness of a Brånemark fixture are about 12 μm for an axial force of 50 N.[1] Compared with the measured deflections of about 230 μm at the same load (Fig 6), these values are of minor importance. The most significant factor to consider in estimating the mobility of the mechanical part of the

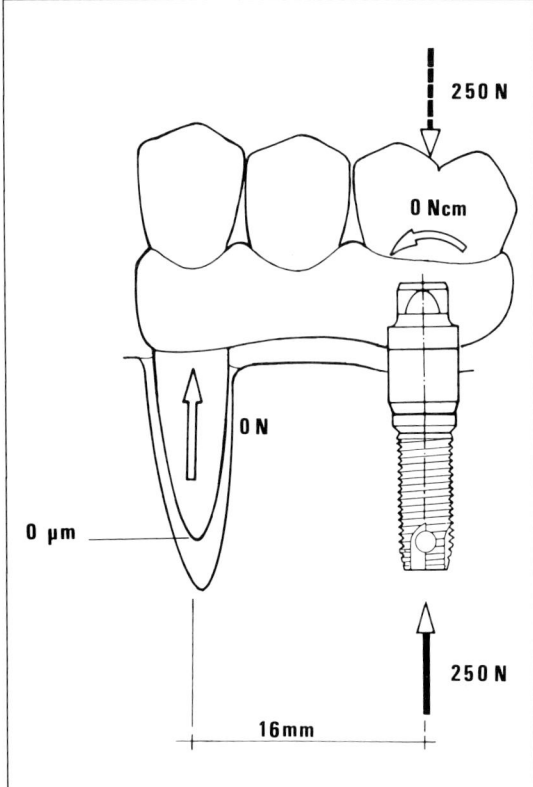

Fig 9 Load distribution with the force exerted on the implant.

implant/prosthesis system is therefore the flexibility of the screw joint.

Evaluation of the circumstances in which the influence of bone flexibility becomes important to the total flexibility of the prosthesis is beyond the scope of this study. However, it is indicated elsewhere[4] that the flexibility of the implant in bone may be significant.

Bending moment versus extension mobility was calculated for the 16-mm extension (Fig 6). The moments can be compared with the maximum moment (gold-screw tensile strength), with the upper moment limit for full reversible deflection (screw-joint yield strength), and with the moment for minimum screw load (screw-joint opening). One inescapable conclusion to be drawn from the diagram is that the bend-

ing moment on the implant at normal vertical tooth mobility (maximum = 50 to 100 μm) is far below the moment required for the joint to open. No fatigue problem need therefore be anticipated when normally mobile teeth are used for support.

These results indicate that with a fixed prosthesis connecting one Brånemark implant to a natural tooth, there is little risk of mechanical implant overload, and that the bending moment on the fixture is limited to about one-third of the maximum mechanical loading capacity of the implant. A consequence of limited mechanical loading is that the stress on the bone is restricted to fall well within the values normally encountered in clinical practice with the Brånemark system.

Vertical force distribution

With the measured data, it is possible to calculate the load distribution on a prosthesis unit for different positions of applied bite force. The three-unit restoration (16-mm extension) may be considered as an example. Tooth mobility is assumed to be 100 μm and bite force 250 N.

Figure 7 shows the situation in which the vertical bite force is at the center of the natural tooth. For a vertical mobility of 100 μm, the bending moment is about 30 Ncm (Fig 8) and the axial force about 20 N. Virtually all load is therefore concentrated at the position of the bite force and an acceptably low bending moment is encountered at the screw joint.

In Fig 8, the bite force is placed between the tooth and the implant, and the force is distributed almost equally between tooth and implant. When the force acts on the implant, the load will be transferred directly to the implant (Fig 9).

It is worthwhile noting that the bending moment on the implant is virtually independent of the bite force as soon as the tooth has reached its bottom position in the alveolus. After that point, the implant and the tooth will have about the same vertical flexibility, depending on the properties of the bone.

Summary

The abutment/gold cylinder screw joint of the Brånemark implant acts as a flexible element in the situation of one implant connected to a natural tooth. Thus when a prosthesis is supported at one end by an implant and at the other end by a natural tooth, the occlusal loads will be well distributed between the supporting units and the loading of the implant screw joint will be well below any fatigue limit if the supporting tooth has normal vertical mobility (50 to 100 μm). The risk of screw loosening of the joint is demonstrated in situations with excessive transverse mobility of the supporting tooth.

References

1. Brunski JB. Biomechanics of oral implants: Future research directions. *J Dent Educ* 1988;52:775–787.
2. Rangert B, Jemt T, Jörneus L. Forces and moments on Brånemark implants. *Int J Oral Maxillofac Implants* 1989;4:241–247.
3. Rangert B, Gunne J, Sullivan DY. Mechanical aspects of a Brånemark implant connected to a natural tooth—An in vitro study. *Int J Oral Maxillofac Implants* 1991;6: 177–186.
4. Sekine H, Komiyama Y, Hotta H, Yoshida K. Mobility characteristics and tactile sensitivity of osseointegrated fixture-supporting systems. pp 326–339 In *Proc Int Congress on Tissue Integration in Oral and Maxillofacial Reconstruction*. Brussels, May 1985, Amsterdam: Excerpta Medica, 1985.

Session I Discussion

G. Niznick (Encino, California): Dr van Steenberghe, you showed a slide and mentioned that
there was increased plaque accumulation on
titanium abutments. What causes that, and
have you considered the fact that the plaque
accumulation might not be due to the titanium
per se, but to the surface roughness of a
machined pure titanium versus the smoothness
of enamel or titanium alloy, which is a hard
material providing a much smoother machined
surface?

D. van Steenberghe (Leuven, Belgium): Your
point is well taken, because I said the most
important factor is the roughness. However,
besides that, surface free energy must be considered. For example, if two different titanium
surfaces with different roughnesses were compared, you would have different results. I would
not be so interested in the quantity of the
plaque, but rather the composition, which is
more important. We do observe this with the
pure titanium surface. The rapid accumulation
of bacteria is in concordance with the majority of
cocci that are observed on that same implant.
We know that cocci multiply themselves very
rapidly every 6 hours. There is a concordance
between the composition and the amount of
plaque. I would not say I would favor enormous
quantities of plaque, but this is nonpathogenic,
ie, the plaque, to a certain degree.

G. Niznick: You showed a conical self-tapping
Nobelpharma implant with bone loss and attrib-

uted it to the polished neck. Scanning electron
microscopic analysis of that implant shows that
the neck is not polished, but machined, the
same as the threads. Perhaps the neck being
wider than the body of the threads and concen-
trating stress in this area are the cause, rather
than surface difference.

D. van Steenberghe: What I meant is that it was
a nonthreaded part. In orthopedics a phenomenon known as stress-shielding is observed. I
cannot give proof that it is stress-shielding.
However, we have observed in an experimental
series that bone apposition remains stable
where the thread started, and it did not remain
stable where no threads existed. It is not a
question of smoothness at the microscopic level
or smoothness at the macroscopic level, ie, the
absence of threads. In my view, that is what
explains the lack of firm bone apposition over
time.

G. Niznick: A study coming out of Stonybrook
University in New York, Department of Periodontics, using a screw-type implant in which
the neck is the same dimension as the thread,
showed only 6/10 to 8/10 of a mm of bone loss in
the first year as measured from the crest of the
ridge, as opposed to systems with wider necks
that show a dramatically higher level of bone
loss. Maybe the bone loss is not due to stress-
shielding but to stress concentrations, which
can be eliminated by matching the neck to the
threads.

R. Baier (Buffalo, New York): Dr O'Leary, it
seems that your artifacts of sectioning and fixa-

Editors' note: A portion of the early discussion for this session was
lost because of faulty recording. The editors offer their sincere
apologies for the omission.

tion were more gentle than most that we have seen over the years. This allowed you to show the reality of this layer that you call periosteum. Beyond having these connective tissue features, do you have any other clues as to periosteumlike qualities, or couldn't this just be a connective tissue zone intervening between implant and adjacent bone? In addition, does your histologic evidence allow you to identify the origin of that lovely bone that you saw at the base of the implant in the marrow space? Was it locally recruited or was it down-welling from the cortex?

T. O'Leary (Indianapolis, Indiana): It was locally recruited. As far as the thin layer of connective tissue on the interface of the bone, I am always skeptical. We sent specimens out to about eight anatomists for review and asked what they thought. They all said it had the characteristics of periosteum.

M. Schwarz (Torrance, California): My comments are relative to Dr van Steenberghe's paper with respect to the microbiology involved with failed or failing implants. We have to be very cautious in drawing conclusions involving microbiology and failing implants for two reasons, one being that there has not been an attempt to separate different types of failed implants.

Even though clinically we cannot completely diagnose the cause of the failure, there are distinctly different types of clinical pictures, ie, the failing implant that gradually fails over time with progressive horizontal bone loss associated with soft tissue inflammation. That should be separated from an implant that has failed with the development of a radiolucency around its entire circumference and mobility with no associated clinical inflammation. When one does research and pools data between dissimilar types of failing implants, there is risk in making wrong interpretations.

Secondly, when an accumulation of pathogens associated with a failed implant is seen, one cannot make conclusions about causation. Because the ecology around failed implants is

going to be completely different, the growth of different types of organisms may be favored. So there may be an association with a particular implant, but the proof of causation is not there as yet.

D. van Steenberghe: Our knowledge from microbiology is so scarce and in pooling different types of implants, with different material surfaces, different causes of failure do indeed exist. For example, an overloaded implant that has become mobile and has become fibrously encapsulated develops a deepened pocket. Then, after a few weeks or few months, colonization with a lot of pathogens occurs. I certainly would not assume that the pathogens caused the failure.

A. Tjellström (Göteborg, Sweden): Dr van Steenberghe mentioned in his presentation that a gingival graft is not a good solution to the problem of gingival granulation tissue and he referred to our work in Göteborg concerning the extraoral application. It is important to have a very thin graft, which is the best solution over an implant extraorally. However, when granulation tissue exists and we are unsuccessful in treating it conservatively and do put a graft in, we have much poorer results with that compared to the normal grafting procedure. The reason for that is hygiene, the bacterial accumulation on the implant surface, and also the distance between the implants. Much more research is needed in this field.

M. Schwarz: If researchers will attempt to separate out different types of failures and investigate that aspect, it may give us a clinical tool for diagnosing the cause of the failure or maybe different microbiota associated with different types of failures.

D. van Steenberghe: We need a few more years for more good longitudinal studies concerning the microbiology around implants. Until then, we do not have all of the answers.

L. Shulman (Boston, Massachusetts): Dr Rangert, could you comment on the effect of proximity of implant to tooth with regard to load sharing and how this relates to clinical treatment planning?

B. Rangert (Göteborg, Sweden): What I showed as a reference was a 16-mm distance. If there is a shorter distance to the supporting tooth, there will be a higher bending moment for the same support type. The question then is whether or not this is a situation of impractical application because in that case, support is not needed since just one freestanding tooth is involved. On the other hand, the longer the extension, the smaller the loads. There are reports stating that the flexibility of bone is important as well, which might also mean that the load levels that I demonstrated are even lower in reality.

D. Harris (Dublin, Ireland): Dr van Steenberghe, you noted in your presentation a different rate and a different volume of bone resorption between a loaded fixture and a sleeping fixture. Have you any information on the rate and extent of bone resorption around sleeping fixtures after the first year, when compared to that which might occur in normal alveolar bone? Is there any evidence that a sleeping fixture might help preserve alveolar bone from the resorption that could occur in response to wearing a denture?

D. van Steenberghe: Bone loss around sleeping fixtures of 0.03 mm or 0.02 mm is what some would consider physiological bone resorption. What is physiological bone resorption? We should consider a piece of jawbone that is not subject to loading by denture or any other means; thus indeed, the bone loss around sleeping fixtures is more or less nil. Whether that means the presence of a sleeping fixture would reduce the physiological rate of bone loss, I could not say. The presence of a fixture loaded by the transfer of force intraosseously reduces the loss of bone when compared to the loss of bone that occurs at the same location when it is loaded by a denture. However, the role of sleeping fixtures in the maintenance of bone height is unknown. The reason for our experiment was to identify the role of loading and the role of exposure to a microbial environment in the ongoing bone loss. So far we are not able to differentiate between the two phenomena.

C. Kopp (Ho-Ho-Kus, New Jersey): Dr Rangert, Professor Brånemark has told us that one of the goals of implant therapy is to require minimal long-term maintenance of the patient. There seems to be a problem with single-tooth implant therapy in that there may be the possibility of needing temporary cements for the natural tooth, having to continually check whether the screws are loosening, and at times needing to replace these screws. I do not see the possibility for using permanent cements for these prostheses. Could you comment on this?

B. Rangert: To some extent it is out of the scope of my study. However, there is an engineering problem in having a single screw keeping all of these forces together. This is just a question of relying on the screw joint not to unscrew in the long run and that has to be studied further before we can recommend that type of connection as a standard procedure.

Preoperative Diagnostic Radiology for the Tissue-Integrated Prosthesis*

M.S. Schwarz, S.L.G. Rothman, N. Chafetz, and B. Stauts

Most of the early work on osseointegration was done on the completely edentulous mandible in which the implants (fixtures) were placed anteriorly between the mental foramina. More recently, however, the largest percentage of patients being treated is partially edentulous. This requires fixtures to be placed into all areas of both the mandible and maxilla. While operating in the posterior region of the jaws, surgeons must place fixtures in close proximity to the maxillary sinuses and the inferior alveolar canal in the mandible. In the anterior maxilla, the exact location and size of the incisive canal must be determined. Furthermore, in the anterior maxilla, esthetic requirements are of high priority. Therefore the surgeon must have a complete understanding of the osseous morphology so that fixtures can be appropriately positioned. In the maxilla especially, the prosthetic teeth are often positioned buccal to the remaining bone so that it is helpful for the surgeon to have an image demonstrating the tooth-to-bone relationship to permit the appropriate fixture angulation.

Preoperative radiographic evaluation has assumed an increasingly important role in treatment planning for implant-supported prostheses. Both external as well as internal bony anatomy should be clearly demonstrated. Accurate radiographic images are required and any magnification must be constant throughout so that direct measurements can be made. In addition, cross-sectional images have become an almost indispensable component of the radio-graphic survey so that anatomic features can be identified in a buccolingual dimension.

Radiographic modalities

Several radiographic modalities are currently being used, including conventional intraoral and extraoral projections, panoramic radiography, axial tomography, computed tomography, and magnetic resonance imaging. Each of these has certain advantages and disadvantages.

The panoramic radiograph can provide a gross display of potential fixture recipient sites, the degree of bone resorption, as well as a general view of the relative position of vital anatomic structures such as the inferior alveolar canal and maxillary sinuses. The panoramic radiograph has several limitations including nonuniform magnification, distortion, and overlapping of structures and ghost images.[1-3] Additionally, information regarding the thickness of the alveolar process is not available with this modality. Accurate assessment of hard tissue morphology and density is impossible because of the differential distortion in various portions of the radiograph.

Lateral cephalometric radiographs provide cross sections of the mandible and maxilla, but only in the midline. The osseous morphology and dimensions are available in the midline but cannot be seen in other portions of the jaws. Even in completely edentulous jaws, bone resorption may be greater lateral to the midline,

*Keynote presentation.

affecting both the height and buccolingual thickness of the bone. Treatment of the partially edentulous patient often involves surgical sites in the posterior quadrants of the jaws where accurate cross-sectional imaging is required to reveal bony dimensions as well as the configuration and location of internal anatomic structures. Therefore, there is a need for cross-sectional imaging throughout the entire potential surgical field. The most useful information displayed by the lateral cephalometric radiograph is the maxillomandibular skeletal relationship.

Conventional x-ray tomograms with special equipment are able to produce radiographic cross sections perpendicular to the alveolar ridge,[4] but they are, by their very nature, blurred images. With this technique, the x-ray tube and film revolve around the patient in opposite directions. The motion blurs all anatomic planes except the single plane at the center of the arc of rotation. Thus, a conventional tomogram produces its planar images by blurring all planes outside the plane of focus. Adjacent extraneous structures decrease image sharpness. Another disadvantage of conventional tomograms is the lack of adequate cross-referencing with standard lateral, frontal, and panoramic radiographs.[5] There are no intrinsic markers to absolutely identify the precise location of each individual slice. Implant positions must be predetermined and stents with radiopaque markers must be fabricated prior to the x-ray film examination (that is, prior to knowing where the most desirable bone is located). Because the stents are used as a guide by the radiographer, only those sites marked will be studied. If the bone is found to be inadequate in any of the marked locations, it may become necessary to recall the patient and radiograph other locations. For complex situations in which multiple fixtures are to be implanted throughout the circumference of the jaw, conventional x-ray tomography is impractical, as it is extremely time-consuming to produce a large number of cross-sectional tomograms. Also, this modality is very technique-sensitive and there are few x-ray technicians who can provide predictable results.

Computed tomography (CT) has the advantage of being easily performed with reproducible results. It can provide images of the entire jaw in any plane desired by the dentist. Several investigators have documented the similarity of mechanical measurements of bone anatomy with measurements obtained from CT images.[6-9] Programs utilizing multiplanar reformation (CT/MPR) have been developed specifically for dental implant surgery (Dentascan, General Electric, Milwaukee, Wisc) and these automatically provide axial, panoramic, and oblique cross-sectional images that are all cross-referenced to one another.[10,11] Earlier problems with artifacts from metallic dental restorations have been eliminated by scanning the patient in the axial plane, thereby avoiding the restorations. The restorations lie in a plane above or below the level of the alveolar bone and therefore do not project onto the axial CT. The artifacts, therefore, project above the plane of the mandibular ridge and below the plane of the maxillary ridge.

A disadvantage of CT is the fact that more radiation is involved than with the other radiographic techniques discussed.[12] While radiation is never desirable, the clinical significance of radiation is related to the type of tissue exposed. The two most sensitive tissues in the head and neck, the corneas of the eyes and the thyroid glands, can be completely avoided by scanning the patient in the axial plane. In addition, with the Dentascan technique, the scanner uses the lowest radiation exposure and the shortest scan time possible.

Magnetic resonance imaging (MRI) has the advantage of no radiation exposure, but has the disadvantage of being much more expensive than any of the other techniques. In addition, ferromagnetic metals distort the magnetic field and compromise the image. At the present time there is no method of cross-referencing images in different planes, making it difficult to identify specific anatomic sites. Finally, MRI does not yield images of cortical bone, a serious limitation in dental implant presurgical evaluations.

Relative to the accuracy of the various radiographic modalities discussed, a recent study[13] compared the measurements made from gross macroscopic specimens with those obtained from periapical and panoramic radiography, hypocycloidal tomography, and computed tomography. With conventional two-dimensional radiographic methods, there were a high number of mandibular canals that could not be detected at all. The results showed that of the techniques investigated, CT gave the most accurate position of the mandibular canal with 94% of the measurements within ±1 mm of the true value. For periapical radiographs, the corresponding figure was 53%, for conventional tomography 39%, and for panoramic radiography 17%.

Bone density estimates can be made with all CT scanners. Each shade of gray on a CT image represents a number corresponding to the absorption of x-rays by that particular volume of tissue. The Hounsfield scale, named after the inventor of CT, arbitrarily defines the radiodensity of water as zero. Fat is less radiodense than water and its values are in the negative range. Very dense bone has attenuation values of above 1,000 units. Each two-dimensional picture element or pixal represents a three-dimensional volume of tissue, usually 1.0 × 0.8 × 0.8 mm. The CT number for each individual pixal or group of pixals can be defined by the scanner and an average CT number calculated. This number is directly related to the bone and fat content of the tissue. There is considerable variation in bone density within each jaw. Medullary bone is very heterogeneous with areas of fatty marrow alternating with areas of more dense trabecular bone. It is possible to define a volume of tissue within the area of a proposed fixture and calculate an average CT number within that volume. It should then be possible to categorize the quality of that bone with respect to its average bone density. It is important to realize that these measurements must be made in a volume of tissue rather than at a point, because the quality of bone varies randomly across the height, width, and breadth of the bone. This information might be of value in predicting the likelihood of osseointegration. It is widely assumed that dense bone is better able to support an implant than is diffuse cancellous bone. However, a preliminary analysis of a series of fixture failures revealed that many of the failures occurred in dense bone and one can speculate that overheating becomes more of a problem as bone becomes more dense.[14] As of this time, there is no definitive answer to the clinical significance of bone density in terms of Hounsfield units.

Radiographic stents

There may be little or no relationship between the position of the prosthetic teeth and that of the remaining bone. The position of the teeth is determined by neuromuscular controls as well as functional and esthetic requirements of the patient. In the anterior maxilla where the teeth are often placed anterior to the edentulous ridge, phonetics, esthetics, and lip support determine tooth position. In the anterior mandible, tooth position is determined by the position of the maxillary anterior teeth as well as the requirements of occlusion and phonetics. In the posterior portion of the jaws, the teeth are located in the "neutral zone" where forces generated by cheek and tongue pressure are in a state of equilibrium.

Because tooth position is not necessarily related to the location of the bone, bony anatomy cannot be used by the surgeon as the only guide for fixture positioning. To achieve the optimum esthetic and functional result, fixtures must often be tipped so that their long axes are different than the long axis of the alveolar processes (ie, the fixtures should be tipped toward the prosthetic teeth). In preoperative treatment planning, it is helpful for the prosthetic teeth to be demonstrated on the radiographic images so that the relative positions of the teeth and the bone can be clearly seen. This is accomplished by utilizing a radiographic stent during the scanning procedure.[5,15] The cross-sectional images obtained from this technology allow the restorative dentist and surgeon to preview the patient's bony anatomy and determine if the potential exists for fixture placement that is consistent with the prosthetic goals.

A primary requirement for the fabrication of any stent is to accurately capture the correct form and position of the intended prosthesis. Thus the first step in this process is the trial arrangement of teeth on accurately mounted casts and, if necessary, oral confirmation of the esthetic and functional appropriateness of the tooth arrangement. When the trial denture is satisfactory, it is replicated to fabricate the stent.

Selection of a radiographic contrast medium to be used with computerized tomography is limited to nonmetallic substances. Metals, particularly those of a high specific gravity, tend to produce radiation scatter on the film, which distorts the image. In addition, the radiopaque material must be compatible with autopolymerizing acrylic resin and not affect the resin's curing time or strength. The contrast material favored by the authors is Hypaque Sodium (Winthrop-Breon Pharmaceuticals, New York, NY). Hypaque Sodium is an iodinated compound (diatrizoate sodium) used in gastrointestinal radiography and is nontoxic. It comes as a fine white powder and mixes easily with clear orthodontic resin. Sharp images are achieved with a contrast powder to acrylic polymer ratio of 1:4. The monomer/polymer ratio way be varied to obtain the flow properties desired by the operator.

Construction of a completely edentulous stent starts with the duplication of either the patient's current denture or the trial denture, whichever represents the desired final prosthesis. Once invested, the prosthesis is removed from the flask and a viscous mix of acrylic resin mixed 4:1 with contrast medium is added to the tooth areas only. The remaining volume of the mold is then filled to excess with clear resin and is processed. Trial insertion of the stent in the patient's oral cavity is required to confirm the fit, occlusion, and correct tooth position.

The partially edentulous stent takes several forms. If the edentulous area is currently restored with a removable partial denture, a mucoadhesion-type stent can be processed on a cast in either the duplicating flask or by simply using an impression tray and irreversible hydrocolloid. The technique is otherwise the same as for the edentulous stent. When the edentulous

area is restored by a fixed partial denture, a provisional restoration will need to be made. Casts of the prepared teeth are obtained and vacuum-formed shells are produced to replicate the desired prosthesis. The tooth-colored provisional and a second provisional utilizing the contrast medium are processed on duplicate casts. These provisionals are trial-seated on the prepared teeth, adjusted, and the tooth positions and form are then confirmed. The radiopaque provisional can be cemented with petroleum jelly while being scanned.

During the CT scan procedure, the patient wears the radiographic stent. It is important to note that in the usual scanning procedure without a stent, axial slices extend just far enough to incorporate the crest of the alveolar processes. Thus, when utilizing a stent, the radiologist and/or radiographic technician must be instructed to scan up through the full extent of the prosthetic teeth.

Use of the described radiopaque stent techniques will produce dramatic images that can greatly enhance communication between the restorative and surgical doctors. Difficult anatomical problems can be predicted and solutions jointly developed by the entire implant team before surgical intervention is attempted. For example, the need for bone augmentation materials or angled abutments can be anticipated and the surgery planned accordingly. Such communication can only provide a much higher quality service for the implant patient (Fig 1).

Vital anatomic structures

Implantation of root-form titanium fixtures into the edentulous mandible has been performed by Brånemark and associates for the past 25 years.[16] Until recently, the Swedish group limited their implant placement to the anterior mandible between the mental foramina.

Initially, six fixtures were placed and later it was found that successful rehabilitation with fixed prostheses could be achieved with five or even four fixtures. Preoperative radiographic

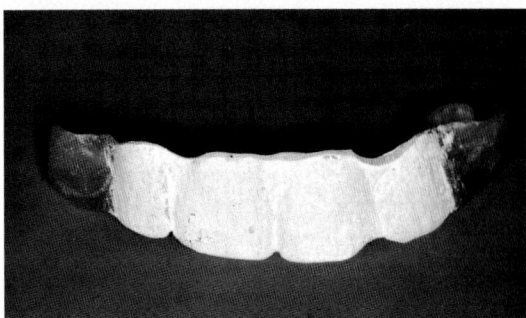

Fig 1a Radiographic stent with radiopaque contrast medium incorporated into crown portions of teeth.

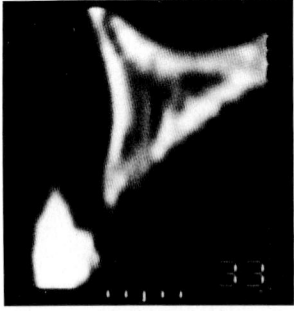

Fig 1b Computed tomographic oblique cross section shows the relationship of the proposed prosthetic tooth to the bone.

evaluation usually involved the use of panoramic and lateral cephalometric radiographs.[16] The images obtained with these methods provided information regarding the height of the available bone as well as the cross-sectional anatomy at the symphysis. However, it failed to demonstrate the cross-sectional anatomy throughout the entire extent of the proposed surgical area. Therefore, in patients with inadequate buccolingual dimension of bone to accommodate root form implants, this condition may not have been discovered until mucoperiosteal flaps were reflected to directly expose the mandible. Additionally, the majority of patients now being treated with implants is partially edentulous and often require fixtures to be placed in the posterior mandible and maxilla. In these situations, the surgeon must have a complete picture of the associated anatomic structures.

In the partially edentulous mandible, posterior quadrant implantation poses the most severe challenge to the surgeon because of the presence of the inferior alveolar neurovascular bundle. Routine radiographic techniques reveal only the distance from the crest of the ridge to the nerve and may not even permit adequate visualization of the canal. When the canal is seen, simply measuring the distance from the crest of the ridge to the canal can be very misleading.[1–3,17–20] Because the ridge may be eccentric, it is impossible to accurately predict what the true relationship of the nerve is to the alveolar bone. This limitation of conventional radiography (panoramic techniques) forces the surgeon to select an implant length that will not involve the inferior alveolar canal, thus precluding anchorage of the "apical" end of the fixture in cortical bone. Because cancellous bone in the posterior mandible is usually very sparse, this limitation of panoramic radiography may significantly contribute to increased failure rates for mandibular posterior implants. CT-guided surgery allows one to visualize the internal osseous morphology in all three dimensions and thus enables the surgeon to plan fixture angulation and length to anchor its "apical" tip into available cortical bone. This could mean extending the fixture inferior to the plane of the nerve so as to anchor it in the cortex on the inferior border of the mandible or to anchor it into the buccal or lingual cortex. If the amount of bone buccal or lingual to the nerve is insufficient to allow passage of an implant, precise measurements from the CT images may allow the surgeon to anchor the fixture into the cortical ceiling of the canal.

The quality of mandibular bone is highly variable and may also impact the success of osseointegration. Demineralization of the edentulous jaw segment may become very profound. It is convenient to define three types of mandibles based on the radiographic appearance of the CT image. In some mandibles there is a large amount of densely ossified bone within the medullary cavity of the mandible. The nerve canal is seen as a well-circumscribed lucent channel within this white bony matrix (Fig 2a).

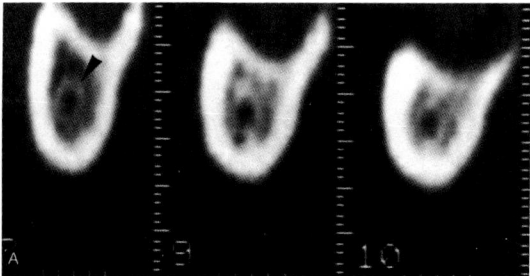

Fig 2a Three sequential cross-sectional oblique views of a mandible with dense bone surrounding the inferior alveolar nerve. (From Rothman SL, et al. CT in the preoperative assessment of the mandible and maxilla for endosseous implant surgery. *Radiology* 1988;168:171–175; with permission.)

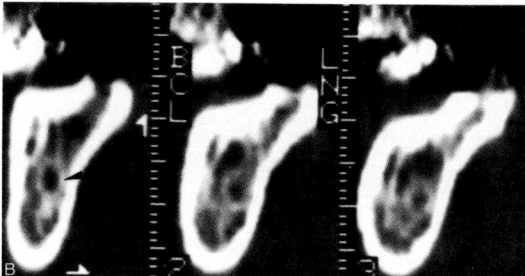

Fig 2b Three sequential cross-sectional oblique views showing fatty marrow surrounding the inferior alveolar nerve. The canal is discernible because of the thin cortical bony rim surrounding it.

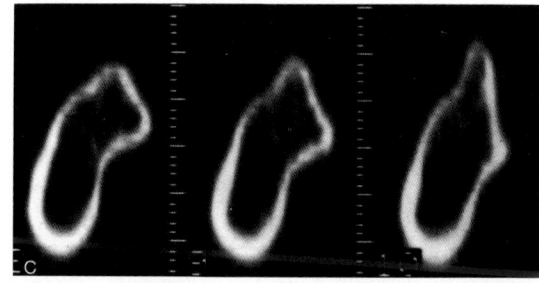

Fig 2c Three sequential cross-sectional oblique views in which the inferior alveolar nerve canal is not demonstrated. The substance of the bone is demineralized to the point that the bone surrounding the nerve canal is not visible on the CT image.

More commonly, the medullary bone is less dense because of a relative decrease in bone trabeculae and an increase in fatty bone marrow. It is common to see a distinct dense bony margin surrounding the nerve within a dark fatty marrow cavity (Fig 2b). In some patients, demineralization and osteoporosis may be so profound that the residual bone matrix is present microscopically but is too small to be resolved by the CT scanner. In these patients, it may be impossible to identify the nerve (Fig 2c). It is unusual for an entire arch to be so demineralized and, therefore, it is usually possible to identify several cross sections where the nerve is visible and several sections in which there is no hint of the bony canal. It may still be possible to derive anatomic information from the CT scan by inference. In our experience, the downward sloping course of the inferior alveolar nerve is very predictable. We have never seen a patient in whom the nerve undulates in a superior to inferior manner.

There does not appear to be any way of predicting the buccolingual position of the nerve within a particular arch. It may lie along the buccal plate, in the center of the bone, or on the lingual side. At some point along its course, it runs obliquely across the bone from its origin on the medial side in the ramus to exit buccally at the mental foramen. With conventional radiography, one can only hope to ascertain the buc-

colingual position of the nerve canal with an occlusal view. The CT program, however, demonstrates the buccolingual position of the nerve in the oblique cross sections at 2-mm intervals.

Even when implanting the anterior edentulous mandible, care must be taken to avoid damaging the inferior alveolar nerve. The terminal fixture on each side should be placed as close to the foramen as possible so as to minimize the length of posterior cantilevers. However, the inferior alveolar canal and its contents customarily loop forward of the mental foramen before exiting in a posterior-superior direction. Our studies have demonstrated the distance of this anterior looping to be quite variable. Computed tomography analysis often demonstrates the extent of the anterior looping and thereby allows for predictably safe placement of the

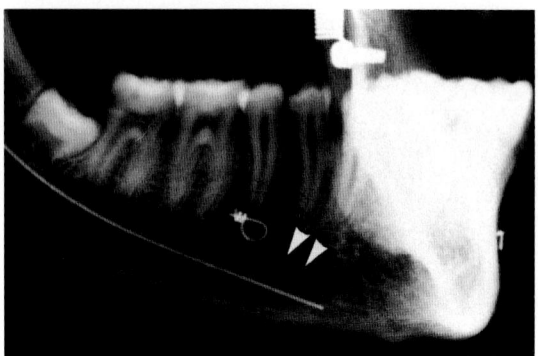

Fig 3a A radiograph of a mandibular specimen with a flexible guide wire placed into the inferior alveolar nerve canal. A second wire loop is placed over the mental foramen. Note that the guide wire projects well forward of the mental foramen, and there is a clearly defined loop projecting backward and labially. This represents an anterior genu of the inferior alveolar nerve.

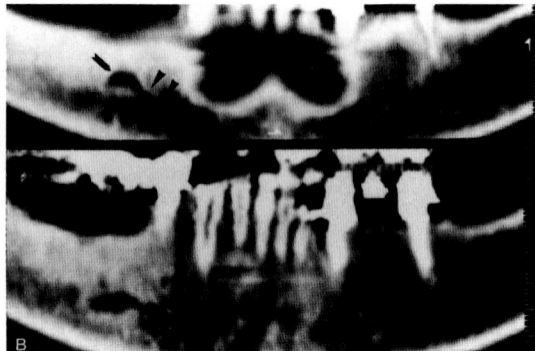

Fig 3b Panoramic CT reformation on a patient, showing the mental foramen *(single arrow)* and the posterior projecting genu of the inferior alveolar nerve *(two arrows)*.

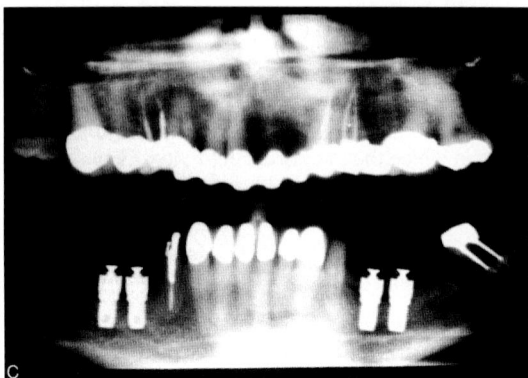

Fig 4 Panoramic dental radiograph showing successful implantation of four fixtures. Note that the implants extend inferior to the plane of the inferior alveolar canal on the left side.

fixtures as posteriorly as possible without encroaching on the nerve (Figs 3a and b).

CT-generated oblique cross-sectional images frequently enhance the placement of implants in the posterior mandible. The ability to view preoperatively the precise location of vital anatomic structures, such as the inferior alveolar nerve, and the ability of the surgeon to make accurate measurements of fixture length and angulation, permit the maximal use of available bone while carefully respecting the integrity of the nerve. With careful technique and CT-guided surgery, some previously untreatable patients may be rehabilitated successfully using short fixtures and proper angulation and by avoiding countersinking (Fig 4).

The maxilla presents a significant challenge to the surgeon because of its quality and quantity of bone. Generally speaking, bone is less dense in the maxilla than in the anterior mandible; therefore, anchoring the "apical" end of the implant into any available cortical bone is especially important. The CT images clearly demonstrate the location of cortical bone in the floor, both of the nasal cavity and the maxillary sinuses. Measurements made directly from the CT images will enable the surgeon to preselect fixture lengths long enough to engage these structures.

In completely edentulous maxillae, ridge resorption and proximity of the maxillary sinuses often preclude placement of implants into the posterior regions. However, it is always desirable to place the terminal implants as far posteriorly as possible without involving the anterior border of the sinuses. The most desirable location for the most posterior implants can be precisely planned preoperatively on CT images and then located surgically in the mouth by simply measuring from the midline.

Computed tomography may reveal maxillary sinus abnormalities that should be recognized by the dentist contemplating implant surgery for the posterior maxilla. The normal maxillary sinus appears totally black on the CT scan, as the schneiderian membrane is thin and cannot be identified. However, CT images may show localized or diffuse areas of thickening of the sinus mucosa, mucosal retention cysts, or areas of active inflammation. Dental pathology, such as end-stage periodontal disease or lesions of endodontic origin associated with maxillary posterior teeth adjacent to the pneumatized sinus, may produce contiguous inflammatory sinus disease. Periapical lesions may totally erode the floor of the maxillary sinus. In such cases, the roots of the teeth will then be seen to be in contact with the swollen sinus mucosa. When mucosal thickening is seen, it is prudent to diagnose and institute appropriate treatment before placement of endosseous implants. Even when active infection and inflammation are eliminated, the radiographic appearance of thickened mucosa is likely to persist.

The incisive canal must be considered when contemplating the placement of fixtures into the central incisor region. The canal varies greatly in size and morphology and may preclude fixture placement. While the full extent of this structure is not seen on conventional two-dimensional radiographs, it can be clearly seen on axial and oblique CT images.

Optimum use of available bone

Preoperative CT evaluation permits maximal use of the available bone; therefore, the number of patients that can be treated with implants is significantly increased. Because the surgeon has access to images of the jaws in all three dimensions throughout the entire circumference of the jaws, identification of the exact location of those sites having maximal amounts of bone is facilitated. Often, in patients who generally have inadequate bone, small areas can usually be identified in which there is enough bone to place

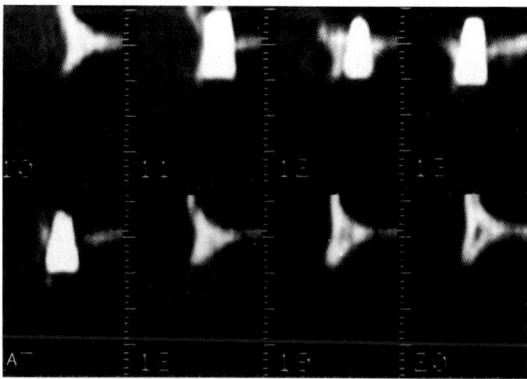

Fig 5 Computed tomographic oblique cross sections showing 7-mm fixture successfully implanted into minimal maxillary bone.

a fixture. These areas of sufficient bone can be precisely located in the mouth by obtaining measurements from known anatomic structures or from radiographic stents (Fig 5).

Treatment that otherwise might not even have been attempted because of the presence of a narrow spiny ridge may be completed successfully. In such patients, the surgeon can visualize the full extent of the osseous topography, which often reveals a significant widening of the buccolingual dimension of the bone in the nasal area. This pyramidal bony wedge may be suitable for implant placement and the spiny ridge can either be removed or it can be left intact with implants being placed from the palatal aspect (Figs 6a and b).

Even with situations in which posterior implant placement is impossible, two to four fixtures can often be placed into the anterior maxilla for the purpose of providing support and retention for an overdenture. However, when anterior ridge resorption is severe, two short implants may not provide adequate support and placement of a third implant into the midline might enhance long-term success. Midline fixture placement may also be advantageous when the curvature of the anterior maxilla is pronounced. A third implant allows the splinting bar to follow more closely the curvature of the arch, whereas with only two fixtures, bar placement might be too far palatal in the midline area.

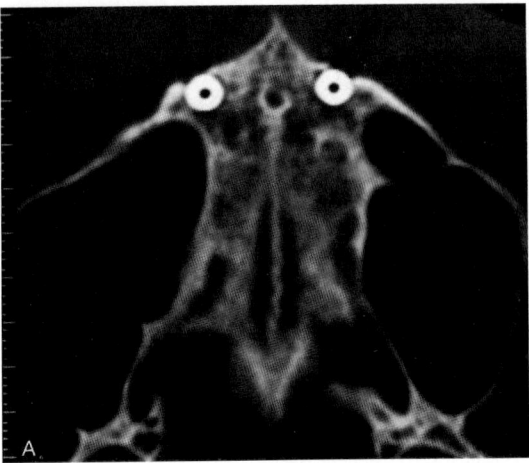

Fig 6a Computed tomographic axial view showing two fixtures placed in the anterior maxilla.

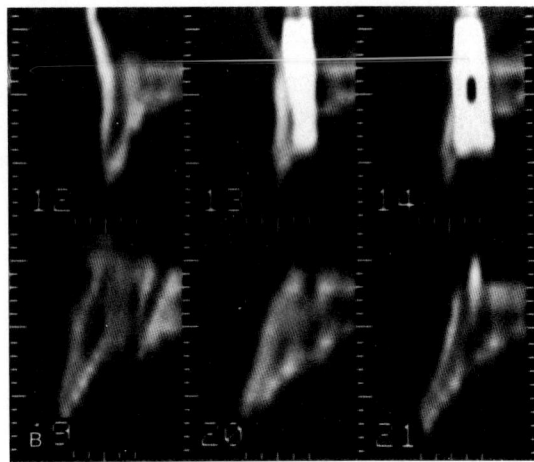

Fig 6b Computed tomographic oblique cross sections showing very narrow anterior ridge with implant fixture inserted lingually into the basal bone.

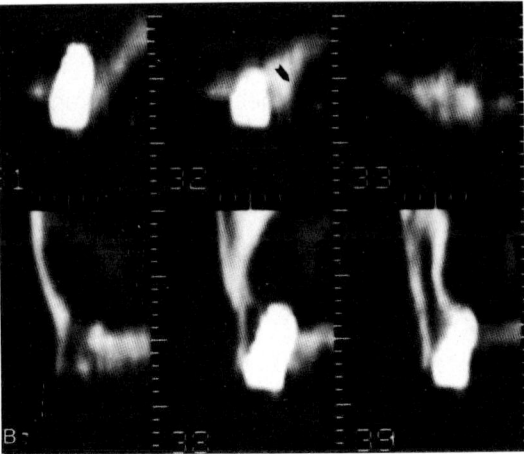

Fig 7a Postoperative oblique cross sections showing successful maxillary midline implant placement labial to the incisive canal. Note presence of the incisive canal in sections no. 31 and no. 32 palatal to the fixture *(arrow)*.

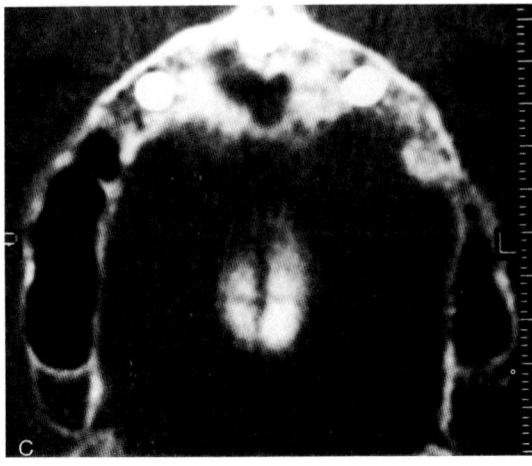

Fig 7b Axial view showing triangulation of three implants with one in the midline.

Another advantage of maxillary midline placement is that bone is very dense in that region. The resulting three implants are much stronger than two because of the triangulation effect, the bone density in the midline, and the 50% increase in total surface area available for osseointegration. Maxillary midline implant placement has not been previously advocated because of the presence of the incisive canal and its contents. However, a CT-generated oblique cross-sectional image in the midline will reveal whether there is adequate bone anterior to the incisive canal to accommodate the placement of an implant (Figs 7a and b).

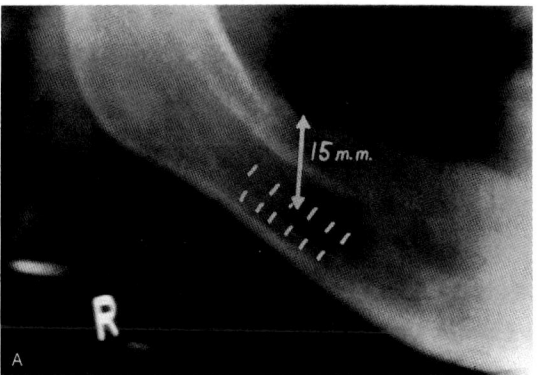

Fig 8a Panoramic radiograph showing 15 mm of bone height from crest of ridge to the inferior alveolar canal.

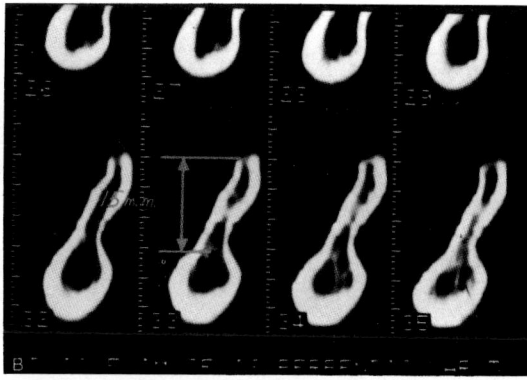

Fig 8b Computed tomographic oblique cross sections showing ridge to be too narrow for successful root form implantation.

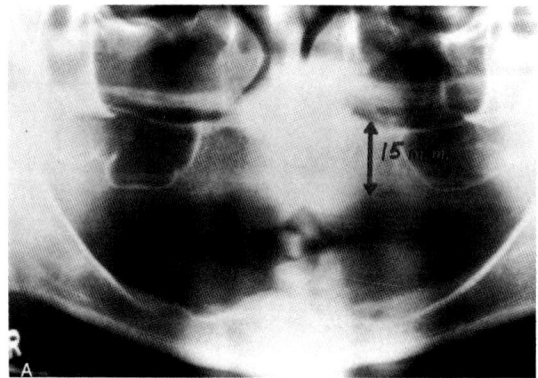

Fig 9a Conventional panoramic radiograph showing more than adequate bone height for implant placement.

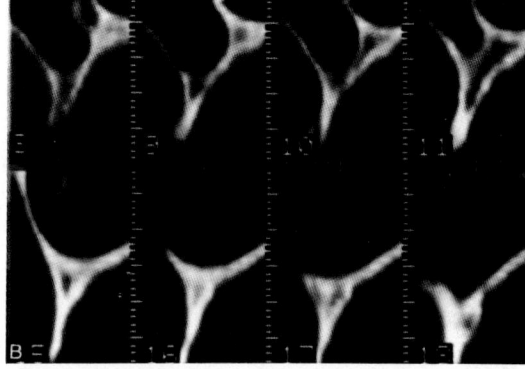

Fig 9b Computed tomographic oblique cross sections showing ridge to be too narrow buccolingually for implant placement.

Preoperative identification of inoperable situations

Preoperative CT assessment of the alveolar process allows the surgeon to avoid operating on patients who cannot be successfully treated. Frequently, bone height is more than adequate, but buccolingually, it is far too narrow for implant placement. Routine two-dimensional radiographs (panoramic or periapical) do not provide diagnostic information concerning ridge thickness. Although the coronal portion of alveolar bony ridge thickness can be measured with calipers and puncture techniques, ridge thickness inferior to the mylohyoid muscle attachment can only be determined preoperatively with oblique cross-sectional images as produced by CT (Figs 8a and b).

Significant edentulous ridge atrophy is a common finding in completely edentulous maxillae following the use of complete dentures over time. The resorption most often occurs in a buccolingual dimension, resulting in significant narrowing of the ridges, which makes implant surgery difficult and, in some cases, impossible. Although buccolingual narrowing of the alveolar ridges cannot be seen on conventional radiographs, it is clearly demonstrated on the

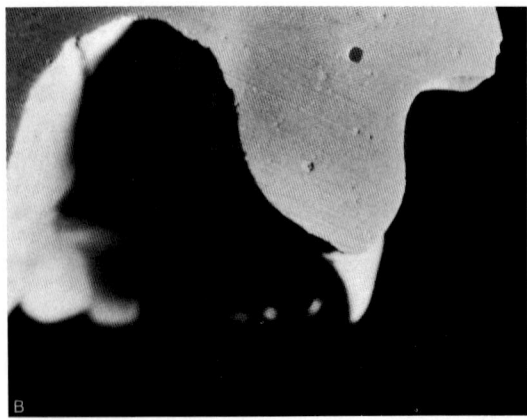

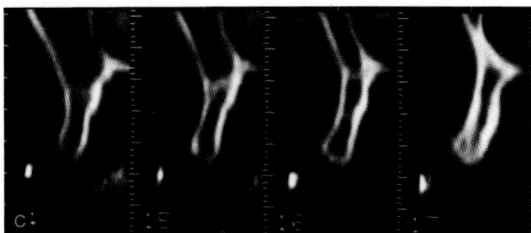

Fig 10b Computed tomographic oblique cross sections demonstrating the alveolar process to be too narrow to accept a root form implant.

Fig 10a Cross section of the study cast of an edentulous ridge at the point at which the implant is to be placed, showing adequate bulk in all dimensions.

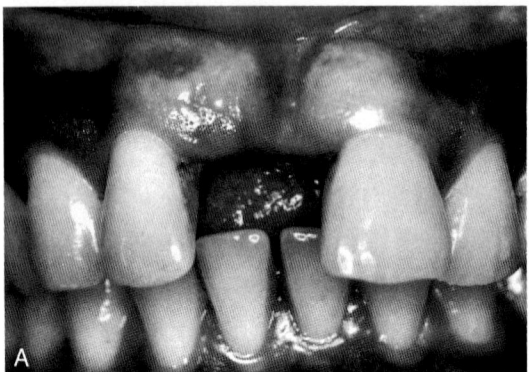

Fig 11a Preoperative photo showing site for proposed single-tooth implant.

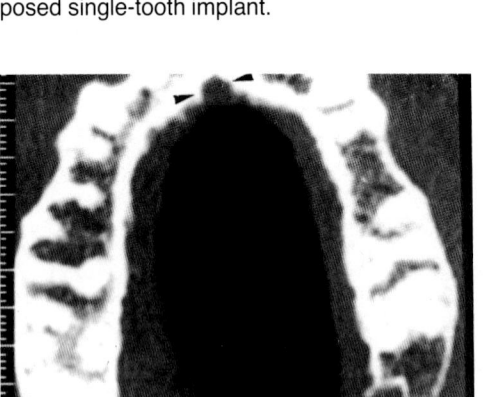

Fig 11c Computed tomographic axial view showing the incisive canal located in the central incisor edentulous area, making implant placement impossible (*arrow*).

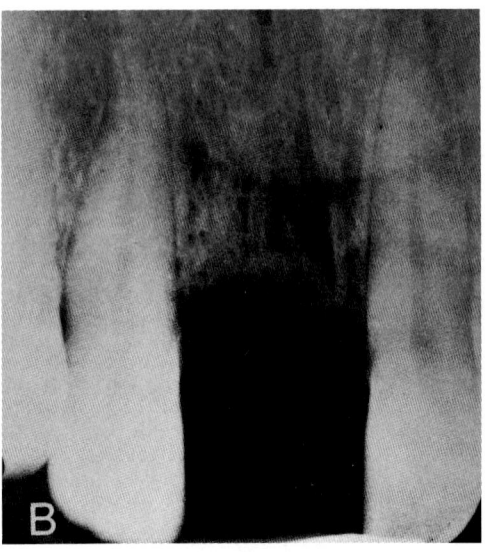

Fig 11b Conventional dental periapical radiograph showing adequate bone for implant placement.

oblique cross-sectional CT images (Figs 9a and b). When viewed on conventional two-dimensional radiographs, some ridges appear to have more than adequate bone for successful implant surgery, but they may not be suitable because of ridge width when viewed in cross section.

Figures 10a and b demonstrate a situation in which clinically, the ridge appears to be large and bulky. However, the CT reveals that the alveolar process is too narrow in cross section to accommodate a root form implant. In another patient (Figs 11a to c), the periapical dental radiograph shows what appears to be an excellent site for a single tooth replacement. The CT scan reveals an incisive canal located in the center of the edentulous space so as to preclude fixture placement.

Conclusion

High-resolution, thin-section CT with cross-sectional oblique and panoramic CT reconstructions have been shown to be excellent media for preoperative evaluation of the mandible and maxilla for dental implant surgery. Oblique cross sections throughout the entire surgical field permit visualization of osseous topography as well as related internal anatomic structures such as the inferior alveolar canal, mental foramina, incisive canal, and the maxillary sinuses. With this diagnostic information, the surgeon/restorative dentist team can plan fixture positioning more effectively, thereby minimizing uncertainties in the operative room and, even more importantly, at the time of restoration.

Acknowledgments

Figs 2b through 11c are reprinted with permission from Schwarz MS, Rothman SLG, Chafetz N, et al. Computed tomography in dental implantation surgery. *Dent Clin North Am* 1989;33:555–597.

References

1. Gratt B. Panoramic radiography/oral radiology: Principles and interpretation. p 314 In P. Goaz, S. White (eds) *Oral Radiology: Principles and Interpretation.* 2nd ed. St Louis: CV Mosby Co, 1987.
2. Samfors K, Welander U. Angle distortion in narrow beam rotation radiography. *Acta Radiol Diagn* 1974; 15:570–576.
3. van Aken J. Panoramic x-ray equipment. *J Am Dent Assoc* 1973;86:1050–1059.
4. Engleman M, Sorensen J, Moy P. Optimum placement of osseointegrated implants. *J Prosthet Dent* 1988; 59:467.
5. Schwarz MS, Rothman SLG, Chafetz N, et al. Computed tomography in dental implantation surgery. *Dent Clin North Am* 1989;33:555–597.
6. Truit H, James R, Boyne P. Noninvasive technique for mandibular subperiosteal implant: A preliminary report. *J Prosthet Dent* 1986;55:494–497.
7. McGivney G, Haughton V, Strandt J, Eichhol J, Lubar D. A comparison of computer-assisted tomography and data-gathering modalities in prosthodontics. *Int J Oral Maxillofac Implants* 1986;1:55–59.
8. Golec TS. CAD-CAM multiplaner diagnostic imaging for subperiosteal implants. *Dent Clin North Am* 1986;30:85–95.
9. Rhodes ML, Kuo YM, Rothman SLG, Woznichk C. An application of computer graphics and networks to anatomic model and prosthesis manufacturing. *IEEE Computer Graphics and Applications* 1987;7:12–25.
10. Schwarz MS, et al. Computed tomography: Part 1. Preoperative assessment of the mandible for endosseous implant surgery. *Int J Oral Maxillofac Implants* 1987;2:137–141.
11. Schwarz MS, et al. Computed tomography: Part 2. Preoperative assessment of the maxilla for endosseous implant surgery. *Int J Oral Maxillofac Implants* 1987;2:143–148.
12. Kelsey C. Essentials of radiology physics. St Louis: Warren H. Green, 1985, p 299.
13. Klinge B, Petersson A, Maly P. Location of the mandibular canal, comparing macroscopical findings, conventional radiography and computed tomography. *Int J Oral Maxillofac Implants* 1989;4:327–332.
14. Rothman SLG. CT evaluation of implant failures. Presented at the Academy of Osseointegration Annual Meeting, Dallas, March 1990.
15. Schwarz MS, Stauts B. Fixture placement. *J Calif Dent Assoc* 1987;15:45–50.
16. Strid K-G. Radiographic procedures. p 318 In P.-I. Brånemark, G.A. Zarb, T. Albrektsson (eds) *Tissue-Integrated Prostheses: Osseointegration in Clinical Dentistry.* Chicago: Quintessence Publ Co, 1985.
17. Lund T, Manson-Hing L. A study of focal troughs of three panoramic dental x-ray machines: 1. The area of sharpness. *Oral Surg* 1975;39:318–328.
18. Lund T, Manson-Hing L. A study of focal troughs of three panoramic dental x-ray machines: 2. Image dimensions. *Oral Surg* 1975;39:647–653.
19. Martinez-Cruz S, Manson-Hing L. Comparison of focal trough dimensions and form by resolution measurements in panoramic radiography. *J Am Dent Assoc* 1987;114:639–642.
20. Rowse C. Notes on interpretation of the orthopantomogram. *Br Dent J* 1971;130:425–434.

Periodontal Aspects of Brånemark and IMZ Implants Supporting Overdentures: A Comparative Study

M. Quirynen, I. Naert, D. van Steenberghe, L. Duchateau, and P. Darius

Both the Brånemark (Nobelpharma AB, Göteborg, Sweden) and the IMZ implant systems (Interpore International, Irvine, Calif) claim osseointegration and high success rates. Brånemark fixtures have been applied successfully for up to 15 years in the anchorage of complete prostheses,[1-3] and for more than 5 years in the anchorage of partial prostheses[4-7] or of overdentures.[8-10] For the IMZ system, two long-term clinical trials up to 10 years have been reported.[11,12] The criteria for success are difficult to compare with those in the aforementioned Brånemark studies.

The successful outcome of any implant procedure depends on a series of parameters[13,14] including: (1) the biocompatibility of the implant material, (2) the macroscopic and microscopic nature of the implant surface,[15,16] (3) the surgical procedure,[17] (4) undisturbed healing,[18,19] and (5) the prosthetic design.

For the two implant systems examined in this paper only the second parameter, the nature of the implant, clearly differs. The IMZ implant is a cylindrical device with a titanium plasma-sprayed grained surface,[11,20] whereas the Brånemark implant is screw-shaped with well-defined surface characteristics.[14] Moreover, the IMZ implants are provided with a viscoelastic abutment that is thought to transfer occlusal forces evenly to the bone.[21] Both implants are made of commercially pure titanium, although the pretreatment of the surface and also the covering oxide layer[16] differ. They are both placed in two stages with special care taken to avoid overheating of the bone, and each has a stress-free healing phase.[11,22] Finally, the prosthetic reconstructions on both implant systems are almost identical.

It was the aim of this study to examine the influence of the implant type on the *peri-implant* tissue reactions when the remaining parameters are kept almost identical.

Materials and methods

Patients

Consecutive overdenture patients, operated on before May 1988 at the Department of Periodontology, Catholic University of Leuven (86 patients) or at another clinical center in Belgium (74 patients), were included in this study. In Leuven, only Brånemark implants were placed, while in the other center only titanium plasma-sprayed IMZ implants were used. All surgical treatment in Leuven was performed according to the instruction manual for the Brånemark implant system and in the other center according to the IMZ manual.

The descriptive statistics for both the Brånemark and the IMZ patient groups are illustrated in Table 1. For patients with overdentures in the mandible, no significant differences between both groups could be found when age, sex, years of edentulism, and antagonistic dental status were compared. The low number of patients receiving treatment in the maxilla did not

Table 1 Descriptive statistics for the Brånemark and IMZ groups

	Brånemark		IMZ	
	Maxilla	Mandible	Maxilla	Mandible
Number of patients	6	80	3 (1)*	70
Age at fixture insertion	53.5 (34–73)	56.9 (32–77)	44.5 (29–59)	57.3 (26–74)
(range)		SD: 10.8		SD: 10.5
Sex: women/men	4/2	58/22	4/0	52/18
Years of edentulism	10.2 (0–18)	8.3 (0–35)	10.0 (3–15)	8.9 (0–39)
Loading time (months)	15.0 (3–38)	17.5 (2–51)	8.5 (5–12)	25.4 (7–49)
			($P = .001$)	
Antagonistic dental status				
% Complete dentures		85.6%		86.6%
% Natural teeth		3.9%		2.7%

*Patient never rehabilitated because of early implant loss.

allow any statistical analysis and are only reported here as preliminary data because of their clinical implications.

The classification of jawbone quality and resorption anatomy was performed in accordance with Lekholm and Zarb[23] using preoperative radiographs (Fig 1). As illustrated in Fig 2, poor bone quality and severe bone resorption were more often recorded in the Brånemark group. However, the difference did not reach the level of significance for both bone quality (2.2 vs 2.1) and quantity (2.3 vs 2.3). The mental foramen was located on the alveolar crest in 29% of the patients in the Brånemark group and in only 15% of the IMZ patients.

Implant and attachment system

In the 80 mandibles and 6 maxillae of the Brånemark group, a total of 175 fixtures (Brånemark) were placed (Table 2). All inserted fixtures were original Brånemark implants and had a diameter of 3.75 mm. In the 70 mandibles and 4 maxillae of the IMZ group, a total of 163 titanium plasma-sprayed implants had been placed. In the mandible, 93% of these implants had a 4-mm diameter, whereas in the maxilla this percentage decreased to 36% because of extreme bone resorption. Various implant lengths were used depending on the anatomic conditions (Table 2). For the mandible, significantly longer implants were used in the IMZ group (13.5 vs 12.8, $P = .01$).

After an undisturbed healing period of 3 (mandible) to 6 (maxilla) months, abutments were placed that extended through the mucoperiosteum. For the Brånemark group, the mean abutment length was 4.4 mm (range 3 to 7 mm) for the mandible and 4 mm (range 3 to 5 mm) for the maxilla. For the IMZ group, the corresponding values for the abutments (DH type) were 3.2 mm (range 2 to 4 mm) and 2.8 mm (range 2 to 4 mm).

The different attachment systems applied in both centers are discussed elsewhere. For 98% of patients in the Brånemark group and 96% of the patients in the IMZ group, the prosthetic design consisted of two implants connected by means of a straight bar located above the alveolar crest and parallel to the hinge axis. The remaining two patients of the Brånemark group had magnet-retained prostheses and the remaining three patients in the IMZ group had support provided by a bar connected to four implants. In the maxillae of the Brånemark group, different attachment systems had been applied to include ball attachments, magnets, or a bar; whereas, for the IMZ group only bars were used except for one patient in whom three ball attachments were used.

The mean loading time for implants in the

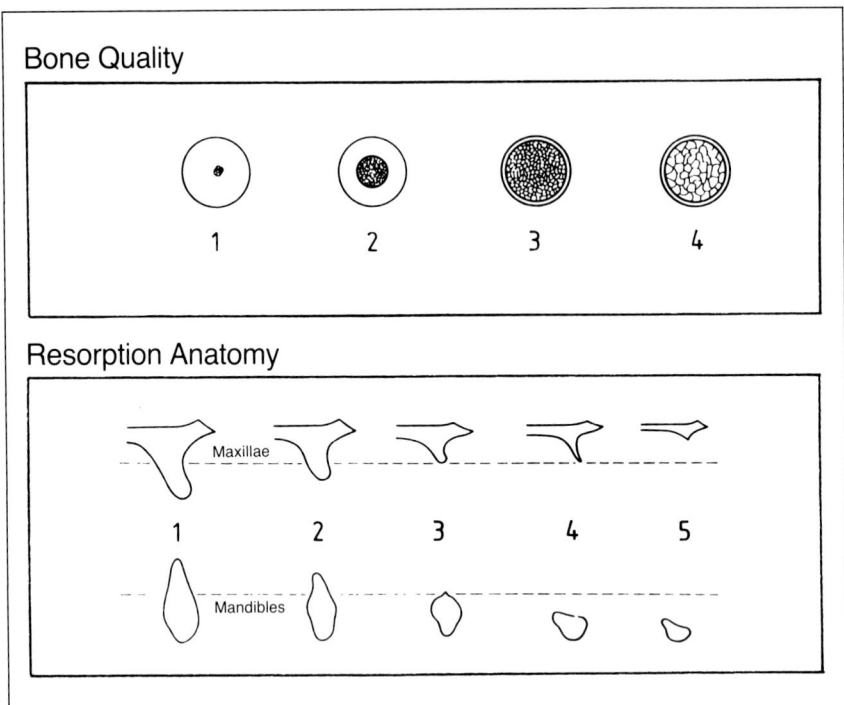

Fig 1 The four categories of jawbone quality (degree of corticalization and mineralization) and the five categories of jawbone resorption.[23]

mandibles and maxillae of the Brånemark group was, respectively, 17.5 months (range 2 to 51 months) and 15.0 months (range 3 to 38 months). For the IMZ group, the corresponding values were 25.4 months (range 7 to 49 months) and 8.5 months (range 5 to 12 months). For the mandible, the loading time was found to be significantly longer for the IMZ group ($P < .01$).

Data collection

All consecutive patients were recalled. Three patients in the Brånemark group and one patient in the IMZ group elected not to return for follow-up because of lack of time or personal reasons. From telephone calls with these four patients and their dentist or periodontist, it was concluded that the implants were still functioning and showed no signs of any complication.

Assessment of osseointegration

An implant was considered nonintegrated: *(1)* if the unconnected implant showed the slightest mobility when tapped backward and forward between two instrument handles, *(2)* if a peri-implant radiographic radiolucency could be detected, or *(3)* if the implant showed signs or symptoms of pain or infection. It is the conviction of the authors that no firm limit can presently be established for an acceptable annual marginal bone loss.

Periodontal parameters

The following clinical parameters were recorded:

1. *The plaque index (PI)* was scored by assessing four sites around the abutment (mesio-

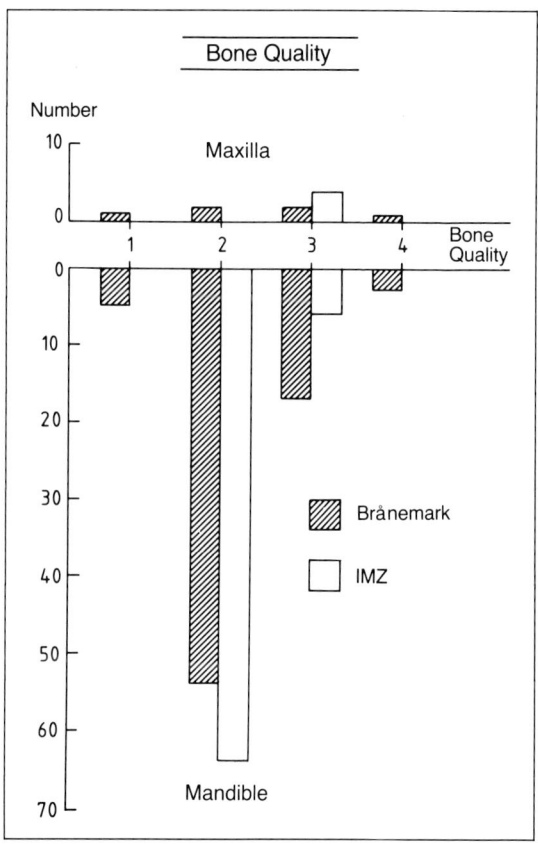

Fig 2a Frequency distribution of the bone quality scores *per* center and *per* jaw.

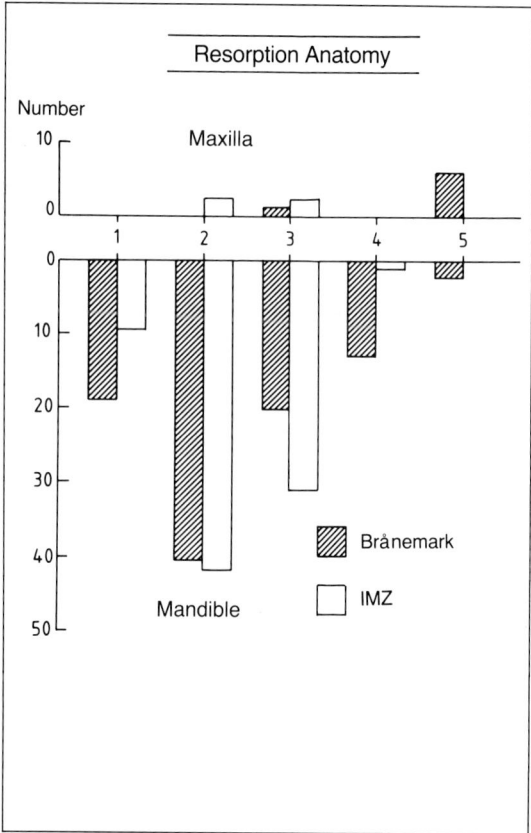

Fig 2b Frequency distribution of the resorption anatomy degrees *per* center and *per* jaw.

buccal, mesiolingual, distobuccal, and distolingual) for the presence or absence of plaque. Since plaque was easily detected (good contrast between white plaque and metallic gray abutment), a disclosing solution was not used.

2. The bleeding tendency of the soft tissues or *gingival index (GI)* surrounding the abutments was assessed at the same locations by running a Merrit-B periodontal probe (Hu-Friedy) around the implant circumference, 1 mm into the gingival pocket and parallel to the margin of the soft tissue. If bleeding was observed within 20 seconds, a positive score was assigned.

3. *The probing pocket depth (PPD)* was measured to the nearest 0.5 mm using a Merrit-B

Table 2 Frequency distribution of the length of loaded implants per jaw and per center

Brånemark fixtures			IMZ implants		
	Maxilla	Mandible		Maxilla	Mandible
Length			Length		
7 mm	0	4	8 mm	0	4
10 mm	11	48 (1)*	10 mm	6 (5)*	3
13 mm	0	55	11 mm	3 (2)*	28
15 mm	1	47 (1)*	13 mm	5	37 (2)*
18 mm	0	6	15 mm	0	77 (1)*
20 mm	0	3			
	12	163		14	149

*Numbers in parentheses signify number of implants lost before loading.

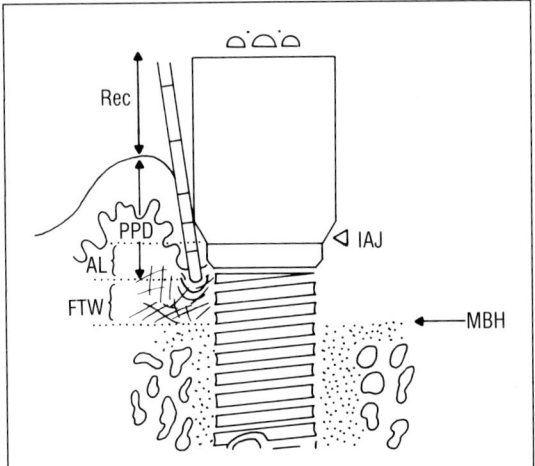

Fig 3 Description of the measurement techniques illustrated for a Brånemark implant. *IAJ* (implant abutment junction) = reference level for bone loss measurements; *Rec* (recession) = distance between the top of the abutment and the marginal border of the soft tissue; *PPD* (probing pocket depth) = distance between the marginal border of the soft tissue and the top of the pocket probe; Attachment level (corresponds with the location of the top of the periodontal probe); *AL* = distance between the IAJ and the attachment level, calculated by the formula: AL = (Rec + PPD) − Abutment length; *MBH* (marginal bone height) = distance between IAJ and the top of the alveolar crest; *FTW* = distance between attachment level and MBH calculated as MBH − AL.

periodontal probe (Fig 3). For each implant, four measurements were made at the aforementioned sites. Special attention was paid to the strict parallelism between the probe and the long axis of the abutment. If necessary, the connection bar was removed.

4. At the same four sites, *the distance between the top of the abutment and the marginal border* of the soft tissue was measured with the same probe and to the nearest 0.5 mm (Fig 3). This distance was called recession (Rec).

5. The location of the so-called *attachment level (AL),* defined as the level at which the top of the periodontol probe stops during probing (Fig 3), was calculated by the formula: **AL = (Rec + PPD) − Abutment**

length. In fact, AL represents the distance between the implant/abutment junction (IAJ) and the attachment level. Finally, the width of the zone (FTW = fibrous tissue width) between the attachment level and the marginal bone level (Fig 3) was calculated.

6. Implant mobility was assessed clinically after removing the interabutment connection. It was also assessed by means of a Periotest (Siemens AG, Bensheim, Germany). This is an electronic device that measures the damping characteristics of the tissue surrounding an implant.[24] The scores are expressed as PTV (Periotest value) scores. For the IMZ implants, the polyoxymethylene intramobile element was replaced by a titanium element to enhance its equivalence with the Brånemark implant wherein the abutment is tightened by means of a titanium abutment screw.

The eventual presence of gingival hyperplasia was recorded on both the mesial and distal sites of the implants. Every augmentation of the gingiva around the abutment up to a distance of 5 mm was scored as hyperplasia. However, hyperplasia that needed treatment because of suppuration, heavy gingivitis, overgrowth of the entire abutment or bar was defined as severe hyperplasia.

At the recall visit, radiographs were obtained for all implants. At the mesial and distal side of each implant, the marginal bone height (MBH), defined as the distance from the implant/abutment junction to the bone crest (Fig 3), was estimated to the nearest 0.5 mm. These observations were compared to the radiographs made at the abutment connection, and the change in marginal bone height (CMBH) during the loading time observed was calculated.

In both centers, for the end-point evaluation, the parallel radiographic technique has been used; however, only in Leuven was a long-cone available. The use of the short-cone in the other center led to a magnification of the image (abutment, implant, and bone loss). Based on the known abutment size, the magnification factor was calculated and the bone loss estimations were corrected. At the abutment placement for the IMZ implants, only orthopantographs were obtained, also necessitating a correction for the magnification factor. The threads on the Brånemark fixtures (with a standard interval of 0.6 mm) and the presence of a straight line as border between the IMZ implant and its' radiolucent intramobile element were useful indicators for the parallelism of the radiographs. In some severely resorbed jaws (<10%), attempts to obtain radiographs of the implant caused extreme discomfort to the patient and ideal radiographs were impossible to obtain.

All measurements were performed by the same investigator (MQ). Part of the radiographs (24 patients from each center) were reestimated by another investigator (DS) so as to calculate the interexaminer reproducibility.

The interexaminer reproducibility (DS vs MQ) of the radiographic examinations is illustrated by the following observations:

- There was a mean deviation for IMZ implants between both examiners of 0.16 and 0.09 mm for the baseline and final radiographic examinations, respectively; this deviation was comparable for the Brånemark implants.
- 82% and 85% of the baseline and final examinations from both investigators were within a range of 0.5 mm for both systems.

Prosthetic considerations and patients' reactions

The prosthetic considerations, the objective and subjective appreciation of the patients are discussed elsewhere.

Statistical analysis

A study of the differences between both groups in age, years of edentulism, bone quality, resorption anatomy, loading time, implant length, and PTV scores included analysis by means of a t-test for equal or unequal variances. The parameters FTW, MBH at the start, PPD, and

AL were examined separately for the mesial and the distal sides by means of the same test.

For an analysis of the bone loss with time, mean bone loss per implant and its loading time were used and a distinction was made between observations for the first year of loading (which is defined as the period of bone healing and remodeling) and later observations. For estimation of bone loss during the first year, only those implants loaded for at least 6 months were analyzed. The comparison between both centers was made by means of a general linear model procedure and a t test for unequal variances. Bone loss during the following years was examined with a regression analysis. An analysis of covariance examined the level of significance for the difference in intercept and slope of the fitted line for the Brånemark and the IMZ groups.

Results

Osseointegration

In the mandibles, 2 of the 163 Brånemark implants (1.2%) and 3 of the 149 IMZ implants (2.0%) were lost, all of them at the abutment connection stage. During prosthesis function, no further implant loss was reported. All lost implants were of medium length (Table 2) and had been placed in jaws with medium bone quality and resorption. In each group one patient needed the insertion of an additional implant before a bar-supported overdenture could be fabricated.

Hydroxyapatite was placed around six IMZ implants to counter severe bone loss. The question, would these implants have lost their integration without this treatment, remains unanswered. Moreover, some other implants in the mandible from the IMZ group showed severe bone loss after loading.

In the maxillae, 0 of the 12 Brånemark implants and 7 of the 14 IMZ implants were lost. In two patients, all IMZ implants (2 and 4, respectively) were lost. These patients had maxillae

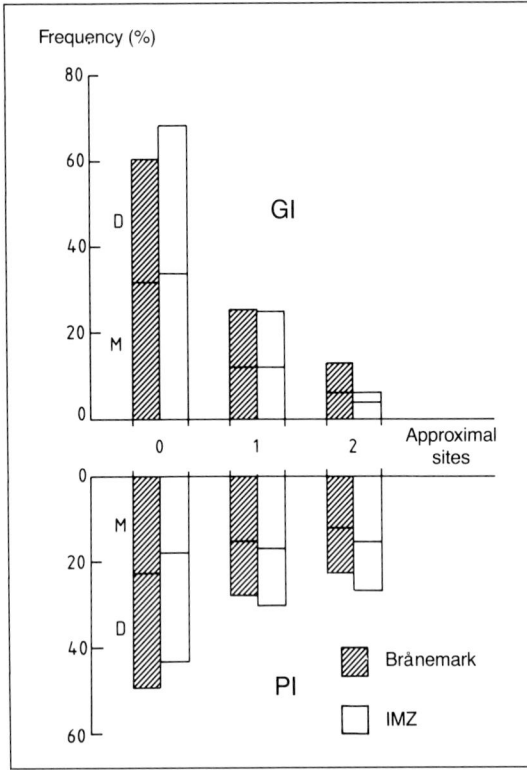

Fig 4 Per implant type, the frequency distribution of mesial or distal approximal sites of mandibular implants covered by plaque or showing clinical signs of gingivitis. *GI* = gingival index; *Pl* = plaque index.

Periodontal parameters

The frequency distribution of approximal surfaces of mandibular abutments from both groups, with 0, 1, or 2 sides covered by plaque or showing marginal gingivitis, is presented in Fig 4. In the IMZ group, the frequency of sites without marginal gingival inflammation is higher than in the Brånemark group (69% vs 61%), although the frequency of plaque-free abutments in the latter group was found to be higher (49% vs 43%).

The frequency distribution of probing pocket depths (PPD) measured around mandibular implants in both groups is depicted in Fig 5. The mean PPD for the IMZ group (3.6 mm) was found to be significantly deeper than for the Brånemark group (2.8 mm), both for mesial and distal sites ($P < .001$). The frequency of pockets deeper than 4.5 mm is 18.4%, and 2% for the IMZ and the Brånemark groups. The mean width of the gingival recession (Rec) is 1.1 mm for the IMZ implants and 2.2 mm for the Brånemark implants.

The significant difference ($P < .001$) in locations of the attachment level (AL) around the implants of both groups is illustrated in Fig 6. In 12.0% and 24.1% of the examinations in the IMZ and Brånemark groups, respectively, the pocket probe could not pass the implant abutment junction (IAJ), and in 12.0% and 1.7% of the examinations, the top of the probe entered the pocket up to 3 mm and more apically of the IAJ.

The distance between the attachment level and marginal bone, called FTW, did not differ significantly ($P > .6$) between the IMZ group (means: mesially 1.11 mm, distally 1.14 mm) and the Brånemark group (means: mesially 1.15 mm, distally 1.26 mm). Figure 7 shows the frequency distribution of the different observations for this parameter. A negative score probably represents an infrabony defect or fibrous tissue that was penetrated by the probe tip.

None of the abutments ever showed signs of the slightest clinical mobility throughout the study. Figure 8 depicts the frequency distribution of all PTV scores for abutments in the

with a score of 3 for both bone quality and resorption. Five of the seven lost IMZ implants had a 3.3-mm diameter. Three IMZ implants were lost before abutment connection, probably because of postoperative infection, and two were lost after the first year of loading. Several implants in the maxillae of both groups showed significant bone loss, indicating that careful monitoring of these implants is warranted. The limited number of patients involved renders every conclusion premature when the maxilla is concerned, but the limited data are presented because it appears, both for the Brånemark and IMZ system, that rehabilitation with overdentures in the maxilla is not comparable to results seen in the mandible.

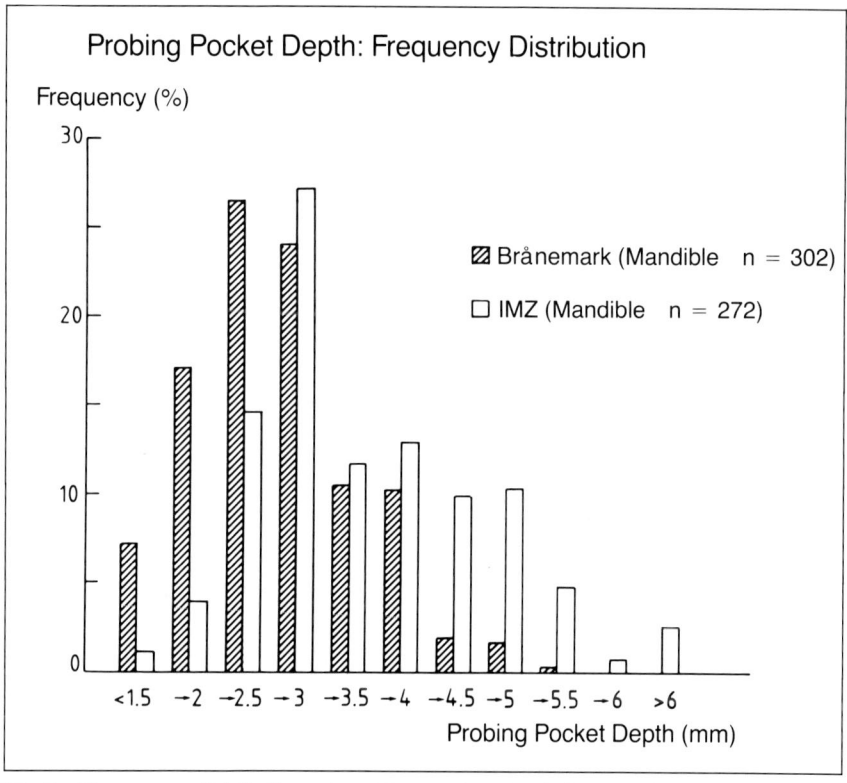

Fig 5 Frequency distribution of probing pocket depth (mean of two mesial or two distal scores) for both the IMZ and the Brånemark groups.

mandible. The mean PTV was −2.2 for the IMZ implants and −1.9 for the implants in the Brånemark group. This difference did not reach a significant level (P = .09).

Gingival hyperplasia was observed mesially and/or distally around 20% of the Brånemark and 14% of the IMZ implants. However, severe hyperplasia for which treatment was indicated was only rarely seen: five patients in the Brånemark group and three patients in the IMZ group.

The radiographic examination at abutment placement showed that, as a mean, marginal bone around the mandibular implants was located 0.70 and 0.90 mm apical to the IAJ for, respectively, the IMZ and Brånemark implants. This parameter did not differ significantly.

Mean bone loss around the IMZ and Brånemark implants, for the period ranging from 6 to 12 months of loading, reached 1.68 and 0.69 mm (P = .004).

The algorithms for the fitted lines representing bone loss after the first year of bone healing and remodeling (Fig 9) are: (1) for IMZ, bone loss in millimeters = +(0.028 × months of loading) + 1.24; (2) for Brånemark, bone loss in millimeters = −(0.012 × months of loading) + 1.10. The slope of the regression lines were significantly different (P = .04).

Table 3 shows the frequency distribution of the CMBH (scored mesially or distally) around the loaded mandibular implants from both groups. In the IMZ group, several implants were found to have a loss of 4 mm or more over the first 2 to 4 years. For the Brånemark implants, bone loss of more than 3 mm during the same periods was never observed.

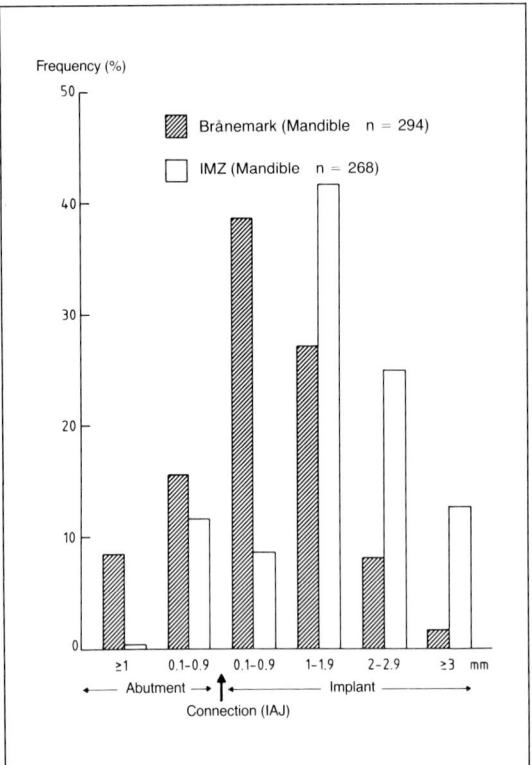

Fig 6 Frequency distribution of the location of the attachment level *(AL)*, mesially or distally, around mandibular IMZ or Brånemark implants.

Discussion

Long-term scientific scrutiny over a 10-year period should be the yardstick for the evaluation of implant-supported restortations.[14] Nevertheless, the present report indicates that differences in bone loss can be detected between two endosseous implant systems both achieving bone apposition. Moreover, a distinction should be made between a failed and a failing implant. A failed implant is an implant that was lost, whereas a failing implant can be an implant that is still functioning but which shows one of the following complications: severe bone loss, untreatable soft tissue irritation, slight mobility, or suppuration.

The small number of observed implants in the maxilla of both groups does not permit the reporting of definite conclusions. However, the failure rate for maxillary implants supporting overdentures, especially for the IMZ implants, is clearly higher than that reported for the mandible. Although specific explanations can be advanced for the loss of several IMZ implants in the present observation, the frequency seems very high. This is in contrast to observations of Kirsch and Ackermann,[11] who reported a lower frequency (3 out of 67) for edentulous maxillae.

Bone loss around both the IMZ and Brånemark maxillary implants was considerable. After a mean loading time of 8.5 and 15 months for the IMZ and the Brånemark groups, respectively, the marginal bone was located 4.3 and 3.5 mm apical to the IAJ. Whether this bone loss was caused by poor bone quality or quantity (see Fig 2), or to the design of the prosthetic restoration (absence of interabutment connection) is not yet understood.

Over this short observation period, the percentage of lost implants in the mandible for the IMZ (2.0%) and the Brånemark groups (1.2%) is remarkably low. However, if ongoing bone loss is considered as leading to failure—although it seems difficult to establish a limit or whether it is a continuous process—the failure rates for the IMZ implants could become higher with time. After 24 months of loading, 20% of the IMZ implants showed an overall bone loss of 4 mm or more. For the Brånemark implants, such bone loss was never observed.

The failure rate for Brånemark implants in the mandible (1.2%) seems to be in contrast to the observations of Engquist and co-workers,[8] who reported a fixture loss of 6% in the mandible with overdentures after 4 years. This may be explained by patient selection and prosthesis design. The Swedish team generally used overdentures when the jawbone was so resorbed that sufficient numbers of fixtures to carry a fixed prosthesis could not be placed (56%) or when such insertion had failed (8%). In the Brånemark population of this study, the percentage of severely resorbed jawbone comprised only 15%. A second explanation may be the overdenture design. Only two fixtures intercon-

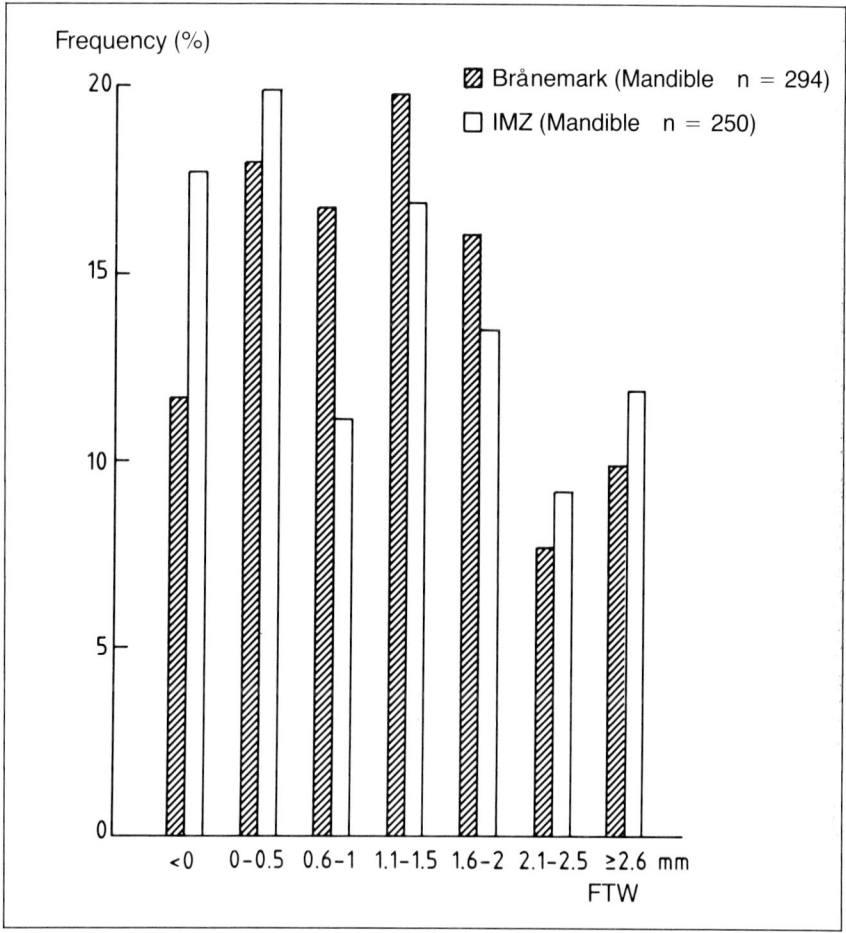

Fig 7 Frequency distribution for the width of the zone between the attachment level and the marginal bone for the mandibular implants in both groups.

nected by a straight bar, parallel to the hinge axis, are used in Leuven. This was not always the case for the patients reported by Engquist and co-workers.[8] Moreover, the Swedish study reported a loss limited to 1% after loading.

The 2% implant loss for the IMZ group in this study is similar to the 1.2% reported by Kirsch and Ackermann[11] or d'Hoedt and Schulte[25] for longer follow-up periods, but using other criteria.

While at abutment connection the bone level for both groups was comparable, the rate of bone loss around the Brånemark implants was significantly lower than for the IMZ implants,

both at the first year of loading and for the following years. After loading of 6 to 12 months, more bone loss was reported for the IMZ than for the Brånemark implants. This higher degree of initial bone loss around the IMZ implants perhaps could be the result of differences in implant design (threads vs cylinder), different interfaces, or the highly polished coronal part of the IMZ implant (2.5 mm in width), which offers completely different surface characteristics than the deeper part.

After 1 year of loading, the bone level around the Brånemark implants seems to be almost stable with time. Some implants even show a

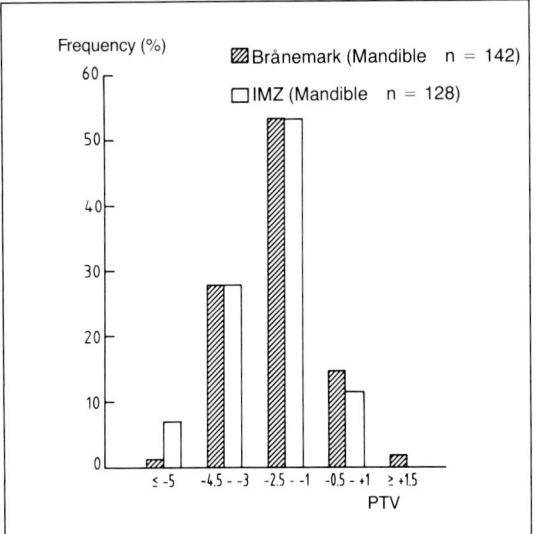

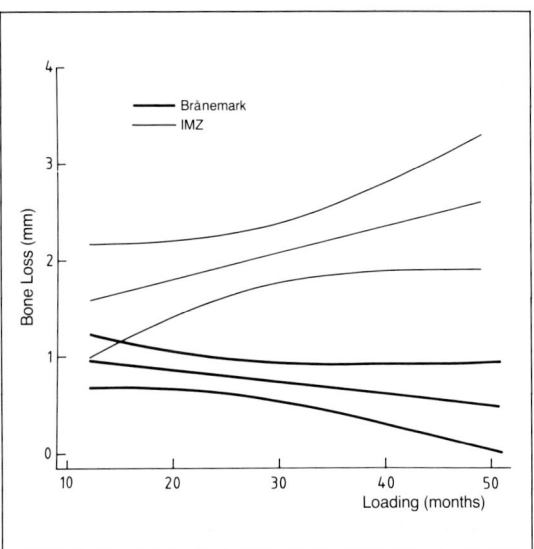

Fig 8 Frequency distribution of Periotest scores for IMZ and Brånemark implants. A score of less than + 10 is comparable with a clinical immobile situation, while for a score of + 10 or more, the mobility can be clinically detected.

Fig 9 Change in marginal bone height with time (mean CMBH per implant) in relation to the loading time. Indicated are the regression lines for the IMZ (n = 90) and the Brånemark implants (n = 47), as well as the 95% confidence interval.

Table 3 Frequency distribution of the change* in marginal bone height (mesially or distally) for loaded fixtures in the mandible

	Frequency distribution (%)							
Months of loading	< -4	-4 to -3.1	-3 to -2.1	-2 to -1.1	-1 to -0.6	-0.5 to -0.1	0	0.1 to $+0.5$	$> +0.5$ mm
4–12 months									
Brånemark (n = 100)	—	—	4.0	17.0	18.0	26.0	23.0	6.0	6.0
IMZ (n = 34)	0.3	14.7	20.5	38.2	8.8	2.9	0	8.8	5.8
13–24 months									
Brånemark (n = 51)	—	—	1.9	27.5	23.5	27.5	15.7	3.9	—
IMZ (n = 78)	3.8	5.1	28.2	29.5	11.5	10.3	7.7	8.9	1.3
>25 months									
Brånemark (n = 42)	—	—	4.7	21.4	11.9	35.7	11.9	9.5	4.7
IMZ (n = 104)	20.1	8.7	18.3	27.9	14.4	5.7	—	2.9	1.9

*Change = bone level at abutment connection − bone level at final examination.

gain in bone especially during the second and third year. Such a gain in bone has also been reported by Cox and Zarb,[26] who used a sophisticated technique to examine the radiographs, and by Quirynen et al,[9] who analyzed consecutive radiographs. This gain in bone, estimated on the radiographs, is probably caused by an increase in corticalization around loaded fixtures.[1] Whether this gain in bone is so important as illustrated in Fig 9, or is partially the result of the cross-sectional character of the data is not clear. However, the 95% confidence interval is small and does not allow large changes. Only a longitudinal study can clarify this problem.

For IMZ implants in the mandible, bone loss after the first year of loading could be predicted by the following equation: $y = ax + b$ (formula for a straight line where y = bone loss in mm, x = years of loading, a = 0.34, and b = 1.24). Whether or not the relation between bone loss and time will remain a straight line after longer observation periods is questionable. It is clear that only a longitudinal study can prove the validity of this formula. These scores are comparable to observations made by Schramm-Scherer and co-workers[12] who found, on a 10-year basis, an annual bone loss of 0.45 mm. Richter and co-workers[27] also noted significant bone loss (1.9 mm) during a 3-year period around IMZ implants supporting overdentures, and for a group of overdentures supported by IMZ implants, Isidor and Kaaber[28] reported small angular defects around 80% of the implants after initial healing and further marginal osseous breakdown around 20% of the implants. However, d'Hoedt and Schulte[25] never observed bone loss ranging to 25% of the implant length in their observation of IMZ implants up to 3.5 years.

Several hypothetical reasons might contribute to the significant bone loss observed around the IMZ implants. Although the baseline bone levels estimated on orthopantographs are less reliable[29] because of less good resolution in bone level determination, the interexaminer agreement was reassuring and the magnification factor had been corrected. Use of the Edlan technique[30] during fixture placement and electrosurgery at the abutment connection might influence the surrounding bone. Another reason could involve the fact that the upper part of IMZ implants (first 2.5 mm highly polished area) does not seem to allow any bone apposition. For the Brånemark implants, this zone is clearly less pronounced (1.5 mm up to the first thread).

Bone loss around the IMZ implants was also reflected in the calculation of the attachment level. As a mean over the full period, the AL was found to be in excess of 1 mm more apically in the IMZ group than in the Brånemark group.

The probing pocket depth (see Fig 5) around implants depends largely on mucoperiosteal trimming at the time of abutment placement and does not have the same significance as around natural teeth. However, when the height of gingival recession and abutment length are taken into consideration, it becomes meaningful. For the IMZ implants, the mean PPD was 3.65 mm and the mean Rec was 1.15 mm for a mean abutment length of only 3.2 mm. In the Brånemark group, the corresponding values were 2.75 mm, 2.2 mm, and 4.4 mm. Even though longer abutments were used in the Brånemark group, the pockets were less deep because the recessions were more important and the bone loss was less severe. In a retrospective study on Brånemark implants,[9] no fixtures with a significant increase in PPD could be found, whereas a study on IMZ implants[25] reported a high frequency of pocket deepening in excess of 3 mm during a 3-year follow-up. Some authors have reported deeper pockets for the Brånemark system[26,31] and less deep pockets for IMZ implants.[32]

The small difference in plaque/gingivitis ratio between the IMZ and Brånemark groups, with more plaque and less gingivitis for the IMZ group, could be the result of different surface characteristics of the abutments resulting in a different plaque quantity and composition.[33,34] Moreover, the application of a tetracycline gel around the intramobile element at each renewal may explain the somewhat reduced pathogenicity of the plaque on the IMZ abutments. Regular remotivation of the patient and repeated oral hygiene instruction seem to be prerequisite for the maintenance of permucosal implants.

The mean PTV scores for the IMZ and Brånemark implants were −2.2 and −1.9, respectively. None of the implants scored higher than +5. Since a PTV score of +10 indicates detectable mobility and a score of +20 indicates visible mobility, it was concluded that all implants were immobile. The small difference between both groups can be explained by the fact that the IMZ implants were, as a mean, significantly longer (13.5 vs 12.9 mm) and their abutments shorter (3.2 vs 4.4 mm). Both parameters have a positive influence on the PTV scores.[9,24] The difference between PTV scores for the IMZ implants in this study and the +1 reported by d'Hoedt and Schramm-Scherer[35] is because of the fact that they did place a suprastructure on top of the abutment, which increased the length of the lever arm.

The higher frequency of hyperplasia in the Brånemark group is the result of using a soft liner (to reduce the open space around the abutments and the bar) in 50% of the overdentures. Aging of this soft liner led to unfavorable conditions for the gingiva.[10]

Conclusion

In conclusion, both the Brånemark and the IMZ implants provide successful support for overdentures over a medium-term period in the mandible, although more bone loss was detected around the IMZ implants. For the maxilla, the small series does not permit any conclusions to be drawn. The high failure rate and/or bone loss in the maxilla necessitates taking a cautious approach with overdentures.

Acknowledgment

The authors are very indebted to the advice and encouragement of the late Professor M. De Clercq, former head of the Prosthetic Department, Catholic University of Leuven, Belgium.

References

1. Adell R, Lekholm U, Rockler B, Brånemark P-I. A 15-year study of osseointegrated implants in the treatment of the edentulous jaw. *Int J Oral Surg* 1981; 10:387–416.
2. Albrektsson T, Bergman B, Folmer T, Henry P, Higuchi K, Klineberg I, et al. A multicenter report on osseointegrated oral implants. *J Prosthet Dent* 1988;60:75–84.
3. Albrektsson T, Dahl E, Enbom L, Engevall S, Engquist B, Eriksson AR, et al. Osseointegrated oral implants. A Swedish multicenter study of 8139 consecutively inserted Nobelpharma implants. *J Periodontol* 1988; 59:287–296.
4. Jemt T, Lekholm U, Adell R. Osseointegrated implants in the treatment of partially edentulous patients: A preliminary study on 876 consecutively placed fixtures. *Int J Oral Maxillofac Implants* 1989;4:211–217.
5. van Steenberghe D, Sullivan D, Listrom R, Balshi T, Henry P, Worthington P, et al. A retrospective multicenter evaluation of the survival rate of osseointegrated fixtures supporting fixed partial prostheses in the treatment of partial edentulism. *J Prosthet Dent* 1988; 61:217–223.
6. Naert I, Quirynen M, Darius P, van Steenberghe D. An up to 6 years follow-up study on 509 consecutively installed Brånemark implants in partial edentulism: Prosthetic aspects. *J Prosthet Dent* 1990 (submitted).
7. Quirynen M, Naert I, van Steenberghe D, Dekeyser C, Callens A. Periodontal aspects of osseointegrated fixtures supporting a partial bridge: An up to 6-years retrospective study. *J Clin Periodontol* 1990; (in press).
8. Engquist B, Bergendal T, Kallus T, Linden U. A retrospective multicenter evaluation of osseointegrated implants supporting overdentures. *Int J Oral Maxillofac Implants* 1988;3:129–134.
9. Quirynen M, Naert I, van Steenberghe D, Teerlinck J, Dekeyser C, Theuniers G. Periodontal aspects of osseointegrated fixtures supporting an overdenture: A 4-year retrospective study. *J Clin Periodontol* 1990; (submitted).
10. Naert I, Quirynen M, Theuniers G, van Steenberghe D. Prosthetic aspects of osseointegrated fixtures supporting overdentures. A 4-year report. *J Prosthet Dent* 1991;65:671–680.
11. Kirsch A, Ackermann KL. The IMZ osteointegrated implant system. *Dent Clin North Am* 1989;33:733–791.
12. Schramm-Scherer B, Behneke N, Reiber T, Tetsch P. Röntgenologische Untersuchungen zur Belastung von Implantaten im Zahnlosen Unterkiefer. *Z Zahnärztl Implantol* 1989;5:185–190.
13. Albrektsson T, Brånemark P-I, Hansson H-A, Lindström J. Osseointegrated titanium implants. Requirements for ensuring a long-lasting, direct bone-to-implant anchorage in man. *Acta Orthop Scand* 1981;52:155–170.
14. Albrektsson T, Zarb G, Worthington P, Eriksson AR. The long-term efficacy of currently used dental implants. A review and proposed criteria of success. *Int J Oral Maxillofac Implants* 1986;1:11–25.
15. Skalak R. Biomechanical considerations in osseointegrated prostheses. *J Prosthet Dent* 1983;49:843–848.
16. Baier RE, Natiella JR, Meyer AE, Carter JM. Impor-

tance of implant surface preparations for biomaterials with different intrinsic properties. pp 13–40 In *Tissue Integration in Oral and Maxillofacial Reconstruction.* Amsterdam: Excerpta Medica, 1986.

17. Eriksson RA, Albrektsson T. The effect of heat on bone regeneration. *J Oral Maxillofac Surg* 1984;42:701–711.

18. Schatzker JG, Horne JG, Sumner-Smith G. The effects of movement on the holding power of screws in bone. *Clin Orthop* 1975;111:257–262.

19. Cameron HU, Pilliar RM, Weatherly GC. The effect of movement on the bonding of porous metal to bone. *J Biomed Mater Res* 1973;7:301–311.

20. Lüthy H, Strub JR, Schärer P. Analysis of plasma flame-sprayed coatings on endosseous oral titanium implants exfoliated in man: Preliminary results. *Int J Oral Maxillofac Implants* 1987;2:197–202.

21. Babbush CA, Kirsch A, Mentag PL, Hill B. Intramobile cylinder (IMZ) two-stage osteointegrated implant system with the intramobile element (IME). Part I. Its rationale and procedure for use. *Int J Oral Maxillofac Implants* 1987;2:203–216.

22. Brånemark P-I. Introduction to osseointegration. pp 11–76 In P.-I. Brånemark, G.A. Zarb, T. Albrektsson (eds) *Tissue-Integrated Prostheses: Osseointegration in Clinical Dentistry.* Chicago: Quintessence Publ Co, 1985.

23. Lekholm U, Zarb GA. Patient selection and preparation. pp 199–209 In P.-I. Brånemark, G.A. Zarb, T. Albrektsson (eds) *Tissue-Integrated Prostheses: Osseointegration in Clinical Dentistry.* Chicago: Quintessence Publ Co, 1985.

24. Teerlinck J, Quirynen M, Darius P, van Steenberghe D. Periotest: An objective clinical diagnosis of bone apposition towards implants. *Int J Oral Maxillofac Implants* 1991;6:55–61.

25. d'Hoedt B, Schulte W. A comparative study of results with various endosseous implant systems. *Int J Oral Maxillofac Implants* 1989;4:95–105.

26. Cox JF, Zarb GA. The longitudinal clinical efficacy of osseointegrated dental implants. A 3-year report. *Int J Oral Maxillofac Implants* 1987;2:91–100.

27. Richter E-J, Jovanovic SA, Spiekermann H. Rein implantatgetragene Brücken—Eine Alternative zur Verbundbrüke? *Z Zahnärztl Implantol* 1990;6:137–144.

28. Isidor F, Kaaber S. Clinical condition of oral mucosa and bone at osseointegrated titanium implants (IMZ). *J Dent Res* 1989;67:769 (abstract).

29. Setz J, Krämer A, Lin W. Vermessung von Orthopantomogrammen in der präimplantären Diagnostik. *Z Zahnärztl Implantol* 1989;5:64–67.

30. Edlan E. Pre-prosthetic surgery. A new technique in the edentulous lower jaw. pp 191–194 In L. Kay (ed) *Oral Surgery.* Transcat IV Int Conf Oral Surg. Copenhagen, 1973.

31. Günay H, Blunck U, Neukam FW, Scheller H. Periimplantäre Befunde bei Brånemark-Implantaten. *Z Zahnärztl Implantol* 1989;5:162–167.

32. Spörlein E, Tetsch P. Sulkusfluidmessung bei Titanimplantaten im zahnlosen Unterkiefer. *Z Zahnärztl Implantol* 1986;5:92–96.

33. Weerkamp AH, Quirynen M, Marechal M, Van Der Mei HC, van Steenberghe D, Busscher HJ. The role of surface free energy in the early in vivo formation of dental plaque on human enamel and polymeric substrata. *Microbial Eco Health Dis* 1989;2:11–18.

34. Quirynen M, Marechal M, Busscher HJ, Weerkamp AH, Darius PL, van Steenberghe D. The influence of surface free energy and surface roughness on early plaque formation. *J Clin Periodontol* 1990;17:138–144.

35. d'Hoedt B, Schramm-Scherer B. Der Periotestwert bei enossalen Implantaten. *Z Zahnärztl Implantol* 1988; 4:89–95.

Mechanical Failure of Porous-Surfaced Ti-6Al-4V Implant Alloy: Mechanisms and Detection Methods

D. H. Kohn, P. Ducheyne, and J. Awerbuch

Dental implants have been used for about 35 years, and it is estimated that as many 300,000 dental implants will be used in the United States by 1992.[1] Despite the history and projected expanded use of these devices, their success can still be evaluated on a qualitative level only.[1] To ensure the success of dental implants, it is imperative that a fundamental understanding of the factors affecting long-term success be well documented.

The concept of osseointegration, for screw-threaded implants,[2] represents a situation of bone *ongrowth*. An alternative method of implant fixation is based on bone *ingrowth* into a three-dimensional porous surface layer.[3,4] Such a composite system has been shown to have a higher bone/metal shear strength than other types of fixation.[5,6] Increased interfacial shear strength results in better stress transfer from the implant to surrounding bone, a more uniform stress distribution between the implant and bone, and lower stresses in the implant.[7,8] In principle, a stronger interfacial bond decreases the propensity for implant loosening.

Three major systems of porous surfaces are in use: powder spheres,[4,6,9–11] fibers,[3,12] or plasma-sprayed coatings,[13,14] all of which are bonded to a dense metallic substrate. The interrelated factors necessary for the success of all classes of porous-surfaced implants may be summarized as follows:

1. Mechanical properties and adhesion of the substrate and porous layer[15–17]
2. Size, shape, and distribution of the pores[5]
3. Viability and mechanical properties of the surrounding tissue[18]
4. Surface state and bone bonding ability of the implant material[18–20]
5. Initial stability and bone ingrowth stimulation[2,18–21]
6. Elastic properties of the substrate, coating, and tissue[8,22–24]
7. Type of loading[5,23,25,26]
8. Implant design[23,24,27]
9. Biocompatibility of the materials[18,19]
10. Considerations for revision surgery, should it become necessary[24]

The long-term success of any implant is therefore determined, in part, by the ability of the material to withstand repetitive loading. The fatigue strength of porous-surfaced Ti-6Al-4V is approximately 75% less than that of uncoated Ti-6Al-4V.[15,16] Based on the magnitude of this reduction in strength, it is important to analyze the parameters affecting fatigue of porous-surfaced materials. In this paper, the results of a series of studies that analyzed the fundamental mechanisms controlling fatigue of porous-surfaced titanium implants are reported. To achieve this objective, a two-phase experimental approach was used. First, the fatigue strength of porous-surfaced Ti-6Al-4V was determined as a function of microstructure. By developing thermochemical treatments, the material parameters contributing to the reduction in fatigue strength were experimentally separated and analyzed. Second, acoustic emission (AE) analysis was employed to detect and monitor fatigue cracking in real time.

Materials and methods

High cycle fatigue testing

The starting material was 15.6-mm-diameter forged-annealed, extra low interstitial (ELI) surgical grade Ti-6Al-4V bar stock. The chemical composition and mechanical properties conformed to the American Society for Testing and Materials (ASTM) F136-84.[28] Fatigue tests were performed on uncoated (U) and porous-coated (PC) Ti-6Al-4V sample groups categorized by one of the following six microstructures: the as-received, equiaxed structure (EA), a β-annealed, lamellar structure (L), two postsintering hydrogen-alloy treated structures conceived in our laboratory (HAT-1, HAT-3),[29] a similar structure (CST, Howmet Turbine Components Corp, Whitehall, Mich),[30] and an acicular structure (BAA) obtained through a more conventional postsintering β-anneal and aging treatment, which does not use hydrogen.[31] These microstructures are shown in Figs 1a to f, respectively. A discussion of the microstructural morphology, physical metallurgy, and phase transformations that produce the microstructures has been presented elsewhere.[29]

After the final heat treatment, uncoated rods were machined into hourglass specimens having a minimum gauge section diameter of 6.25 mm. Specimens were polished in the longitudinal direction to 400 grit. The maximum surface roughness was 0.4 μm. For the porous-surfaced specimens, following final polishing, the substrate was alkaline cleaned, glass bead blasted, and cleaned again. A 750-μm-thick porous surface was then deposited onto a 25-mm length of the gauge section by a β-sintering treatment. The porous surface consisted of three layers of commercially pure titanium powder spheres, with a mean pore size of 280 μm and a mean volume porosity of 46.7%.[32]

The average diameter of the porous-surfaced specimens was 7.8 mm. Stresses were calculated based upon the substrate cross-sectional area, since the maximum stress occurs at the porous surface/substrate interface.

A control group of uncoated specimens that were machined, polished, and bead blasted prior to β-annealing (U-L-M) was also tested. These specimens were prepared in the same manner as the porous-coated samples were, except that no porous surface was deposited. Testing this group therefore enabled one-parameter analyses of the geometric effects of the porous surface (PC-L vs U-L-M) and surface effects of β-annealing (S-L vs U-L-M).

Rotating beam (R = −1) high-cycle fatigue tests were performed on an RBF-200 testing machine (Fatigue Dynamics, Inc, Dearborn, Mich). Testing was conducted in air, at room temperature, at 100 to 130 Hz. Fifteen samples per treatment condition were tested by the staircase method to determine a mean fatigue strength at 10^7 cycles.[33] A stress increment, d, of 17.25 MPa (2.5 ksi) was used. Fracture morphologies were investigated using scanning electron microscopy (SEM) (Phillips Model 500, Eindhoven, Netherlands).

Acoustic emission analysis

Specimens were obtained from 3.2-mm-thick forged-annealed, extra low interstitial (ELI) Ti-6Al-4V plate material with an equiaxed $\alpha + \beta$ microstructure. Specimens were machined so that the direction of loading was parallel to the rolling axis of the plate. Specimens had nominal gauge section dimensions of 237.5 mm × 37.5 mm, with a 25-mm-long reduced gauge section, having a net to gross gauge section ratio of 0.67.

Two types of reduced gauge sections were tested: uncoated and porous coated. For the porous-coated specimens, the porous surface was sintered along the length and thickness of the reduced gauge section. The morphology of the porous surface and sintering conditions are as described in the previous section. A control group of uncoated specimens was sub-

Figs 1a to f Light micrographs of Ti-6Al-4V.

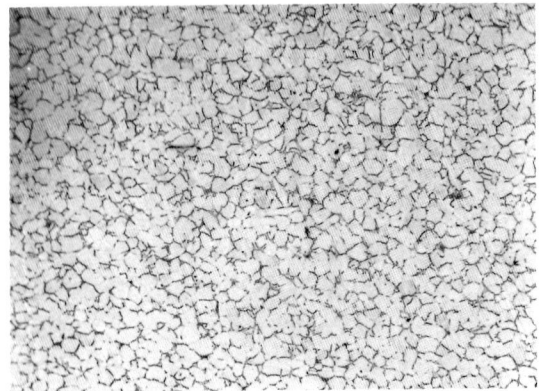

Fig 1a Equiaxed (×200).

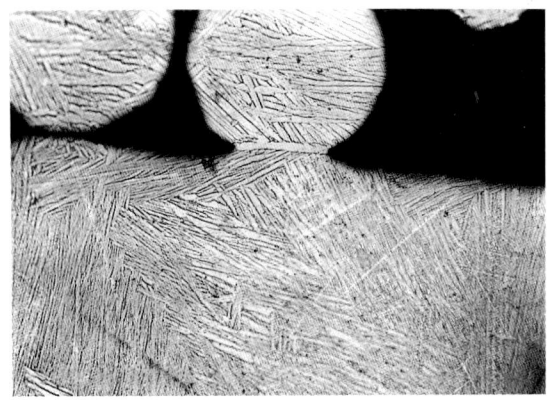

Fig 1b (Porous-surfaced) lamellar (×200).

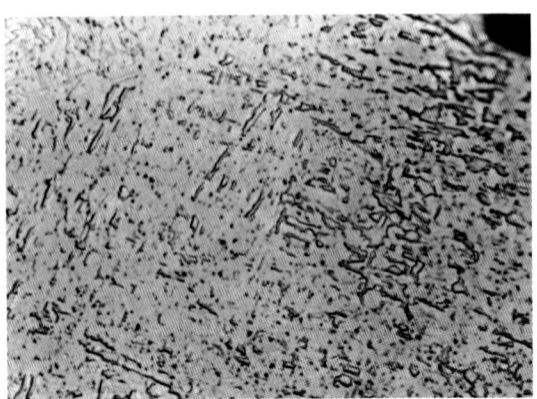

Fig 1c HAT-1 (×1,000).

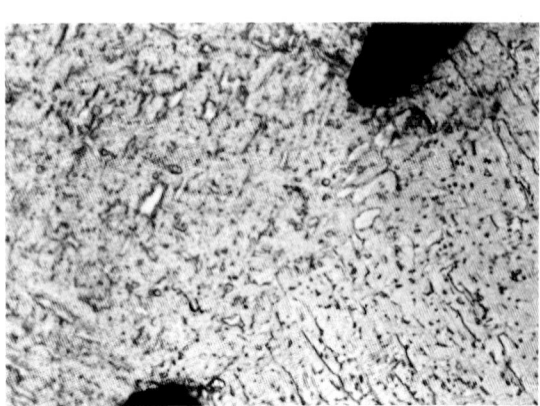

Fig 1d HAT-3 (×1,000).

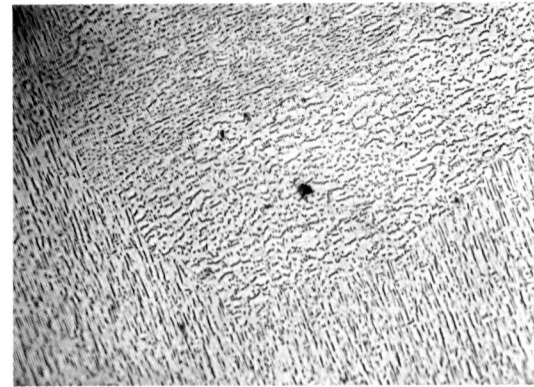

Fig 1e CSTR (×500).

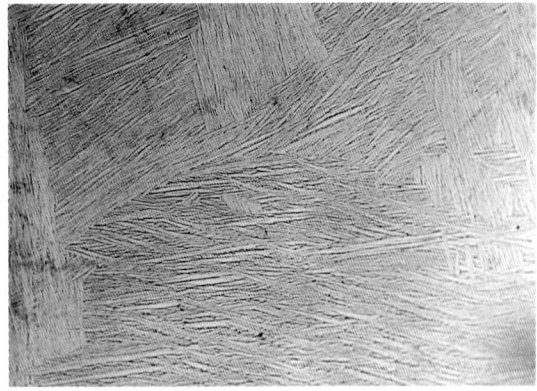

Fig 1f BAA (×200).

jected to the same annealing treatment as the porous-surfaced specimens. Thus, both coated and uncoated specimens had a lamellar microstructure.

Tension-tension fatigue tests ($R = 0.1$) were performed on a closed loop servohydraulic mechanical testing machine (Instron Model 1331, Canton, Mass). Tests were conducted under load control, with a sinusoidal load cycle, at a frequency of 1.0 Hz. The applied stress was equal to 70% of the ultimate strength of the material (730 MPa). Prior to the first fatigue cycle, the specimens were statically loaded (0.05 mm/min) to determine if there were any flaws in the material that might be AE sources.

Two transducers were mounted symmetrically onto the two neck regions of the specimens, 250 mm apart. Acoustic emission was monitored with PAC 3000/3004 (Physical Acoustics Corp, Princeton, NJ) and D/E 3000 (Dunegan/Endevco, San Juan Capistrano, Calif) acoustic emission instrumentation simultaneously on each specimen. The pertinent operating parameters for systems are described elsewhere.[34] The D/E system performed real-time data analysis of AE event characteristics, while the PAC system was used for detailed post-test analyses of event intensities. The specific data analysis techniques employed to filter and relate AE event characteristics to material variables and failure mechanisms are also described elsewhere.[34,35]

Monitoring of fatigue crack propagation was also performed optically through a closed circuit television system (CCTV). A video camera (Panasonic Intralux 6000, 30 frames/s, Secaucus, NJ) with a high magnification ($\times 125$) microscope zoom lens was used to observe fatigue crack propagation. The camera was mounted on an electronically controlled, movable platform that had a 25-mm vertical span and a 50-mm horizontal span. By moving the camera during the course of a test, the full width and reduced gauge length of the specimen could be visually inspected for surface cracks. Acoustic emission sensitivity to incipient fatigue cracking was established by relating the cycle number of the first AE event to the cycle number of the first visual evidence of a fatigue crack observed on the CCTV. Fatigue crack propagation was recorded onto a videocassette for post-test correspondence with the AE results. Fatigue fracture surfaces were analyzed under the SEM and related to AE event accumulation rates and intensities.

Results

High cycle fatigue properties

The results of high cycle fatigue testing are shown in Tables 1 and 2. Also shown are the results of Student's t tests, determining the level of significance between the mean fatigue strengths of the different microstructures with respect to the fatigue strengths of the lamellar sample groups.

The fatigue strengths of uncoated Ti-6Al-4V depend on fatigue crack initiation resistance and are related to the developed microstructures via a Hall-Petch relationship, with fatigue strengths being inversely proportional to the α-grain size (Fig 2). The fatigue strengths of the HAT microstructures were 29% to 35% greater than the fatigue strength of the lamellar microstructure, and they were also 9% to 13% greater than the fatigue strength of the equiaxed microstructure. These results are explained by the fact that post-β-annealing treatments using hydrogen completely refined the lamellar microstructure to produce a homogeneous structure consisting of refined α-grains in a matrix of discontinuous β. The α-grain sizes of the hydrogen-alloy treated microstructures (0.91 to 1.26 μm) were made smaller than the α-grain sizes of both the lamellar (4.0 μm) and equiaxed microstructures (3.4 μm).

The fatigue strengths of the different porous-surfaced microstructural groups, however, were in the range of 177 to 233 MPa, with no statistical significance between the values. This result can be explained by analyzing the factors affecting the fatigue strength of porous-surfaced

Table 1 Fatigue strengths of uncoated Ti-6Al-4V of different microstructures*

Sample group	σ_{fat} (MPa)	95% CI (MPa)	Level of significance of the difference with U-L
U-EA	590 (9)	[572<μ<609]	P<.001
U-L	497 (7)	[484<μ<510]	——
U-HAT-1	669 (51)	[570<μ<769]	P<.1
U-HAT-3	643 (7)	[629<μ<658]	P<.001
U-CST	638†		
U-BAA	538‡		
U-L-M	453 (15)	[424<μ<483]	P<.05

*Standard deviations appear in parentheses; NS = not significant at P = .05.
†Data from reference 30, for comparison with data in Tables 1 and 2.
‡Data from reference 31, for comparison with data in Tables 1 and 2.

Table 2 Fatigue strengths of porous-surfaced Ti-6Al-4V of different microstructures*

Sample group	σ_{fat} (MPa)	95% CI (MPa)	Level of significance of the difference with PC-L
PC-L	218 (8)	[202<μ<235]	——
PC-HAT-3	177 (9)	[159<μ<194]	P<.025
PC-CST	198 (19)	[162<μ<235]	NS
PC-BAA	233 (10)	[213<μ<253]	NS

*Standard deviations appear in parentheses; NS = not significant at P = .05.

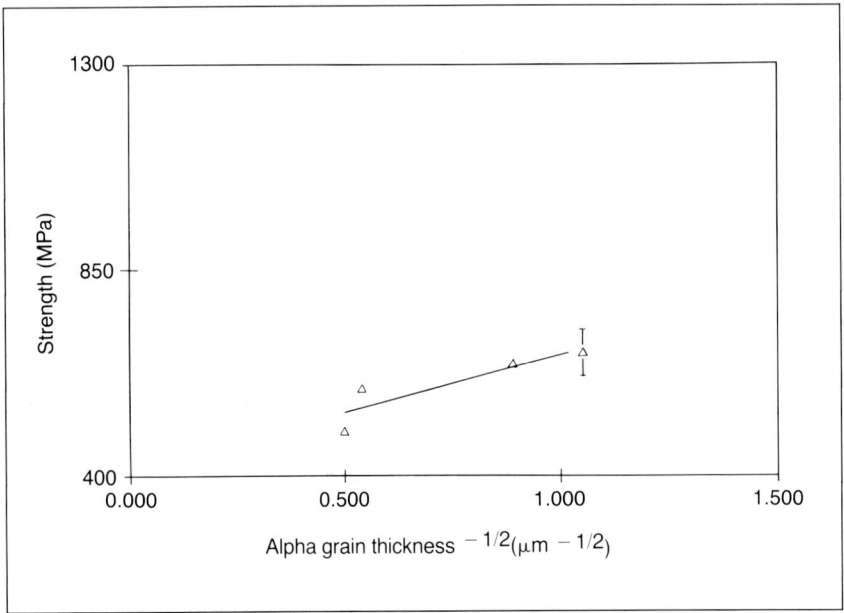

Fig 2 Plot of fatigue strength as a function of α-grain thickness for Ti-6Al-4V.

Table 3 Parametric effects on fatigue strength of porous-surfaced Ti-6Al-4V

Parameter	Effect on fatigue strength (%)	Groups compared
Total effect of porous coating	− 63	U-EA vs PC-L
	− 57	U-BAA vs PC-BAA
	− 69	U-CST vs PC-CST
	− 72	U-HAT-3 vs PC-HAT-3
	− 56	U-L vs PC-L
Effect of sintering: Microstructure surface effects	− 16	U-EA vs U-L
	− 9	U-L vs U-L-M
Effect of postsintering treatments: Microstructure	+ 35	U-L vs U-HAT-1
	+ 29	U-L vs U-HAT-3
	+ 28	U-L vs U-CST
	+ 8	U-L vs U-BAA
Effect of geometry (minimum)	− 52	U-L-M vs PC-L

Ti-6Al-4V. The effects of the porous surface geometry, microstructure, and surface changes related to β-annealing were determined one-parametrically (Table 3). The differences in fatigue strength are significant at the $P < .05$ level or better.

The fatigue strength of as-sintered, porous-surfaced Ti-6Al-4V was 63% less than the fatigue strength of as-received, uncoated Ti-6Al-4V. This reduction was caused by the effects of: *(1)* the porous surface (52%), *(2)* the transformation of the bulk microstructure from equiaxed to lamellar (16%), and *(3)* the combination of surface asperities and changes in surface composition during sintering (9%). In interpreting these effects, it must be kept in mind that they are not necessarily additive.

Although the HAT-3 and CST microstructures are similar (see Fig 1), the environments during thermochemical cycling were different, resulting in a different α-case thickness. However, since there was no significant difference between the fatigue strengths of the PC-HAT-3 and PC-CST groups, it can be concluded that surface chemical effects did not contribute significantly to the difference in fatigue strength between the PC-L and PC-HAT-3 samples.

Comparing the fatigue data for the porous-surfaced samples, it is clear that a refined α-grain size has no effect on, and in fact may reduce, the fatigue strength of porous-surfaced Ti-6Al-4V. Since postsintering microstructural refinements do not increase the fatigue strength of porous-surfaced Ti-6Al-4V, it can be concluded that microstructural changes are overridden by geometric considerations. Since microstructural and surface chemical effects are overridden by surface geometry, the reduction in fatigue strength due solely to geometry (52%), determined by comparing the PC-L and U-L-M sample groups, represents a minimum percent reduction.

The reason the fatigue strength of porous-coated Ti-6Al-4V is insensitive to changes in microstructure is because the notch effect of the surface porosity does not allow the material to take advantage of the superior fatigue crack initiation resistance of a refined α-grain size. Thus, sinternecks act as initiated microcracks. Therefore, the critical stage of fatigue of porous-surfaced Ti-6Al-4V is crack propagation rather than crack initiation.

Since fatigue crack propagation is the governing phase of fatigue of porous-surfaced Ti-6Al-4V, it is important to consider not only fatigue crack initiation (FCI), but also the various stages of fatigue crack propagation—short (SFCP) and long fatigue crack propagation (LFCP)—and relate these stages to the different microstructures of interest. This analysis

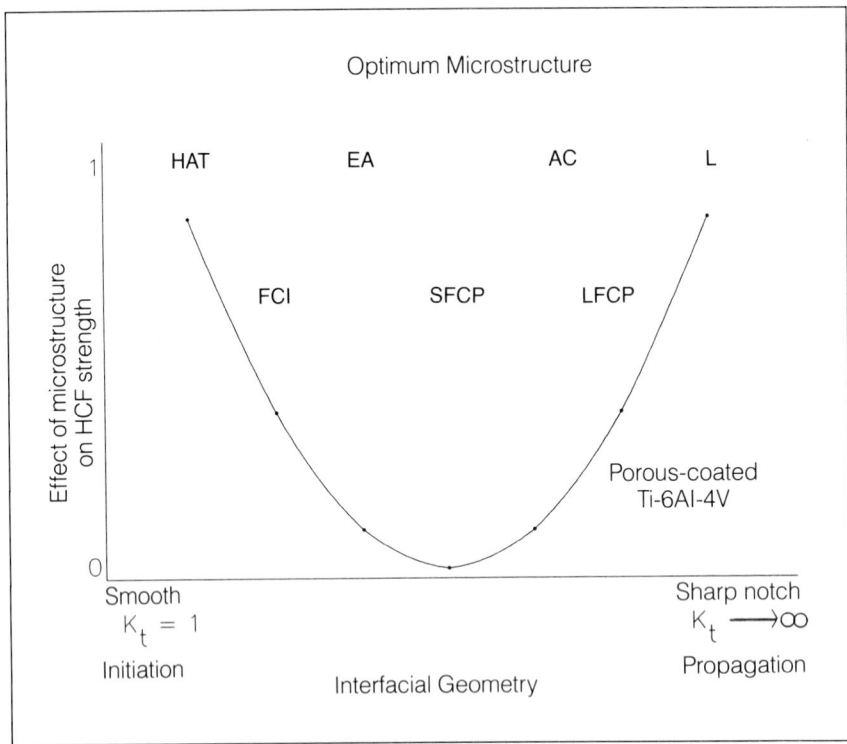

Fig 3 Schematic of Ti-6AI-4V fatigue strength and governing stages of fatigue (*FCI* = fatigue crack initiation, *SFCP* = short fatigue crack propagation, *LFCP* = long fatigue crack propagation) as functions of microstructure (*HAT* = hydrogen alloy treated, *EA* = equiaxed, *AC* = acicular, *L* = lamellar) and interfacial geometry.

helps explain the ineffectiveness of microstructural alterations on the fatigue strength of porous-coated Ti-6AI-4V.

High cycle fatigue strength as a function of microstructure and interfacial geometry is depicted schematically (Fig 3). As stress concentration increases, the controlling stage of fatigue changes from fatigue crack initiation to short fatigue crack propagation to long fatigue crack propagation. Similarly, as the governing stage of fatigue changes, the microstructure that maximizes the resistance to damage accumulation during that particular stage also changes. At low stress concentrations ($K_t = 1$), fatigue crack initiation is the governing stage of fatigue, and microstructures with small α-grains (equiaxed and hydrogen-alloy treated microstructures) possess the greatest high cycle fatigue strength.[36,37] At higher stress concentra-

tions ($K_t > 3.5$), fatigue is governed by long crack propagation, and coarse lamellar microstructures possess the greatest high cycle fatigue strength.[36,38] However, at intermediate stress concentrations, such as the likely stress concentrations at porous surface/substrate interfaces, there is no effect of microstructure, since the total fatigue life is equally dependent on the different phases of fatigue.

Current porous implant surfaces, which affect fatigue strength in the same manner as notches do, lie in the crack growth region of Fig 3. Only upon reducing the stress concentrations at the porous surface/substrate interface will the merits of postsintering treatments on porous-surfaced Ti-6AI-4V be achieved. It should be noted that the stress concentrations within a coating may vary[39] and different types of porous surfaces may have different stress concentra-

Table 4 Summary of acoustic emission (AE) and closed circuit television system sensitivity for fatigue tests

Specimen no. 1*	$\sigma_{max}:\sigma$UTS	σ_{max}(MPa)	f(Hz)	Cycle no. of 1st AE event		Cycle no. of 1st optical observation	Crack length at 1st optical observation	Cycles to failure	Total events at failure
N-1	0.8	717	0.01	10		13	10 μm	14	11
N-2	0.7	607	0.01	88		88	32 μm	415	200
N-3	0.7	607	0.01	8		102	56 μm	175†	267
N-4	0.6	530	1.0	74		133	40 μm	171	40
N-5	0.5	453	1.0	2		24	10 μm	790	125
U-1	0.7	730	1.0	22		2130	1.2 mm	8190	2012
U-2‡	0.7	730	1.0	1		1	3.2 mm	100†	188
PC-1§	0.7	730	1.0	28	T:	96	200 μm	7776	5935
					D:	1200	80 μm		
					S:	4260	480 μm		
PC-2	0.7	730	1.0	60	T:	590	200 μm	6492	2026
					D:	600	80 μm		
					S:	5250	10 μm		

*N = notched, U = unnotched, PC = porous-surfaced.
†Specimen not tested to failure.
‡Crack initiated at imperfection during initial static loading.
§For porous-surfaced specimens: T = transverse crack in coating, D = interfacial debonding, S = substrate cracking.

tions. However, the fatigue strengths of different titanium porous surfaces are similar,[15,40] and therefore the conclusions drawn from this study can be extended to include the other types of titanium porous surfaces currently in use.

Incipient fatigue failure: Physical detection method and local failures

Any design criterion is based upon a limiting stress, below which a component can be safely subjected to in-service. In the case of fatigue, it is generally thought that this stress is best determined by the onset of fatigue crack initiation. For smooth-surfaced components, the initiation phase of fatigue takes up over 95% of the components' total fatigue life, and therefore, it would appear as though the fatigue strength is a good criterion for designing against fatigue failure. However, for components with irregular surface geometries, such as porous-surfaced implants, in which the propagation phase of fatigue is much more of a factor in the total fatigue life, a knowledge of the fatigue strength itself is no longer sufficient for design purposes.

Although a working knowledge of the fatigue strength certainly provides a safety margin against failure, it does not give insight into the mechanisms controlling fatigue crack initiation. Therefore, a technique of determining the onset of fatigue crack initiation is needed. Acoustic emission analysis can serve this purpose.[34] Moreover, as is presented here, AE also offers the ability to analyze the fundamental mechanisms affecting fatigue.

Correspondences between the onset of AE and the onset of fatigue cracking as determined optically were made for all specimens (Table 4). The results determined for notched specimens and reported previously[34] are reported again for comparison with porous-surfaced specimens. The smallest crack lengths that could be reliably detected in notched Ti-6Al-4V were approximately 10 μm. In the porous-surfaced specimens, optical observations revealed incipient transverse cracks approximately 200 μm long through the porous surface, and cracks approximately 80 μm long between adjacent spheres and at sphere/substrate interfaces. Because of the spherical nature and porosity of the surface, these crack lengths represent the limits of reso-

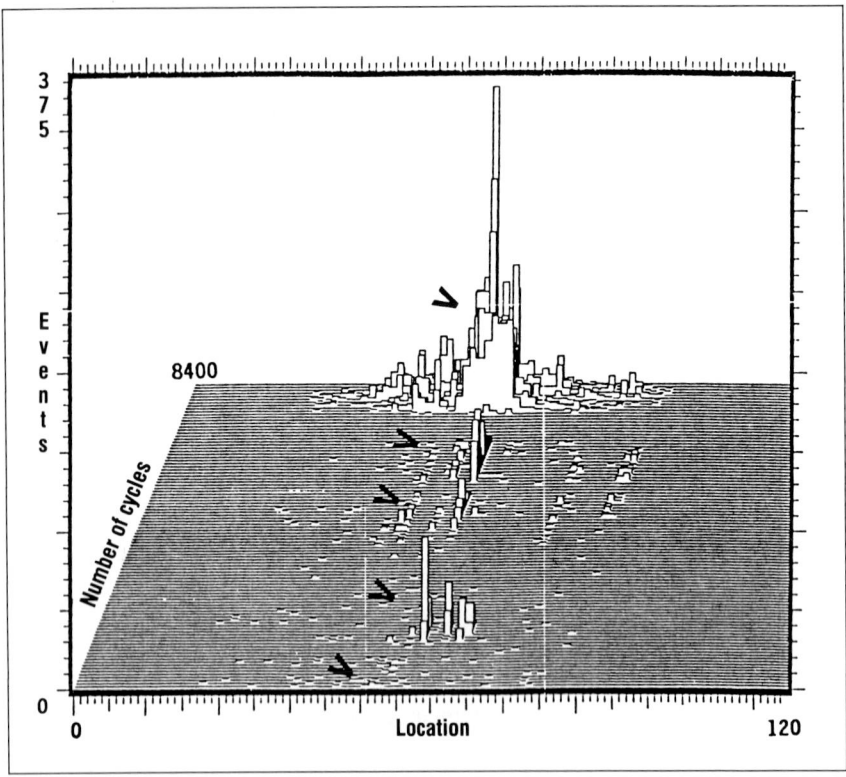

Fig 4a Location distribution histogram (LDH).

lution on the CCTV for porous surfaces. In all specimens tested (porous and nonporous), however, AE initiated prior to the optical detection of fatigue crack initiation. Optical observations revealed only surface damage, whereas AE was generated throughout the thickness of the specimen. Therefore, the AE technique can serve as a sensitive early warning device for detecting incipient fatigue cracks even smaller than 10 μm in length.

For the porous-surfaced specimens, most events occurred in the region of the porous surface and surges in emission occurred at specific fatigue cycle ranges. The location where AE was generated is deduced from the location distribution histogram (LDH) (Fig 4a). The rate of AE generation increased at specific fatigue cycle numbers (N = 28; 1,170; 4,140; 5,070; 6,790), as is depicted on the curve of cumulative num-

ber of events vs number of fatigue cycles (E-N curve) (Fig 4b). These cycle numbers correspond to the surges in AE seen in the LDH.

The surges in AE correspond to the fatigue cycle numbers at which different modes of fatigue damage were first observed (Table 4). For each porous-surfaced specimen, three forms of fatigue cracking were observed optically in the following sequence: (1) transverse cracking in the spherical powder coating, (2) sphere/sphere and sphere/substrate debonding, and (3) substrate cracking. Therefore, a multimode fracture process occurs in porous-surfaced Ti-6Al-4V and this sequence can be detected by changes in AE event rate. Assuming AE sensitivity to incipient fatigue cracking in porous-coated specimens is equivalent to the sensitivity in notched specimens (ie, 10 μm), the fact that optical observations of crack lengths much

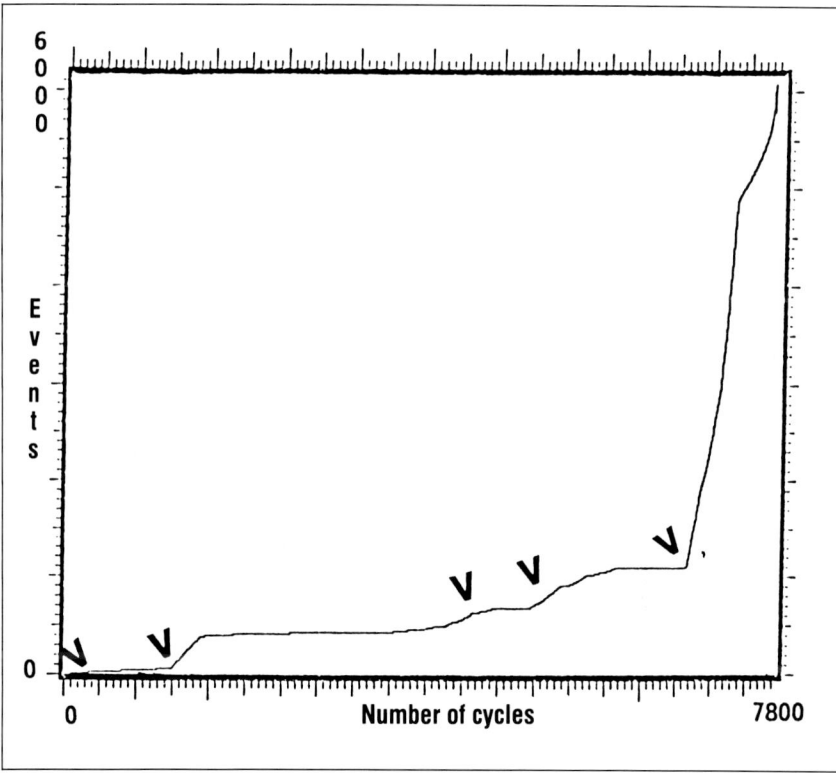

Fig 4b Cumulative number of events versus number of fatigue cycles (E-N curve) for porous-coated specimen PC-L-1, showing surges in emission at five cycle ranges. Increases in emission occurred at five cycles of the E-N curve, corresponding to the surges in the LDH.

greater than 10 μm soon followed the onset of emission means that cracks rapidly propagated through the porous surface.

Fatigue cracks in the spherical coating and interfacial cracks sometimes became blunted in the surface porosity (Figs 5a and b). As a result of crack arrest in the surface macroporosity, fatigue failures in neighboring spheres may be independent of each other. Therefore, it can be concluded that the AE generated in porous-surfaced Ti-6Al-4V is intermittent because of the discontinuous nature of the porous surface. The discontinuous nature of the AE in porous-surfaced specimens becomes more apparent by comparing the E-N curves of the coated (Fig 4b) and uncoated specimens (Fig 6). Other cracks at the porous surface/substrate interface changed direction and propagated into the substrate (Fig 5b), rather than blunting, causing catastrophic fracture of the substrate. Once a fatigue crack propagated into the substrate of a porous-surfaced material, changes in AE event rate (Fig 4b) paralleled the changes in event rate detected on uncoated samples (Fig 6). Therefore, in total, the sequential process of fatigue fracture in porous-surfaced Ti-6Al-4V includes: cracking in the surface, interfacial debonding, substrate fatigue crack initiation, and slow and rapid substrate fatigue crack propagation. All of these phenomena are detectable with AE.

Discussion: Clinical significance

Clinically, the reduction in fatigue strength of porous-surfaced implants has the potential to manifest itself in one of three ways: *(1)* fatigue

103

Figs 5a and b SEM photographs of fractures within the porous coating of specimen PC-L-1.

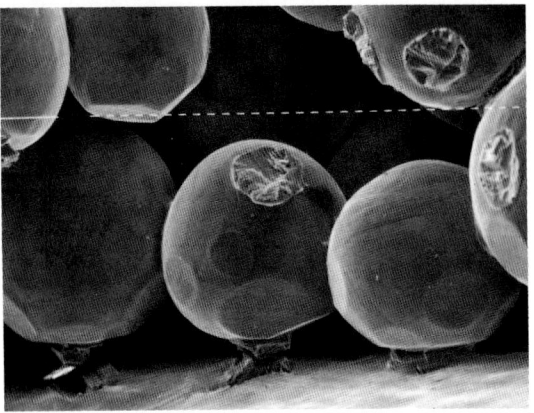

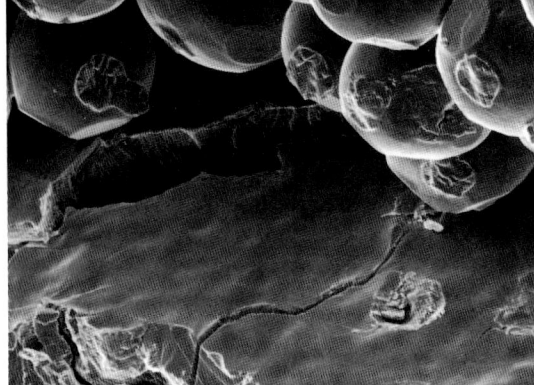

Fig 5a ×640.

Fig 5b ×160.

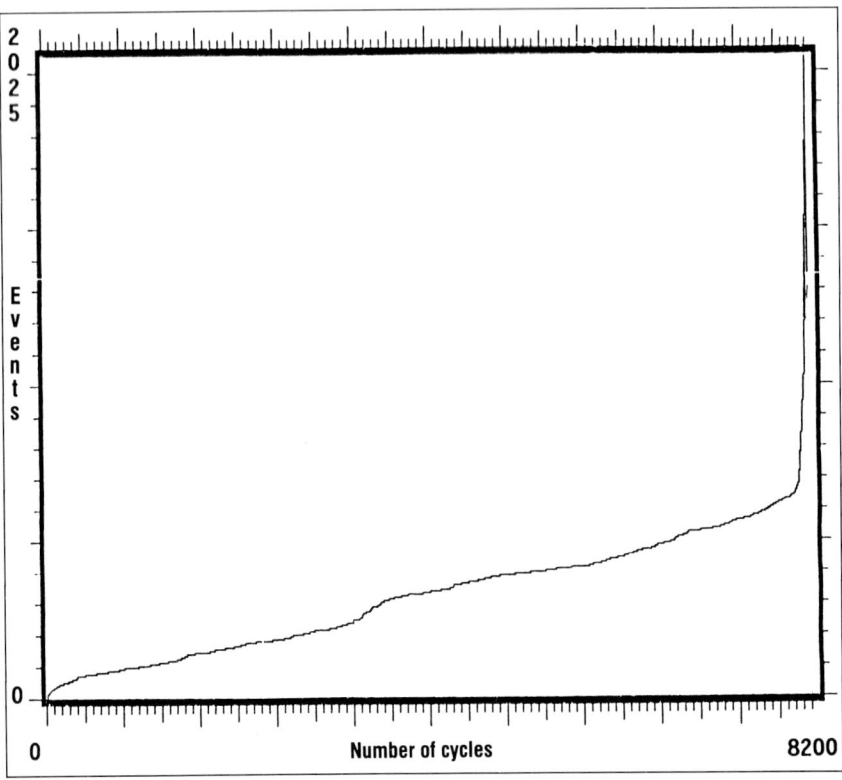

Fig 6 Cumulative number of events versus number of fatigue cycles for uncoated lamellar specimen U-L-1 (from reference 35).

fracture of the substrate, (2) debonding of the porous surface from the substrate, and (3) indirectly, in the form of bone remodeling, since implants are made bulkier to compensate for the reduced fatigue strength. Although substrate fracture is rare, it does occur.[41-43] However, there are many more reports of adverse bone remodeling[24,44] and a growing number of observations of coatings debonding from the substrate of dental and orthopedic implants in vivo.[14,43,45,46]

The causes of porous surfaces fracturing in vivo have not been conclusively established. One reason for the occurrence of these in-service fractures may be that the fatigue strength of the porous surface/substrate interface is less than the fatigue strength of the porous surface/bone interface. The combined stress concentration at the surface notches and surface tractions placed on the coating caused by "micromotion" at the implant/tissue interface may also be a cause of coating detachment. Additionally, since porous surfaces are equivalent to notches, fatigue crack growth can occur under far-field compressive loading.[47] It is interesting to note that many of the observed loose coatings occurred in regions of macroscopic compressive loading. Furthermore, the different modes of material failure observed and detected in vitro have also been observed in vivo.[14,43,45,46] Based on the sequential nature of failure observed and detected in these in vitro studies, local in vivo shear failures should be documented.

These studies underscore that to eliminate material failures, the mechanisms governing fatigue in porous-surfaced materials must be well understood. In particular, studies of shear fatigue of porous surface/substrate interfaces are warranted, as are retrieval analyses aimed at establishing mechanisms of in vivo material failures.

Summary and conclusions

This study has documented the factors controlling fatigue of porous-surfaced titanium implants by testing an extensive set of material and surface conditions and by using AE as a highly sensitive method of detecting microcracks in these complex surfaces. Hydrogen-alloy treatments significantly increase the fatigue strength of smooth-surfaced Ti-6Al-4V by as much as 35% over β-annealed Ti-6Al-4V and as much as 13% over equiaxed Ti-6Al-4V. These increases in fatigue strength are explained by the resultant decrease in α-grain size and aspect ratio. The fatigue strength of current types of porous-surfaced Ti-6Al-4V is independent of microstructure and is propagation-controlled.

Acoustic emission provides the ability to spatially and temporally locate multiple fatigue cracks of 10 μm or less, in real time. Fatigue of porous-surfaced Ti-6Al-4V is governed by a sequential, multimode fracture process of transverse fracture in the porous surface, sphere/sphere and sphere/substrate debonding, substrate fatigue crack initiation, and slow and rapid substrate fatigue crack propagation. Because of the discontinuity of the porous surface, the first three modes of fracture occur in a discontinuous fashion. Therefore, the AE generated is intermittent and the onset of each mode can be detected, in real time, by changes in AE event rate. Porous-surfaced implants have fractured in vivo. Some of the modes of in vivo failure are analogous to the modes of failure observed and detected in vitro.

References

1. National Institutes of Heath Consensus Development Conference Statement on Dental Implants. *J Dent Ed* 1988;52:824–827.
2. Brånemark P-I, Hansson BO, Adell R, Breine U, Lindström J, Hallen O, et al. Osseointegrated implants in the treatment of the edentulous jaw. Experience from a 10-year period. *Scand J Plast Reconstr Surg* 1977; 11(suppl 16):1–132.
3. Galante J, Rostoker W, Lueck R, Ray RD. Sintered fiber metal composites as a basis for attachment of implants to bone. *J Bone Joint Surg* 1971;53A:101–114.
4. Welsh RP, Pilliar RM, Macnab I. Surgical implants: The role of surface porosity in fixation to bone and acrylic. *J Bone Joint Surg* 1971;53A:963–977.

5. Bobyn JD, Pilliar RM, Cameron HU, Weatherly GC. The optimum pore size for the fixation of porous-surfaced metal implants by the ingrowth of bone. *Clin Orthop* 1980;150: 263–270.
6. Maniatopoulos C, Pilliar RM, Smith DC. Threaded versus porous-surfaced designs for implant stabilization in bone-endodontic implant model. *J Biomed Mater Res* 1986;20:1309–1333.
7. Pilliar RM, Cameron HU, Macnab I. Porous surfaced layered prosthetic devices. *Biomed Eng* 1975;10: 126–131.
8. Huiskes R. Design, fixation and stress analysis of permanent orthopaedic implants: The hip joint. pp 121–162 In P. Ducheyne, G.W. Hastings (eds) *Functional Behavior of Orthopaedic Biomaterials, vol. II—Applications.* Boca Raton, Fla: CRC Press, 1984.
9. Klawitter JJ, Weinstein AM, Peterson LJ. Fabrication and characterization of porous-rooted cobalt-chromium-molybdenum (co-cr-mo) alloy dental implants. *J Dent Res* 1977;56:474–480.
10. Young F, Kresch C, Spector M. Porous titanium tooth roots: Clinical evaluation. *J Prosthet Dent* 1979;41: 561–565.
11. Deporter DA, Friedland B, Warson PA, Pilliar RM, Howley TP, Abdulla D, et al. A clinical and radiographic assessment of a porous-surfaced titanium alloy dental implant system in dogs. *J Dent Res* 1986;65:1071–1077.
12. Weiss MB, Restoker W. Development of a new endosseous dental implant. Part I: Animal studies. *J Prosthet Dent* 1981;46:646–651.
13. Johnson WA, Kopatz NE, Yoder EB. Fine powders produced by plasma processing. *Progress in Powder Metallurgy,* Metal Powder Industries Federation (MPIF) 1986;42:775.
14. Luthy H, Strub JR, Schärer P. Analysis of plasma flame-sprayed coatings on endosseous oral titanium implants exfoliated in man: Preliminary results. *Int J Oral Maxillofac Implants* 1987;2:197–202.
15. Yue S, Pilliar RM, Weatherly GC. The fatigue strength of porous-coated Ti-6%AI-4%V implant alloy. *J Biomed Mater Res* 1984;18:1043–1058.
16. Cook SD, Georgette FS, Skinner HB, Haddad RJ. Fatigue properties of carbon- and porous-coated Ti-6AI-4V alloy. *J Biomed Mater Res* 1984;18:497–512.
17. Anderson P, Levine DL. Adhesion of fiber metal coatings. pp 7–15 In J.E. Lemons (ed) *Quantitative Characterization and Performance of Porous Implants for Hard Tissue Applications,* ASTM STP 953. Philadelphia: ASTM, 1987.
18. Albrektsson T, Brånemark P-I, Hansson HA, Kasemo B, Larsson K, Lundstrom I, et al. The interface zone of inorganic implants in vivo: Titanium implants in bone. *Ann Bioeng* 1983;11:1–27.
19. Ducheyne P, Healy KE. Surface spectroscopy of calcium phosphate ceramic and titanium implant materials. In B. Ratner (ed) *Surface Characterization of Biomaterials.* Amsterdam: Elsevier, 1988.
20. Ducheyne P, Hench LL, Kagan A, Martens M, Bursens A, Mulier JC. Effect of hydroxyapatite impregnation on skeletal bonding of porous coated implants. *J Biomed Mater Res* 1980;14:225–237.
21. Delport P, Ducheyne P, Martens M. The initial stability of porous coated total knee prostheses. pp 43–48 In P.

Ducheyne, G. Van der Perre, A.E. Aubert (eds) *Biomaterials and Biomechanics 1983.* Amsterdam: Elsevier, 1984.
22. Ducheyne P, Aernoudt E, De Meester P, Martens M, Mulier JC, Van Leeuwen D. Factors governing the mechanical behavior of the implant-porous coating-trabecular bone interface. *J Biomech* 1978;11:297–307.
23. Brunski JB, Hipp JA. In vivo forces on endosteal implants: A measurement system and biomechanical considerations. *J Prosthet Dent* 1984;51:82–90.
24. Engh CA, Bobyn JD. The influence of stem size and extent of porous coating on femoral bone resorption after primary cementless hip arthroplasty. *Clin Orthop* 1988;231:7–28.
25. Ducheyne P, De Meester P, Aernoudt E, Martens M, Mulier JC. Influence of functional dynamic loading on bone ingrowth into surface pores of orthopedic implants. *J Biomed Mater Res* 1977;11:811–838.
26. Brunski JB, Moccia AF, Pollock SR, Korostoff E, Trachtenberg DI. The influence of functional use of endosseous dental implants on the tissue-implant interface. I. Histological aspects. *J Dent Res* 1979;58:1953–1969.
27. Bobyn JD, Pilliar RM, Binnington AG, Szivek JA. The effect of proximally and fully porous-coated canine hip stem design on bone modeling. *J Orthop Res* 1987; 5:393–408.
28. ASTM standard specification for wrought titanium 6AI-4V ELI alloy for surgical implant applications, *Annual Book of ASTM Standards, vol. 13.01:Medical Devices,* Designation: F136–84. 1987, pp 28–30.
29. Kohn DH, Ducheyne P. Microstructural refinement of β-sintered and porous coated Ti-6AI-4V by temporary alloying with hydrogen. *J Mater Sci* 1991;26:534–544.
30. Soltesz SM, Smickley RJ, Dardi LE. Non traditional thermal processing of HIP'ed investment cast Ti-6AI-4V alloy. pp 187–194 In G. Lutjering, U. Zwicker, W. Bunk (eds) *Titanium, Science and Technology.* Proc 5th Int Conf on Titanium, Oberursel, West Germany: Deutsche Gesellschaft Fur Metallkunde, 1985.
31. Ducheyne P, Kohn D, Smith TS. Fatigue properties of cast and heat treated Ti-6AI-4V alloy for anatomic hip prostheses. *Biomaterials* 1987;8:223–227.
32. Smith TS. Morphological characterization of porous coatings. pp 92–102 In J.E. Lemons (ed) *Quantitative Characterization and Performance of Porous Implants for Hard Tissue Applications,* ASTM STP 953. Philadelphia: ASTM, 1987.
33. *ASTM Special Technical Publication 91-A.* A guide for fatigue testing and the statistical analysis of fatigue data, Philadelphia: ASTM, 1963.
34. Kohn DH, Ducheyne P, Awerbuch J. Acoustic emission during fatigue of Ti-6AI-4V: Incipient fatigue crack detection limits and generalized data analysis methodology. *J Mater Sci* (in press).
35. Kohn DH, Ducheyne P, Awerbuch J. The sources of acoustic emission during fatigue of Ti-6AI-4V: Effect of microstructure. *J Mater Sci* (in press).
36. Margolin H, Williams JC, Chesnutt JC, Lutjering G. A review of the fracture and fatigue behavior of ti alloys. pp 169–216 In H. Kimura, O. Izumi (eds) *Titanium '80 Science and Technology,* Proc. 4th Int Conf on Titanium. Warrendale, Pa: The Metallurgical Society of AIME, 1980.

37. Kohn DH, Ducheyne P. Tensile and fatigue strength of hydrogen-treated Ti-6Al-4V alloy. *J Mater Sci* 1991;26:328–334.

38. Eylon D, Pierce CM. Effect of microstructure on notch fatigue properties of Ti-6Al-4V. *Met Trans A* 1976; 7A:111–121.

39. Wolfarth D, Filiaggi M, Ducheyne P. Parametric analysis of interfacial stress concentrations in porous coated implants. *J Appl Biomat* 1990;1:3–12.

40. *Zimmer Technical Publication,* Fatigue and porous coated implants. Warsaw, Ind: Zimmer, Inc, 1984.

41. Parr GR, Steflik DE, Sisk AL, Aguero A. Clinical and histological observations of failed two-stage titanium basket implants. *Int J Oral Maxifillofac Implants* 1988;3:49–56.

42. Cook SD, Thomas KA. Mechanical failure of nonce-mented human porous coated implants. *Trans Soc for Biomat* 1990;16:272.

43. Morrey BF, Chao EYS. Fracture of the porous-coated metal tray of a biologically fixed knee prosthesis. *Clin Orthop* 1988;228:182–189.

44. Young FA, Keller, JC. Porous titanium dental implants in primates and humans. *Eng Med* 1984;13:203–206.

45. Luthy H, Strub JR. Thickness of plasma flame-sprayed coatings on titanium implants exfoliated in dogs. *Int J Oral Maxillofac Implants* 1988;3:269–273.

46. Heck DA, Chao EY, Sim FH, Pritchard DJ, Shives TC. Titanium fiber-metal segmental prostheses: A radiographic analysis and review of current status. *Clin Orthop* 1986;204:266–273.

47. Hubbard HP. Crack growth under cyclic compression. *Trans ASME J Basic Eng* 1969;625–631.

Forces on Dental Implants and Interfacial Stress Transfer*

J.B. Brunski

To be successful, all tissue-integrated implants, whether oral, maxillofacial, or orthopedic, must support in vivo loads and deliver them to surrounding interfacial tissues in a safe and effective manner. While this is obvious for a dental implant that supports dental prostheses and for an extraoral maxillofacial implant that attaches a prosthesis to the facial skeleton, it is also true for an orthopedic implant such as a femoral or knee prosthesis that reconstructs a synovial joint. In view of this common biomechanical purpose of all implants in bone, there are two key problems that implant designers must confront.

First, there is the problem of knowing the loading of implants in vivo. For dental implants, the problem is complicated by the fact that several implants may be used to support a prosthesis, which in turn means that there will be load sharing among the implants. So far, this "load partitioning" problem has not been completely solved, although significant progress toward a solution has been made. It is now possible to identify key variables in the problem and to examine load partitioning among dental implants via theoretical and experimental approaches. However, as yet no in vivo validation of these predictions has been provided.

Second, there is the problem of understanding interfacial stress transfer. This is a difficult two-part problem. The first part is a stress analysis problem in mechanics: What are the details of stress transfer from implant to interfacial tissues? In view of the variety of shapes and sizes of available dental implants, as well as the different bone types into which dental implants are being inserted, it should be evident that this problem is both time-consuming and technically involved. However, an additional aspect of this problem involves the biology of the interface: What is the biological significance of the solution to the stress analysis problem just described? Even if it were possible to accurately predict the stresses and strains everywhere in the tissue-implant interface, what would be the biological significance of these results? What makes this problem difficult are the significant gaps in our understanding of the structure and properties of interfacial tissues as well as the mechanisms of biological responses to interfacial stress transfer.

This paper will focus on the following aspects of dental implant biomechanics: (1) What are the in vivo loads on dental implants? What data are available and what modeling approaches are being used to predict the loadings, especially in the case of multiple implants supporting prostheses? (2) What information is available to guide our understanding of stress transfer at the bone/dental implant interface and its biological significance?

Problem no. 1: In vivo loadings on dental implants

Under equilibrium conditions, the loading of a dental prosthesis must be counterbalanced by

*Keynote presentation.

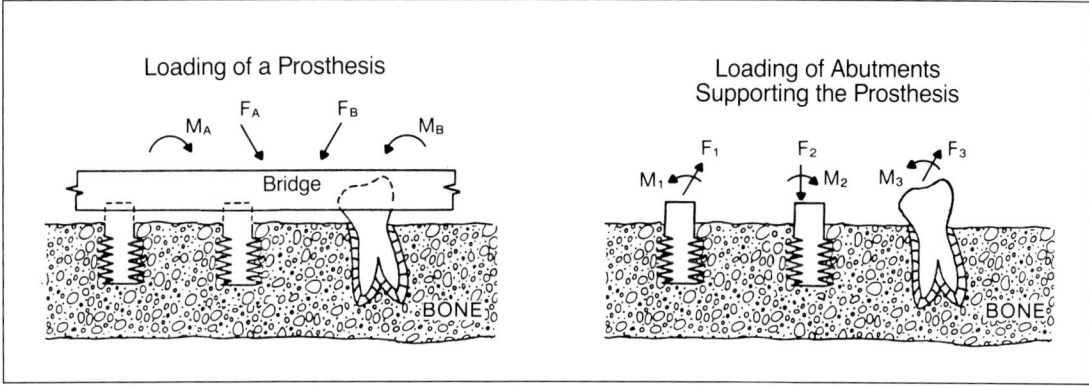

Fig 1 In vivo, a dental prosthesis will be exposed to forces and moments acting at various locations. In general, the individual abutments that support the prosthesis will not experience the same loadings as the prosthesis.

reactions (forces and moments) in the abutments that support it (Fig 1). The abutments could all be implants or a mixture of natural teeth and implants. The goal is to understand how these reactions are distributed among the abutments and to realize that the reactions depend on a number of factors, including:

1. The magnitude, direction, and location of all intraoral loadings on the prosthesis
2. The geometry and mechanical properties of the prosthesis
3. The nature of the connections between abutments and prosthesis
4. The number, location, and angulation of the implants
5. The mechanical properties of the implants and abutments
6. The mechanical properties ("stiffness") of the abutment and its interface with tissue
7. Jaw and skull deformability

Unfortunately, information is lacking about the majority of these factors. An exception is factor no. 1. Data are available on biting forces on teeth and restorations under various in vivo conditions. A recent study, for instance, showed that young human males could exert maximal vertical biting forces of about 500 N, 400 N, and 200 N on natural molars, premolars, and inci-

sors, respectively, while complete denture wearers (without dental implants) exerted maximal biting forces of only 46 to 62 N, with no differences between molar and incisal regions.[1] However, for patients with complete dentures in the maxilla and an implant-supported prosthesis in the mandible, biting forces were on the order of 300 N.[2] A more complete discussion of masticatory physiology, bite forces, and related data is found in additional references.[3–6]

For the remaining factors affecting abutment loadings, conclusive data are scarce. At present, theoretical and experimental models have been used to predict the load distribution among implants supporting a prosthesis, although these have not yet been completely validated in vivo.

Starting with the simple case of two abutments supporting a rigid prosthesis loaded by a single vertical load, it is possible, using methods of two-dimensional rigid body mechanics, to estimate the loadings on each abutment. Rangert et al[7] developed a "see saw" analogy for this problem. Their approach isolates a pair of implants in a distribution and neglects the contributions from any implants in the remainder of the arch (Fig 2). The model illustrates how the interimplant spacing can affect loads on the implants. For a vertical force P at the distal end of a prosthesis with a cantilever of length a

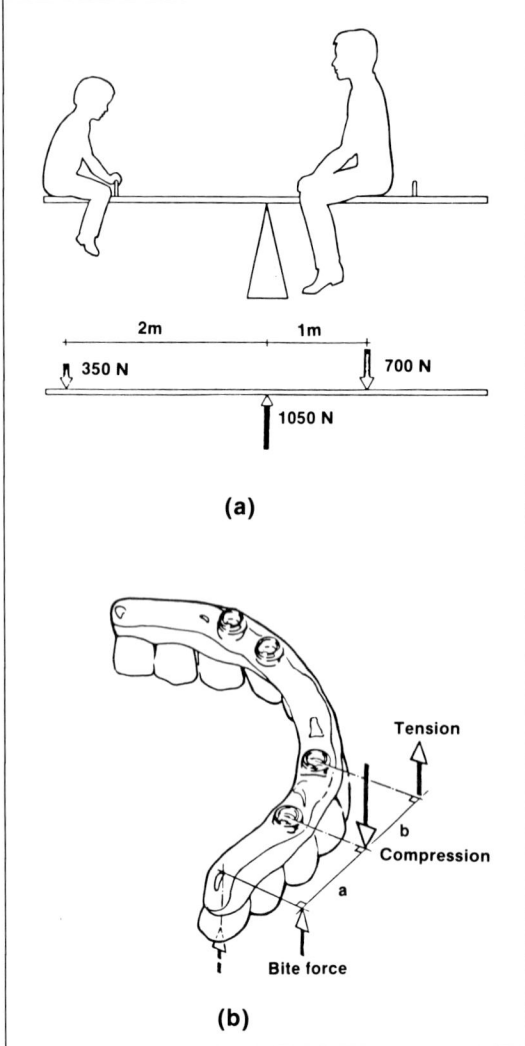

(a)

(b)

Fig 2 The model of Rangert et al draws an analogy between a child's seesaw and the loading of implants supporting a prosthesis. (From reference 7.)

and an implant spacing *b,* the force on the implant nearest the cantilever is predicted to be compressive and of a magnitude equal to $(1 + a/b)P$. The force on the implant farthest from the cantilever should be tensile and of a magnitude equal to $(a/b)P$. Consequently, this model predicts that for a constant cantilever length *a,* the loadings on the abutments will increase as the interimplant spacing, *b,* decreases. This model has been used to give

clinicians an intuitive "feel" for implant loading and the factors affecting loading.

However, for the more general problem of predicting the loadings on *all* implants or teeth supporting a prosthesis, this problem becomes a statically indeterminant problem in mechanics; the loadings on the individual abutments cannot be calculated using the methods of rigid body statics alone. Additional information is needed to solve such a problem and may include known or assumed properties of the prosthesis, implants, and/or interfacial tissues, for example, elastic modulus and geometry of the prosthesis, or the "stiffnesses" of implant and natural tooth abutments.

Skalak's model[8] represents the first solution to this statically indeterminant problem. He used an approach patterned after a method for predicting the load distribution among bolts or rivets connecting structural members in engineering.[9] It is assumed in his model that the prosthesis and bone are perfectly rigid, while the implants are linearly elastic studs that are rigidly connected to the prosthesis and bone. For a prosthesis supported by N implants and subjected to vertical and horizontal loads, the model provides equations for horizontal and vertical force components on each of the N-supporting implants. A useful feature of the model is that it can separately deal with vertical and horizontal prosthesis loads by resolving the applied loading on the prosthesis into horizontal and vertical components, the effects of which are computed separately in the analysis (see reference 8 for details).

The following example situations illustrate the types of predictions that can be made with Skalak's model.[10] Consider the case of four versus six implants symmetrically distributed about the midline of a semicircular mandible (22-mm radius) over an arc of 112.5°. The implants support a prosthesis that is loaded unilaterally at the distal cantilever region (Fig 3). This geometry corresponds approximately to four or six implants placed between the mental foramina in the human mandible.

For the six-implant case, a vertical force of 30 N applied distally at the cantilever region of the

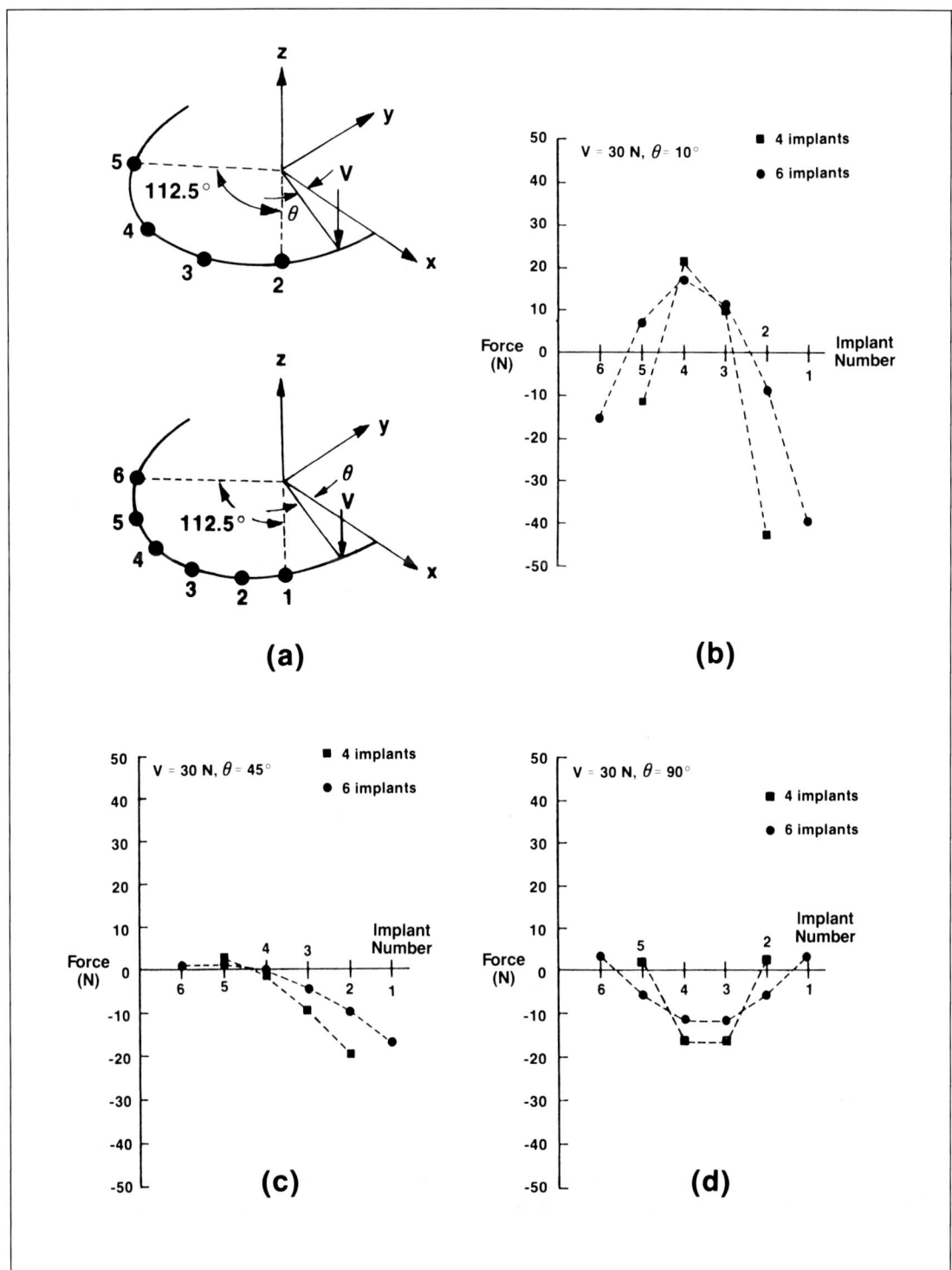

Fig 3 Sample results based on the Skalak model for a four- versus a six-implant arrangement of implants supporting a prosthesis. In both cases the implants span the same angular arc of 112.5°. (See text for details.)

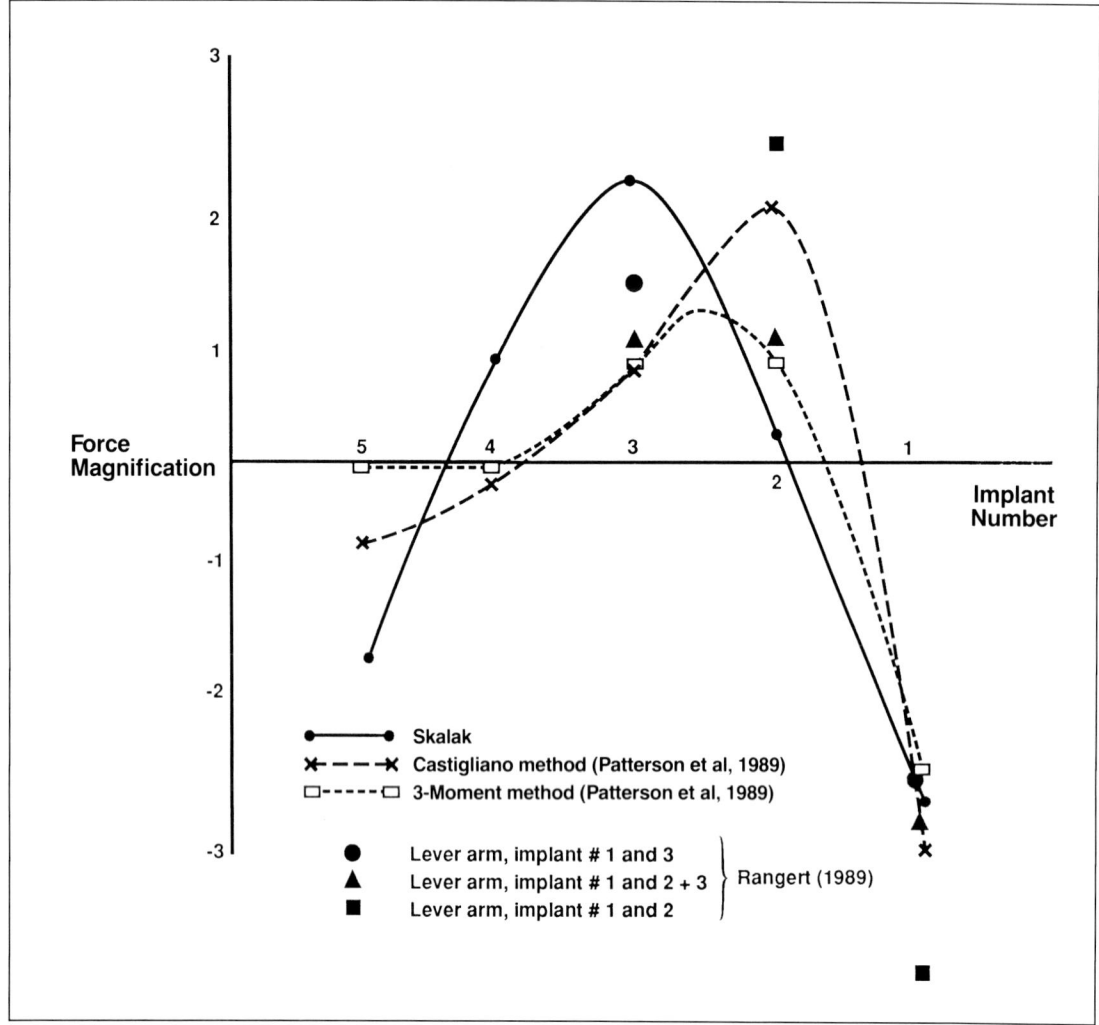

Fig 4 A five-implant case analyzed by the models of Skalak, Patterson, et al, and Rangert et al; generally, the models predict different loads on the implants, although the qualitative load distributions are similar.

prosthesis produces compressive forces on the implants nearest the applied load (implants no. 1 and no. 2 in Fig 3), and on the implant farthest away (implant no. 6 in Fig 3). At the same time, this applied loading on the prosthesis causes tensile loading on implants no. 3, no. 4, and no. 5. This results from the tendency of the entire rigid prosthesis to tip (when loaded distally) about an axis of rotation that runs approximately buccolingually between the most distal implants (no. 1, no. 2, and no. 6) and the most mesial

implants (no. 3, no. 4, and no. 5). In Skalak's model, the size, shape, and material properties of the prosthesis and jaw do not enter into the calculations; the prosthesis and jaw are idealized as being perfectly rigid. The implants represent the only deformable elements in the model.

In comparison with the six-implant case, the Skalak model for four implants over the same 112.5° arc (Fig 3) predicts that the vertical forces on the most distal implants (no. 2 and no. 4) are comparable to those on the most distal implants in the six-implant case (ie, implants no. 1 and no. 6). When the prosthesis is loaded more toward the midline of the jaw, the results also tend to be similar for the four- and six-implant cases. Therefore, according to these calculations there is evidently little biomechanical difference between using four versus six implants to support a prosthesis, provided that the four or six implants are distributed over the same 112.5° arc. This follows from the fact that the magnitudes of the vertical forces on each implant are about the same in each case. (Note: There is a difference if the four implants are distributed over a smaller arc.[10] Significantly, the largest load on any single implant in either example is about 1 to 2 times the force applied to the prosthesis. However, in a five-implant distribution (see Fig 4, discussed shortly) it is possible to generate loads on an individual implant as large as 3 P, where P is the load applied to the prosthesis. The loads on any one implant depend strongly on how the prosthesis is loaded and the implant's location in the distribution.

Another useful feature of Skalak's model is that it is linear in the load P on the prosthesis. This means that the aforementioned numerical examples for an applied force P = 30 N may be scaled to any other applied force P' by simply multiplying the results in the appropriate graph by the ratio P'/P.

Recent models by Brooke-Smith and Patterson[11,12] differ from Skalak's and Rangert et al by incorporating the elastic rigidity of the prosthesis. The rigidity is EI, where E is Young's elastic modulus and I is the second moment of area of the prosthesis cross section. Brooke-Smith and Patterson used two different approaches in their models, namely one based on Castigliano's theorem and one based on the so-called "three-moment method" in strength of materials.[13] Sample results are illustrated for the case of five implants supporting a distally loaded prosthesis (Fig 4). Plotted in this same figure are results computed with the Skalak and Rangert et al models for the same five-implant problem. It can be seen that when the prosthesis is not assumed to be infinitely rigid, but instead has a finite rigidity, there remain higher loads on the

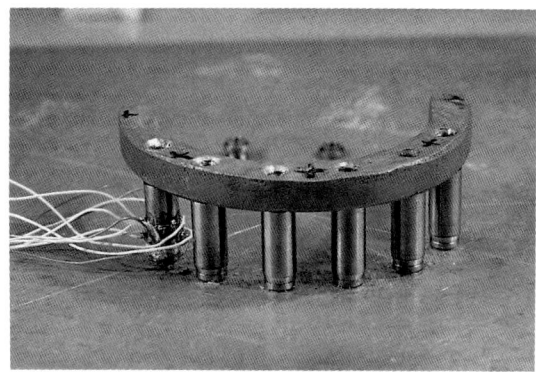

Fig 5 A laboratory model of six fixtures supporting a dental alloy prosthesis. The Brånemark fixtures are placed in a semicircular array in a 1-inch-thick aluminum block. A strain-gauged abutment cylinder (ie, a load cell) is seen connected to the third fixture from the left. (The implants in the background are for a similar study of a four-implant distribution.)

implants nearest the loading point on the prosthesis (ie, implants no. 1 and no. 2 in Fig 4), and lower loads on implants farthest away (ie, implants no. 3, no. 4, and no. 5 in Fig 4), relative to the Skalak model results. The main difference between the Brooke-Smith-Patterson results and the Skalak-Rangert results is that the implants nearest the loading point tend to experience larger loads in the former model.

The obvious question about the models mentioned is which is most realistic in vivo. Experiments will be needed to answer this question, since as yet there are no suitable in vivo data against which to compare theory and experiment. One experimental approach (in progress) is to construct models of prostheses and implants in the laboratory, record implant loadings under specific loading conditions, then compare measurements with theoretical predictions, as will be illustrated shortly, and extend these methods to in vivo trials.

An experimental test case consisted of six Brånemark fixtures threaded into a 1-in.-thick aluminum plate in the same semicircular arc used in the calculations with the Skalak model (Fig 5). Two semicircular dental prostheses of equal dimensions (approximately 6 mm in

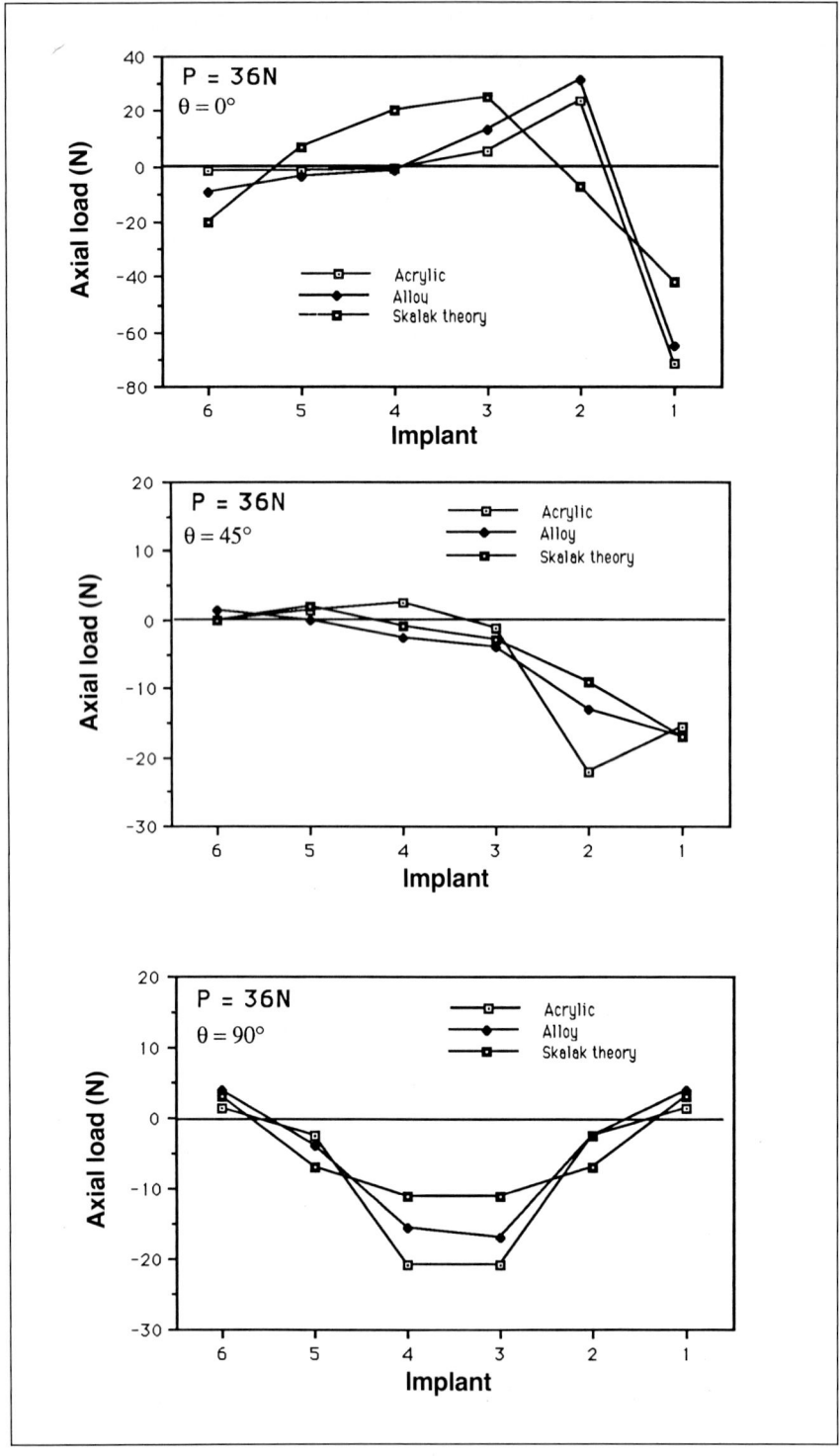

Fig 6 Sample data from tests of acrylic resin and dental alloy prostheses attached to the implants as shown in the laboratory model in Fig 5.

height, 6 mm in width) but different elastic moduli were considered: one prosthesis was dental acrylic resin (Duralay Reliance Dental Mfg Co, Worth, Ill) and the other was a cast silver-palladium metal framework per the Brånemark prosthetic technique. Prostheses were fabricated using a direct pattern method (with self-curing acrylic resin) to assure a passive fit of the final prosthesis. Standard Brånemark abutments were strain-gauged to permit measurement of vertical loads on each abutment.[14] Prostheses were then attached by the usual Brånemark gold cylinders and gold screws. Three loading cases were considered, all involving a single vertical load of 36 N applied at three different locations: distal (Θ = 10°), intermediate (Θ = 45°), and at the midline (Θ = 90°). (The angle Θ refers to the angle that defines where the force was applied to the prosthesis; see Fig 3.)

The results (Fig 6) revealed that there were deviations from the Skalak theory; the theory underpredicted the vertical forces on abutments closest to the loading point and overpredicted the forces on abutments farthest away. This finding was more pronounced for the acrylic resin prosthesis, which has a lower elastic modulus, but also occurred to a lesser extent with the metallic alloy prosthesis. It seems likely that prosthesis deformability needs to be considered to help explain these results, as suggested by the Brooke-Smith-Patterson approach. However, whether this effect will also be seen in vivo remains to be seen. It is probable that the bone/implant interface in vivo confers a stiffness much less than that for implants in an aluminum plate, which may shift the results back toward those from the Skalak treatment.

In summary, the data, theories, and experiments described here have not yet permitted a complete solution to problem no. 1—determining in vivo loads on dental implants. However, the available research on biting forces, together with evolving theoretical and experimental work, will eventually provide a more complete solution. An important goal for future research will be the development of proper in vivo methods for checking theory against experiment.

Problem no. 2: Biological significance of interfacial stress transfer

Since all dental implants will ultimately be loaded in vivo, as discussed under problem no. 1, the following question arises: How should implants be designed to create "appropriate" stress transfer conditions at the interface and thereby engender "appropriate" biological responses? Many implant systems are now available that differ substantially in shape, size, biomaterial, and surface texture.[15] Considering these differences, should one expect a difference in the way these implants perform biologically, and if so, why? Steinemann's aphorism about implant performance continues to be the best statement of a design philosophy for implants: "Even if it works, ask why!"[16]

A first step in considering the biological significance of interfacial stress transfer is to examine what can be considered as the worst case scenario, in other words, single cycle overload. Assuming that an implant has been successfully placed in bone and allowed to heal or "osseointegrate" under minimal loading condidions, after the implant is put into function, what force would it take to fail the interface by overload in one loading cycle?

While this appears to be a simple question, it is not. Overloading could occur as a result of axial or lateral forces, or both. However, to simplify the problem, it is useful to define "single cycle overload" to mean mechanical failure of the interface caused by one loading cycle of vertical force. (Such an overload would be analogous to an ultimate tensile strength of an engineering structure.) Unfortunately, few conclusive data exist about this type of overload failure in vivo, although anecdotal reports of such failures continue to be heard. In the absence of such data, some insight can be derived from the results of push-out tests, which have been used for many years as a way to measure the shear strength of the interface of candidate implant materials in bone. (A recent exchange of letters and editorial comments concerning the nature

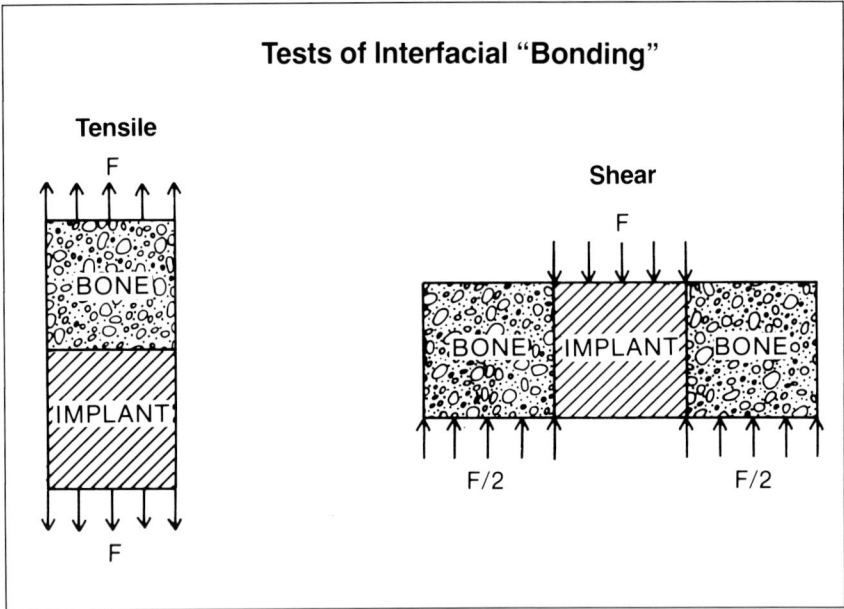

Fig 7 Schematic diagrams illustrating the nature of tensile versus shear (push-out) tests of bone/implant interfaces.

of push-out tests and their limitations appears in reference 17.)

In a typical push-out test, cylindrical plugs of candidate implant materials are placed transcortically or intramedullarly in dog femurs and allowed to heal for periods ranging from 4 to 32 weeks. The bone-implant samples are then harvested en bloc and tested mechanically as depicted schematically in Fig 7. When the implant is pushed (or pulled) out, measurements are made of the force required to fail the bone/implant interface. Typically, the failure force is defined as the maximum force on the force-displacement plot. The interfacial shear strength is then computed by dividing the failure force by the bone-implant contact area. This area is usually a nominal or a measured area. Two limitations to this computation of interfacial shear strength are: *(1)* the nominal or measured areas may not be accurate, and *(2)* the interfacial stress state is not necessarily as simple as implied by the use of the term "shear." The latter is evident in recent finite element stress analyses that show that the actual interfacial stress

fields can differ considerably, depending on boundary conditions of the test set-up and geometry of the implant during a push-out test.[18] Thus it is not correct to imply that the interface fails in shear when in reality there are also tensile or compressive stresses at the interface; the exact stress field will depend on implant geometry and surface roughness, the presence or absence of "bonding," and so forth.

Despite these complications in performing push-out tests, push-out test data in Tables 1 and 2 provide some insight into the likelihood of interface failure of candidate fixation rationales for implants by single cycle overload. The data in these tables are values of interface strengths in units of stress. To obtain an estimate of the *force* required to cause interface failure in each case, the failure stresses may be converted to failure forces by multiplying by the known or estimated areas of bone-implant contact in each case (see footnote to Table 1).

The fixation rationales in Tables 1 and 2 can be conveniently divided into: *(1)* "macrointerlock," eg, implants with macroporous coat-

Table 1   Macrointerlock fixation: Interfacial shear strengths and failure loads

Implant material	Fixation rationale	Shear strength (MPa)	Failure load* (N)	Implant period (weeks)	Animal, site	Test method	Reference
Co-Cr-Mo	Porous, beads, pore size 50–400 μm	17.2 ± 1.4	729	8	Dog femora, transcortical	Push-out	19
Ti-6Al-4V	Porous, beads, pore size 125 μm	16.7 ± 0.4	622	4	Dog, monkey femur, transcortical	Push-out	20
Polyethylene	Porous, beads, pore size 250 μm	16.5 ± 2.7	614	16	Dog, monkey femur, transcortical	Push-out	20
Ti(CP)†	Porous, beads, pore size 200 μm, sintered onto Ti-6Al-4V	21.9 ± 4.6	1238	32	Dog femora, transcortical	Push-out	21
Carbon-coated Ti	Porous, beads, pore size 200 μm, sintered onto Ti-6Al-4V	27.1 ± 4.8	1532	32	Dog femora, transcortical	Push-out	22
Co-Cr-Mo	Porous, beads, pore size 155–350 μm	21 (mean)	1187	12	Dog femora, transcortical	Push-out	23
Ti(CP)	Brånemark fixture	30.6 ± 1.45	1010	Freshly inserted	Dog tibia, transcortical	Pull-out	24
Ti + HA coating	Circumferential grooves, 750-μm deep, 75-μm HA coating on CP Ti	12.12 ± 2.43	685	32	Dog femora, transcortical	Push-out	25
Ti(CP)	Same as above, but no coating	10.53 ± 3.29	595	32	Dog femora, transcortical	Push-out	25

*Failure loads calculated based on maximal bone/implant interfacial area = πDL, where D = average implant diameter, L = average length of implant in bone; L is taken as 3 mm for the femoral cortical thickness in all cases except the case of the Brånemark fixture in canine tibia, where L = 2 mm.
†CP = Commercially pure.

ings or large threads or grooves cut into the surface; *(2)* "microinterlock," eg, implants with special surface textures created by plasma spraying or sandblasting; or *(3)* "bioactive" attachment of bone to implant, eg, implants with hydroxyapatite (HA) or other calcium phosphate coatings. Some implants could derive fixation from a combination of all three of these fixation methods. However, the key question is: How strong are each of these fixation rationales, particularly in comparison to bite forces?

First, for macrointerlock implant samples without "bioactive" coatings[19–24] (Table 1), the shear strengths (stresses) range from about 5 to 30 MPa. These stresses are estimated to correspond to failure forces of about 622 to 1532 N. Interestingly, the strength of Brånemark screws freshly inserted into about a 2-mm thickness of *dead* cortical bone[24] exceeds the strengths for implants that had been permitted to heal in *living* cortical bone before testing. This illustrates the point that, if one simply wants the most retention, then one should use an implant shape that affords the largest mechanical retention, which, based on the aforementioned comparison, seems to be the screw geometry.

Second, for macrointerlock systems with "bioactive" calcium phosphate coatings[25] (Table 1), data from the transcortical dog femur model show 32-week strengths of 10.53 ± 3.29 MPa

Table 2 Microinterlock fixation: Interfacial shear strengths and failure loads

Implant material	Fixation rationale	Shear strength (MPa) (at 8 mos)	Failure load* (N)	Implant period (weeks)	Animal, site	Test method	Reference
PMMA	Polished, uncoated	4.07 ± 1.27	230	32	Dog femur, transcortical	Push-out	26
PMMA	Polished, carbon-coated	2.08 ± 0.88	118	32	Dog femur, transcortical	Push-out	26
Carbon	As deposited	2.26 ± 0.58	128	32	Dog femur, transcortical	Push-out	26
Carbon	Polished	1.34 ± 0.37	75.8	32	Dog femur, transcortical	Push-out	26
Ti(CP)†	Polished, uncoated	2.00 ± 0.84	113	32	Dog femur, transcortical	Push-out	26
Ti(CP)	Polished, carbon-coated	1.67 ± 1.52	94.4	32	Dog femur, transcortical	Push-out	26
Ti(CP)	Grit-blasted, uncoated	2.85 ± 1.35	161	32	Dog femur, transcortical	Push-out	26
Ti(CP)	Grit-blasted, carbon-coated	2.47 ± 0.43	140	32	Dog femur, transcortical	Push-out	26
Al_2O_3	Polished, uncoated	2.48 ± 1.30	140	32	Dog femur, transcortical	Push-out	26
Al_2O_3	Polished, carbon-coated	2.65 ± 1.21	150	32	Dog femur, transcortical	Push-out	26
Al_2O_3	Grit-blasted, uncoated	2.92 ± 0.76	165	32	Dog femur, transcortical	Push-out	26
Al_2O_3	Grit-blasted, carbon-coated	2.74 ± 0.90	155	32	Dog femur, transcortical	Push-out	26
Ti(CP)	Bead-blasted, uncoated	1.21 ± 0.77	68.4	32	Dog femur, transcortical	Push-out	27
Ti-6Al-4V	HA-coating	6.07 ± 1.29‡	343	32	Dog femur, transcortical	Push-out	27

*Failure loads calculated as per Table 1.
†CP = Commercially pure.
‡Push-out failures occurred almost entirely (90%) at the HA-titanium substrate interface.

to 12.12 ± 2.43 MPa for uncoated versus HA-coated titanium implants, respectively. (These implants had 750-μm-deep circumferential grooves in the overall cylindrical geometry.) The failure strengths correspond to forces of about 595 to 685 N. These strength and force values are toward the low end of the range quoted previously for macrointerlock systems having no "bioactive" coatings.

Third, for microinterlock systems without "bioactive" coatings[26] (Table 2), the shear strength values are approximately equivalent over a broad range of materials and surface textures at 32 weeks in the dog transcortical model; the range of interfacial shear strengths is about 1 to 4 MPa. The corresponding failure forces are 68 to 230 N. Note that these strength and force values are much less than those for macrointerlock systems listed in Table 1.

Finally, consider sample test data on HA-coated microinterlock systems[27] (Table 2). Cook's et al data from the dog transcortical model system at 32 weeks reveal shear strengths of 1.21 ± 0.77 MPa for uncoated pure titanium versus 6.07 ± 1.29 MPa for HA-coated Ti-6Al-4V alloy. These stresses correspond to failure forces of about 68 N for titanium versus 343 N for HA-coated Ti-6Al-4V. (For the HA-coated samples, the strength was limited by the strength of adherence of the HA to the substrate metal. This interface was the site of failure in about 90% of the tests.) Notably, the failure forces for both uncoated and coated samples are small in comparison with the values reported for macrointerlock systems.

What is the interpretation of these data in terms of the original question of resistance to single cycle overload failure of implants? Assuming that the data can be extrapolated to implant systems in humans—and there are concerns about the validity of this extrapolation—these failure forces should be compared to expected biting forces in humans.

To make this comparison, a convenient rule of thumb is useful: based on the Skalak model, the largest axial forces on dental implants tend to occur when a cantilever prosthesis is loaded by a vertical load P applied at the end of the cantilever. Specifically, the axial force on the most distal implant nearest the loading point on the cantilever can be about 2 to 3 P (depending on prosthesis loading, implant locations, etc), while the next nearest implant will experience a tensile force of about 1 to 2 P. Therefore, a patient who bites with a typical axial force of 300 N could conceivably load an individual implant in axial tension or compression up to a maximum of about 600 to 900 N.

This range of vertical forces, that is, 600 to 900 N, exceeds the failure forces of all microinterlock systems in Table 2, including the HA-coated titanium alloy. Moreover, even for the macrointerlock systems, the Co-Cr-Mo, Ti-6Al-4V, and polyethylene (PE) porous-coated implants, as well as the grooved titanium implants, might also fail under this range of biting forces. Evidently, only a few implant fixation rationales, including the Brånemark screws and some of the porous systems, should be able to resist axial biting forces greater than 1,000 N.

However, as cautioned earlier, there are reasons to question the wisdom of extrapolating the aforementioned push-out data from animal models to human situations. First, it is questionable if push-out data from tests of implants in purely *cortical* bone of animals apply to dental implants in the mixtures of cancellous and cortical bone more typical of implant sites in humans. This is an important point because it is well known that the mechanical properties of cancellous bone are generally inferior to those of cortical bone; for example, the compressive strength of cortical bone is about 250 MPa, whereas that of cancellous bone is about 10 MPa.[28] As an indication of what this could mean, preliminary results from a series of pull-outs of Brånemark fixtures in samples of fresh bovine cancellous bone gave an average pull-out force of 414 ± 173 N (m = 80; range 163 to 976 N).[29] This average pull-out force is considerably less than that measured for the same size Brånemark fixtures freshly inserted into cadaveric cortical bone of the dog, ie, on the order of 1,500 N.[24] Therefore, it seems likely that push-out tests of implants in cortical bone of animals might actually *overestimate* the failure forces for implants in human bone of a mixed cortico-cancellous nature. This issue remains to be resolved.

Another caution about extrapolating single cycle overload data from cortical bone in animal models to in vivo cases in humans is that these tests do not directly investigate another conceivable failure mode in vivo, ie, interface failure by fatigue. It is possible that bone/implant interfaces might fail because of repetitive loading at otherwise "safe" loads, analogous to fatigue failures of conventional engineering materials at "safe" levels of stress. This possibility needs to be considered in vivo, since it is known that accumulated damage develops in bone in vivo.[30] Whether this process occurs around dental implants and contributes to interface failures in vivo is simply unknown at present.

A final concern about extrapolating these push-out data from animals to humans is that the published studies have not ordinarily used implants of exactly the same dimensions as clinical dental implants. For example, Cook's et al[27] tests of HA-coated Ti-6Al-4V plugs were conducted with 6-mm-diameter cylinders, whereas commercially available HA-coated dental implants can have outside diameters of about 4 mm. It is therefore possible that the interface failure forces expected for actual implants in humans might be less than those suggested by Cook's et al results from animal experiments.

Moving beyond this worst case scenario of single cycle overload and the related possibility of fatigue failure, a perplexing but important remaining problem concerns the biological significance of stress transfer at loading levels below those that cause frank overload or fatigue damage. The key questions are: What is the biological significance of these nondestructive interfacial stresses in bone around implants? How does bone respond to interfacial stresses; what mechanisms are involved?

Answers to these questions require an understanding of the biology of bone response to implant placement. This understanding must begin with basic wound healing of bone and also incorporate subsequent steps in maturation and modeling/remodeling of the healing site, plus the possibility that these normal events might be significantly affected by implant placement and loading, as follows.

Once an oral implant is placed, a phase of bone healing occurs subsequent to the trauma of the surgical procedure. The healing response will depend on the type of bone, animal or human, its original anatomy, and the degree of damage, among other factors. It would be expected that, under optimal conditions, the early stages of this healing response would eventually merge into a later stage of bone modeling and remodeling, which in turn would reach a steady state after about 6 to 12 months.[31–33] The most important point to emphasize is that the placement and presence of an implant can cause perturbations in normal bone healing and remodeling as a result of surgical, biomaterial, and biomechanical factors. Discussion here is restricted to biomechanical factors and their effects on bone response at the interface.

What is meant by the word "interface"? The interface is a region or zone of interaction that can include the oxide surface of the implant (assuming for the moment that the implant is metal) as well as the surrounding tissue af-

fected by the presence of the implant.[34,35] Therefore, the interface that develops after the implantation of a titanium implant in bone begins within the oxide layer on the metal surface and extends out into the tissue up to a region that can be considered normal or indistinguishable from bone typical for the implantation site. While imprecise, this definition allows for the fact that the interface is a *region of interaction* that can involve a substantial volume of the tissue, ranging from nanometers up to millimeters in dimension.

Which biomechanical factors are most important to consider in relation to the early healing period and the interface? One key factor is "relative motion," or "micromotion," at the bone/implant interface.[34,36] This can be defined as relative displacements including sliding, opening of gaps, etc, that occur between the implant and bone adjacent to the implant. The evidence is persuasive that micromotion is biologically significant; the supporting data come from both orthopedics and dentistry. Micromotion can affect both the type and organization of tissues at the interface, especially if the micromotion begins soon after implantation. Sir John Charnley[37] as well as Uhthoff[38] and Cameron[39] reported that mobile screws in bone were surrounded by fibrous tissue that caused a loss of holding power. Uhthoff also pointed out that the absence of micromotion, or at least the minimization thereof, permitted a "solid incorporation of the screw by bone." (Currently, this "solid incorporation . . . in bone" finding would probably be called osseointegration.) Likewise, research on porous implant fixation has reinforced the aforementioned conclusions.[40,41] At present, the general view in orthopedics is that implant stability in bone during healing, ie, the absence of micromotion, is a prerequisite for secure bone ingrowth.[42] Moreover, in the dental implant literature, a similar line of evidence about micromotion has developed.

Brunski et al[43] studied smooth-surfaced pure titanium blade-vent dental implants under two different biomechanical situations in dog mandibles; one implant per animal was always protected from biting forces while the contralateral implant partially supported a three-unit fixed partial denture that was exposed to loading immediately. Histological analyses revealed major amounts (up to 0.5 mm thick) of collagen-rich, vascularized fibrous connective tissue that was only found at the interfaces of the functionally loaded implants. In contrast, the interfaces of the protected implants developed bone in direct, or nearly direct, apposition to the titanium implants (ie, osseointegration). The interpretation was that because of the relatively nonretentive shape of the blade-vent implant and its connection to a loaded prosthesis, there was micromotion at the interface of the loaded implants. In this study it was probably limited to the range of occlusoapical tooth mobility of the teeth to which the prosthesis was splinted.

Few other studies have investigated how micromotion leads to interfacial fibrous tissue. However, a review of many previous publications on dental implants.[34,43] suggests that micromotion of the implant in the healing bone predisposed the interface toward formation of fibrous tissue rather than bone. Moreover, this observation seems to hold irrespective of the implant biomaterial.[44]

An unresolved question involving micromotion concerns the biological mechanisms whereby micromotion at the interface leads to the development of fibrous tissue. One possibility is that the fibrous tissue is a type of repair or scar tissue that forms in reaction to the continuous disruption of the tissue stroma during bone healing at the site.[42] Others hypothesize that the stress and strain states in the developing tissues might affect cell shape and physiology and, in turn, the types of interfacial tissues that form.[45] It also remains unclear whether an implant that does have a certain amount of initial stability in bone (eg, by virtue of its shape or placement in bone) can be loaded immediately after implantation without the formation of fibrous tissue. The basic question is how much micromotion can be tolerated before fibrous tissue will start to develop. Interestingly, current research with single-stage implants such as the ITI Benefit (Institute Straumann AG, Waldenberg, Switzerland) Swiss screw[46] indicates that fibrous tissue does not form even when there are loads on the implant immediately after its placement in bone. Perhaps by virtue of its surface texture and geometry, this type of implant is stable enough in bone so that appreciable micromotion does not occur even when the implant is loaded, albeit to a limited extent, early after its placement.

Assuming that fibrous tissue has been avoided at the interface and that direct bone-implant apposition has been achieved through a period of unloaded healing, as in the case of a two-stage implant, then the major remaining question concerns the response of bone at the interface when the implant is finally put into function. New stress and strain conditions will develop at the interface when an implant is loaded after this period of undisturbed healing under nonloaded conditions. What occurs in terms of bone response?

There are a number of possibilities after loading starts. If the applied loadings are excessive, interfacial bone failure may occur through frank overload or perhaps fatigue, as discussed earlier. However, before overload occurs, there is the question of stress and strain distribution that develops in the interfacial tissues when the implant is loaded, and whether these have any significant biological effects. While it might be presumed that they would, on the basis of general recognition of form-function relationships in bone, this issue is far from being settled.

For the same loading on two different implants, a screw versus a smooth cylindrical dental implant for example, the spatial distribution of stress and strain in interfacial bone will depend primarily on the geometry of the implant, the mechanical properties of the implant and the bone, whether there is bonding or just apposition at the interface (boundary condition), and the amount of bone that actually exists around the implant. The influence of these factors is conveniently illustrated by results from recent finite element (FE) computer models.

In regard to implant geometry and boundary conditions, work by Siegele and Soltesz[47] illustrates that screw-shaped and cylindrically shaped implants will both produce stress con-

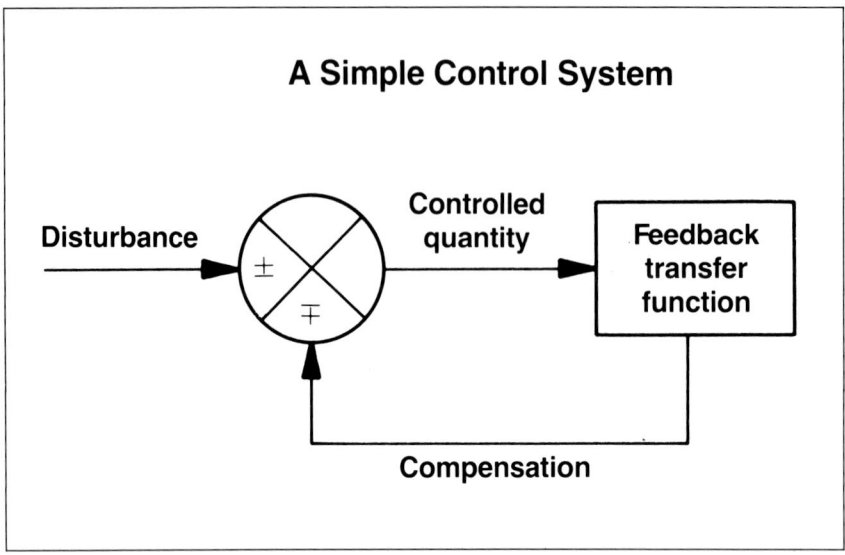

A Simple Control System

Disturbance ± Controlled quantity Feedback transfer function Compensation

Fig 8 A functional block diagram illustrating a typical physiological control system.

centrations in bone, but at different locations. These occur at the tips of the threads of the screw shape and at the blunted apex of the cylindrical shape. Furthermore, this study, as well as that of Hipp et al,[48] demonstrates that the nature of the boundary conditions that are assumed for the bone-implant junction can make a major difference in the model results; the stress distributions differ for the case of a bonded interface versus a sliding interface. (The latter interface is one that cannot support tensile or shear forces.) Other FE studies have investigated how implant elastic modulus and the type of interfacial bone, cortical or cancellous, affect the interfacial stress fields around dental implants.[49,50]

The biological meaning of the results from all of the aforementioned FE studies has yet to be clearly defined. Some researchers suggest that *high* stresses in bone near the neck of implants promotes bone resorption,[51] while others suggest that *low* stresses in bone at the neck region may contribute to bone loss because of a stress-shielding effect.[52] It may be that these apparently conflicting views can be resolved once it is better understood how bone responds to mechanical loading in vivo.

A variable that almost certainly affects FE testing results, but which has not been systematically studied, is the amount of bone that is actually in contact with dental implants in vivo. Most FE models assume that bone completely surrounds the implant, although histological data from animal and human studies indicate that this is probably not the general case in vivo.[53] Therefore, FE models that assume 100% bone contact are probably not very realistic; they may be significantly underestimating the stresses and strains in bone around implants. Contrariwise, as long as such models are used in some comparative sense, they may be useful.

In summary of these FE studies, no completely agreed-upon guidelines for the clinician have emerged about optimal shape, modulus, interface bonding, bone-implant coverage, and interfacial stress/strain fields for dental implants. It is likely that this will continue to be an important area requiring more research in view of the many different shapes, sizes, and surface coatings of implants now being placed into sites of varying quantity and quality of bone in human patients.

Finally, in considering the biological significance of interfacial stress transfer, the question arises: When interfacial bone is subjected to stresses and strains, what mechanisms may be stimulated and lead to changes in bone structure? There is a long-standing hypothesis that bone activity is governed by some type of mechanically sensitive control system. This idea has a long history in both orthopedics and dentistry, and is known as Wolff's Law.[54] According to this control system concept (Fig 8), a disturbance in the ambient state of bone is first detected in some way by the biological system. The control system evaluates this disturbance and enacts some type of compensatory response that can diminish the disturbance and thereby return the system to normal. While many researchers postulate that such a system operates in bone, the problem is to identify the biomechanical mechanisms underlying the model. To date, this identification problem remains largely unsolved. Consequently, it is not possible to give detailed design rules for implants. Firm knowledge of the mechanisms underlying the control system are simply not known.

Acknowledgment

This study was supported by the National Institute of Dental Research Training Grant 5-T32-DE07054-13.

References

1. Blamphin CNJ, Brafield TR, Jobbins B, et al. A simple instrument for the measurement of maximum occlusal force in human dentition. *Proc Inst Mech Eng* 1990;204:129–131.
2. Falk H, Laurell L, Lundgren D. Occlusal force pattern in dentitions with mandibular implant-supported fixed cantilever prostheses occluded with complete dentures. *Int J Oral Maxillofac Implants* 1989;4:55–62.
3. Bates JF, Stafford GD, Harrison A. Masticatory function—A review of the literature. 2. Speed of movement of the mandible, rate of chewing and forces developed in chewing. *J Oral Rehabil* 1975;2:349–361.
4. Carr AB, Laney WR. Maximum occlusal force levels in patients with osseointegrated oral implant prostheses and patients with complete dentures. *Int J Oral Maxillofac Implants* 1987;2:101–108.
5. Brunski JB. Biomaterials and biomechanics in the design of dental implants. *Int J Oral Maxillofac Implants* 1988;3:85–97.
6. Carlsson GE, Haraldson T. Functional response. pp 155–163 In P.-I. Brånemark, G.A. Zarb, T. Albrektsson (eds) *Tissue Integrated Prostheses: Osseointegration in Clinical Dentistry.* Chicago: Quintessence Publ Co, 1985.
7. Rangert B, Jemt T, Jorneus L. Forces and moments on Brånemark implants. *Int J Oral Maxillofac Implants* 1989;4:241–247.
8. Skalak R. Aspects of biomechanical considerations. pp 117–128 In P.-I. Brånemark, G.A. Zarb, T. Albrektsson (eds) *Tissue Integrated Prostheses: Osseointegration in Clinical Dentistry.* Chicago: Quintessence Publ Co, 1985.
9. McGuire W. *Steel Structures.* Englewood Cliffs, NJ: Prentice Hall, 1968.
10. Brunski JB, Deutsch JE. Numerical analysis of load distribution among dental implants. *J Dent Res* 1989;68:225. Abstract.
11. Brooke-Smith M. A study of the fatigue life of small gold locating screws used in the osseointegrated implant technique. Master's Thesis. Sheffield University, 1988.
12. Patterson EA, Brooke-Smith M, Johns RB. Estimation of the fatigue life of gold studs in a dental prosthesis. pp 892–893 In *Proc 12th Canadian Conference of Applied Mechanics.* vol. 2. Ottawa, Ontario: Carleton University, 1989.
13. Timoshenko SP, MacCullough GH. *Elements of Strength of Materials.* 3rd ed. New York: Van Nostrand, 1949.
14. Ng A. Design of load-sensing abutment for use as a bite force transducer with Brånemark fixtures. Master's Thesis. Troy, NY: Rensselaer Polytechnic Institute, 1991.
15. English CE. An overview of implant hardware. *J Am Dent Assoc* 1990;121:360–368.
16. Steinemann SG. Surface phenomena and tissue attachment. *J Dent Res* 1988;67:106. Abstract.
17. Black J. Editorial: 'Push-out' tests (plus exchange of letters). *J Biomed Mater Res* 1989;23:1243–1245.
18. Shirazi-Adl A. A stress continuous finite element formulation—Application to biomechanics of a push-out test with attached interface. pp 311–314 In S.A. Goldstein (ed) *Advances in Bioengineering,* BED-vol 17. New York: American Society of Mechanical Engineers, 1990.
19. Bobyn JD, Pilliar RM, Cameron HU, Weatherly GC. The optimum pore size for the fixation of porous-surfaced metal implants by the ingrowth of bone. *Clin Orthop* 1980;150:263–270.
20. Young FA, Kresch CH, Spector M. Mechanical properties of the bone-implant interface for porous titanium and porous polyethylene dental implants. p 407 In G.W. Hastings, D.F. Williams (eds) *Mechanical Properties of Biomaterials.* New York: John Wiley & Sons, 1980.
21. Clemow AJT, Weinstein AM, Klawitter JJ, et al. Interface mechanics of porous titanium implants. *J Biomed Mater Res* 1981;15:73–82.
22. Anderson RC, Cook SD, Weinstein AM, Haddad RJ. An evaluation of skeletal attachment to LTI pyrolitic carbon, porous titanium, and carbon-coated porous

titanium implants. *Clin Orthop* 1984;182:242.

23. Cook SD, Walsh KA, Haddad RJ. Interface mechanics and bone ingrowth into porous Co-Cr-Mo alloy. *Clin Orthop* 1985;183:271–280.

24. Hoshaw SJ, Brunski JB, Cochran GVB. Pull-out and fatigue failure of bone dental implant interfaces. pp 205–208 In P.A. Torzilli, M.H. Friedman (eds) *1989 Biomechanics Symposium.* New York: American Society of Mechanical Engineers, 1989.

25. Thomas KA, Kay JF, Cook SD, Jarcho M. The effect of surface microtexture and hydroxyapatite coating on the mechanical strengths and histologic profiles of titanium implant materials. *J Biomed Mater Res* 1987;21:1395–1414.

26. Thomas KA, Cook SD. An evaluation of variables influencing implant fixation by direct bone apposition. *J Biomed Mater Res* 1985;19:875–901.

27. Cook SD, Kay JF, Thomas KA, Jarcho M. Interface mechanics and histology of titanium and hydroxyapatite-coated titanium for dental implant applications. *Int J Oral Maxillofac Implants* 1987;2:15.

28. Gibson LJ. The mechanical behaviour of cancellous bone. *J Biomech* 1985;18:317–328.

29. Balon B. Strength of the bone-fixture interface in bovine cancellous bone in vitro. Master's Thesis. Troy, NY: Rensselaer Polytechnic Institute, 1991.

30. Burr DB, Martin RB, Shaffler B, Radin E. Bone remodeling in response to in vivo fatigue microdamage. *J Biomech* 1985;18:189–200.

31. Albrektsson T. Bone tissue response. pp 129–143 In P.-I. Brånemark, G.A. Zarb, T. Albrektsson (eds) *Tissue Integrated Prostheses: Osseointegration in Clinical Dentistry.* Chicago: Quintessence Publ Co, 1985.

32. Roberts WE, Turley PK, Brezniak N, Fielder PJ. Bone physiology and metabolism. *CDA Journal* 1987;15: 54–63.

33. Gross U, Kinne R, Schmitz H-J, and Strunz V. The response of bone to surface-active glasses/glass-ceramics. *CRC Crit Rev Biocomp* 1988;4:155–179.

34. Brunski JB. The influence of force, motion and related quantities on the response of bone to implants. pp 7–21 In R.F. Fitzgerald, Jr. (ed) *Non-Cemented Total Hip Arthroplasty.* New York: Raven Press, 1988.

35. Kasemo B, Lausmaa J. Biomaterials from a surface science perspective. In B.D. Ratner (ed) *Surface Characterization of Biomaterials.* New York: Elsevier, 1988.

36. Brunski JB, Hipp JA, Cochran GVB. The influence of biomechanical factors at the tissue-biomaterial interface. pp 505–515 In J.S. Hanker, B.L. Giammara (eds) *Biomedical Materials and Devices, Materials Research Society Symposium Proceedings.* Vol 110. Pittsburgh: Materials Research Society, 1989.

37. Charnley J. The fixation of prostheses in living bone. p 52 In D.C. Swanson (ed) *Modern Trends in Orthopedics.* New York: Appleton Century-Crofts, 1970.

38. Uhthoff HK. Mechanical factors affecting the holding power of screws in compact bone. *J Bone Joint Surg* 1973;55B:633.

39. Cameron HU, Pilliar RM, MacNab I. The effect of movement on the bonding of porous metal to bone. *J Biomed Mater Res* 1973;7:301.

40. Schatzker JG, Horne JG, Sumner-Smith G. The effects of movement on the holding power of screws in bone. *Clin Orthop* 1975;111:257.

41. Pilliar RM, Lee JM, Maniatopoulos C. Observations on the effect of movement on bone ingrowth into porous-surfaced implants. *Clin Orthop* 1986;208:108.

42. Spector M. Current concepts of bony ingrowth and remodeling. pp 69–86 In R.F. Fitzgerald, Jr. (ed) *Noncemented Total Hip Arthroplasty.* New York: Raven Press, 1988.

43. Brunski JB, Moccia AF, Pollack SR, et al. The influence of functional use of endosseous dental implants on the tissue-implant interface. I. Histological aspects. *J Dent Res* 1979;58:1953.

44. Nishihara K, Akagawa T, Hara H, Nakagiri S. Stress analysis related to artificial roots of connective tissue-adhesive type. Abstract, *First World Congress of Biomechanics.* Vol II, p 114. San Diego: University of California, 1990.

45. Carter DR, Giori NJ. The effect of mechanical stress on tissue differentiation in the bony implant bed. In J.E. Davies (ed) *The Bone-Biomaterial Interface.* Toronto: University of Toronto Press (in press).

46. Buser D, Weber HP, Bragger U. The treatment of partially edentulous patients with ITI hollow screw implants: Presurgical evaluation and surgical procedures. *Int J Oral Maxillofac Implants* 1990;5:165–174.

47. Siegele D; Soltesz U. Numerical investigations of the influence of implant shape on stress distribution in the jaw bone. *Int J Oral Maxillofac Implants* 1989;4:333–340.

48. Hipp JA, Brunski JB, Shephard MS, Cochran GVB. Finite element models for implants in bone: Interfacial assumptions. pp 447–452 In E. Schneider, S.A. Perren (eds) *Biomechanics: Current Interdisciplinary Research.* Dordrecht: Martinus Nijohoff Publishers, 1985.

49. Cook SD, Klawitter JJ, Weinstein AM. The influence of implant elastic modulus on the stress distribution around LTI carbon and aluminum oxide dental implants. *J Biomed Mater Res* 1981;15:879–887.

50. Lavernia CJ, Cook SD, Weinstein AM, Klawitter JJ. An analysis of stresses in a dental implant system. *J Biomech* 1981;14:555–560.

51. Soltesz U, Siegele D, Riedemuller J, Schulz P. Stress concentration and bone resorption in the jaw for dental implants with shoulders. pp 115–122 In A.J.C. Lee, T. Albrektsson, P.-I. Brånemark (eds) *Clinical Applications of Biomaterials.* New York: John Wiley & Sons, 1982.

52. Cook SD, Weinstein AM, Klawitter JJ. Parameters affecting the stress distribution around LTI carbon and aluminum oxide dental implants. *J Biomed Mater Res* 1982;16:875–885.

53. Brunski JB. Biomechanics of dental implants: Future research directions. *J Dent Educ* 1988;52:775–787.

54. Treharne RW. Review of Wolff's law and its proposed means of operation. *Orthop Rev* 1981;10:35.

Interfacial Bond Strengths of Ti-6Al-4V and Hydroxyapatite-coated Ti-6Al-4V Implants in Cortical Bone

J.L. Taylor, J.B. Brunski, S.J. Hoshaw, G.V.B. Cochran, and K.W. Higuchi

Growing interest in "bioactive" coatings such as hydroxyapatite (HA) for oral and orthopedic implants has been encouraged by results of biomechanical "push-out" tests. In a typical push-out test,[1,2] a candidate biomaterial in the form of a small cylinder with a specific surface coating or texture is implanted into a slightly undersized hole drilled in cortical bone (usually canine femur) and allowed to heal for a particular time. Then, upon animal sacrifice, the bone is excised and the cylindrical plug is pushed out of the bone site. An "interfacial shear strength" is calculated by measuring the push-out force and dividing it by the nominal or measured implant-bone contact area.

Although this test has been widely used and apparently accepted as a convenient measure of interfacial bonding between implant materials and bone, recent editorials and letter exchanges have examined the factors affecting the results and interpretation of such tests.[3] Some of these factors are: specimen dimensions, surface geometry and roughness, surface preparation and cleaning, implant site preparation and the initial tightness of fit of the cylinder in the prepared hole, and animal age and tissue handling. Equally important, others[4–6] have pointed out that push-out tests involve a shearing of the implant relative to the interfacial bone, which can make it more difficult to distinguish contributions of surface roughness versus physical-chemical bone-implant bonding to interfacial strength. Moreover, recent finite element analyses of the influence of support conditions in the loading fixture on interfacial stress states in push-out tests indicate that the interfacial stress states can be highly irregular, depending more on the loading jig support conditions than intrinsic sample properties, at least in some cases.[7]

Therefore, Gross et al[5,6] and Steinemann et al[4] have proposed tensile tests of the bone/implant interface, not necessarily as an alternative to push-out tests, but perhaps as a more sensitive test mode in which to investigate fundamental aspects of bonding between implant and bone. It can be imagined that, in the limit of perfect smoothness of the implant surface, there would no longer be sufficient roughness to allow microscopic interlocking of tissue and implant, in which case a direct measurement could be made of any physical-chemical bonding between implant and bone. Gross et al utilized cylindrical samples with a flattened portion that rested against cancellous bone. Steinemann et al used a disc inserted into a well cut into cortical bone. The present study reports on a test method similar to Steinemann's et al. It was used to measure bone/implant interfacial tensile pull-off forces for samples of Ti-6Al-4V and hydroxyapatite (HA)-coated Ti-6Al-4V prepared with comparable surface roughness.

Materials and methods

The implants utilized in this study were made of Ti-6Al-4V alloy and machined to a washer shape with an 8.9-mm outer diameter, 4.9-mm

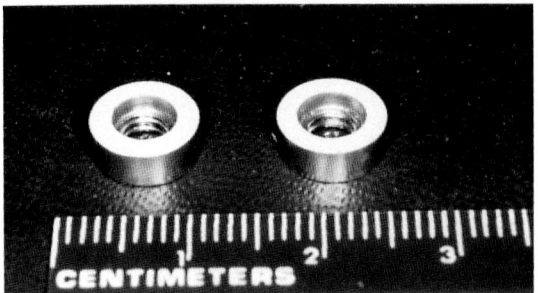

Fig 1 HA-coated Ti-6Al-4V washers, as-received surfaces.

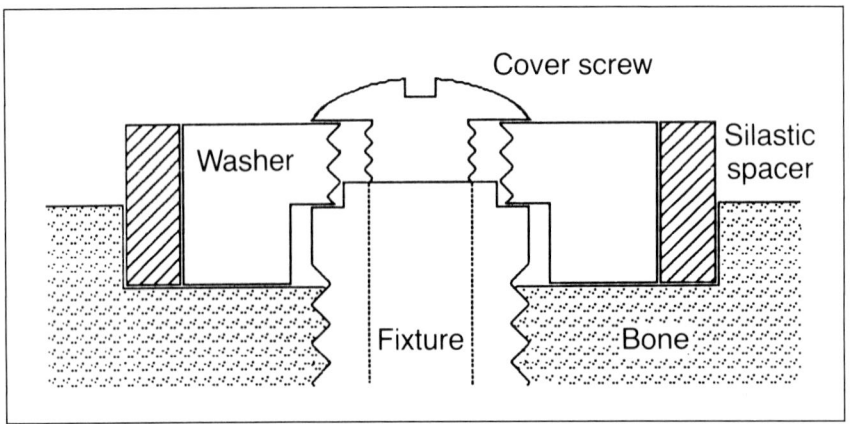

Fig 2a Schematic illustration (cross-sectional view) of the method by which washers were held down into the wells cut in cortical bone.

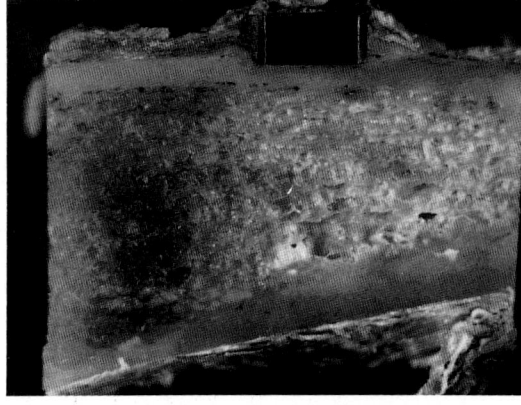

Fig 2b Histological view corresponding approximately to the schematic diagram in Fig 2a.

inner diameter, and 3-mm thickness (Fig 1). In one group of 12 titanium washers, the underside of each washer was prepared by metallographic polishing using 600 grit SiC paper (Buehler no. 30-5160), sonification in distilled water, 6 μm diamond paste (Metadi II, Buehler no. 40–6250, nylon cloth no. 40-7052, no lubrication), sonification in ethanol, and 0.3 μm alumina-water slurry (Buehler no. 40–6352, microcloth no. 40–7052). This was followed by sonification in trichloro-ethylene (two times) and ethanol (two times), distilled water rinses, and steam autoclaving with the samples in Petri dishes inside sterilization bags. A second group of 12 washers was HA-coated via plasma spraying (Bio-Interfaces,

Inc, San Diego, Calif) to form a 60-μm layer on the undersides of the washers. The coating was confined to the undersides of the washers by masking the other surfaces during plasma spraying. The HA surfaces were then polished, cleaned, and autoclaved in a manner identical to that of the titanium alloy washers.

Both washer types were implanted in the femurs of four coonhounds. Each femur contained three washers placed in the lateral, mid-diaphyseal cortex and spaced approximately 10 mm apart. A modified brad-point drill (custom made for this study) was used to prepare shallow, flat-bottomed wells (10-mm diameter, 1-mm depth) in the cortical bone to receive the washers. Drilling was performed at 100 rpm with saline irrigation. Individual washers were secured in the flat-bottomed wells by a Brånemark (Nobelpharma USA, Inc, Chicago, Ill) cover screw threaded with a maximum torque of 13 N-cm into a titanium Brånemark fixture (7 mm long, 3.75-mm diameter), which was placed in the center of the implantation site (Figs 2a and b). A thin Silastic (Dow Chemical, Midland, Mich) spacer covered the side surface of each washer to prevent tissue attachment other than at the bottom surface.

Following sample collection at 66 days (one dog), 110 days (one dog), and 301 days (two dogs), seven uncoated titanium and eight HA-coated washers were tested in tensile pull-off tests. The remaining washers were saved for histological and other analyses. In a typical tensile pull-off test, the cover screw was first gently removed from the Brånemark fixture and a pin from the actuator of an MTS 858 Bionix load frame was carefully threaded into the washer while the test bone was stabilized in the loading jig (Fig 3). Axiality of the loading axis with respect to the washer was adjusted and confirmed by an orientation jig. Tensile tests were conducted at 1 mm/min until pull-off occurred. All washers were originally scheduled for a 300-day implantation period; however, dogs died at 66 days and 110 days due to complications. Samples from the two shorter-term dogs were tested fresh-frozen and thawed, while samples from the two dogs at 301 days were tested fresh.

Table 1 Data from tensile tests

	Pull-off load (N)	
Time (d)	Ti-6Al-4V	HA-coated Ti-6Al-4V
66	0	100
	0	151
110	0	66
	0	2*
301	0	95
	40.7	74
	34.4	129
	—	133

*Questionable value; not used in the t test.

Results

Data collected in the tensile tests (Table 1) revealed a significant difference ($P < .001$) between the mean pull-off load of 107 ± 32.1 N for the HA-coated washers and 10.1 ± 18.3 N for the titanium group.

A more extensive analysis of the failure modes at bone/titanium and bone/HA interfaces is currently underway; at present, the following qualitative observations can be made. Interfacial failures in the tests of the HA-coated group were mixed-mode; there was often a combination of fracture within the coating itself and fracture of the coating from the titanium substrate. In the first type of fracture, portions of the HA coating remained on the surfaces of both the implant and the bone of the implantation site (Figs 4a and b). In the second type of fracture, exposed titanium metal suggested that failure had occurred at the HA coating/implant interface (Figs 5a and b). In the HA-coated group there were no cases showing evidence of tensile fracture of the bone adjacent to the HA coating. In general, more of the HA coating remained on the titanium washer substrate at 66 days and 110 days than at 301 days. However, because of the small sample size, it was not possible to identify any clear trends with implantation time in the HA pull-off loads.

All washers in the uncoated titanium group had 0 N pull-off loads at 66 days and 110 days.

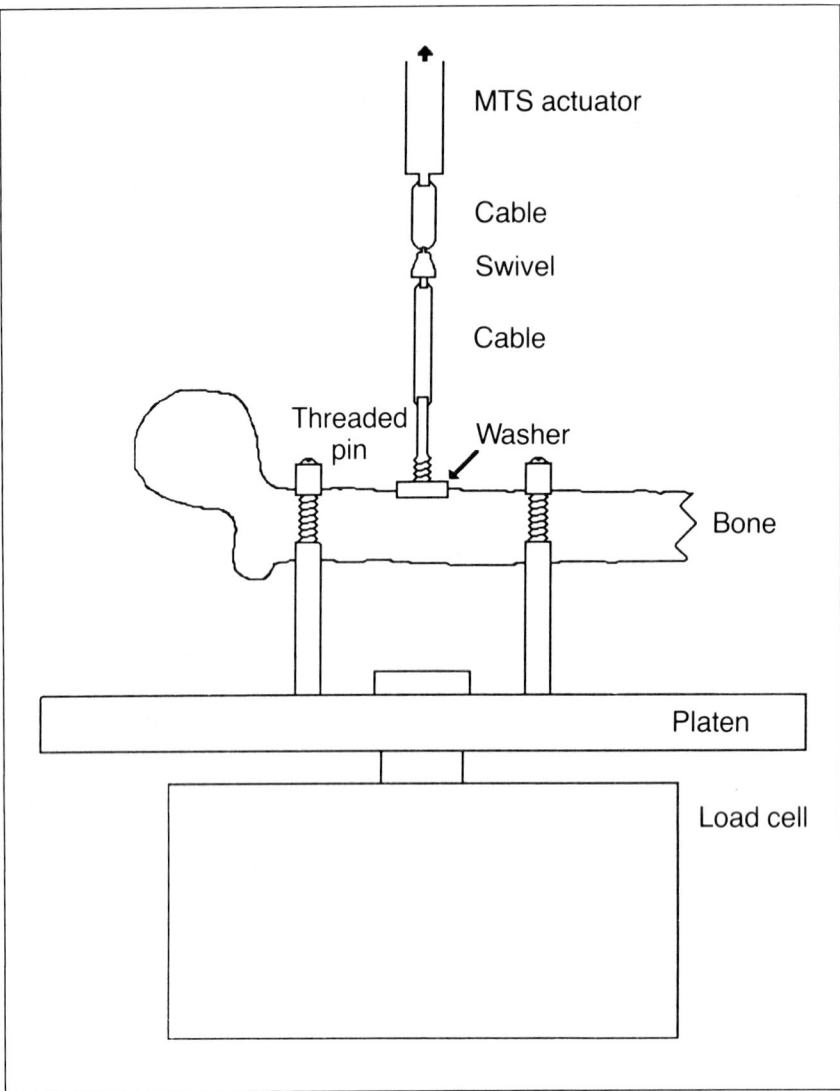

Fig 3 Schematic diagram of the tensile testing setup.

Washers either fell off during preparations for tensile testing or simply lifted off the bone with essentially zero load at the beginning of the test. This was also true for one washer at 301 days. However, significant forces were required to remove two of the titanium group washers from their implantation sites at 301 days (see Table 1). In general, there was no evidence, at least at this macroscopic level of analysis, of tissue or other biological deposits on the surfaces of the uncoated titanium washers (Figs 6a and b).

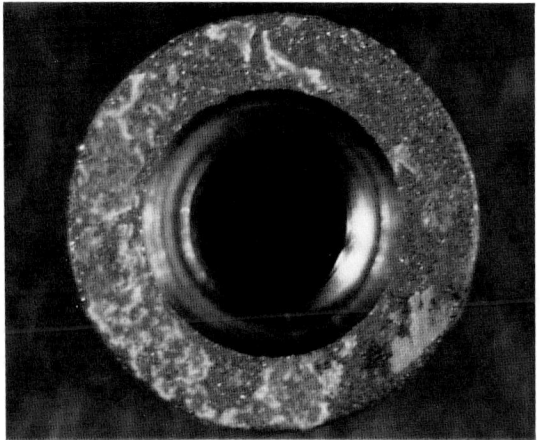

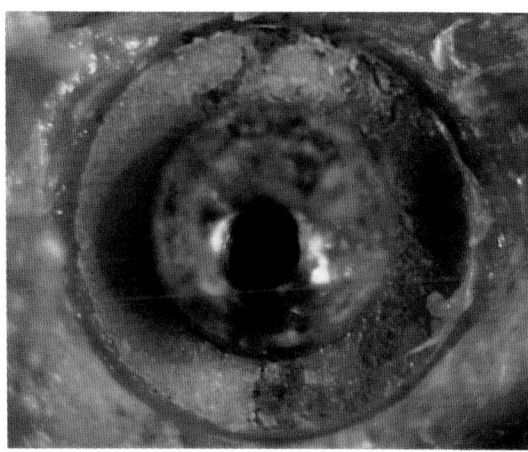

Fig 4a Macrophotograph of the test surface of HA-coated washer after the pull-off test. Note remnants of HA coating left on the surface of the metallic substrate.

Fig 4b Macrophotograph of the well in bone that held the washer in Fig 4a. Note the HA remnants still attached to the bone in the well.

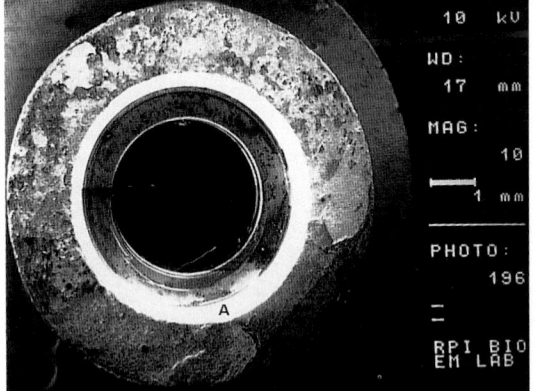

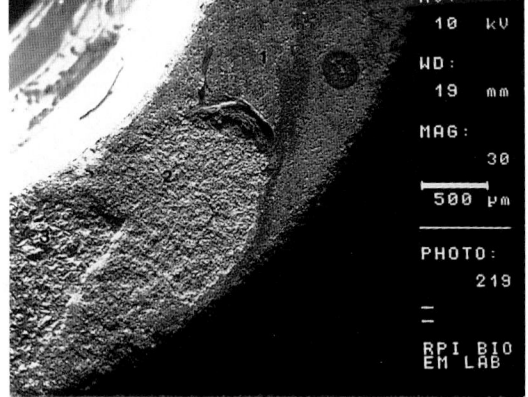

Fig 5a Scanning electron micrograph (secondary mode) of the test surface of an HA-coated washer after a pull-off test; the view corresponds to that in Fig 4a and shows remnants of the HA coating.

Fig 5b Higher magnification of region A in Fig 5a; three regions can be identified: 1 is intact HA coating; 2 is the region of intracoating fracture; 3 shows metal substrate from which the HA has come off during the tensile test. Note that HA in region 1 is relatively smooth compared to as-received HA coating, although there is some evidence of surface microporosity, even in this polished sample.

Discussion

The principal findings of this study were that HA-coated washers required higher pull-off loads than uncoated titanium washers, and that failures in the HA group occurred by separation of the HA coating from the substrate and fracture within the HA coating itself. Based on nominal bone-washer contact area (39.2 mm^2), the mean interfacial tensile strengths were 2.7 $\pm$ 0.82 MPa and 0.27 $\pm$ 0.47 MPa for the HA-coated and uncoated titanium washers, respectively.

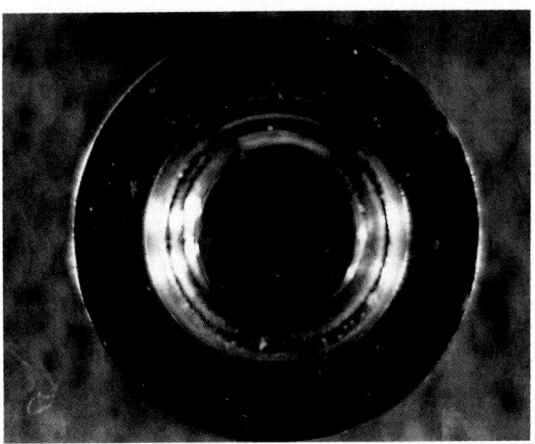

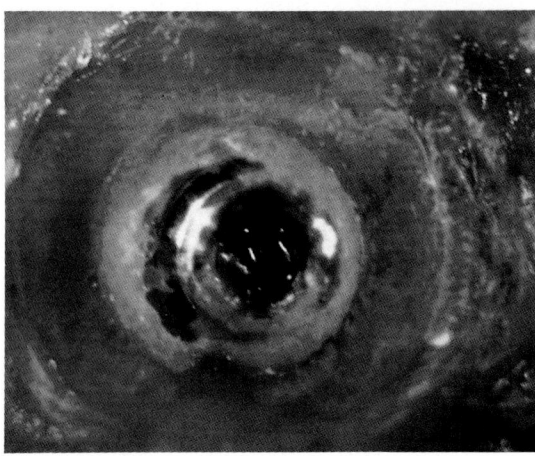

Fig 6a Macrophotograph of the test surface of a Ti-6Al-4V alloy washer after the pull-off test. Note absence of tissue remnants.

Fig 6b Corresponding view of the bone site in which the titanium washer was held.

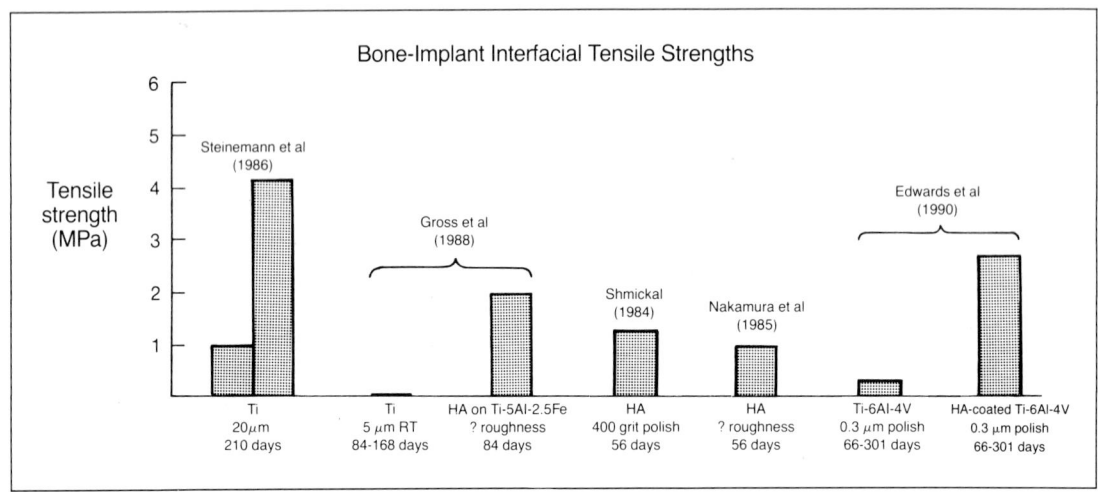

Fig 7 Bar chart showing data on interfacial tensile strengths for various biomaterials and surface roughness.

An explanation for the difference in mean pull-off loads and interfacial stresses between the two groups is of primary concern. Before attributing the difference solely to unlike surface chemistries of the two implant types, it is useful to consider the role of surface roughness. According to previous work, surface roughness can affect the results of tensile pull-off tests of both metallic and ceramic biomaterials in vivo, as discussed shortly.

Data from previous tensile pull-off experiments[4-6,8,9] involving metals and ceramics is compared with results from the present study in Fig 7. The peak-to-valley roughness of samples in the present study was nominally 0.68 μm, which is on the order of the size of the alumina polishing particles. The only group to test titanium metals with comparably smooth surfaces was that of Gross et al.[6] They reported 0 MPa for the tensile strength between cancellous bone and pure titanium having a roughness (R_t) of 5 μm (84 to 168 days, chinchilla rabbit model). They also measured interfacial tensile strengths equal to 0 MPa for samples of Ti-6Al-4V having a roughness (R_t) of 5 μm in the same model at 168 days. Significantly, in 168-day tests with Ti-6Al-4V and Ti-5Al-2.5Fe alloys, Gross et al reported that the interfacial tensile strengths increased from 0 MPa at 5 μm R_t to as much as 1.81 MPa for Ti-6Al-4V and 1.7 MPa for Ti-5Al-2.5Fe at 47 to 57 and 37 to 42 μm R_t values, respectively. These results indicate that surface roughness plays a role in the bond strength measured for bone/implant interfaces.

Based on the data above, the uncoated titanium samples of nominal roughness 0.68 μm in this study would have been expected to show 0 MPa for the interfacial tensile strength. In fact, five of the seven samples did have zero pull-off loads, but two of the three pull-off specimens at 301 days required significant pull-off loads (34.4 and 40.7 N). When included in the averaging, these results were responsible for the nonzero mean strength of 0.27 MPa. The pattern of these data resembles that reported by Steinemann et al,[4] who measured no bone/titanium interfacial tensile strength until 100 days after implantation, even with rough plasma-coated and sand-blasted titanium surfaces ("roughness depth" of 20 μm). Steinemann et al suggested that a minimum time may be required before any interfacial tensile strength can develop between pure titanium and bone. However, the Steinemann et al study did not distinguish whether this might be a result caused by the time needed for bone ingrowth into even small surface roughness, or for "bone-bonding" to the implant surface by as yet undetermined physical-chemical bonding, or both. Thus, in the present study, it is not clear what interactions between bone and titanium might have caused

the nonzero pull-off forces in two of the three samples at 301 days.

Turning now to the HA-coated washers, Gross et al[5,6] also suggested a relationship between roughness and bone/implant interfacial strength for bioactive ceramics. For example, with KG Ceravital (Ernst Leitz & Co, Wetzlar, Germany), the 84-day interfacial tensile strength increased from 0.82 ± 0.08 MPa to 1.11 ± 0.11 Mpa as the roughness (R_t) increased form 0.06 to 52 μm.[6] In addition to this, Gross et al reported a value of 1.97 MPa for HA coated onto Ti-5Al-2.5Fe, but quoted no roughness measure. The interfacial tensile strength of HA-coated washers from the present study (2.7 MPa) slightly exceeds this value as well as those reported by Shmickal[8] and Nakamura et al,[9] who used bulk HA (Fig 7). Unfortunately, pertinent roughness data are not sufficient to complete the comparison of these results with those of the present study. Scanning electron photomicrographs of HA samples from the present study (eg, Fig 5b) suggest some degree of microporosity of the polished HA surface even after polishing to a nominal 0.68 μm finish. This might contribute to bone-HA attachment. As a result, this study is currently not able to separate the contributions of surface roughness versus surface chemistry in the development of interfacial tensile bond strengths between cortical bone and the HA-coated washers.

Failures of HA coatings in this experiment typically involved fracture from within the HA coating and HA separation from the metal substrate. Evidently, the data represent a mixture of failure strengths for the HA-titanium substrate bond and the coated HA. It is notable that the tensile stress values for the HA-coated washers in this study are much less than those reported in the literature for the HA-substrate bond strength in vitro. Kay et al[10] and Geesink et al[11] reported values of 26 to 40 MPa to 85 MPa, respectively, for HA on titanium. The reasons for the discrepancy between these data and the results of the present study are unclear, but the different mechanical test setups and environmental conditions in the in vitro versus in vivo tests may have been factors. It is possible that in the present study, lower values were measured because of in vivo degradation of the HA coating itself and/or the HA-titanium bond.

Finally, all interfacial stress values in this study were based on a nominal washer-bone contact area of 39.2 mm^2, calculated from the washer geometry and an assumption that the entire washer surface was in contact with bone. However, this assumption is likely to be incorrect for two reasons. First, the implantation wells cut in the bone were not always perfectly dimensioned. Preliminary observations of some wells reveal that the areas of contact with the washers could have been less than 39.2 mm,^{2} particularly in cases when the limited cortical thickness and pronounced surface curvature of the dog femur prevented drilling the well to a sufficient depth. Second, even if it were always possible to cut perfect wells, the actual bone-washer contact also depends on the microstructural details of the bone at the interface. Vascular spaces in the bone, such as haversian and Volkmann's canals, would diminish the actual bone-implant contact area. However, this would seem to be a minor effect relative to other uncertainties. Nevertheless, for these reasons, the reported interfacial tensile strength values should be interpreted as conservative stress estimates, because it is likely that less-than-nominal washer-bone contact areas existed in vivo.

Conclusion

In view of the concerns just discussed, particularly surface roughness and its role in interfacial tensile strength, it is not yet possible to make a final conclusion about the reasons for higher mean pull-off loads with the HA-coated washers. However, the results are consistent with the hypothesis that unlike surface physical-chemical properties of HA versus titanium contribute to the difference. Moreover, the findings indicate that the interfacial tensile strengths of the HA-coated titanium washers were limited by properties of the coating and substrate, and not by the strength of the adjacent bone.

Acknowledgments

This study was supported by research grant 5 T32 DE 07054–12 from the National Institute of Dental Research, and by grant from the Veterans Administration RR & D project no. 160.

References

1. Anderson RC, Cook SD, Weinstein AM, Haddad RJ Jr. An evaluation of skeletal attachment to LTI pyrolitic carbon, porous titanium, and carbon-coated porous titanium implants. Clin Orthop 1984;182:242–247.
2. Thomas KA, Kay JF Cook SD, Jarcho M. The effect of surface microtexture and hydroxylapatite coating on the mechanical strengths and histologic profiles of titanium implant materials. J Biomed Mater Res 1987;21:1395–1414.
3. Black J. "Push-out" tests. J Biomed Mater Res 1989; 23:1243–1245. Editorial.
4. Steinemann SG, Eulenberger J, Maeusli P-A, Schroeder A. Adhesion of bone to titanium. pp 409–414 In P. Christel, A. Meunier, A.J.C. Lee (eds) Biological and Biomechanical Behavior of Biomaterials. Amsterdam: Elsevier Science, 1986.
5. Gross U, Roggendorf W, Schmitz H-J, Strunz V. Biomechanical and morphometric testing methods for porous and surface reactive biomaterials. pp 330–346 In J.E. Lemons (ed) Quantitative Characterization and Performance of Porous Implants for Hard Tissue Applications, ASTM STP 953. Philadelphia: American Society for Testing and Materials, 1987.
6. Gross U, Schmitz H-J, Strunz V. Surface activities of bioactive glasses, aluminum oxide and titanium in a living environment. pp 211–226 In P. Ducheyne, J.E. Lemons (eds) Bioceramics: Materials Characterization Versus In Vivo Behavior. Vol. 52. New York: Annals NY Academy of Science, 1988.
7. Harrigan TP, Kareh J, Harris WH. The influence of support conditions in the loading fixture on failure mechanics in the push-out test: A finite element analysis. J Orthop Res 1990;8:678–684.
8. Schmickal T. Inaugural dissertation thesis. Cologne: University of Cologne, 1984.
9. Nakamura T, Yamamuro T, Higashi S, Kokubo T. A new glass-ceramic for bone replacement: Evaluation of its bonding to bone tissue. J Biomed Mater Res 1985;19:685–698.
10. Kay JF, Jarcho M, Logan G, Embry J, Stinner C. Physical and chemical characteristics of hydroxylapatite coatings on metal. J Dent Res 1986;65. Abstract no. 472.
11. Geesink RGT, De Groot K, Klein CPAT. Bonding of bone to apatite-coated implants. J Bone Joint Surg [Br] 1988;70B:17–22.

Tooth-to-Implant Fixed Prostheses: Biomechanics Based on In Vitro and In Vivo Measurements

E.-J. Richter, H. Spiekermann, and S.A. Jovanovic

Osseointegrated implants are successfully used in severely resorbed edentulous mandibles and serve as abutments for fixed prostheses.[1,2] In the partially edentulous jaw, implants may be added to complete a shortened dental arch. The fixed restoration in these situations either is fully implant-supported or a tooth-implant connecting restoration. The latter type is associated with some potential problems based on the different stiffnesses of implants and natural teeth.[3–8]

Appropriate implant mechanics,[4,8,9] as well as suitable prosthodontic attachment types[4,8,10–13] have been discussed and clinically tested. Lundgren and co-workers published detailed information concerning vertical loads on implants,[14] but there is little quantitative information about lateral[15] or horizontal forces.[16] These can be significant for a tooth-to-implant–supported fixed prosthesis located in the chewing center. During mastication the swinging movement of the mandible into centric occlusion creates forces in a buccolingual direction, thus producing a bending moment in the implant around a mesiodistal axis. This load is similar to the horizontal chewing forces on teeth and it cannot be essentially reduced.

During chewing and swallowing, the vertical force arising on a mobile tooth causes a second bending moment in the implant around a buccolingual axis with a lever arm as long as the prosthesis. If this moment is greater than the first, it must be considered critical and will affect treatment.[7] To compare both types of loads, first the bending moment on the implant caused by lateral forces during chewing was measured and secondly, in a laboratory model, the moment caused by intrusion of the natural abutment tooth was determined.

Materials and methods

Lateral implant loads (in vivo measurements)

Ten tooth-to-implant fixed prostheses in the mandibles of nine different patients were examined (one patient had bilateral tooth-implant restorations). The type 3 IMZ (Interpore International, Irvine, Calif) implants (3-mm diameter) were located in the molar region with a restoration connecting the first or second premolar. The intramobile element (IME) was replaced by a measuring device with strain gauges of the same size, which produced signals only for buccolingual loading (Fig 1). After placement, no change in the pattern of occlusal stops could be found and the patients felt no difference in the commonly used jaw relation (Figs 2a and b). After fixation of the abutment screws, the measuring device was calibrated. The chewing signals were recorded in a personal computer.

Crackers, carrots, sausages, and "jelly babies" were the patients' test food. Three chewing cycles with each food were gathered (Fig 3). Prosthodontic procedures utilized in the

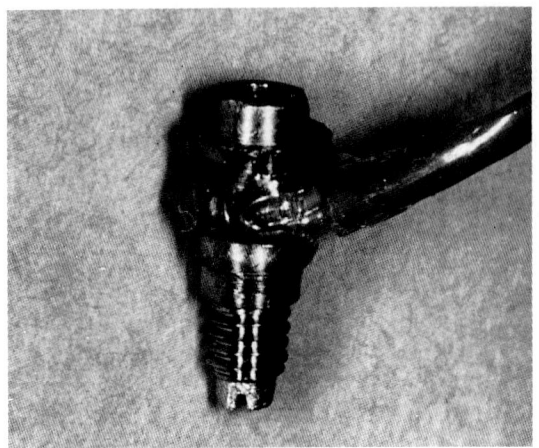

Fig 1 The intraoral measuring device replacing the intramobile element (IME) and the transmucosal implant extension (TIE)

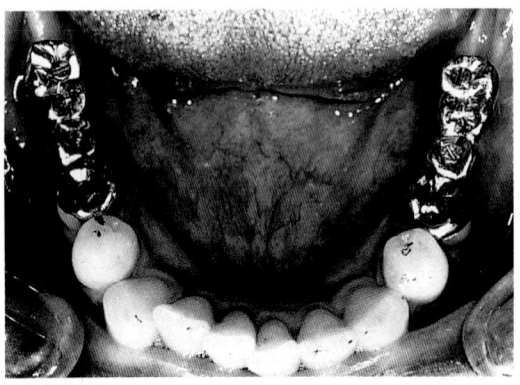

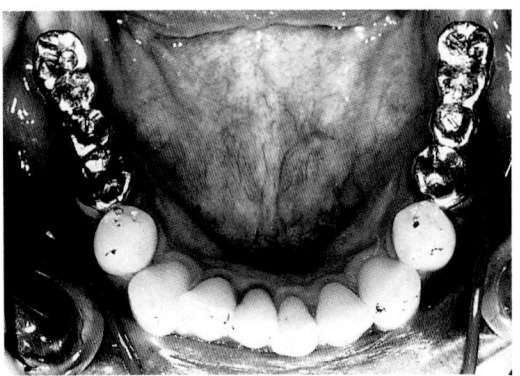

Figs 2a and b The pattern of occlusal stops, marked by an 8-μm occlusion foil, is similar in both the common clinical restoration (a) and the restoration fixed on the implants incorporating the measuring devices (b).

prostheses were as follows: rather than narrow tooth chewing surfaces in the buccolingual dimension (Fig 2), a flat cuspid-fissure relief with diminished occlusal contacts on the implant restoration and canine guidance with distinct disocclusion in the articulation position of the mandible were used. Computerized calculation of the bending moment was performed without any peri-implant angular bone loss.

Axial tooth loads (in vitro measurements)

The tooth-to-implant prosthesis was imitated in the following test setting. The identical micromovement of an IMZ implant was used as measured intraorally by the Periotest (Siemens AG, Bensheim, Germany).[17] Two-phase tooth mobility was simulated by springs (Fig 4) and for the connecting restoration (length 16 mm, cross section 6.25 mm × 3.25 mm), a nonprecious metal alloy (Wiron 88, Fa. Bego, D 2800 Bremen, Germany) with a Young's modulus of 2.10^5 N/mm^2 was used. The vertical load on the "tooth" was limited to 12 N, but the linear characteristic enabled a quantification of the bending moment for higher loads. Four different types of connecting devices between the prosthesis and implant were fastened with a moment of 100 Nmm and tested. The types were an IME, an intramobile connector (IMC), a titanium metal IME, and a mobile test device. The moment was measured by strain gauges located near the implant end of the prosthesis.

Results

Lateral implant loads (in vivo measurements)

Intraoral measurements of the bending moment in a buccolingual direction were summarized as follows:

1. In 7 of 10 patients, the mean maximum load-

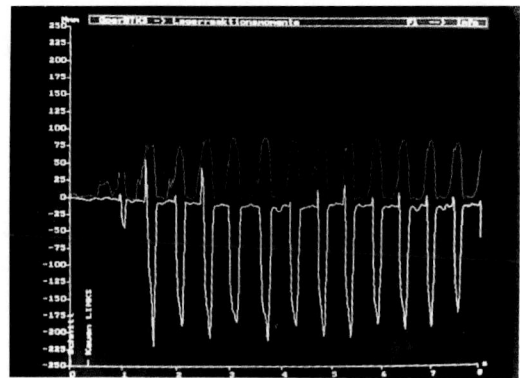

Fig 3 Simultaneous registration of the load levels for two implants when chewing a piece of carrot.

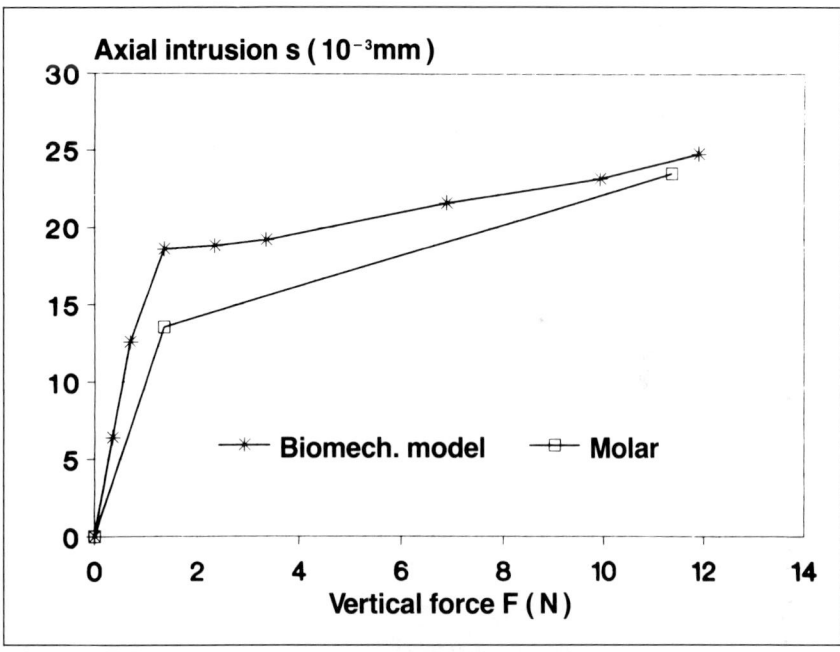

Fig 4 The relations of vertical force F and axial intrusions comparing the biomechanical test "tooth" with measurements of a natural molar.

ing when clenching in centric occlusion was higher than the mean maximum stress during chewing (Figs 5 and 6).

2. In 9 of 10 patients, stress while chewing was higher to the buccal than to the lingual side (Fig 6).

3. Of those five patients in whom lingual forces were seen in centric occlusion (Fig 5), a predominance of this load level was registered during mastication for only one patient (no. 3 in Fig 6).

4. The mean load level (integrated load peaks

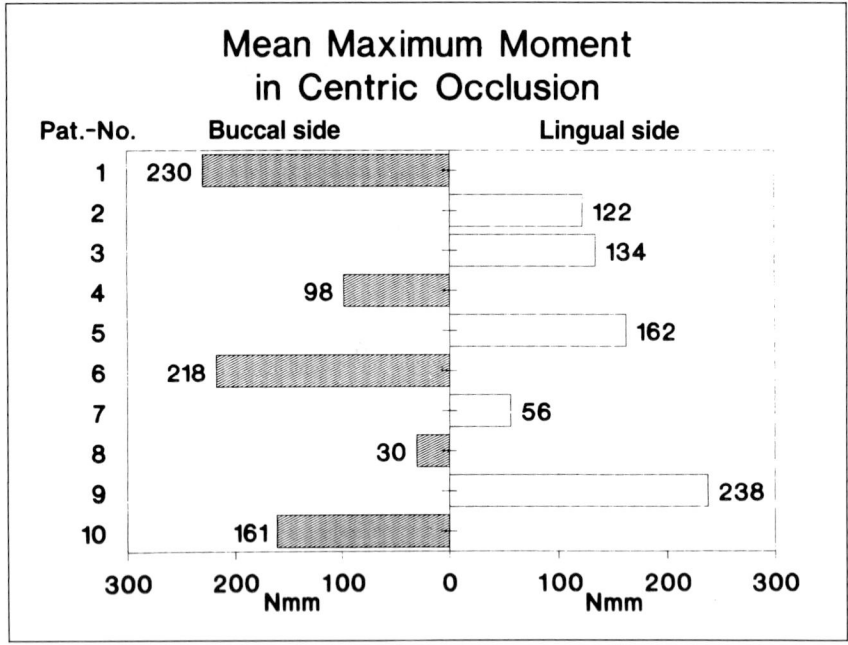

Fig 5 The mean maximum moment in a buccolingual direction during clenching as strong as possible in centric occlusion.

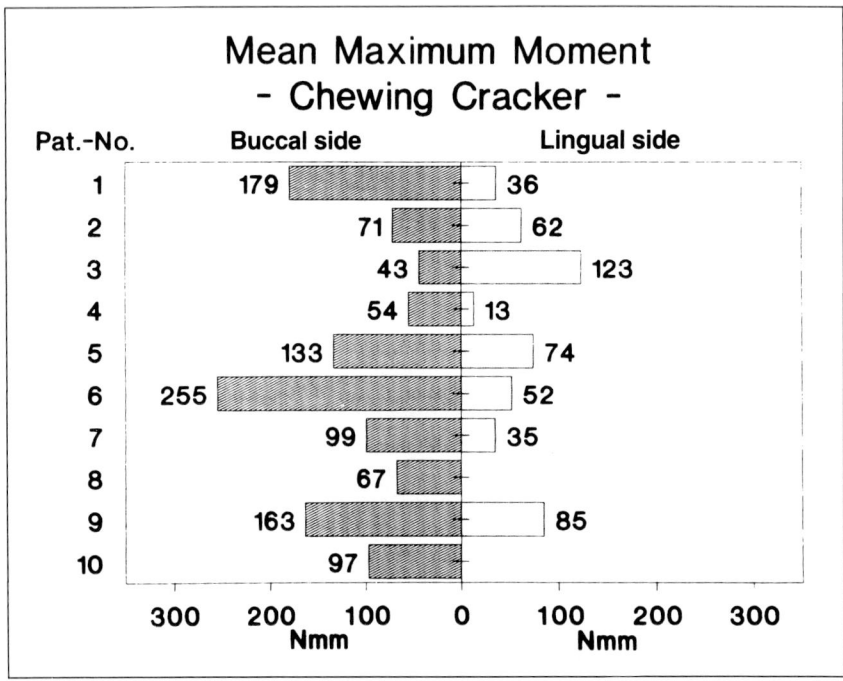

Fig 6 The mean maximum moment in buccolingual direction during chewing of crackers.

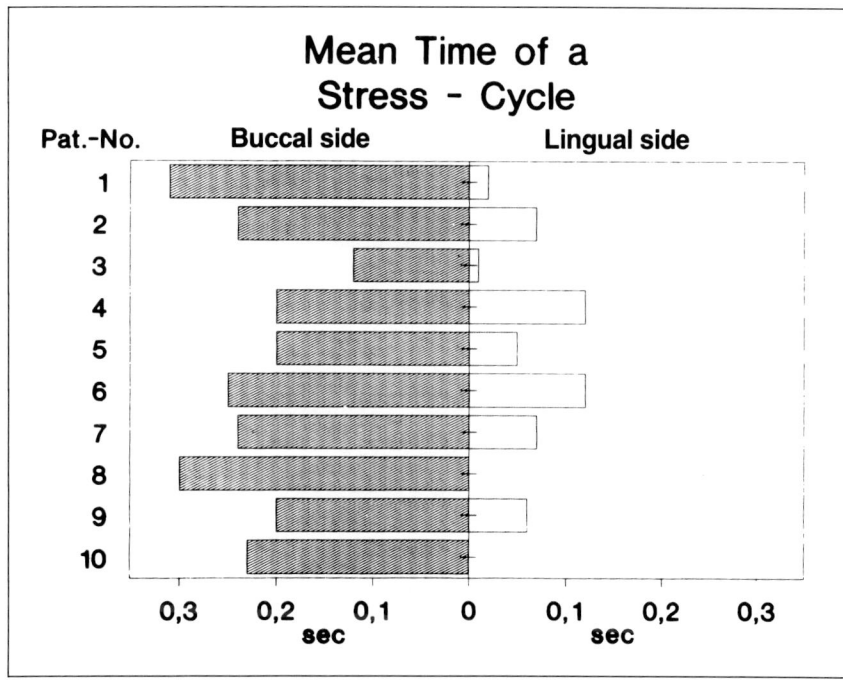

Fig 7 The duration of an implant-stress cycle regularly lasted longer on the buccal side.

and temporally averaged) was about half of the mean maximum load.

5. The highest stress was measured for "jelly babies"; all other food types caused bending moments of nearly the same height.

6. In only 6 of the 34 registrations that could be evaluated, was an increased load to the buccal side found.

7. In only 2 of the 34 patients was the duration of the load per chewing cycle longer to the lingual than to the buccal side. Regularly, the mean stress-duration per cycle was much longer in the buccal direction (Fig 7).

8. Stress during swallowing was slightly less than during chewing.

Axial tooth loads (in vitro measurements)

Vertical loads on the "tooth" greater than about 1.5 N (according to the secondary phase of tooth mobility) caused a linear increasing bending moment in the implant around a buccolingual axis

with every connecting device (Fig 8). The highest moment of 160 Nmm for a test load of 10 N without a mesial abutment was lowered as follows when a tooth with normal resilience carried the load: the maximum bending moment was 40% of the highest stress using a metal IME, 25% with the IME, 15% with the IMC, and only 14% for the test device.

Discussion

To compare the bending stress level of the implant buccolingually and mesiodistally, the maximum vertical load during chewing on a tooth in the chewing center must be determined. Similar data have been reported by other authors (Table 1). It is known that the load level on a single tooth depends mainly on the measuring device and modus itself, its type of occlusal surface, the occlusal adjustment, and the com-

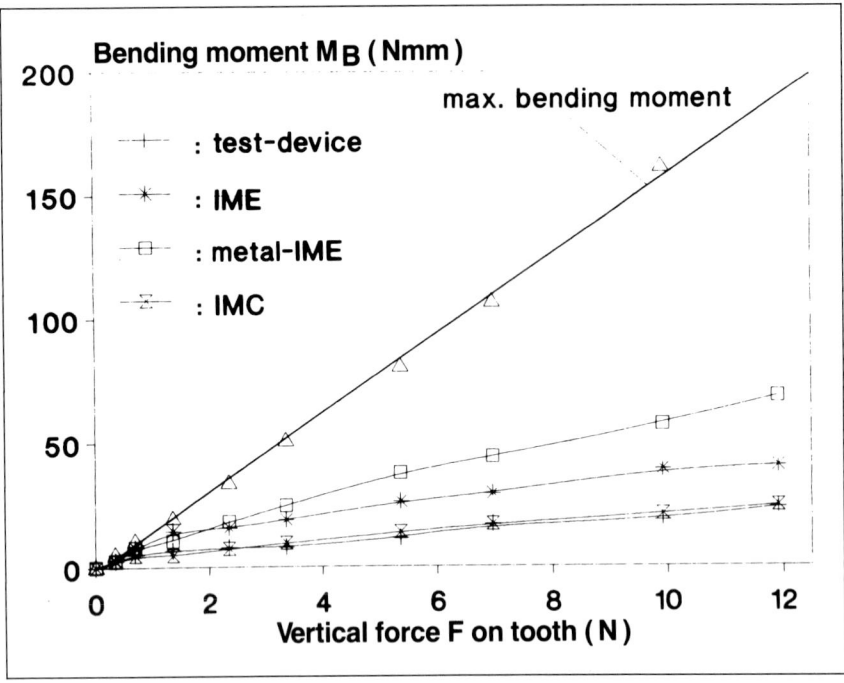

Fig 8 The bending moment raised in the implant of a tooth-to-implant fixed restoration: the maximum moment is lowered differently by various connecting devices (see text for details).

Table 1 The maximum axial load on a tooth or an implant in the premolar or molar position

Load (N)	Tooth or implant	Reference	Comments
244	T	Körber and Ludwig[18]	Mean value German lit
306	T ♀	Röhrle and	Calcul. muscle
227	T ♂	Sollbach[13]	Cross section
90	T	Lundgren D et al[7]	Maxillary denture
210	T	Lundgren D et al[19]	Mandibular denture
60	I	Haraldson T et al[20]	Maxillary denture
144	I	Haraldson T et al[11]	Maxillary denture

monly used chewing side. Using these factors, the mean maximum vertical load on a premolar during mastication is difficult to determine. Based on our own measurements and the literature data, 100 N seems to be a low value for the maximum axial force.

A calculation of maximum bending moments in the implant in a mesiodistal direction results in the following data:

Metal IME ("rigid" implant)	640 Nmm
IME	400 Nmm
IMC	240 Nmm
Test device	224 Nmm

The highest buccolingual stress level caused by mastication in this series of patients was 255 Nmm. This amount of bending moment may be regarded as physiologic loading of the teeth as well, because its origin is essentially combined with the arcing-chewing movement of the mandible. Higher moments for the rigid implant, as well as the implant using the IME, must be considered critical because they are nearly twice as high. This may represent a biomechanical reason for the higher level of bone loss with tooth-to-implant fixed prostheses compared to only implant-retained restorations.[7]

Our clinical experience with patients having two implants in the interforaminal area of the mandible, a bar attachment, and an overdenture, who suffer less angular peri-implant osteolysis than patients with tooth-to-implant fixed prostheses may confirm this hypothesis. The patients who were treated with completely implant-supported restorations showed better results than those with tooth-implant supported restorations.[7]

The results of our measurements reveal that completely implant-supported prostheses are advantageous. If a shortened dental arch cannot be completed with more than one implant, a resilient connecting device inside the implant with mobility qualities similar to or better than the IMC seem to be suitable.

References

1. Adell R, Lekholm U, Rockler B, Brånemark P-I. A 15-year study of osseointegrated implants in the treatment of the edentulous jaw. *Int J Oral Surg* 1981; 10:387.

2. Albrektsson T, Dahl E, Enbom L, Engevall S, Engquist B, Eriksson AR, et al. Osteointegrated oral implants: A Swedish multicenter study of 8139 consecutively inserted Nobelpharma implants. *J Periodontol* 1988; 5:287.

3. Skalak R. Aspects of biomechanical considerations. pp 123–126 In P.I. Brånemark, G.A. Zarb, T. Albrektsson (eds) *Tissue-Integrated Prostheses: Osseointegration in Clinical Dentistry.* Chicago: Quintessence Publ Co, 1985.

4. Brunski JB. Biomechanics of oral implants: Future research directions. *J Dent Educ* 1988;52:775–787.

5. English C-E. Questions need answering. *CDA J* 1988;1:26-34.

6. Ericsson I, Lekholm U, Brånemark P-I, Lindhe J, Glantz P-O, Nyman S. A clinical evaluation of fixed-bridge restorations supported by the combination of teeth and osseointegrated titanium implants. *J Clin Periodontol* 1986;13:307–312.

7. Lundgren D, Laurell L, Falk J, Ericsson I. Distribution of occlusal forces in a dentition unilaterally restored with a bridge construction supported on osseointegrated titanium implants. Amsterdam: Excerpta Medica 1985, pp 333–339.

8. Richter E-J, Jovanovic SA, Spiekermann H. Rein—Implantatgetragene Brücken—eine Alternative zur Verbundbrücke? *Z Zahnärztl Implantol* 1990;6:137–144.

9. Spiekermann H. Implantatprothetik, München—Wien, Hanser 1989, Fortschritte der Zahnärztlichen Prothetik und Werkstoffkunde IV, pp 241–272.

10. Ericsson I, Lekholm U. Evaluation of clinical function and marginal tissue reactions at tooth tissue-integrated reconstructions: Tissue integration in oral and maxillo-facial reconstruction. Amsterdam: Excerpta Medica 1985, pp 309–319.

11. Haraldson T, Carlsson GE. Bite force and oral function in patients with osseointegrated oral implants. *Scand J Dent Res* 1977;85:200–208.

12. Richter E-J. Basic biomechanics of dental implants in prosthetic dentistry. *J Prosthet Dent* 1989;61:602–609.

13. Röhrle H, Sollbach W. Kraftflußberechnungen von Zahn—und Wurzelimplantaten. *BMFT Forschungsbericht T* 1985, pp 85–137.

14. Falk H, Laurell L, Lundgren D. Occlusal interferences and cantilever joint stress in implant-supported prostheses occluding with complete dentures. *Int J Oral Maxillofac Implants* 1990;5:70–77.

15. Graf H. Bruxism. *Dent Clin North Am* 1969;13:659.

16. Spiekermann H. Implantatprothetik, München—Wien, Hanser 1980, Fortschritte der Zahnärztlichen Prothetik und Werkstofffkunde I, pp 253–258.

17. d'Hoedt B, Schramen-Scherer B. Der Periotestwert bei enossalen Implantaten. *Z Zahnärztl Implantol* 1989; 4:89.

18. Körber KH, Ludwig K. Maximale Kaukraft als Berechnungsfaktor zahntechnischer Konstruktionen. *Dent Lab* 1983;31:55–60.

19. Lundgren D, Laurell L, Bergendal T. Occlusal force pattern in dentitions restored with mandibular bridges supported on osseointegrated implants. *Swed Dent J* 1985;28(suppl):107–115.

20. Haraldson T, Carlsson GE, Ingervall B. Functional state, bite force and postural muscle activity in patients with osseointegrated oral implant bridges. *Acta Odontol Scand* 1979;37:195–206.

Plasma-Sprayed Ceramometal Interface Characterization: Interface Fracture Toughness and Tensile Bond Strength

R.M. Pilliar and M. Filiaggi

The use of plasma-sprayed hydroxyapatite (HA) coatings over titanium and titanium alloy substrates for dental implants has attracted wide attention as a possible method for enhancing implant-to-bone fixation. It is assumed that the "bioactive" hydroxyapatite surface layer will result in strong bonding of bone tissue to the implant surface, thereby allowing reliable stress transfer between the implant and the bone. Animal studies have been reported that demonstrate the strong bonding that can develop at the bone/hydroxyapatite interface, both as evidenced by interfacial shear[1,2] and tensile[3] bond strength measurements. The use of plasma-sprayed hydroxyapatite coatings is being applied to dental[4] and orthopedic[5] implants currently in human use.

For these load-bearing applications, it is equally important that a strong and reliable bond be achieved and maintained at the hydroxyapatite/metal substrate interface. In fact, since this interface is nonviable and thus prone to irreversible breakdown processes such as mechanical fatigue, it is even more critical that a strong, fracture-resistant interface be formed between the metal and the ceramic coating. Only if good bonding is maintained between the ceramic coating and the metal substrate will the implant function as an effective load-bearing unit. Unfortunately, this interface has received far less attention for hydroxyapatite-coated titanium and titanium alloy implant systems, partly because of the primary need to develop a well-bonded bone/hydroxyapatite interface in the first instance, but partly, too, because of problems in characterizing plasma-sprayed ceramic coatings on metal substrates in general. Some studies of shear and tensile bond strengths of plasma-sprayed hydroxyapatite coatings on titanium and Ti-6Al-4V alloy substrates have been reported.[6,7] The results of the different studies vary considerably, however, suggesting the need for careful examination of testing conditions and possibly the development of new testing strategies.

The objective of our study was to critically assess the mechanical testing of plasma-sprayed ceramic coatings on metal substrates, specifically HA coatings on Ti-6Al-4V substrates. The use in humans of calcium phosphate plasma-sprayed coatings over titanium and titanium alloy implants and reports of mechanical spalling of the coating from the titanium substrate[8] inspired these studies. In addition to using a traditional approach to strength characterization of the interface (tensile bond strength measurement), it was also our intent to develop a test method based on fracture mechanics principles to assess the interfacial fracture toughness (K_{Icint}) of this interface. It was hypothesized that such a test might prove more sensitive for assessing the effect of varying processing parameters and exposure to biological media on the interface fracture characteristics.

Materials and methods

Ti-6Al-4V alloy bar stock supplied in the mill-annealed condition and conforming in chemical composition to American Society for Testing and Materials (ASTM) specification F136-84 for surgical grade extra low interstitial (ELI) Ti-6Al-4V alloy was used as the substrate for plasma spraying. The hydroxyapatite powders used for plasma spraying were supplied by a commercial implant manufacturer (Zimmer Inc, Warsaw, Ind) who unfortunately could not disclose details of the starting powders because of proprietary considerations. Plasma spraying was done by Zimmer using their in-house plasma spray facility.

The substrate surfaces were prepared in our laboratories prior to sending samples out for plasma spraying. The specific surface roughening procedures used are defined shortly. After surface roughening, all samples were given a 10% nitric acid bath for 30 minutes to form a passive oxide layer on the titanium alloy and then cleaned ultrasonically in acetone for 30 minutes.

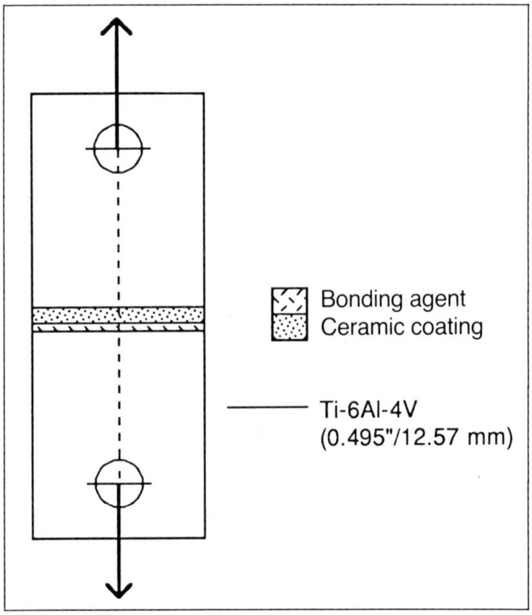

Fig 1 Schematic of the tensile bond test specimen.

Interface tensile bond strength specimen description and testing conditions

The specimen geometry used (Fig 1) corresponded closely to the specifications outlined in ASTM C633 for adhesive or cohesive strength testing of flame-sprayed coatings. The actual specimen diameter was slightly undersized (23 mm) because of available bar stock, and the coating thickness was less than the specified lower limit of 380 μm since thinner coatings normally are used on implants (typically 50 to 100 μm). To form the test specimen, two specimen halves of approximately 2.54 cm in length were machined in the form shown in Fig 1. The surfaces of samples to receive well-bonded plasma spray coatings were roughened by gritblasting. Other surfaces intended to mimic poorly bonded regions on the fracture toughness specimens (the weakly bonded "outer regions"[9] referred to shortly), were also prepared.

After plasma-spray coating with a nominally 100-μm-thick HA layer, the specimen halves were "coupled" by bonding the carefully aligned halves (one half with an HA coating and the other half roughened but uncoated) using a relatively high viscosity dental bonding agent (Concise, 3M, St Paul, Minn). The reason for the use of the high viscosity Concise was to minimize penetration of the adhesive through the somewhat porous, plasma-spray coating layer since it was thought that such penetration could lead to artificially high values of interfacial tensile bond strength. Prior to this bonding operation, great care was taken to ensure exact specimen half alignment (using a custom-made alignment jig), and low pressure was used to develop a consistently thin glue line. Excess bonding agent was removed circumferentially prior to adhesive curing since any overlapping of bonding agent over the surfaces of the two half sections would contribute to artificially high values of measured tensile bond strength.

Tensile testing was performed using an Instron (Instron Corp, Canton, Mass) universal test machine with special gripping adapters to allow specimen loading. Specimens were loaded in tension at 0.1 cm/min crosshead speed and the maximum load was recorded. All

141

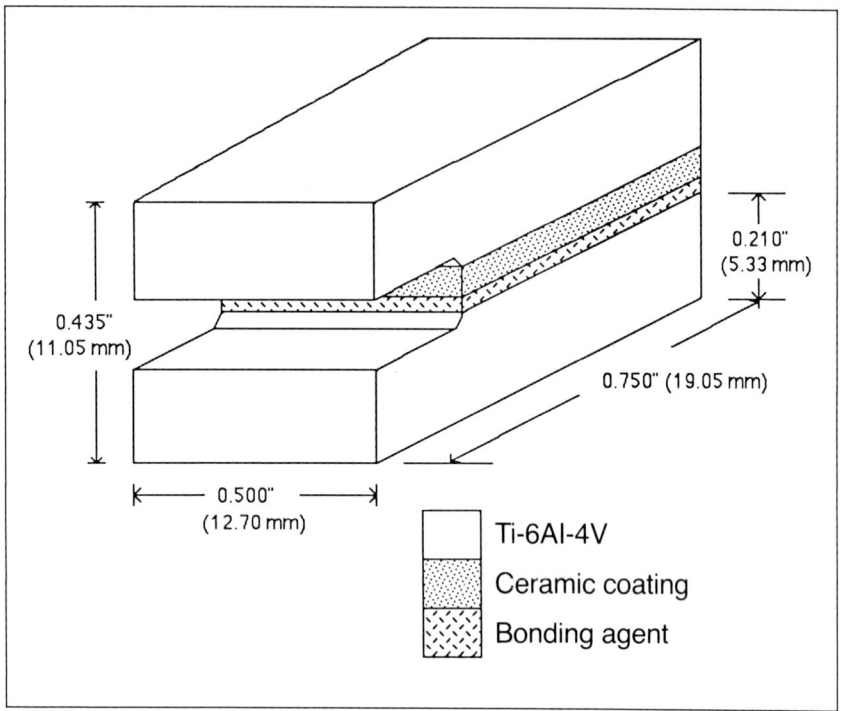

0.435"
(11.05 mm)

0.210"
(5.33 mm)

0.750" (19.05 mm)

0.500"
(12.70 mm)

Ti-6Al-4V

Ceramic coating

Bonding agent

Fig 2a Schematic of the modified composite short bar specimen.

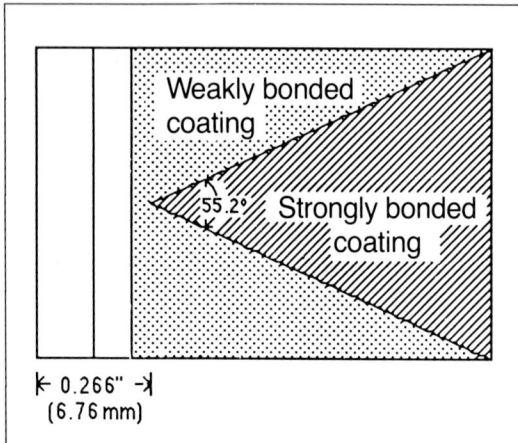

Weakly bonded coating

55.2° Strongly bonded coating

0.266"
(6.76 mm)

Fig 2b Top view of a coated short bar half showing regions of weakly and strongly bonded coating.

testing was done at room temperature in air. To determine bond strengths, the maximum load recorded during the test was divided by the cross-sectional area of the specimen. Only specimens in which adhesive failure occurred at the metal/ceramic interface were considered to give valid interfacial tensile bond strengths and specimens showing mixed mode fracture (adhesive + cohesive) were ignored.

Interfacial fracture toughness specimen description and testing conditions

The interfacial fracture toughness test specimen design was based on the short bar test specimen developed by Barker.[10] This homogeneous test specimen is described in ASTM B771 for testing of cemented carbides. A modified short rod specimen has been described for evaluating the interfacial fracture toughness of composite specimens.[11,12] In extending this approach to testing the interface of plasma-sprayed ceramic coatings on metal substrates (particularly the relatively thin coatings used in implant applications), the problem arises of propagating a crack consistently along the inter-

142

face of interest. A novel approach was developed to deal with this issue.

As with the interface tensile bond strength specimens, two specimen halves were coupled together using Concise to form the specimen design shown in Fig 2. To ensure crack initiation and continued propagation at the hydroxyapatite/Ti-6Al-4V interface, the surface of the specimen half to be plasma spray coated was prepared as shown in Fig 2 with a properly roughened "inner" chevron region (to which good bonding was intended) and a smoother "outer" region in which poor bonding of the HA plasma-sprayed coating to the metal substrate occurred. For some specimens, complete elimination of any bonding was achieved by using a plasma-spray resistant tape applied over this outer region. As with the tensile specimen halves that were plasma spray coated, the titanium alloy surfaces for coating were roughened, passivated using a 10% nitric acid solution, and rigorously cleaned ultrasonically using acetone. After plasma spray coating the surface of one specimen half with an approximate 100-μm-thick HA coating, it was mated to a roughened but uncoated second half. This "complete" short rod specimen was loaded in mode I loading according to the procedures outlined in ASTM B771 for short bar/rod testing of cemented carbides. For all specimens tested, the peak load was measured and used to calculate the interfacial fracture toughness using the relation described by ASTM B771:

$$K_{IcSB} = \frac{A_m P_c}{B^{3/2}} C_c$$

where K_{IcSB} is the plane strain fracture toughness determined using short bar specimens and in our case equal to K_{IcInt}, B is the specimen breadth (12.70 mm), A_m is the dimensionless calibration constant (22 for homogeneous short bar specimens of scaled geometry equal to that of our specimen), P_c is the peak load, and C_c is a correction factor for some out-of-tolerance dimensions for the specimen. Full details of the testing procedure have been published elsewhere.[9]

Failure analysis

In addition to the mechanical testing described previously, tested specimens were examined using scanning electron microscopy and x-ray microanalysis to determine the failure mode and whether or not fracture had occurred at the HA/titanium alloy interface.

Coating structural characterization

To determine the structure of the as-prepared plasma spray-coated samples, some specimen halves were ground and polished normal to the coating/substrate interface and examined by scanning electron microscopy to detect voids, cracks, and other imperfections in the coating. Image analysis of some of these sections allowed a quantitative assessment of coating density.

Results

The results of the mechanical testing are summarized in Tables 1 and 2. In Table 2 (K_{IcInt} determinations), the "corrected" K_{IcInt} values correspond to the use of the factor "C_c" to account for out-of-tolerance a_o and O values.

The interfacial tensile bond strength values reported in Table 1 for the "well-bonded" plasma spray-coated interfaces show values consistently in the range of 6 to 10 MPa. These are far less than the values reported previously by de Groot et al[6] and Kay et al[7] for HA/Ti-6Al-4V interfaces. In a supplementary study investigating the use of Concise rather than a lower viscosity, higher strength epoxy for bonding specimen halves, it was shown that samples prepared at the University of Leiden, the Netherlands, and bonded together using Concise, gave lower values (10.3 MPa) than other specimens bonded using the higher strength, lower viscosity epoxy adhesive. These results appeared to support our contention that the bonding agent contributed to the previously reported

Table 1 Tensile bond strength data:
Hydroxyapatite coated Ti-6Al-4V

Group	Surface	Coating thickness (μm)	No. samples	Bond strength (MPa)
HA-1	Gritblasted	135 ± 30	12	6.7 ± 1.5
HA-1	Bead-gritblasted	120 ± 20	5	3.7 ± 1.2

Table 2 K_{IcSB} determinations: Hydroxyapatite coated Ti-6Al-4V

Group	Coating thickness (μm)	Outer region preparation	No. samples	K_{IcSB} (MPa$\sqrt{m}$)	"Corrected" K_{IcSB}
HA-1	110 ± 20	Bead-gritblasted	6	1.31 ± 0.09	1.41 ± 0.10
HA-2	95 ± 10	Bead-gritblasted	3	0.60 ± 0.05	0.60 ± 0.05
HA-2	95 ± 25	Tape	2	0.66 ± 0.01	0.62
HA-3	130 ± 10	Tape	2	0.95 ± 0.09	0.93 ± 0.11

high tensile bond strength values reported by de Groot et al.[6] Also reported in Table 1 are the bond strengths corresponding to plasma spray coating over smoother substrate surfaces (0.9 to 1.4 μm arithmetic average roughness). As expected, these values were lower but nevertheless indicated a significant bond strength, a finding that raised some concern over the absolute values of our K_{IcInt} determinations. This is discussed further.

The K_{IcInt} values reported in Table 2 are, to the best of our knowledge, the first ever reported for a plasma spray-coated HA/Ti-6Al-4V interface. The results show that there was some variation in interfacial fracture toughness from one batch of specimens to another, but within any one batch, the results were fairly consistent. This suggested that variations (uncontrolled) in either preparation of surfaces for plasma coating or in the plasma spray conditions per se could have been responsible for the interbatch variation. Fortunately, the fractures that occurred with all these specimens after K_{IcInt} testing were

very clean and occurred along the HA/Ti-6Al-4V interface so that surface roughness values for the three batches could be measured after testing. As noted in Table 3, significant differences were found from one batch to another, caused, we believe, by variation in the gritblasting medium used for the different batches. The smoother surfaces gave lower values of K_{IcInt}, as would be expected. This inadvertent experimental variable in these studies served to demonstrate the sensitivity of the fracture toughness testing for assessing the effects of processing variables.

Overall, the K_{IcInt} values measured were low, indicating that the HA/Ti-6Al-4V interface was prone to easy fracture for these samples.

Because of the potential contribution of a poorly bonded outer region to the measured fracture toughness for the interface, some test specimens were included in which a special, heat-resistant tape was used to mask this outer region. This ensured no bonding of the HA to the metal substrate in this region. The results of

Table 3 Surface roughness variability

Batch	Surface roughness (chevron) μin (μm)	Surface roughness (outer) μin (μm)	K_{IcSB} (MPa$\sqrt{m}$)
HA-1	140–160 (3.6–4.1)	45–55 (1.1–1.4)	1.41 ± 0.10
HA-2	110–130 (2.8–3.3)	35–40 (0.9–1.0)	0.60 ± 0.05
HA-2	80–120 (2.0–3.0)	—	0.62
HA-3	110–130 (2.8–3.3)	—	0.93 ± 0.11

specimens so prepared are also included in Table 2. They indicate that this smoother outer region did not appear to significantly affect the K_{IcInt} determinations.

Hydroxyapatite coating structure

Examination of the plasma-sprayed HA coatings by scanning electron microscopy indicated a lamellar structure corresponding presumably to the individual HA particles in molten form splatting onto the substrate surface and onto successive layers of rapidly solidified HA particles (Fig 3). This structure is fairly typical of plasma-sprayed ceramic coatings and shows that some porosity invariably is present in these coatings both within individual particles and between particles. This interparticle porosity is rather irregular and often takes the form of interlamellar channels that can result in interconnected pores through the full thickness of the plasma coating layer. It is this type of interconnected porosity that raises concerns with adhesive penetration during both tensile and fracture toughness test specimen preparation and was the reason for our choice of a high viscosity bonding agent for mating sample halves to form specimens for our testing. Using quantitative microscopy, the average porosity in representative cross-sectional micrographs of plasma-sprayed layers was determined to be

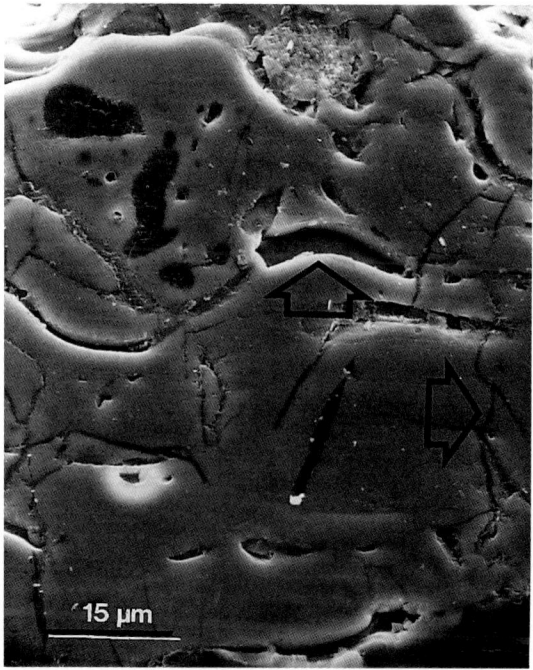

Fig 3 The as-sprayed coating cross section, showing extensive channel-like porosity and microcracks *(arrows)*.

8.4%. This measurement was made using limited numbers of sections so that a proper statistical evaluation of percent porosity was not possible. However, the observations did give some qualitative feel for the extent of intrinsic porosity in the as-sprayed coatings.

Examination of the interface showed the nature of the mechanical interlock that developed at the HA/titanium alloy interface (Fig 4). This represents what is considered to be the major source of bond formation at plasma-sprayed metal/ceramic interfaces.[13] The sectioning methods used resulted in some artefactual separation at the HA/Ti-6Al-4V interface as seen in the figure. However, the close proximity of the interfacial profiles of the ceramic and metal mating surfaces attest to the close apposition that occurs on plasma spraying. It is thought that thermal contraction effects result in "keying" of the ceramic particles onto asperities on the roughened metal substrate.

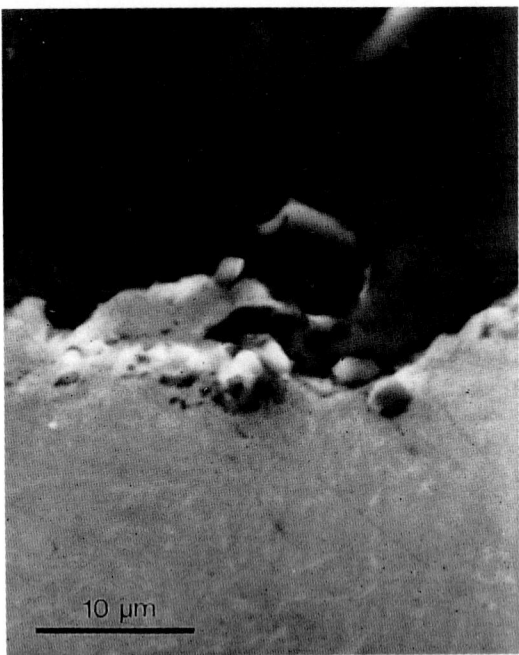

Fig 4 The plasma sprayed HA/titanium alloy interface, revealing the mechanical interlocking that occurs at the interface.

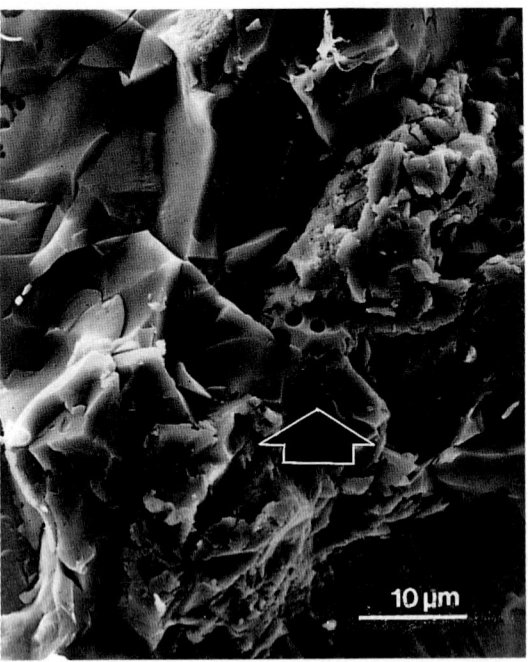

Fig 5 A typical fracture surface of a tested HA-coated short bar specimen, showing some isolated retention of the coating *(arrow)* in the gritblasted grooves of the metal substrate surface.

Fracture surface appearance

A representative fracture surface of a tested interfacial fracture toughness specimen taken from the chevron region is shown in Fig 5. It is similar to that observed for the tensile bond test specimens. The scanning electron fractographs indicate that failures occurred predominantly at the metal/ceramic interface with only isolated regions of cohesive failure within the HA particles adhered to the titanium alloy surface being observed (see arrow, Fig 5). Although mechanical interlock, as evidenced by the HA particle retained, is no doubt the major bonding mechanism involved at this interface, x-ray microanalysis and electron spectroscopic imaging reported elsewhere[9,14] of the interface zone showed that there is at least some chemical bonding because of P ion diffusion into the titanium alloy (or titanium oxide) surface layer occurring during the plasma spraying process. This result is consistent with a report published earlier[15] on studies of diffusion of P from plasma-sprayed HA coatings into titanium (or titanium oxide) surfaces. This chemical bonding, however, is considered a secondary bonding mechanism that does not contribute greatly to the overall bond strength. Minimal bonding would result, for example, on a highly polished, smooth substrate surface, a result supported by the observed trend to lower bond strength values for coatings sprayed onto smoother substrate surfaces (see Table 1).

Discussion

The measured interfacial mechanical properties for these plasma-sprayed HA coatings on titanium alloy substrates indicate relatively low interface properties. The tensile bond strengths recorded are significantly lower than values reported by others.[6,7] We believe that adhesive penetration can result in the measurement of artificially high bond strengths for plasma-sprayed HA coatings.

The observed fracture surface for the failed tensile bond strength specimens (adhesive at the HA/Ti-6Al-4V interface) indicated that this interface was the weakest link of this system. However, it should be noted that the main objective of this study was not the improvement of the HA/titanium alloy interface but, rather, the development of reliable test methods for assessing the mechanical properties of this interface. The tensile bond strength and interfacial fracture toughness values determined in the study represent baseline values that could be used for studying effects of material and process variation on interface fracture resistance.

Our interfacial fracture toughness test results must be treated as giving relative values at this time. To establish absolute values for K_{IcInt} would require the determination of a compliance calibration curve for the composite test specimens used. This was attempted in our studies but difficulties in stabilization of an extensometer modified to suit the specimen geometry and loading conditions prevented completion of this part of the study. Thus, the results for K_{IcInt} must be considered preliminary at this time. Additionally, a load-unload test sequence coupled with proper specimen mouth opening displacement measurements as outlined by Barker[16] for elastic-plastic analysis of specimens should be completed to verify the assumption of linear elastic behavior. Despite these limitations, the small scatter observed in measuring K_{IcInt} by the methods developed is encouraging. The test method is fairly straightforward. Should significantly higher interface toughnesses be developed through appropriate processing variations, a problem could potentially arise in choosing a sufficiently high viscosity adhesive of much higher strength. Of course, such an improvement could also be related to the formation of a less defective coating layer (ie, lower porosity), in which case adhesive penetration might be less of a problem.

Conclusion

A method for forming interfacial tensile bond strength test specimens has been described in which a high viscosity bonding agent is used to mate specimen halves for testing by accepted methods. The result of this modification to specimen fabrication was the determination of lower interfacial tensile bond strengths that the authors believe represent true values for the plasma-sprayed HA/Ti-6Al-4V interface.

A method for determining the fracture toughness of the plasma-sprayed HA/titanium alloy interface has also been developed. The results of preliminary tests have demonstrated the ability of this test method to detect the effect of variations in the plasma coating process (specifically substrate surface preparation) on interface toughness properties.

Acknowledgments

This study was supported by funding from the Premier's Council Technology Fund of the Ministry of Industry, Trade and Technology (Ontario), and the Ontario Centre for Materials Research. In addition, the assistance of Zimmer Mfg Co (Warsaw, Ind) and Dr K. de Groot (University of Leiden) is gratefully acknowledged.

References

1. Cook SD, Thomas KA, Kay JF, Jarcho M. Hydroxy-apatite-coated titanium for orthopaedic implant applications. *Clin Orthop* 1988;232:225–243.
2. De lange GL, Donath K. Interface between bone tissue and implants of solid hydroxyapatite and hydroxyapatite-coated implants. *Biomaterials* 1989;10:121–125.
3. Spivak JM, Ricci JL, Blumenthal NC, Alexander HA. A new canine model to evaluate the biological response of intermedullary bone to implant materials and surfaces. Paper presented at 16th Annual Meeting, Society for Biomaterials, 1990, p 212.
4. Benjamin LS, Block MS. Histologic evaluation of re-

trieved human HA-coated subperiosteal implant: Report of a case. *Int J Maxillofac Implants* 1989;4:63–66.

5. Geesink RG, de Groot K, Klein CP. Chemical implant fixation using hydroxyl-apatite coatings. *Clin Orthop* 1987;225:147–170.

6. de Groot K, Geesink RG, Klein CP, Serekian P. Plasma sprayed coatings of hydroxyapatite. *J Biomed Mater Res* 1987;21:1375–1381.

7. Kay J, Jarcho M, Logan G, Liu ST. The structure and properties of hydroxyapatite coatings on metal. Paper presented at 12th Annual Meeting, Society for Biomaterials, 1986, p 13.

8. Edge MJ. In vivo fracture of the tricalcium phosphate coating from the titanium body of an osseointegrating-type dental implant: A case report. *Int J Maxillofac Implants* 1988;3:57,58.

9. Filiaggi MJ, Coombs NA, Pilliar RM. Characterization of the interface in the plasma sprayed HA coating Ti-6Al-4V implant system. *J Biomed Mater Res* 1991 (in press).

10. Barker LM. A simplified method for measuring plane

11. Mecholsky JJ, Barker LM. A chevron-notched specimen for fracture toughness measurement of ceramic-metal interfaces. ASTM STP 855, 1984, pp 324–336.

12. Wang T, Pilliar RM. Bone cement bonding—Interfacial fracture toughness determination. *Clin Mater* 1989; 4:135–153.

13. Brown SD. Medical-physiological potential of plasma-sprayed ceramic coating. Thin Solid Films 1984;119:127–139.

14. Filiaggi MJ, Coombs NA, Pilliar RM. Mechanical and chemical characterization of a metal-bioceramic interface. *Mat Res Soc Symp Proc* 1989;153:377–382.

15. Ducheyne P, Healy KE. The effect of plasma-sprayed calcium phosphate ceramic coatings on the metal ion release from porous titanium and cobalt-chrome alloys. *J Biomed Mater Res* 1988;22:1137–1163.

16. Barker LM. Theory for determining K_{lc} for small, non-LEFM specimens, supported by experiments on aluminum. *Int J Frac* 1979;15:515–536.

strain fracture toughness. *Eng Fract Mech* 1977;9:361–369.

Biomechanical Aspects of Implant-Supported Prostheses for Edentulous Jaws

H. Weber and U. Benzing

Many factors contribute to the long-term success of an implant-supported oral prosthesis. Once the implants have healed, the bacterial impact and the functional loading of the implant prosthesis probably remain as the major factors determining the survival time of the implants.

This paper included discussion of some biomechanical aspects of different clinical restorations for the edentulous maxilla and mandible. The investigations included the strain gauge measurements recorded in vivo from the transmucosal implant extension (TIE) of the IMZ System. It is shown that stress loading of the implant begins with fixation of the suprastructure. The different stress patterns occurring under function are related to the distribution of implants as well as to the type of suprastructure. These findings can be used to optimize theoretical mathematical models that are needed to predict the appropriate implant-prosthetic solution for clinical cases.

Assessment of Interface Biomechanics of Hydroxyapatite-Coated Endosseous Implants Biovent, Integral, IMZ (Hydroxyapatite- and Titanium-Plasma–Coated) in Rabbit Cancellous Bone

H.-J. Schmitz, S.A. Jovanovic, and J. Krauser*

To elucidate biomechanical qualities of different endosseous implants with various surface coatings, implants were placed into the cancellous bone of rabbit distal femur. Biological characterization of surface structures was achieved by shear and tensile testing after an 84-day period, together with histomorphometrical analysis. Commercially available hydroxyapatite-coated Biovent and Integral implants, and IMZ system implants with titanium-plasma coating and hydroxyapatite coating were studied. In immediate ex vivo testing, IMZ specimens yielded initial shear strength of 0.3 N/mm; after an 84-day period of healing without functional loading, shear strength increased in titanium-plasma–coated specimens to 2.82 ±0.65 N/mm and tensile strength amounted to 1.4 ±0.31 N/mm. Hydroxyapatite-coated specimens more quickly developed the capability to transfer interfacial loads, showing shear strength of 3.98 ±0.7 N/mm after 84 days and tensile strength of 2.24 ±0.27 N/mm. A comparison of the influences of different hydroxyapatite-coatings in additional Biovent and Integral implants in terms of biomechanics, histomorphometry, and scanning electron microscopy is presented.

*Keynote speaker.

Session II Discussion

G. Niznick: Dr Quirynen, is the bone loss related to the polished neck of the IMZ implant or the inability of a cylinder to distribute stress as well as the screw? Where did you take your bone measurements from—both from the crest or were the measurements for the Brånemark implant from the base of the countersink and the measurement for the IMZ implant from the crest of the ridge?

M. Quirynen (Leuven, Belgium): Both bone height measurements were taken from the implant/abutment junction. The answer to your first question, the polished part of IMZ implants was early found no longer covered with bone. Bone loss of about 2.5 mm was seen during the first year and that includes 2 mm for the polished side and just 0.5 mm for the coated side. After the first year, bone loss continued and was located more than 2 mm apically to the implant/abutment junction located at the coated side of the IMZ implant.

C. Berman (New York, New York): I have a question for Dr Quirynen. What was the surface of these IMZ implants? Were they plasma-sprayed or hydroxyapatite-coated?

M. Quirynen: They were plasma-sprayed.

R. Baier: Dr Kohn, with regard to the acoustic emission monitoring, I did not ascertain from your method description whether you did this in air or some liquid fill media. Is it equally applicable in any medium and how would one assure that the porosities were filled if the testing were done in liquid? Would you speculate on the influence the degree of liquid fill, particularly in the in situ case, versus the degree of filling of the pores of a real implant, would have on the mechanical-chemical response that an acoustic emission is capable of measuring?

D. Kohn (Ann Arbor, Michigan): My testing was done in air. The testing could conceivably be done in solution, but it would be a bit more difficult. The physical premise behind acoustic emission is just atomistic motion and if there is a large enough atomistic motion in setting a fracture, such as a slip plane or something, there will be a threshold above which we adhere. Anything we do to complicate the testing situation, the much more difficult the task is to interpret. But it could conceivably be done.

In vivo, what may be more important than actual solutions would be the effect of the relative motion of the bone on the coating. It has been postulated, at least for orthopedic implants, that if there is so-called micromotion, the result is an added surface traction on the coating and some people believe that is actually the reason that some of these coatings are debonding in service. The mechanical effect of the physiological fluids ... I do not know if that would necessarily add a high enough surface traction to play a role. More of the solid-solid contact from the bone riding against the coating could be a factor mechanically.

C. Kopp: Dr Schwarz, in your presentation

many cases were shown in which a computed tomography scan was used to determine diagnostically those patients who should not be treated due to lack of bone quantity. You stated that tooth position dictates implant position and, by example, showed that tooth position may dictate implant position in situations of maximal bone quantity through use of a template. However, in situations of minimal bone, rather than the tooth dictating the position, it is actually the bone itself that will dictate implant position. Do you use templates in situations of minimal bone quantity to dictate implant placement?

M. Schwarz: I think that we are in agreement. What we are trying to achieve is a functional, comfortable, and esthetic prosthesis and rather than focus on the hardware, it is best to look more at the software in determining how to position an implant to give the patient a more comfortable result. The final prosthesis or the position of the prosthetic teeth should be used as a guide for fixture positioning, which is a little bit different than dictating the position of the fixture. In cases of minimal bone, the surgeon does not have the latitude to tip the fixture and one has to take full advantage of what remaining bone there is. The anatomy of the bone in those cases is going to dictate fixture position.

B. Rangert: Dr Brunski, what knowledge is there today to demonstrate the difference between a cylindrical implant and a threaded implant, as concerns marginal bone resorption from a biomechanical point of view?

J. Brunski (Troy, New York): There is not a lot of evidence that would really answer that question for sure. There are only a few biological processes that we would anticipate occurring and, in the case of an implant in cortical bone, one would have to be careful to distinguish between the type of resorption that is part of the normal biological remodeling process creating new osteons, etc, as opposed to some sort of resorption that is stimulated by frank damage to the bone. There has been speculation attempting to ascertain what kind of frank microscopic dam-

age in bone will provoke a microscopic healing event, the subsequent resorptive stages, and then replenishment of that bone. All I can say is that we do not have good evidence on that.

M. Block (New Orleans, Louisiana): Dr Schwarz, I have a couple of questions concerning placing the implants between the nerve and the cortical plate. How many paresthesias have resulted from that procedure and also when attempting to engage the roof of the canal? Since it has been our experience that there are difficulties in doing that, we now reposition the nerve. Do you have any comments about that?

D. Tolman for M. Schwarz: Dr Schwarz indicates no comment.

R. Pilliar (Toronto, Ontario, Canada): Dr Quirynen, it is of concern to see the linear relationship that you reported for the IMZ implant. What type of mechanism do you think is acting to create this sort of thing? The interpretation of your results is that all of these implants will ultimately fail for whatever reason with that linear bone loss relationship. Would you comment on that and perhaps speculate a mechanism?

M. Quirynen: I had no comment and did not speculate on the reason for this observation or for this difference. In fact we were surprised at this finding. It would be better to delay 3 to 4 years and see if this effect is really ongoing. If it is, then in the next 10 or 15 years, all of these IMZ implants will be failures. I cannot give you any reason for that except the type of implant, of course.

C. Berman: Dr Schwarz, as I understand it you are currently working with General Electric scanners. Will it be possible to get some numerical readouts regarding bone quality or bone density on the reformatted images using the General Electric scanning machines? Will the Dentascan be able to do this in the reformatted images? I realize it can do it on the axial images now, but what about the reformed images?

Since the determination of bone quality is

currently one of the major issues, we need to be able to presurgically document data as to which implants work best in poor quality bone. If we had a technique to do this, it would be very helpful in research and perhaps in developing some prognostic guidelines.

M. Schwarz: I am not currently involved with any work on the Dentascan system and am not aware of anything that is being done on reformatted images. When we first got into developing Dentascan, readings of bone density were also contemplated. One of the problems is that there is so much variation in bone density from one point of the mandible to another, and, even in the volume of one single implant fixture, if one wants to get a reading on bone density, it is necessary to define the volume of bone that the proposed implant is going to occupy and then get an average bone density for that entire volume. But, specifically related to your questions, I am just not aware of any work that is being done with reformatted images.

C. Berman: The Siemens group of scanners can do this now. The main reason being that they have a very rapid call-up speed. When the signal goes in to make a cut at a certain spot, within about 6 or 8 seconds, the image will be brought up; whereas the General Electric scanners, from what I understand, take about 4 or 5 minutes to do the same thing and it is much more laborious to get "reformats by hand."

M. Schwarz: At present, I am not sure that even if we had a reading of bone density we would know what the clinical relevance of that was. However, if studies were done of failed implants related to bone density, with enough data, there may be some prognostic value.

T. West (Columbia University, New York): Dr Weber, there seemed to be a lot of variation in the strain gauge charts at the point in time where you screwed the bar down. Is that true?

H. Weber (Tübingen, Germany): That's true.

T. West: You claim that the strain which you are showing is related to bone density. Have you looked at a correlation to some very minor variations, possibly in the way the bar fit?

H. Weber: In this group I have been talking about, everything remained the same. The bars were unscrewed several times. Each measurement was made several times on each patient and the difference reported was the difference between two patients having the same bar length, the same height of transmucosal implant extension, and the same length and diameter of implant. Everything remained the same as far as these parameters were concerned. Thus we felt that due to our measurements, which could be repeated several times, the only explanation for the difference in the stress buildup could be due to the type of bone. We then compared the radiographs and went back again to our calculation and chose another Young's modulus for the bone. As a result we could approach these findings.

T. West: But these are two different bars between two different patients, even though you have tried to control that. There can be minor casting errors, which means that where you place the screw in one bar might not fit quite as well as the next bar.

H. Weber: We published this discussion as part of our results in the *International Journal of Oral & Maxillofacial Implants,* saying that due to an inherent mismatch, which is always inherent with dental castings, a stress buildup is generated. This stress buildup might be even higher during the fixation than it is during chewing.

R. Kraut (Einstein Medical School, New York): Dr Weber, we heard from Dr Quirynen earlier about significant bone loss around the IMZ implants when used for Dolder bars—rather alarming results were reported there. You have now shown other aspects of that system. Would you comment on whether your experience with bone loss has been the same as his?

H. Weber: The Belgium group was comparing two different groups that had been treated in two different centers. As far as our findings are concerned, and I have mainly been using the IMZ system for 10 years, I cannot support the findings that have been given by the Belgium group.

R. Riley (Carlsbad, California): Dr Pilliar, did you attempt to measure the amount of penetration of the coating with your Concise cement as compared to REN 32/62 or FM 1000?

R. Pilliar: With regard to the penetration of the Concise, with that we looked at the fractured surface and analyzed it to see whether any remnants of cement had gotten through to that fracture and we could not see any. With that observation and the low values found, we feel that we did not penetrate through with the use of that adhesive.

R. Riley: Did you do it on a comparative basis?

R. Pilliar: I have only given you results of the Concise that we used in this particular test. One of the other things that happened during the course of this experimentation was that we went to DeGroot's group in Holland and had them plasma-coat some specimens for us. A student who also went over stayed and tested the system that they had prepared with our Concise. We then compared it to their testing with their adhesive. We had the lower values with our system, so there was a comparison of systems there done exactly the same way.

R. Riley: Can I pursue that a little further, Dr Pilliar? Is it possible to add a dye or something to detect the penetration of the low viscosity into it and look at it?

R. Pilliar: That would be nice to do. We thought that we would have it just by using the ESKE analysis of the surface. We did not see it there. This could be done in a quality control lab to be able to say yes, this is a valid test. Of course, the adhesive can do more than just come through, penetrate, and contact the metal surface. It can serve within the thin ceramic layer to completely change the nature of that because it effectively bonds the whole ceramic layer together. So it can do other things as well as just penetrate and adhere to the metal substrate.

A. Fenton (Toronto, Ontario, Canada): Dr Pilliar, if the adhesive could affect the ceramic surface, what can the bony interface do to that surface? Could it then create a stronger film attachment under a biological situation?

R. Pilliar: Once bone grows into this layer, it can certainly affect the properties of that layer. We are not talking about something akin to pores in porous-coated systems in which there are pores that are greater than 50 μm before you get bone penetration and ingrowth into those pores. These are much finer, so extensive bone growth right through that 50-μm layer would likely not occur. There might be a few spicules attaching to the upper surface, but that is about all. That probably would not contribute to the strength of the ceramic-to-metal interface.

E. Chao (Rochester, Minnesota): There were a couple of papers in this session mentioning in vivo measurements of a bending moment. Their data indicated tremendous bending loads for these fixtures during swallowing activities. Could the authors explain how that could happen?

H. Weber: The only answer I can give is that obviously the teeth are in contact when those patients swallow. In edentulous patients, one might assume that the tongue by itself could exert some force as well.

J. Brunski: Dr Krauser, in the tensile testing mode for the coatings and the titanium surfaces, could you say anything about the mode of failure in the hydroxyapatite cases?

J. Krauser (North Palm Beach, Florida): No, I could not. Let me call on my colleague, Dr Schmitz.

H. Schmitz (Aachen, Germany): To denote the significance of this paper, for the first time we showed that there are two different modes of healing of these implants. With the smooth titanium implant, a frame of bone is formed and by this frame the implant is attached in the bone and is retained in the bone. With hydroxyapatite over the rough structuring, there is a different mode of single or multitrabecular incorporation. When the coating was addressed, we found that in most cases the failure occurred between bone and coating. However, in the histological slides, in some instances, this was also dependent on the way the specimens were coated. There was a detachment of the layer from the substrate material and this was especially notable on coatings that were not as well prepared. In other coatings that were better prepared, we did not observe this detachment of the coating itself. However, in our experiments there was no loosening or detachment at the bone interface. The detachment and cracking occurred between the coating and the bone itself. Only in histological sections was there the appearance of crack formation between the coating and substrate material.

G. Niznick: Dr Krauser, were the scanning electron micrographs that you showed on the various coatings prepared by you as part of this study, or were they prepared by Calcitek?

J. Krauser: Those coatings were given to me by Calcitek and they were the same coatings of the implants that were tested in our study.

C. Kopp: Dr Richter, in the clinical environment, do you utilize single implant-single tooth support for a three-unit bridge? Also, have you seen any long-term progressive bone loss around this type of implant arrangement?

E. Richter (Aachen, Germany): We use the IMZ implant in combination with a tooth for a tooth-to-implant fixed bridge. We normally do not use it for single-tooth reconstruction. Normally, with fixed prostheses we use the Brånemark implant for fully implant-borne prostheses as well as single-tooth reconstruction.

Your second question concerns bone loss around the implant. We see bone loss around those implants (IMZ) in situations where they were connected to teeth. As far as fully implant-borne restorations, I cannot say whether there is more or less bone loss because we have worked with this system for just 3 years. When connecting natural teeth to implants with fixed prostheses, we normally use the intermobile element as the system was introduced with. In my opinion, this kind of bone loss is greater than the bone loss seen with the IMZ implant in the edentulous lower jaw using a bar attachment. One aspect surely must be the force that is put on the implant.

Another aspect is that this kind of bone loss appears on the other side because of the spaces between the components that are put on the implant. We found that the original intermobile element, the IME, generates some spaces between the element and the implant. Our results with those elder implants after 5 years were as follows. Implants with the intermobile element more in the gingival tissue position in the beginning had a rather high level of bone loss. After 5 years, with this bone loss the intermobile element came more extragingivally. Then we saw regeneration of the soft tissue and the situation looked better. So the problem is those spaces between the implant and the intermobile element. With this background, the company has changed this intermobile system to the intermobile connector with a goal to have a solid, rigid implant extension on it that probably will provide better results. We are going to publish the results of our comparison of the titanium plasma-sprayed screw implant to the IMZ implant in the edentulous lower jaw, both supporting bars. Our findings were that both implant types experienced some degree of bone loss; slightly more bone loss with the IMZ implant. This kind of bone loss was not as great as that reported by the Belgium group after a period of 3 years.

R. Shuken (Reseda, California): Dr Krauser, after how many days were the animals sacrificed?

J. Krauser: Eighty-four days for all the animals.

R. Shuken: To a clinician, what is the significance of your data as it relates to the Brånemark system as far as you analyzed? Your presentation included percentages of osseointegration and removal forces using different techniques.

How significant is that information to me when the Swedish protocol calls for a minimum number of 120 days before it is even loaded; what does 84 mean?

J. Krauser: Basically, 84 days is 3 months. Since a previous two-part study done with the titanium plasma-sprayed-IMZ and the hydroxyapatite-IMZ implants gave reasonable data, we just included other implant systems in this animal model with that particular time frame. The rabbit does have a more rapid interface development than the human, so a 3-month healing period I believe is at least equivalent to approximately 6 months in the human model. There is some similarity there. We also showed that the interface is different on a threaded design versus the bioactive hydroxyapatite coatings. As far as clinical significance, I do not think that pullout has that much significance. However, tensile, which is a more laterally or perpendicularly oriented force, has a lot of significance. A thread design implant does well in pullout, but poorly in tensile testing. If one is dealing with soft spongy bone, there may be some negative connotation. There are no pure lateral forces in the mouth either. All the forces seen in clinical function represent groupings of forces. We presented the data as it was, but tensile is more clinically relevant than the pullout.

Biomechanical Analysis of a Simulated Tooth-and-Implant–Supported Fixed Partial Denture

E.A. McGlumphy, S.C. Jacks, and D.A. Mendel

It has been suggested that there is a unique set of biomechanical problems associated with joining an implant and a natural tooth with a fixed partial denture. Common clinical manifestations of this problem may include fracture or loosening of the implant prosthetic components. The authors undertook a series of investigations to simulate a tooth-and-implant–supported fixed partial denture during function in order to compare the relevant physical properties of contemporary implant prosthetic components. This paper summarized the results of studies that have evaluated the properties of stress transfer, resistance to fatigue, and resistance to ultimate failure force in many of the most popular implant systems. In addition, comparisons of the biomechanical differences between rigid and resilient internal elements, as well as the effect of torque on the loosening of prosthetic components in function, were described and discussed.

Implant-Prosthetic Treatment Concepts for the Edentulous Jaw

H. Spiekermann, S.A. Jovanovic, and E.-J. Richter

Since the introduction of "osseointegrated" implants, there has been an increasing interest in the field of dental implants. Implant-supported dental restorations have proved to be of great therapeutic value in the treatment of the edentulous jaw. At present, endosseous dental implants are increasingly recommended as artificial abutments for oral reconstructions.[1-4] As this is no longer the treatment of last resort, the endosseous implant is now finding a place in routine dental care. The absolute indication described for the osseointegrated dental implant remains the edentulous, atrophic mandible; relative indications are the edentulous maxilla, the partially edentulous jaw, the single-tooth replacement, and maxillofacial applications.

Treatment of the edentulous jaw

There are two different concepts for the prosthetic rehabilitation of edentulous patients: an implant-retained overdenture and a fixed bone-anchored prosthesis. Until the mid-1980s in the German speaking countries, the main implant modality was the implant-retained overdenture. Since that time, an increasing application of treatment with fixed prostheses in the edentulous jaw has been observed because of the results presented by the Brånemark group using the principle of implant osseointegration.[5-8]

The implant-retained overdenture and fixed prostheses provide a number of advantages and disadvantages.

Advantages of fixed prosthesis:

1. The prosthesis is absolutely stable and offers almost normal chewing efficacy and bite force.
2. Because of the endosseous fixation, forces generated within the jaw have a stimulating effect.
3. Since the prosthesis is fixed, there is a psychological advantage for the patient.

Disadvantages of fixed prosthesis:

1. Some patients complain of the escape of air and saliva beneath the prosthesis (especially in the maxilla), which can compromise phonetics, esthetics, and lip support.
2. The treatment is far more time-consuming and expensive, and the skills of the dentist and the dental technician must be greater.
3. Oral hygiene procedures are more difficult for the patient (especially important with elderly patients).

Treatment of the edentulous jaw with implants as overdenture abutments provides a number of advantages. Implant-supported overdentures will satisfy the functional and esthetic needs of the patient when a minimally to moderately resorbed jaw is present and when the patient presents with relative denture problems.

Patients who have been treated with implant-retained overdentures and who continue to present with complaints can be treated by placing more implants to serve as additional abutments for a fixed-implant prosthesis. In these cases, an overdenture can serve as a provisional denture during the prosthetic phase of the fixed restoration.

Advantages of overdenture treatment:

1. An overdenture is less demanding than a fixed prosthesis and fewer implants are needed, resulting in a more economical plan for the patient and less risks for elderly and health-compromised patients.[9–12]
2. Patients with extremely resorbed ridges, who are unsuitable for the placement of five to six implants needed to support a fixed restoration, can be treated.
3. Unfavorable jaw relationships can be treated more effectively.
4. Lip support, esthetics, and phonetics are improved because of conventional prosthesis flange extension.
5. Dental hygiene procedures are easier to perform.

Disadvantages of the overdenture treatment:

1. The fact that the denture is still removable may result in a possible negative psychological factor for the patient.
2. Functional compressive factors will exist in the edentulous areas on the underlying mucosa and bone because of the mucosal support of the overdenture. Continued bone resorption is anticipated and relining of the prosthesis will be necessary.

This paper describes implant-prosthetic treatment concepts for the edentulous jaw in an attempt to simplify the large versatility in implant prosthetic reconstructions. A schematic classification of four treatment concepts for constructing an implant-retained overdenture or a fixed bone-anchored prosthesis is presented.

Treatment concepts for the edentulous mandible

During treatment planning for a patient with an

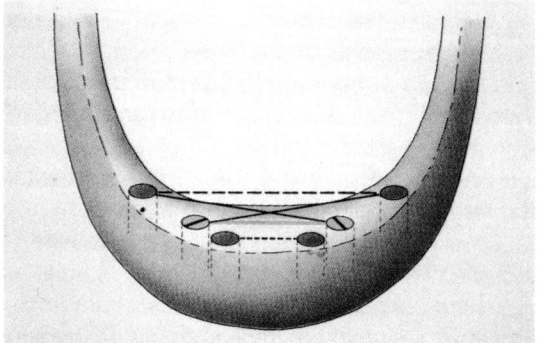

Fig 1 Bars, which are placed nonparallel to the lingual or to the buccal side, can introduce such problems as restriction of tongue movement, mucosal irritation, excessive force on implants, etc. The ideal contour of the bar is demonstrated by the central line, located between the implants inserted in the canine region.

edentulous mandible, the described implant-prosthetic classification has proven its efficacy.

Class I

Two endosseous implants are placed in the symphyseal area of the mandible. The position of both implants should be in the anterior residual crest at its largest dimension, and the straight line connection between the two sites should be as parallel as possible to the terminal mandibular hinge axis. In almost all cases the preferred site is the canine region. The straight bar should have a length between 17 and 20 mm and the placement of the bar should not interfere or restrict the space for the tongue. Figure 1 demonstrates schematically the correct and incorrect position of implants in the frontal region of the mandible. The implants are connected with a round or a pear-shaped solid gold alloy bar. The overdenture receives its stability from the retention wings of the matrix or clip, which can be activated if necessary. The denture can freely rotate around the bar when load is applied in the posterior area of the denture. Using this treatment plan, the denture will be implant-retained and partially supported in the anterior, and totally tissue-supported in the posterior segments of the mandible.

When the anterior region of the mandible is shaped so that the implants must be inserted more toward the midline, the prosthetic concept is changed from an active retention to a passive stabilization. This alternative is necessary because of the short bar and limited active retention of a clip with a decreased length. Stabilization of the denture in this situation is achieved by a swing-lock, which obtains its retention by engaging the lower portion of the bar.

Advantages of bar attachments:

1. Splinting the implants helps distribute the load between them.
2. The attachment has adequate retention.

Disadvantages of using bar attachments:

1. Each one must be individually fabricated and its use depends on the implants being located in a usable position.
2. Adequate oral hygiene is more difficult to maintain.

As an alternative technique in this treatment concept, individual prefabricated attachments such as O-rings or magnets can be used. They have the advantage of being easier to clean and are more economical.

This class I treatment concept is indicated for patients with minimally to moderately resorbed mandibles and for patients with a relative lack of retention and function of their conventional complete mandibular dentures. In general, the placement of two implants with the bar-and-clip retention system provides improved comfort and function. This treatment concept provides a very economical restoration.

Class II

Four endosseous implants are placed anterior to the mental foramina. Most frequently, one-stage implants are used for this treatment concept. The four implants are equally distributed

between the mental foramina. Immediately after placement of the implants, a bar is incorporated to stabilize the pergingival implants during the healing period. After the postoperative edema has subsided, the matrix or clip of the bar is polymerized into the denture. The bar attachment can be round (Hader bar), pear-shaped (Dolder bar), or telescopic. The denture is stabilized by three bar-and-clip attachments and cannot rotate freely over the bar. Using this treatment concept, the denture will be implant-supported in the anterior, and totally tissue-supported in the posterior segments of the mandible.

The class II treatment concept with four one-stage implants is indicated for patients with minimally to extremely resorbed mandibles, for patients who present with narrow, Gothic-arch-shaped mandibles, and for patients who have experienced a total lack of retention with their conventional complete mandibular dentures. Another practical advantage of this concept is that if an existing denture does not demonstrate any functional or esthetic compromises, clips can be incorporated in the denture as soon as the postoperative edema has subsided. The patient then receives an immediate postoperative improvement in retention.[13,14]

Class III

The placement of four or five endosseous implants is performed in the interforaminal region of the mandible. These implants are connected with an individually fabricated distal extension bar. The distal cantilever extensions do not exceed more than 12 mm from the distal aspect of the most posterior implant. The removable denture obtains stability and retention through clips, O-ring attachments, Ceka-attachments, or magnets. The overdenture is totally implant-supported, and rotation over the bar is not possible. This treatment concept is indicated for patients with moderate to advanced mandibular resorption, for patients with severe posterior mandibular atrophy with neuropathy symptoms, and for patients with a total lack of retention of their complete mandibular dentures. The advantages of this treatment over the former two concepts are increased stability, bite force, and chewing efficacy with minimal risk of dislodgment of the overdenture. The primary disadvantage remains in the removable character of the prosthesis.

Class IV

Surgical placement of five to six implants is accomplished in the usual manner between the mental foramina, and a mandibular fixed bone-anchored prosthesis is fabricated. The type of implant-supported fixed suprastructure depends on the hard and soft tissue status and the vertical jaw dimensions of the patient. The framework is distally extended from the most posterior implant a maximum of 15 mm, and acrylic resin teeth are used to dampen the masticatory stress delivered to the supporting implants.

The fixed treatment concept is indicated for patients with minimally to extremely resorbed mandibles, for patients with severe posterior mandibular atrophy and neuropathy symptoms, as well as for patients desiring a fixed prosthesis. As an alternative to the acrylic resin–veneered metal prosthesis, a porcelain-fused-to-metal restoration can be fabricated on optimally placed implants to enhance the esthetic appearance of the implant prosthesis.

Treatment concepts for the edentulous maxilla

The greatest problem that occurs in treatment planning for the maxilla is patient selection. Patients with minimal ridge resorption are amenable to complete denture therapy as well as implant therapy. Usually, a well-made denture will be successful. Those patients with nonresorbed residual ridges who do pursue implant treatment often do so for psychological reasons. Patients with resorbed ridges are less

amenable to complete denture therapy because of decreased denture retention and stability. However, they also become significantly less amenable to implant therapy because of the increased risk of implant failure. Most patients who are candidates for implants in the maxillary arch want to eliminate the palatal portion of their maxillary dentures. However, when the palatal portion of a maxillary denture is removed, denture retention is sacrificed. Mandibular ridge class IV treatment concepts have also evolved for the implant-prosthetic reconstruction of the edentulous maxillary ridge.

Class I

Surgical placement of two implants is performed in the maxillary canine regions. The implants are stabilized by a round or a pear-shaped solid gold alloy bar. The denture will be implant-retained in the anterior and totally tissue-supported in the posterior region of the maxilla. Only in patients with an extreme gag reflex can the palatal extension be shortened. The use of single free-standing implants with individual attachments is contraindicated for mechanical reasons. Patients with an extremely advanced resorption of the maxillary ridge are candidates for this treatment concept because of the available bone volume, which allows only the placement of two implants. These patients should also be considered for alternative treatment utilizing an autogenous bone grafting procedure.

Class II

The surgical placement of three or four implants should be considered for the routine rehabilitation of an edentulous maxilla. The implants are connected with a round, pear-shaped, or telescopic solid gold alloy bar. When 7- or 10-mm implants are placed in the maxilla, no cantilever extensions should be made during the first year of implant function. After an uncomplicated first year of use, the cantilever can be extended to 5 mm to acquire more retentive area for the clip.

Plastic or gold clips are polymerized into the denture base to provide the retentive character of the attachment. The anterior portion of the denture is implant-supported and the posterior portion is totally tissue-supported. The palatal portion of the maxillary prosthesis can be reduced if the denture has sufficient retention from the bar-and-clip attachment. Patients with moderate to extreme maxillary ridge resorption are good candidates for this treatment concept.

Class III

Four to six implants are placed into the anterior and, if possible, in the middle region of the maxillary ridge. The implants are connected by an individually fabricated distally extended bar (maximum cantilever extension is 10 mm). The totally implant-supported overdenture is retained by clips, O-ring attachments, Ceka attachments, or magnets. The palatal portion of the maxillary prostheses can be completely eliminated. The use of single free-standing implants with individual attachments is contraindicated for mechanical reasons. The indication for concept class III is apparent for those patients who desire considerable stability and retention of their dentures and a chewing pattern that closely resembles the natural dentition, but who are not opposed to a removable prosthesis.

Class IV

The placement of five to six implants is accomplished in the anterior and, if possible, in the middle region of the edentulous maxilla. Many fabrication methods for fixed bone-anchored prostheses have been introduced, but the most widely used is the "high-water" design, acrylic resin–veneered metal framework. Since the completely bone-anchored prosthesis may not obturate the space between the prosthesis and residual tissues, the air flow pattern produced during speech is unimpeded. This can present problems for the patient if there has been advanced resorption of the maxilla. Phonetics,

esthetics, and lip support may be compromised. These problems can be overcome in some way by the fabrication of a removable gingival epithesis.

Alternative prosthodontic techniques for this fixed treatment concept include a porcelain-fused-to-metal restoration and a two-piece casting with an acrylic resin–veneered metal framework. With a two-piece casting, esthetic and phonetic requirements dictate that the tissue surface of the primary casting contacts the gingiva in a manner similar to that of the pontic-to-gingiva contact found in conventional fixed partial dentures.

The secondary telescopic acrylic resin–veneered metal prosthesis is screwed into the primary framework. The advantages of this design are the elimination of occlusal screw-access holes, redirection of malaligned implants, and fabrication of more esthetic and phonetic prostheses. Because of the very complex factors involved in the fabrication of the maxillary fixed prosthesis, the diagnostic workup requires a more comprehensive process that must include a wax trial denture. The esthetic and phonetic anterior tooth arrangement should be pre-established. Posterior tooth positioning for the proper location of the occlusal plane should also be determined. Following the tooth arrangement, if there is no need for lip support from the denture flange, the use of a fixed prosthesis may be a good option for patients with mild to advanced resorption of the maxillary ridge.[8,15]

Summary

The described classification of four different prosthetic treatment implant concepts for the edentulous jaw has been developed following conventional prosthodontic principles. Therefore, it has not been our goal to incorporate diverse important implant success factors such as bone equality and quantity, jaw relationships, and the various implant systems. Although certain overlap is inevitable among these treatment concepts (especially among concepts I to III), this schematic prosthetic approach has demonstrated efficacy in clinical use.

References

1. Albrektsson T, Zarb GA, Worthington P, Eriksson AR. The long-term efficacy of currently used dental implants: A review and proposed criteria of success. *Int J Oral Maxillofac Implants* 1986;1:11–25.
2. Brånemark P-I, Zarb GA, Albrektsson T. Tissue integrated prostheses. Osseointegration in clinical dentistry. Chicago: Quintessence Publ Co, 1985.
3. Davis DM. The role of implants in the treatment of edentulous patients. *Int J Prosthodont* 1990;3:42–50.
4. Engquist B, Bergendal T, Kallus T, Linden U. A retrospective multicenter evaluation of osseointegrated implants supporting overdentures. *Int J Oral Maxillofac Implants* 1988;3:129.
5. Falk H, Laurell L, Lundgren D. Occlusal force pattern in dentitions with mandibular implant-supported fixed cantilever prostheses occluded with complete dentures. *Int J Oral Maxillofac Implants* 1989;4:55–62.
6. Kondell PA, Landt H, Nordenram A, et al. The tissue integrated prosthesis in the treatment of edentulous patients. *Swed Dent J* 1988;12:11–16.
7. Krauser JT. Case planning and treatment plan recommendations for the totally edentulous mandible. *Florida Dent J* 1989;60:4–7,60–62,65.
8. Lindquist LW, Rockler B, Carlsson GE. Bone resorption around fixtures in edentulous patients treated with mandibular fixed tissue-integrated prostheses. *J Prosthet Dent* 1988;59:69.
9. Haraldson T, Stalblad PA, Jemt T. Oral function subjects with mandibular overdentures supported by osseointegrated implants. *J Oral Rehabil* 1988;15:181.
10. Misch C. Implant overdentures relieve discomfort for the edentulous. *Dentist* 1989;67:37–38.
11. Parel SM. Implants and overdentures: The osseointegrated approach with conventional and compromised applications. *Int J Oral Maxillofac Implants* 1986;1:93.
12. Spiekermann H. Implantatprothetik. In *Voss/Meiner: Fortschritte der Zahnärztl. Prothetik und Werkstoffkunde Bd.* I to IV. München: Carl Hanser Verlag, 1980, 1984, 1987, 1989.
13. Babbush CA, Kent JN, Misiek DJ. Titanium plasma sprayed (TPS) screw implants for the reconstruction of the edentulous mandible. *J Oral Maxillofac Surg* 1986;44:274.
14. Ledermann PD. Das TPS-Schraubenimplantat nach siebenjähriger Anwendung. *Quintessenz* 1984; 11:2031.
15. Balshi TJ. Resolving aesthetic complications with osseointegration: Using a double-casting prosthesis. *Quintessence Int* 1986;17:281–287.

Oral Implants Used to Stabilize Hypermobile Teeth

D. Lundgren and L. Laurell

Currently, endosseous oral implants are routinely used to support oral prostheses in both totally and partially edentulous jaws. Experience has demonstrated that natural teeth and osseointegrated implants with good long-term prognosis can be "stiffly" connected via a conventional fixed partial denture, provided that certain requirements are fulfilled. In these studies, the natural teeth were reported to exhibit a "normal" mobility.

This report evaluates the results of permanent stabilization of hypermobile teeth or tooth-supported fixed prostheses by the aid of jawbone-anchored endosseous implants.

Materials and methods

Six partially edentulous individuals between 45 and 66 years of age were included in the study. They were supplied with one to four Brånemark implants (Nobelpharma AB, Göteborg, Sweden) according to the technique and time schedule recommended for that implant system. Following adequate healing time, the implants were connected to pre-existing hypermobile fixed partial dentures.

Two types of connections were utilized. Type 1 was lateral locking to reduce lateral tooth hypermobility. This connection consisted of a male part protruding from the implant-supported fixed prosthesis to lock the female part of the tooth-supported prosthesis with a close fit, but without any screw connection. Type 2 used screw coupling to reduce axial and lateral tooth hypermobility.

The type 1 connection was used in four patients who underwent observation periods from 1 to 5 years. The type 2 connection was used in two patients who underwent observation periods from 2 to 4 years.

The baseline and follow-up examinations included clinical measurements of tooth and implant mobility, as well as radiographic evaluations of their supporting tissues. The amplitude of the tooth mobility was measured by the aid of thin foils of known thickness placed between the connection units. During application of the foils, a laterally or coronally directed force of about 10 N was applied to the tooth-supported unit.

The radiographic evaluations of implants and teeth were performed on intraoral standard films using conventional criteria.

Results

Table 1 (type 1 cases) shows the results for lateral deflection of the tooth-supported units after application of a laterally directed force of about 10 N. The individual values at baseline registration, ie, at the time of delivery of the prosthesis, varied from 0.40 to 0.85 mm, whereas the corresponding value at the 1-year followup examination varied from 0.20 to 0.50 mm. This corresponds to a percentage mobility reduction for the individual tooth-supported unit varying between 30% and 50%.

Table 1 Type 1 connections*

Patient	Baseline	1 year	Mobility reduction (%)
A	0.85	0.50	41
B	0.70	0.45	36
C	0.65	0.45	30
D	0.40	0.20	50

*Lateral deflection (mm) of tooth-supported units at baseline examination and after 1 year in service when a laterally directed force of about 10 N is applied.

Table 2 Type 2 connections*

Patient	Baseline	1 year	Mobility reduction (%)
A	0.60	0.06	90
B	0.80	0.14	83

*Coronal deflection (mm) of tooth-supported units at baseline examination and after 1 year in service when a coronally directed force of about 10 N is applied.

Table 2 (type 2 cases) shows the results for coronal deflection of the tooth-supported unit after application of a coronally directed force of about 10 N. The values at baseline registration were 0.60 and 0.80 mm. The corresponding values at the 1-year followup examination were 0.06 and 0.14 mm. This means a percentage mobility reduction of 90% and 83%, respec-

tively. No major alterations in tooth mobility compared to the 1-year results have been observed in those patients who have been subjected to additional follow-ups.

All implants exhibited signs of clinical osseointegration and there were no radiographic signs of discrepant marginal bone loss or radiolucent diastases at the baseline or at the follow-up examinations.

At the baseline examination, the hypermobile teeth that supported the fixed prostheses showed evident radiographic signs of periodontal ligament widening, which was especially pronounced in the type 2 connection cases. These teeth exhibited clear-cut radiographic signs of periodontal ligament narrowing at the followup examinations.

Discussion

Obviously, jawbone-anchored, osseointegrated implants can be utilized not only to decisively contribute to the support of fixed prostheses on natural teeth with "normal" mobility, but also to stabilize hypermobile teeth or abutments without jeopardizing the osseointegration of the implants. Several factors might influence the outcome of such a stabilizing function, for instance: number and location of implants; quality of osseointegration; number, location, and mobility of natural teeth; and, not least, the occlusal force pattern.

Impact of Osseointegration on Prosthodontics*

G.A. Zarb

In one of his essays in *The Lives of a Cell: Notes of a Biology Watcher,* Lewis Thomas[1] observed that with clinical scientists:

> It has been our perpetual habit to try anything, on the slimmest of chances, the thinnest of hopes, empirically and wishfully, and we have proved to ourselves over and over again that the approach doesn't work well. Bleeding, cupping, and purging are the classical illustrations, but we have plenty of more recent examples to be embarrassed about. We have been hoaxed along by comparable substitutes for technology right up to the present. There is no question about our good intentions in this matter: we all hanker, collectively, to become applied scientists as soon as we can, overnight if possible.

Up to a decade ago, the field of dental implants was largely regarded as an example of the "try anything" approach that Thomas was referring to. Consequently, implant therapy languished at the low end of the scientific heap, as clinical specialists and educators demanded basic science and therapy effectiveness outcome studies before implants could be seriously considered. Luckily the topic was not to remain marooned, and in 1982 the technique of osseointegration was introduced to North American dental educators at the Toronto Conference by the Göteborg group. The authentic, electric shock of the new was administered, and almost overnight an entirely new "think" became incorporated into the dental therapeutic repertoire.

An assessment of the impact of osseintegration suggests the late Marshall McLuhan's analogy of a journey in the automobile of progress, as it heads relentlessly, if sometimes recklessly, toward a more perfect future of enriched life quality for our patients. McLuhan had cautioned that any such journey would probably be far more significant if the rear view mirror was always kept in sight. The driver would then remember where he's coming from, and what he's left behind. Hence our ongoing concern in the discipline of prosthodontics with the relationship of an implant system to a reduced burden of illness for our patients. My objective, in this brief presentation, is to assess the impact of the osseointegration technique in the context of certain stated prosthodontic objectives, and to take a long hard look at what might have been left behind.

Biomechanical objectives

It is proposed that the induction of an attachment mechanism for dental implants should fulfill three criteria:

1. Elicit a safe and predictable interfacial response
2. Provide support that sustains long-term loading
3. Allow for versatility and diversity of prosthetic applications.

*Keynote presentation.

Predictability and longevity

The first two criteria, comprising safe predictability and long-term function, will be discussed together since they are essentially inseparable. An analogous attachment mechanism for alloplastic tooth roots demands comparison with a periodontal ligament. This ligament evolved in mammals to subserve quantitative and qualitative functions, functions that presumably require replication in a periodontal ligament replacement. It is a very forgiving attachment mechanism, since its innervation, resiliency, and osteogenic potential make it so adaptable. Obvious examples are the way it copes with traumatic occlusion, or the controlled trauma of orthodontic movement. In fact, one could argue that in the absence of local irritation or inflammation, trauma could be accommodated almost indefinitely.

The periodontal ligament is vulnerable to putative factors such as pathogenic microorganisms in plaque. The osseointegrated response suggests a process whereby clinically asymptomatic rigid fixation of alloplastic materials in bone is achieved and maintained during functional loading. This documented ankylosis-like response has proven to be a very worthy clinical substitute for the well-documented quantitative-cum-qualitative role of the periodontal ligament. However, it is *not* a compliant interfacial response, since it is not derived from the same embryological source as the periodontal ligament. The absence of a shock-absorbing role with the osseointegration technique has not been regarded as a deterrent for a range of prosthodontic therapies. In fact, a 1989 Consensus Report on the Current State of Implant Prosthodontics[2] stated: "The role of the host/implant interface is paramount. Concepts about the nature of this interface are evolving in response to laboratory and clinical research. Of the documented biologic interfacial responses that are associated with long-term patient care, the most predictable is so-called 'osseointegration.' It is concluded that an acceptable biologic rationale exists for implant-stabilized prostheses."

This conclusion resulted from stock-taking of salient publications, which indicated the following: (1) the induced bone fixation appears resistant to long-term tensile and shear forces associated with occlusal loading[3]; (2) patients' problems of prostheses-related maladaptation, pain, and compromised life quality were dramatically reduced[4,5]; (3) reported morbidity appears to be minimal and virtually innocuous, and the system offers ample scope for retrievability where required.[6,7] The only apparent trade-off, from a treatment outcome point of view, has been the absence of a compliant interface, but this has not precluded clinical longitudinal success as evidenced by several studies. This has prompted the inevitable question: Should we not begin to regard osseointegration as cause for a requiem for the periodontal ligament? Perhaps we will have an answer at the next Congress. Furthermore, it could be argued that osseointegration results in significant associated bone responses, since reports indicate a relative retardation of bone resorption around implants.[8] Two preliminary reports also suggest that osseointegration may even minimize, or in some cases, counteract residual ridge resorption[9] and particularly physiologic age-related bone mineral content loss, which leads to osteoporosis.[10]

Many opinions have also been expressed about specific disciplines' viewpoints on osseointegration. While these opinions are certainly well-intentioned, they may tend to narrow the scope of the clinical technique and the dentist's interpretation of the process. Such opinions inadvertently perpetuate borrowed convictions or observations from the dentulous oral cavity and presume that the same must happen in mouths with osseointegrated implants. This attitude is reinforced by evidence that the microenvironment of tooth and implant sulci may be quite similar,[11] hence the appearance of frequent references in periodontal literature regarding the necessity for a perimucosal seal of the soft tissues to the implant surface. One distinguished colleague[12] has observed that failure to achieve or maintain this seal results in apical migration of the epithelium into the implant/bone interface and fibrous encapsulation of the endosseous or root portion of the implant system. This is a throwback to the predicament of the old blade vent implant era, when the hoped for circumferential seal around the transepithelial extension was regarded as an implant's Achilles' heel.

Given the differences between a periodontal ligament and an induced interfacial lock between titanium implants and host bone, the pathogenesis of periodontal disease is unlikely to be identical to the interfacial breakdown that can lead to implant loosening. Consequently, one must feel inclined to state: no periodontal ligament, no periodontal disease. It is also tempting to suggest that traditional prosthodontic-periodontic criteria as contributors to the process of implant loss is not particularly enlightened thinking. Which is not to suggest that soft tissue concerns, vis-à-vis prosthesis design or patient home care, are irrelevant. We have documented the "nuisance value" of soft tissue complications in osseointegration.[13] But these largely iatrogenically induced problems are not causes of implant failure (at least within the time framework of reported observations). They appear to be just a nuisance—no more and no less. Admittedly some implant system manufacturers regard periodontal-like disease around their implants as consequential.[14,15] I suspect that this says more about those implant systems themselves than it does about the nature of implant failure per se.

Current research indicates that host factors play a major role in periodontal disease susceptibility, and the identification of high-risk groups has assumed considerable importance. It is not unreasonable to presume that some of the many edentulous patients successfully treated with osseointegrated implants lost their dentitions because of periodontal disease susceptibility, but have in turn proven nonsusceptible to implant failure.

At this stage of limited understanding of the peri-implant mucosal response to implant longevity, it appears that traditional interpretations of gingival behavior around natural teeth do not necessarily apply to the implant model. Observed results appear to endorse the absence of a measure of mucosal health from proposed criteria for implant success.[16] Perhaps osseoin-

tegration and mucosal integration are mutually inclusive, at least with the Swedish oral implant system.

It is readily conceded that there appears to be microbiological variance between edentulous and partially edentulous patients.[17] This is probably the result of the large variety of bacteria harbored in pockets around teeth. These pockets act as a reservoir of periodontal pathogens that contaminate the implant sites, hence the argument that success with implant-treated edentulous patients is related to a reduced intraoral microbiological challenge. Furthermore, the presence of such pathogens may in turn hasten subsequent peri-implant disease if the site is not well maintained. The profession's apparent assumption of quasi-identical sulcular environments demands preimplant periodontal therapy, followed by periodic plaque removal, and impeccable oral and occlusal hygiene. We must not presume, however, that plaque and occlusal stresses are the exclusive etiologic factors in implant failure, therefore requiring related therapeutic initiatives. This may be a convenient, and is in fact a prudent, clinical attitude to adopt, given the established fact that periodontal diseases are caused by bacteria in plaque. Hence, with teeth, no matter which course the disease process may follow, it begins with gingivitis. But clinical evidence and experience to date do not support the automatic identification of a tooth root with its osseointegrated analogue. Hence the urge or temptation to describe a new disease, eg, peri-implantitis, must be resisted. We must avoid falling into a similar trap to the one associated with the handling of temporomandibular joint disorders—developing diverse treatment methods in search of a disease. Clearly as Dr van Steenberghe pointed out in his elegant and comprehensive overview [see pp 41 to 47], much more research is needed in this fascinating area.

The definition of a clinical success formula in most aspects of dental treatment has tended to depend on both subjective and objective criteria. Like the proverbial two sides of a coin, these criteria can be looked at separately, although they are an integral part of the same scientific currency. Regrettably, and perhaps inevitably, given the previous lack of reliable longitudinal documentation for the implant method, considerable reliance on subjective criteria has dominated this field. Consequently, anecdotal reporting of the "success by default" variety has abounded.

The very nature of the clinical objective of a functional attachment mechanism for an implant tends to preclude investigation at the cellular and intracellular level. As in orthopedic implant research, serial sampling of the host site response is not feasible since biopsies are difficult to obtain and are taxing to the donor. Clinical success has therefore been frequently based on artifact material, and a history of clinical performance extrapolated from one or two points in time. I am therefore not convinced that the availability of research tools and techniques plus compelling documentation have been successfully applied to this topic. Nor have a multitude of research trails finally converged in reasonably precise knowledge of the longitudinal response of different host sites to diverse prosthodontic applications of the implant technique.

A scrutiny of presumed components of the well-attested-to Swedish success formula has enabled the proposal of a set of criteria that may be used as a reliable yardstick for both review bodies, and researchers, in assessing current and newer implants. Above all, this yardstick protects the patient. An informed consent when undertaking implant therapy should include knowledge of the highest standards of service that are currently available. The following conditions for criteria applications are recommended: *(1)* that only individual, osseointegrated implants should be evaluated; *(2)* that the implants must have been in functional use at the time of testing; and *(3)* that introgenic complications (eg, sinus or nasal cavity intrusion, mandibular canal impingement, prosthesis fracture, etc) be considered separately and not included in a percentile success computation.

Published reports, together with personal long-term experience with the Brånemark implant system (Nobelpharma AB, Göteborg, Sweden), has led to the proposal of a series of clinically determined criteria.[18] When considered together, this criteria package may be interpreted to describe a clinical osseointegration success formula. This formula includes the following:

1. An individual, unattached implant is immobile when tested clinically.
2. There is no evidence of peri-implant radiolucency as assessed on undistorted periapical radiographs.
3. The total mean vertical bone loss should preferably be less than 0.2 mm annually following the first year of service.
4. There should be no persistent pain or discomfort attributable to the implant.
5. The implant design should not preclude placement of a crown or prosthesis with an appearance satisfactory to the patient and dentist.
6. In the context of the above, a success rate of 68% at the end of a 10-year period should be the minimum.

These criteria evolved as a result of prospective edentulous patients' studies and are intended to form a reasonable basis for dental implant assessment. They must however be fine-tuned or modified as clinical quantification techniques are refined, or as different systems, eg, compliant interfacial ones, are developed. For example, in establishing limits for bone loss, the guidance must come from the lowest level of bone loss from an adequately documented study. Since documentation demonstrates that a mean bone loss of no more than 0.2 mm per year after the first year is attainable, this figure should serve as a valid criterion for success. It is important that this proposed 0.2-mm figure not be applied literally to individual implants. Clinical experience reveals that marginal bone loss of a rapid and usually self-limiting nature may occur, if infrequently. Such cervical bone reduction has been attributed to localized mechanical overload, or to mechanical injury of the soft tissue seal with bacteria-initiated disease. In these cases, bone loss can easily exceed the 0.2-mm figure, and once the adverse exacerbation is over, the marginal bone level restabilizes without the implant's mobility criterion ever having been seriously challenged. Since such an anomalous situation is infrequently encountered, the feasibility and practicality of our relevant proposed criterion seems reasonable.

Versatility and diversity of application

The biomechanical objectives of the osseointegration technique—safe predictability, long-term efficacy, retrievability—are compellingly documented in published retrospective and prospective studies on the treatment of edentulous populations with fixed prostheses. However, while extremely promising, diverse treatment possibilities with osseointegration techniques remain unproven in longitudinally documented evaluations. One cannot help observing that the apparent single-minded approach of fixed prosthesis treatment for edentulous patients militated against the evolution of diverse yet parallel treatment and research endeavors. Furthermore, the gradual realization by the dentist that osseointegration could become a routine preprosthetic surgical technique—an adjunct for solving prosthodontic problems—now demands a more active role by both dentist and specialist alike in placing the technique in a more universal didactic and applied context. This explains the recent initiatives in implant prescriptions for supporting overdentures,[19] as well as single or multiple tooth replacements in partially edentulous patients. It should be pointed out that the reported edentulous successes need not automatically translate to the partially dentate treatment ones,[20] since different host zone sites may behave differently. The work of Jemt et al[21] is of course noteworthy in this regard, but long-term multicenter results are still ongoing, and until they are available, we cannot yet subsume the routine application of the technique. Nonetheless a very large number of clinical case histories can be described that underscore the enormous potential of this technique.

Some prosthodontic research considerations

Several questions remain unanswered—questions that continue to spawn controversy. These questions make up a sort of "wish list" of research topics for graduate students in clinical dentistry, and include:

1. Patient selection considerations: age, health, periodontal status
2. Imaging techniques: pre- and posttreatment considerations
3. Selection of host sites
4. Prosthodontic aspects: techniques, designs, materials
5. Educational considerations
6. Cost effectiveness

Each one of the listed points deserves additional comments.

Patient selection considerations

Young patients with congenitally compromised dentitions or craniofacial growth could benefit considerably from interventions that provide anchorage for protraction of the facial bones and for the movement of teeth. Preliminary research in this area appears promising[22–24] and can only benefit overall treatment planning for such patients. Congenitally missing teeth could also be readily replaced, thus precluding the risk of intraoral ecologic upset that may be associated with traditional prosthetic methods. Elderly edentulous patients have already benefited immeasurably since the advent of osseointegration.[25,26] The overdenture technique appears to offer great scope for these patients, particularly in the context of home care maintenance for those patients who are incapable of taking care of themselves, eg, Alzheimer's patients. The interfacial response to senescent changes, especially where metabolic disease has been, or is present, deserves study, especially since increased longevity of the elderly is today a global trend.[27]

The periodontally compromised patient deserves a treatment planning reevaluation. Traditionally this patient has been a candidate for the periodontal/prosthesis method (if this could be afforded). While dramatic and frequently beneficial, this treatment may also prove to be a heroic undertaking and fraught with risks. Many of these patients would probably be better off if teeth with dubious prognosis were extracted to make room for implants with a better prognosis, particularly if favorable bone sites are selected. Osseointegration offers considerable scope for reparative procedures to cope with the sequellae of tissue loss. But perhaps osseointegration should also be seen in the context of tissue conservation or the avoidance of decline, eg, residual ridge resorption. Immediate implant placement for such patients also deserves clinical trials since this is where they are needed most.

Imaging techniques

An understandable predilection for computerized axial tomography (CAT) scan techniques has been expressed. However this is not practical for the many dentists who do not have access to such equipment. Adapting standard tomographic methods appears reasonable, and while not as reliable, recent publications plus multicenter clinical experiences attest to the efficacy of the method.[28] We are lacking simple and readily accessible methods for determining bone quality in a manner that minimizes variables in treatment planning. Furthermore the radiographic techniques for monitoring implant success provide a relatively crude resolution level, and it would be most advantageous if improved quantification methods were available.

Host sites

The ingenuity of our surgical colleagues has led to the exploration of "extra-site" terrain for implant placement. The selection of the pterygoid plates area is a notable location,[29] but long-term

and diverse loading situations need to be analyzed. The application of grafting techniques seems to offer promise for those patients whose residual bone levels are so severely undermined that pathologic fractures are a risk. Here too, results are promising, if somewhat preliminary. The recent introduction of membrane techniques to generate new bone around implants is also laudatory and is bound to yield exciting new therapeutic directions.[30]

Prosthodontic aspects

The prosthodontic aspect of osseointegration has been largely empirical and has borrowed from traditional prosthodontic methods that are themselves largely empirical. Consequently the entire prosthetic application of the technique—the reconciliation of numbers and length of fixtures, the nature of the opposing dentition, the choice of materials, the size of the occlusal table or number of occluding units, the magnitude, duration, and frequency of occlusal loading, etc—offers fertile scope for research. Several authors[29–31] have already risen to this challenge and more scientific guidelines for the prosthetic endeavors are anticipated.

Education

Introduction of the osseointegration technique into undergraduate curricula is now a pressing concern. The major problem is how to change the bathwater without hurting the baby that's in it. The risk is the two extreme positions; one, that educators may inadvertently throw out the baby with the bathwater, and two, that the technique's introduction is resisted and educational obsolescence will result.

Cost effectiveness

Finally it should be possible to plan treatment and prescribe implant-supported prostheses in a manner that does not deny treatment to those who need it most. The majority of elderly patients are on fixed incomes, a fiscal predicament that is likely to preclude "state-of-the-science" dentistry. It should be emphasized that the hallmark of a health service is not only the intelligence underscoring its therapeutic innovations, but also the universality of its application. Anything short of such an objective usurps the true notion of a health profession.

Conclusion

Swedish and other publications on long-term clinical research in the field of osseointegrated dental implants clearly offer considerable optimism for this clinical technique. In fact, we are dealing with a very significant advance that has had a profound impact on prosthodontic treatment.

The salvage procedures routinely employed in prosthodontics already enable the clinician to cope with a large range of morphofunctional challenges. However, detailed scrutiny of clinical results does reveal varying degrees of success, along with the infrequently acknowledged treatment failures. In response to the inherent difficulties we confront clinically, plus the shortcomings of our prosthodontic services per se, we have developed a wide and ingenious range of clinical and laboratory procedures. Marrying these procedures to the osseointegration technique has already enabled us to enrich the quality of our patients' lives. When the remaining pieces of the fascinating research puzzle finally come together, osseointegration is likely to become prosthodontics' most significant therapeutic method.

References

1. Thomas L. *The Lives of a Cell: Notes of a Biology Watcher.* New York: Bantam Books, Inc, 1974.
2. Zarb GA. Prologue and epilogue: Consensus report from the International College of Prosthodontists panel on the current state of implant prosthodontics. *Int J Prosthodont* 1991;3:11,51–52.
3. Albrektsson T, Albrektsson B. Osseointegration of bone implants. *Acta Orthop Scand* 1987;58:567–577.
4. Zarb GA, Schmitt A. The longitudinal clinical effectiveness of osseointegrated dental implants: The Toronto study. Part II: The prosthetic results. *J Prosthet Dent* 1990;64:53–61.
5. Blomberg S, Lindquist LW. Psychological reactions to edentulousness and treatment with jawbone-anchored bridges. *Acta Psychiatr Scand* 1983;68:251.
6. Worthington P, Bolender C, Taylor T. The Swedish system of osseointegrated implants: Problems and complications encountered during a four-year trial period. *Int J Oral Maxillofac Implants* 1987;2:77–84.
7. Zarb GA, Schmitt A. The longitudinal clinical effectiveness of osseointegrated dental implants: The Toronto study. Part III. *J Prosthet Dent* 1990;64:234.
8. Chaytor D, Zarb GA, Schmitt A, Lewis D. The longitudinal effectiveness of osseointegrated dental implants. The Toronto study: Bone level changes. *Int J Periodont Rest Dent* 1991;11:113–126.
9. Sennerby L, Carlsson GE, Bergman B, Warfvinge J. Mandibular bone resorption in patients treated with tissue-integrated prostheses and in complete denture wearers. *Acta Odontol Scand* 1988;46:135–140.
10. Wowern von N, Harder F, Hjørting-Hansen E, Gotfredsen K. ITI implants with overdentures: A prevention of bone loss in edentulous mandibles? *Int J Oral Maxillofac Implants* 1990;5:135–139.
11. Apse P, Ellen RP, Overall CM, Zarb GA. Microbiota and crevicular fluid collagenase activity in the osseointegrated dental implant sulcus: A comparison of sites in edentulous and partially edentulous patients. *J Periodont Res* 1989;24:96–105.
12. Meffert RM. The soft tissue interface in dental implantology. *J Dent Educ* 1988;52:810–811.
13. Apse P, Zarb GA, Schmitt A, Lewis D. The longitudinal clinical effectiveness of osseointegrated dental implants: The Toronto study: Peri-implant mucosal assessment. Submitted for publication, 1990.
14. Kirsch A, Mentag P. The IMZ endosseous two phase implant system: A complete oral rehabilitation treatment concept. *J Oral Implant* 1986;12:576–589.
15. Block MS, Kenty JN, Finger IM. Factors associated with tissue compromise with endosseous dental implants. *J Dent Res* 1990;69(special issue):267. Abstract no. 1268.
16. Smith D, Zarb GA. Criteria for success for osseointegrated endosseous implants. *J Prosthet Dent* 1989;62:567–572.
17. Apse P, Zarb GA, Schmitt A, Lewis D. The longitudinal effectiveness of osseointegrated dental implants. The Toronto study: Peri-implant mucosal response. *Int J Periodont Rest Dent* 1991;11:95–111.
18. Albrektsson T, Zarb GA, Worthington P, Eriksson AR. The long-term efficacy of currently used dental implants: A review and proposed criteria of success. *Int J Oral Maxillofac Implants* 1986;1:11–25.
19. Zarb GA, Schmitt A. The longitudinal clinical effectiveness of osseointegrated implant-supported overdentures: A preliminary report on the Toronto study. In E. Schepers, I. Naert, G. Theuniers (eds) *Overdentures*

on Oral Implants (EOTC). Leuven, Belgium: Leuven University Press, 1991.

20. Smith DE. A review of endosseous implants for partially edentulous patients. Int J Prosthodont 1990;3:12.

21. Jemt T, Lekholm U, Adell R. Osseointegrated implants in the treatment of partially edentulous patients: A preliminary study on 876 consecutively placed fixtures. Int J Oral Maxillofac Implants 1989;4:3.

22. Smalley WM, Shapiro PA, Hohl TH, Kokich VG, Brånemark P-I. Osseointegrated titanium implants for maxillofacial protraction in monkeys. Am J Orthod Dentofac Orthop 1988;94:285–295.

23. Roberts WE, Smith RK, Zilberman Y, Mozsary PG, Smith RS. Osseous adaptation to continuous loading of rigid endosseous implants. Am J Orthod 1984; 86:95–111.

24. Ödman J, Lekholm U, Jemt T, Brånemark P-I, Thilander B. Osseointegrated titanium implants—A new approach in orthodontic treatment. Eur J Orthod 1988; 10:98–105.

25. Zarb GA, Schmitt A. Terminal dentition in elderly patients and implant therapy alternatives. Int Dent J 1990;40:67–73.

26. Köndell PA, Nordenram A, Landt H. Titanium implants in the treatment of edentulousness: Influence of patient's age on prognosis. Gerodontics 1988;4:280–284.

27. Matthiessen PC. Demography—Impact of an expanding elderly population. p 365 In P. Holm-Pederson, H. Löe (eds) Geriatric Dentistry. Copenhagen: Munksgaard, 1986.

28. Klinge B, Petersson A, Maly P. Location of the mandibular canal: Comparison of macroscopic findings, conventional radiography, and computed tomography. Int J Oral Maxillofac Implants 1989;4:327–332.

29. Tulasne JF. Implant treatment of missing posterior dentition. In T. Albrektsson, G.A. Zarb (eds) The Brånemark Osseointegrated Implant. Chicago: Quintessence Publ Co, 1989.

30. Dahlin G, Sennerby L, Lekholm U, Linde A, Nyman S. Generation of new bone around titanium implants using a membrane technique: An experimental study in rabbits. Int J Oral Maxillofac Implants 1989;4:19–25.

31. Falk H. On occlusal forces in dentitions with implant-supported fixed cantilever prostheses. Swed Dent J 1990;69(supplement).

32. Davis DM, Rimrott R, Zarb GA. Studies on frameworks for osseointegrated prostheses: Part 2. The effect of adding acrylic resin or porcelain to form the occlusal superstructure. Int J Oral Maxillofac Implants 1988; 3:275–280.

33. Rangert B, Jemt T, Lars L. Forces and moments on Brånemark implants. Int J Oral Maxillofac Implants 1989;4:241–247.

Tissue-Integrated Implants Ad Modum Brånemark in the Rehabilitation of Partially Edentulous Jaws

I. Ericsson, P.-O. Glantz, and P.-I. Brånemark

Tooth loss may cause disturbances of masticatory function and comfort as well as psychological disturbances. Until recently the methods of choice for rehabilitation involved conventional fixed prostheses, removable partial dentures, and/or in some patients, orthodontic tooth movements.[1] Some of these methods are, however, associated with disadvantages such as loss of tooth substance and a potential risk for loss of tooth vitality. Some patients present severe retention problems for a fixed restoration and/or a removable partial denture. In addition, the prognosis for prosthetic treatment can be complicated by carious lesions, progression of periodontal disease, or technical failures, such as loss of retention and fracture of bridge components or abutment teeth.[2–5]

In the treatment of severe periodontal disease, destruction of the supporting tissues has often reached a level where extraction of several teeth cannot be avoided. This means that in following periodontal treatment for such patients, only a few teeth may remain—teeth that not only have reduced periodontal tissue support but also may exhibit pronounced hypermobility.[4,6] There may be an obvious need for prosthetic treatment to restore lost oral functions, improve esthetics, and stabilize mobile teeth. The fixed prosthesis is well suited to fulfill these requirements.[2,6–8]

In 1926, Ante's law[9] was published. This law states that "the combined pericemental area of the abutment teeth should be equal to or greater than that of the teeth to be replaced" with the use of fixed prostheses. A consequence of Ante's law has been that partially dentate jaws, especially in cases where the abutment teeth are unfavorably distributed in relation to the fabrication of a fixed restoration, have usually been treated with removable partial dentures. During the last two decades a series of studies have been published demonstrating the long-term success of treatment, which includes both periodontal and prosthodontic measures in patients with advanced loss of periodontal tissues.[2,6–8] These prosthodontically restored dentitions have thus definitely not fulfilled the demands originally outlined in Ante's law.[9] One reason for extending the indications for fixed prostheses is that the fixed restoration can more favorably distribute the masticatory forces to the remaining periodontium than a removable partial denture. In addition, most patients find a fixed prosthesis much more comfortable than a removable one.

Potential risks incurred with the use of extensive fixed prostheses include loss of retention between an abutment and the restoration as well as fractures of the metal component of the prosthesis or of abutment teeth.[3–5] In 1982, Nyman and Ericsson[7] stated that "the limitations for fixed bridgework in patients with few abutment teeth and reduced periodontal tissue support around these teeth are related to the technical and biomechanical problems involved in the fabrication of the bridges rather than to the biological capacity of the remaining periodontium to support the bridges successfully." Sometimes there may be a need to use implants as additional abutments for fixed pros-

Table 1 Partially dentate jaws

Type I: Separate units
Type II: Integrated into tooth-supported
          restorations
          A. Rigid one-piece prosthesis
          B. Implant- and tooth-supported
             segments are joined together through
             incorporation of precision-type
             attachments

thodontic restorations. Patients who have lost all teeth posterior to the canine can be candidates for such treatment, especially when the goal is to place a cross-arch prosthesis following appropriate periodontal treatment. Furthermore, patients with one or both jaws totally edentulous have been treated (under secure and predictable conditions) during the last 20 to 25 years with fixed prostheses using osseointegrated titanium implants ad modum Brånemark as abutments.[10–13]

The encouraging results regarding tissue-integrated titanium implants to support fixed restorations in edentulous jaws for long periods of time have prompted us to use such implants as additional abutments for fixed prostheses in partially edentulous patients.

The purpose of this report is to describe different designs of restorations using osseointegrated titanium fixtures as additional abutments for fixed prostheses in partially dentate jaws.

Patient selection

For this type of rehabilitation, the prerestorative periodontal treatment phase must be successful. Thus, the only patients who can be considered for implant placement are those for whom such treatment has been carried out with optimal results.

In addition to a lasting successful clinical result of the periodontal treatment, a second requirement is the presence of critical amounts of healthy bone in which to place the implants. The criteria used for this evaluation have been presented in detail by Lekholm and Zarb.[14]

The surgical and prosthodontic techniques do not differ from the well-known approach described by Brånemark and collaborators.[15] The presence of teeth can, however, offer certain additional difficulties, particularly in the selection of implant locations and directions.

Types of restorations

Implant-supported fixed partial dentures can be designed as separate units (type I) or integrated into tooth-supported restorations (type II) (Table 1). Type I cases generally exhibit biomechanically less complicated situations than type II cases and are also easier to handle from a clinical-technical point of view. Consequently, type I designs are preferred whenever the remaining abutment teeth exhibit no or only minor reduction in alveolar bone support, and where no splinting of the remaining teeth is required (Figs 1a and b). The ultimate type I reconstruction is that which replaces a single missing tooth (15).

In patients with marked reduction of the supporting alveolar bone and hypermobile teeth, the connected type II prosthesis should be used. The reason for this is the obvious risk that with time chewing forces may tilt the remaining natural teeth buccally or lingually. In the type II group there are two fundamentally different designs (A and B). Type II A is the rigid one-piece design (Figs 2a and b). Type II B is the prosthesis in which the implant and tooth-supported segments are joined through incorporation of precision-type attachments (Figs 3a to d).

The choice between rigid one-piece and attachment-connected multipiece prostheses is often based on an evaluation of the positions and status of the remaining teeth. The introduction of attachments between the implant and tooth-supported segments facilitates elimination of some of the functional stresses that are created as a result of the inherent biomechanical variations between nonmobile implants and hypermobile teeth with reduced periodontal support. The use of attachments can therefore

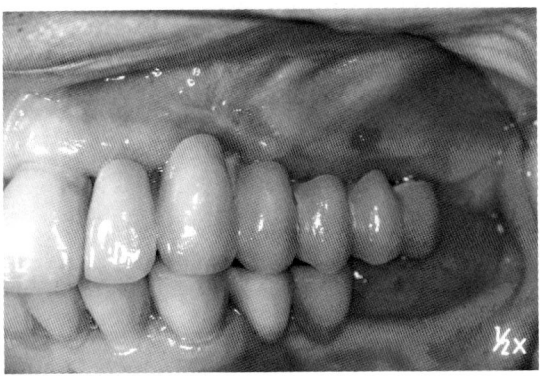
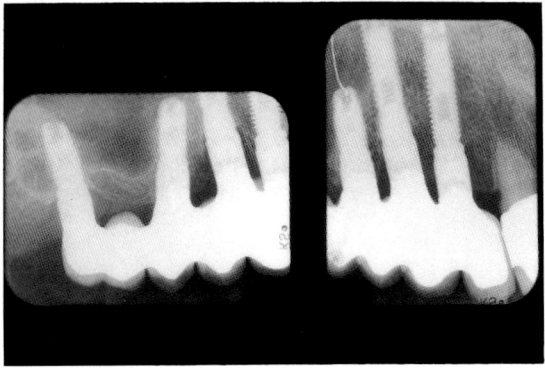

Figs 1a and b The clinical and radiographic appearance 1 year following placement of a type I prosthesis extending from tooth 17 to tooth 12 and supported by four implants.

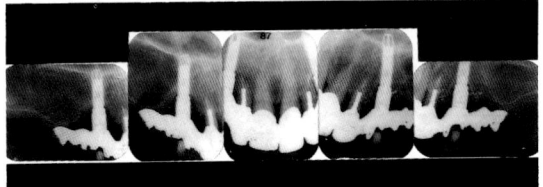
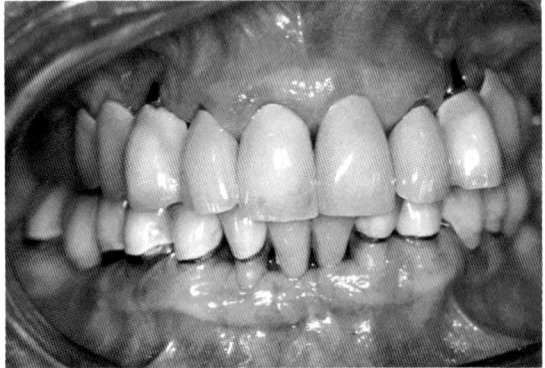

Figs 2a and b The clinical and radiographic appearance of a type II A prosthesis 3 years following insertion. The patient has an extensive maxillary sinus, making it impossible to place more than one implant on each side distally to teeth 12 and 22, respectively. Teeth 12, 11, 21, and 22 are together with the two implants serving as abutments for the fixed cross-arch restoration extending from tooth 15 to tooth 25.

be looked upon as a safety measure in cases that are difficult to prognosticate accurately.

For both technical and clinical reasons there are limited opportunities to incorporate attachments where teeth and implants are mixed in the same area of the treated jaws. In such cases, rigid one-piece prostheses with a complex, and thus not easily definable, biomechanical functional pattern have to be used. In some patients, unexpected bone resorption around the implants has been reported.[16]

Conclusion

When evaluated with clinical criteria, during the initial 8 to 10 years following treatment, a satisfactory outcome of the use of a combination of osseointegrated titanium implants and teeth as abutments for fixed prosthetic reconstructions has been achieved.[16–19] No failures of significance have occurred so far in the patient material. If the encouraging results persist, it seems likely that the basic principle applied in the

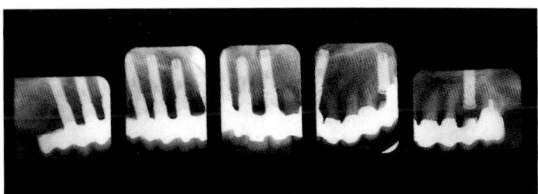
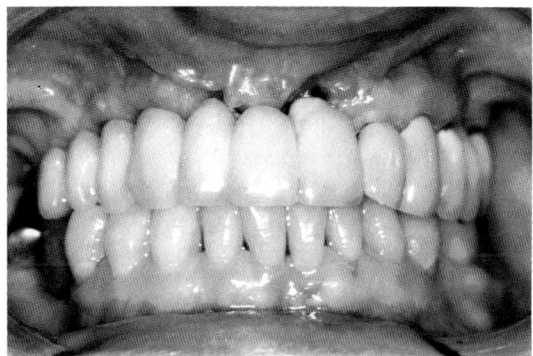
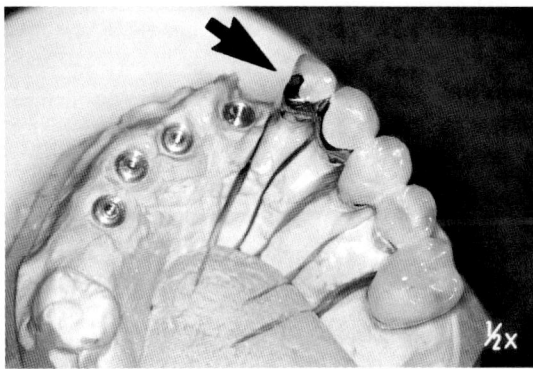
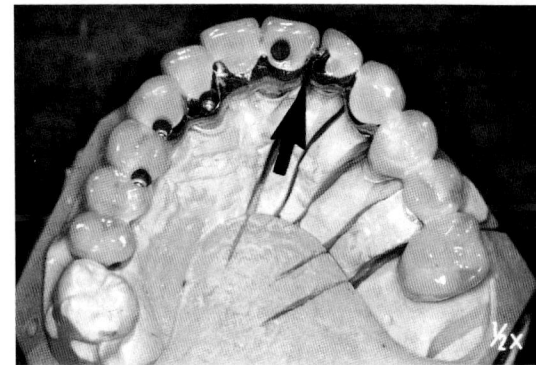

Figs 3a to d The clinical and radiographic appearance of a type II B prosthesis (fabricated in porcelain-fused-to-gold) immediately following insertion. In the "first quadrant" (teeth 15 to 21), four fixtures were placed, while in the second quadrant, following proper periodontal treatment, four abutment teeth were present. An attachment of Boos type *(arrow in c and d)* is placed in the contact area between the tooth- and the fixture-supported segments.

treatment of these patients can be accepted as further advancement of the indications for fixed prosthodontic restorations.

There is presently a rapid trend to extend the use of implants. Many improved or new implant systems have recently been introduced.[20-21] Provided that the implant systems used exhibit the favorable long-term clinical results demonstrated with the Brånemark system, it is likely that in the future, other types of implants will provide an additional means to increase the clinical, functional life of teeth with markedly reduced periodontal support.

References

1. Follin M. Orthodontic movement of maxillary incisor into the midline. A case report. *Swed Dent J* 1985;9:9–13.
2. Nyman S, Lindhe J. A longitudinal study of combined periodontal and prosthetic treatment of patients with advanced periodontal disease. *J Periodontol* 1970;50: 163–169.
3. Glantz PO, Nyman S. Technical and biophysical aspects of fixed partial dentures for patients with reduced periodontal support. *J Prosthet Dent* 1982;47:47–51.
4. Glantz PO, Nyman S. Technical and biophysical aspects of crown and bridge therapy. pp 549–562 In J. Lindhe (ed) *Textbook of Clinical Periodontology*, 2nd ed. Copenhagen: Munksgaard, 1989.
5. Randow K, Glantz PO, Zöger B. Technical failures and some related clinical complications in extensive fixed

prosthodontics. An epidemiological study of long-term clinical quality. *Acta Odontol Scand* 1986;44:241–255.

6. Lindhe J, Nyman S. Occlusal therapy. pp 534–548 In J. Lindhe (ed) *Textbook of Clinical Periodontology,* 2nd ed. Copenhagen: Munksgaard, 1989.

7. Nyman S, Ericsson I. The capacity of reduced periodontal tissues to support fixed bridgework. *J Clin Periodontol* 1982;50:163–169.

8. Nyman S, Lindhe J, Lundgren D. The role of occlusion for the stability of fixed bridges in patients with reduced periodontal tissue support. *J Clin Periodontol* 1975; 2:53–66.

9. Ante IH. The fundamental principles of abutments. Thesis. *Michigan State Dental Society Bulletin* 1926; 8:14–23.

10. Brånemark P-I, Hansson BO, Adell R, Breine U, Lindström J, Hallén O, et al. Osseointegrated implants in the treatment of the edentulous jaw. Experience from a 10-year period. *Scand J Plast Reconstr Surg* 1977;11(suppl 16).

11. Adell R, Lekholm U, Rockler B, Brånemark P-I. A 15-year study of osseointegrated implants in the treatment of the edentulous jaw. *Int J Oral Surg* 1981;6:387–416.

12. Adell R. Long-term results. pp 175–186 In P.-I. Brånemark, G.A. Zarb, T. Albrektsson (eds) *Tissue-Integrated Prostheses: Osseointegration in Clinical Dentistry.* Chicago: Quintessence Publ Co, 1985.

13. Lindquist LW, Carlsson GE, Glantz PO. Rehabilitation of the edentulous mandible with a tissue-integrated fixed prosthesis: A six year longitudinal study. *Quintessence Int* 1987;18:89–96.

14. Lekholm U, Zarb GA. Patient selection and preparation. pp 199–209 In P.-I. Brånemark, G.A. Zarb, T. Albrektsson (eds) *Tissue-Integrated Prostheses: Osseointegration in Clinical Dentistry.* Chicago: Quintessence Publ Co, 1985.

15. Brånemark P-I, Zarb GA, Albrektsson T (eds) *Tissue-Integrated Prostheses: Osseointegration in Clinical Dentistry.* Chicago: Quintessence Publ Co, 1985.

16. Ericsson I, Lekholm U, Brånemark P-I, Lindhe J, Glantz PO, Nyman S. A clinical evaluation of fixed-bridge restorations supported by the combination of teeth and osseointegrated titanium implants. *J Clin Periodontol* 1986;13:307–312.

17. Ericsson I, Glantz PO, Brånemark P-I. Use of implants in restorative therapy in patients with reduced periodontal tissue support. *Quintessence Int* 1988;19: 801–807.

18. van Steenberghe D, et al. A retrospective multicenter evaluation of the survival rate of osseointegrated fixtures supporting fixed partial dentures in the treatment of partial edentulism. *J Prosthet Dent* 1989;61: 217–223.

19. Jemt T, Lekholm U, Adell R. Osseointegrated implants in the treatment of partially edentulous patients: A preliminary study on 876 consecutively placed fixtures. *Int J Oral Maxillofac Implants* 1989;4:211–217.

20. Albrektsson T, Zarb GA, Worthington P, Eriksson AR. The long-term efficacy of currently used dental implants: A review and proposed criteria of success. *Int J Oral Maxillofac Implants* 1986;1:11–25.

21. Arvidson K, Bystedt H, Ericsson I. Histometric and ultrastructural studies of tissues surrounding Astra dental implants in dogs. *Int J Oral Maxillofac Implants* 1990;5:127–134.

A Comparative Study Between Brånemark and IMZ Implants Supporting Overdentures: Prosthetic Considerations

I. Naert, M. Quirynen, D. van Steenberghe, and P. Darius

Complete dentures can fulfill the aim of esthetic oral rehabilitation by means of replacing the teeth and providing soft tissue support. However, complete dentures have not been equally successful for restoring oral function. Reduction of stability, retention, and load-bearing capacity[1] have been considered major factors in this compromised functional capacity. Edentulousness can lead to feelings of insecurity and considerable psychosocial problems.[2] Although phonetic and esthetic problems may be more easily managed with overdentures than with a fixed bridge, the predominant motivation for choosing overdenture therapy is generally economical and morphological in nature. The functional benefits of complete dentures supported and retained by natural tooth roots[3] and implants[4,5] have been documented. It is tempting therefore to adapt the osseointegration concept to the overdenture method in patients who accept wearing removable dentures but who will not or cannot afford much treatment expense.

From long-term studies of Brånemark implants supporting fixed protheses, it appears that failures are concentrated at the time of abutment surgery or during the first year.[6] Since the same experience seems to apply for overdentures, one can cautiously extrapolate the overdenture data in a long-term perspective. However, there are clinical differences between overdentures and fixed bridges. Preliminary results[7,8] and medium-term results[9–11] indicate the good potential of this technique using Brånemark implants. Although the IMZ implant has been available for about 10 years,[12] documented comparative followup studies of its use are scarce.[13] The most remarkable differences between these implants is the micro- (microgrooved versus micro-grained) and macroscopic (screw shaped versus cylindrical) surface and the use of an elastic intramobile element (IME), reported to function as a shock absorbing device designed to simulate the function of the periodontal ligament.[14] Both implants are made of commercially pure titanium but differences at the molecular level cannot be fully assessed with the presently available technology.[15]

The aim of the present study was to determine whether, from a prosthetic point of view, the same success can be expected for overdentures supported by IMZ implants as compared to Brånemark implants. Moreover, prosthetic factors have been investigated to explain differences in the rate of marginal bone loss between both systems as reported elsewhere in a companion paper concerned with the periodontal aspects.[16]

Materials

Patients

From November 1984 to May 1988, two Brånemark implants (Nobelpharma AB, Göteborg, Sweden) were placed in either the maxillae or mandibles of 86 consecutive patients at the

Table 1 Descriptive statistics for the Brånemark and the IMZ group

	Brånemark		IMZ	
	Maxilla	Mandible	Maxilla	Mandible
No. patients	6	80	3 (1)*	70
No. loaded implants	12	161{2}‡	9{5}	146{3}
Age at implant insertion, NS	53.5 (34–73)†	56.9 (32–77) SD:10.8	44.5 (29–59)	57.3 (26–74) SD:10.5
Sex: women/men	4/2	58/22	4/0	52/18
Bone quality NS	2.5 (1–4) SD:1	2.17 (1–4) SD:0.6	3(/) SD:0	2.1 (2–3) SD:0.3
Resorption anatomy NS	4.7 (3–5) SD:0.8	2.3 (1–5) SD:1.0	2.5 (2–3) SD:0.5	2.3 (1–4) SD:0.7
Antagonistic dental status				
Complete dentures %	—	85.6	—	86.6
Partial dentures %	—	12.2	—	13.4
Implant bridge %	—	2.2	—	—

*Patient never rehabilitated because of early implant loss.
†Numbers in parentheses indicate a range.
‡Numbers in braces indicate implants lost before loading.
NS = not significant for mandibles.

University Clinic, Leuven, Belgium. The surgery was performed according to the principles of osseointegration and the instruction manual for the Brånemark Implant System. In another clinical center in Belgium, two to four IMZ implants (Friedrichsfeld GmbH, Mannheim, Germany) were placed in one of the jaws of 74 consecutive patients during approximately the same period. The surgical and prosthetic procedures that followed were those written in the instruction manual (Das IMZ Manual, A. Kirsch and K.L. Ackerman, Germany).

The descriptive statistics are summarized in Table 1. Statistical analysis revealed no significant difference between the two groups for parameters such as age, sex, antagonistic dental status, bone quality, and resorption anatomy.[17] In both centers, the bone quality of the patients treated was moderate for both maxillae and mandibles and the resorption degree was moderate for the mandible and moderate to severe for the maxilla.[16] The frequency distribution of the number of years of edentulousness for the mandibles for different age categories and for both groups is reported in Fig 1. The mean time of edentulousness for the Brånemark group and

the IMZ group was 8.3 years (SD = 9.7) and 8.9 years (SD = 8.9), respectively; (P = .6). The mental foramen was located on the crest of the alveolar ridge in 29% and in 15% of the patients for the Brånemark and the IMZ groups, respectively. Distribution of the number of patients by number of previous complete mandibular dentures for different age categories for both groups is depicted in Fig 2. The mean number of previous complete dentures for the Brånemark group was 2.5 (SD = 2.1, range 0 to 6) and 1.6 for the IMZ group (SD = 1.3, range 0 to 6).

The main complaints with the old mandibular dentures were functional in 67.6% and 94.6%, cosmetic in 6.8% and 1.8%, and psychosocial in 25.7% and 3.6% for the Brånemark and the IMZ groups, respectively. In both centers, for the mandible the original rehabilitation plan consisted of an overdenture. For the Brånemark group, only two implants per maxilla could be placed because of the lack of sufficient bone to place more for the support of a fixed prosthesis.

Implants

A total of 175 Brånemark implants, 12 in the

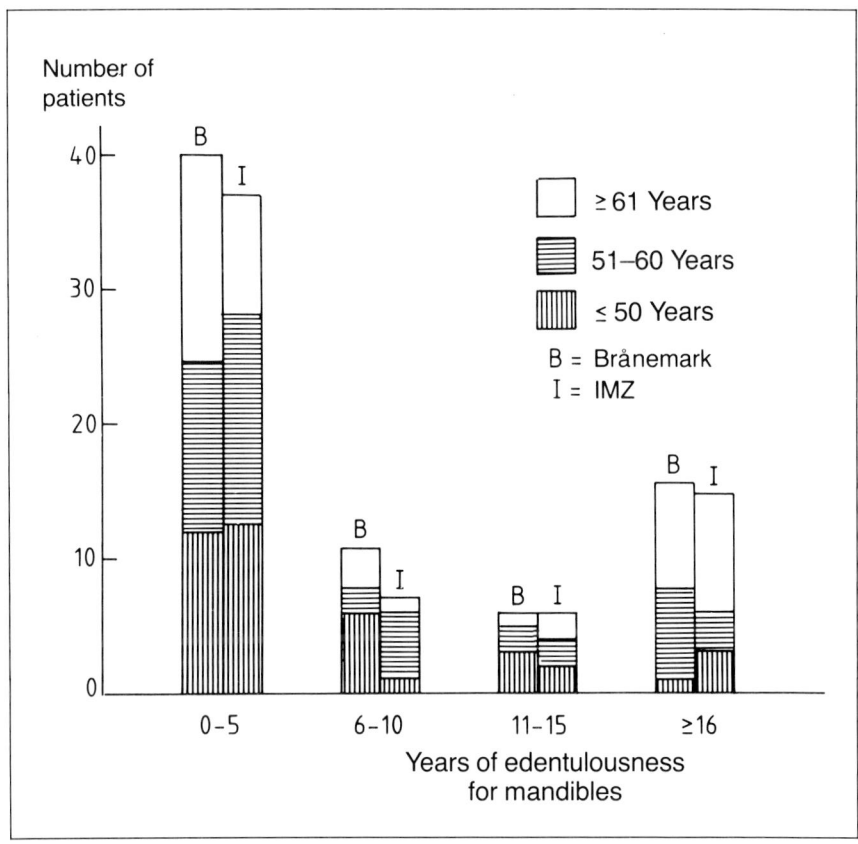

Fig 1 Frequency distribution of the number of years of edentulousness for the mandibles in different age categories and centers.

maxillae and 163 in the mandibles have been placed. One hundred sixty-three IMZ implants were inserted, of which 14 were in maxillae and 149 in mandibles. Mean implant lengths in the mandible for the Brånemark implants and the IMZ implants were 12.9 mm (SD = 2.6) and 13.5 mm (SD = 2.6) (P = .02), respectively. Distribution of the length of the loaded implants by center is summarized elsewhere.[16]

All Brånemark implants had a diameter of 3.75 mm, whereas the diameter of the IMZ implants was either 3.3 or 4 mm. The choice of implant diameter depended on the bone width. Four-millimeter IMZ implants were used in the maxilla in 36% of the patients and in 93% of the mandibles.

The frequency distribution of mandibular overdentures by year is depicted in Fig 3. The mean loading time for Brånemark implants in both maxillae and mandibles was 15 months (SD = 14.4, range 3 to 38) and 17.5 months (SD = 11.9, range 2 to 51), respectively. For the IMZ group, the mean loading time in the maxillae and mandibles was 8.5 months (SD = 3.4, range 5 to 12) and 25.4 months (SD = 11.6, range 7 to 49), respectively. The IMZ implants in mandibles had been loaded significantly longer (P < .01). The low number of patients with implants in the maxillae did not allow any statistical analysis between the two groups.

For both systems, in the mandible two implants were placed in the parasymphyseal area (the canine region in more than 95% of the patients) and connected by a line parallel to the

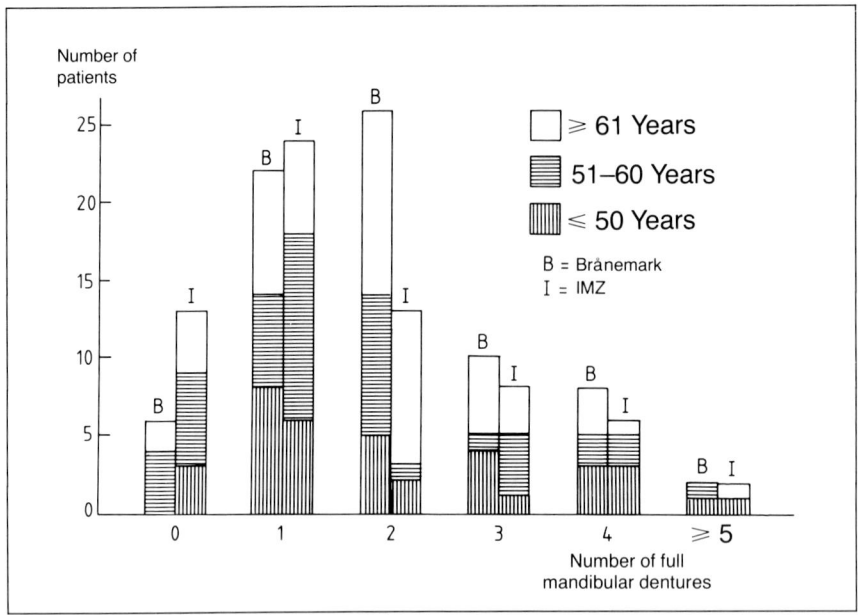

Fig 2 Distribution of the number of patients by number of previous complete mandibular dentures in different age categories and centers.

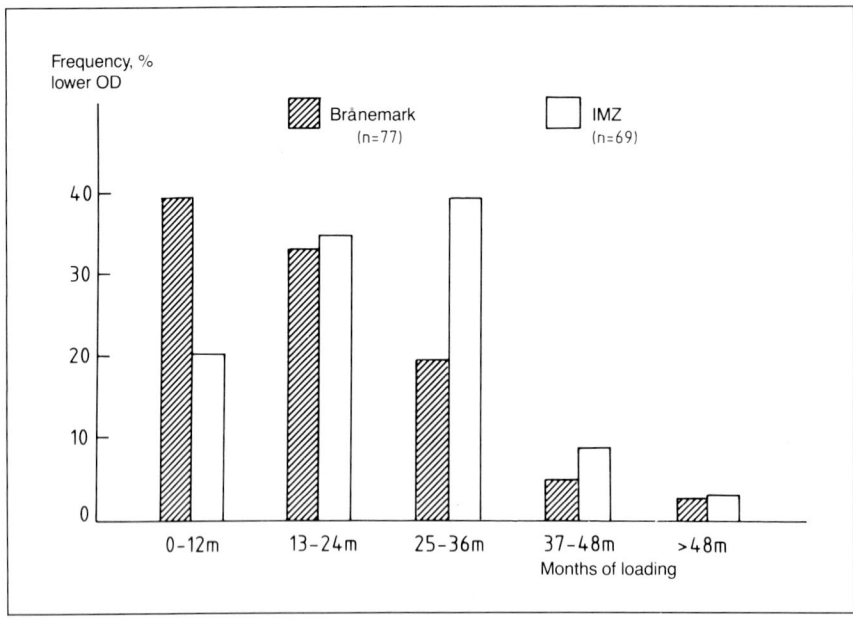

Fig 3 Frequency distribution of loaded mandibular overdentures by year for both centers (*OD* = overdentures).

Table 2 Different attachment systems per jaw and per center

Attachment system	Implant type	Number of patients		Implants per patient	
		Maxilla	Mandible	Maxilla	Mandible
Bar	Brånemark	1	78	2	2
	IMZ	1 (1*/1†)	70	4	2{67}‡ or 4{3}
Ball attachment	Brånemark	4	—	2	—
	IMZ	1	—	3	—
Magnets	Brånemark	1	2	2	2{1} or 3{1}
	IMZ	—	—	—	—

*Planned, but not performed due to implant loss.
†Not examined because of implant loss before final examination.
‡Numbers in braces indicate number of jaws within which implants were placed.

terminal mandibular hinge axis. Three to four implants were placed in the other mandibles. The mean interabutment distances in the mandible for the Brånemark group and the IMZ group were 20 mm (SD = 4.4, range 8 to 29) and 21.5 mm (SD = 4.8, range 10 to 35), respectively. In the maxilla, only two implants per jaw were inserted in the Brånemark group, while four were used for the IMZ group.

Attachment system

Table 2 summarizes the different attachment systems used in each center. In the mandible, bars were used on two implants in all but two patients in the Brånemark group and in all but three patients in the IMZ group, for whom four implants were used. In the Brånemark group, Dolder-type bars (no. 53.01.2, Cendres et Metaux SA, Biel, Switzerland) and in the IMZ group, Ackerman-type bars (no. 55.01.2, Cendres et Metaux SA, Biel, Switzerland) were used. The length of the retention clip (10 to 18 mm) in the Brånemark group and the number of the retention clips (two to three) in the IMZ group depended upon interabutment distance. A space maintainer of 0.75 mm for the Brånemark group and 0.50 mm for the IMZ group was placed between the bar and the retention clip before processing the overdenture. For the maxillae, in all but two patients nonsplinted attachments were used, eg, ball-attachments (Nobelpharma AB, Göteborg, Sweden; Friedrichsfeld GmbH, Mannheim, Germany) and rare earth Jackson magnets (Solid State Inn, Inc, Mount Airy, NC).

Prosthetic design

In this study all but five overdentures had a resilient design, which permitted free rotation during occlusal loading. This scheme resulted in a twist-free load transmission to the implants in a nearly axial direction.[8] A nonresilient design was used when four implants were utilized. All overdentures were made according to traditional removable prosthodontic principles and techniques on a semi-adjustable articulator (Dentatus ARH, Stockholm, Sweden). The teeth used on the overdenture were acrylic resin (Ivoclar AG, Lichtenstein). All mandibular overdentures in the Brånemark group were reinforced by a chrome-cobalt framework (Fig 4); no reinforcement was used in the IMZ group.

The principles of occlusion and articulation used in both centers were the same. This meant equal and simultaneous contact in centric relation without interfering premature contacts and a balanced articulation without anterior contact. At the insertion of the complete dentures, occlusion and articulation were refined and new jaw relation records were made when necessary.

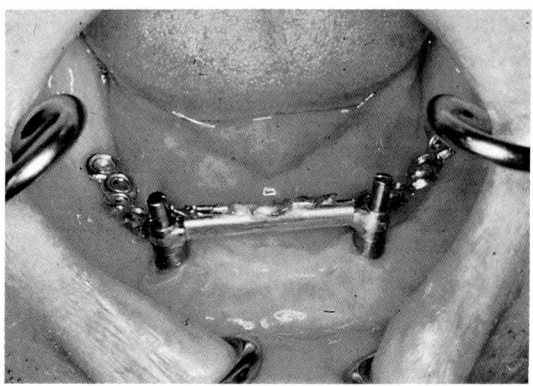

Fig 4 For the Brånemark group, the mandibular resin base was reinforced by a Cr-Co framework, to which the retention clip was soldered.

The retention clips were adjusted at insertion of the overdenture to prevent dislodgment by extra wide mouth opening and extreme tongue movement.

One-fifth of the patients in the Brånemark group and half of the patients in the IMZ group had not worn a conversion prosthesis between the time of implant placement and abutment connection.

Methods

Data collection

All consecutive patients (86) treated with an overdenture supported by Brånemark implants or IMZ implants (74), who were operated on before May 1988 were recalled. Three patients in the Brånemark group and one patient in the IMZ group did not respond because they preferred to remain with their own dentist who did the regular followup. The treatment results of these patients were discussed with the colleagues by telephone. The other patients were all seen by the same prosthodontist (IN) and periodontist (MQ).

Osseointegration and marginal bone loss

A well-known definition[18] of implant success provides for an annual bone loss of less than 0.2 mm after the first year and has been used as a criterion in the present study. However, a higher annual bone loss does not necessarily imply failure, even in the long term, should this process be continuous. From a previous study, it is known that in some patients the mean change in marginal bone height was somewhat higher than 0.2 mm/year for the Brånemark group, but was compatible with long-term survival.[11] An implant was considered to be a failure: *(1)* when a freely standing implant showed the slightest sign of mobility, *(2)* when a peri-implant radiolucency could be detected radiographically, and finally, *(3)* if the implant showed any sign or symptom of pain or infection. Close bone apposition was assessed clinically and radiographically. After detaching the bars, implant mobility was also measured by means of the Periotest (Siemens AG, Bensheim, West Germany).[19,20] This is an electronic device that is used to quantify the damping characteristics of the implant and the surrounding tissues. At the recall visit, intraoral radiographs were taken, using the paralleling technique to evaluate the close bone apposition for each individual implant, and the marginal bone level was scored. Bone height was defined as the mean distance between the fixture-abutment connection and the marginal bone level mesially and distally from the implant, and was estimated to the nearest 0.5 mm.[16] The change of marginal bone height was estimated by comparing these radiographs with those taken at the time of abutment connection.

Prosthetic parameters

The following prosthetic parameters were considered: occlusion and articulation, number of relines, and all complications with implant components and overdentures that had arisen between recall visits.

Retentive force for the mandibular overdenture was quantified by means of a dynamometer (Correx, Bern, Switzerland) with a maximal capacity of 20 N (1 kgf = 9.807 N). A metal loop was fixed onto the mandibular overdenture just above the bar. This loop was fixed to the dynamometer by a wire. A vertical force was applied to dislodge the overdenture (Fig 5). Three measurements were made for each overdenture and the mean score was calculated. Interinvestigator (IN and MQ) and intrainvestigator reproducibility was statistically assessed and the confidence interval calculated.

To investigate in vivo the differences in lateral stress breaking effect between the polyoxymethylene IME (type DH) and the titanium IME, as well as the aging effect of the former, the Periotest values (PTV) of these devices were determined. On top of the IME a 3-mm gold cylinder was tightened, toward which the rod of the Periotest was directed. To prevent fracture of the old IME (an IME in function for at least 6 months) during unscrewing, the Periotest value with the latter in place was first measured. The mean of two repeated scores was calculated. Soft tissue complications such as mucositis and traumatic ulcerations, soreness, and hyperplasia were also registered.

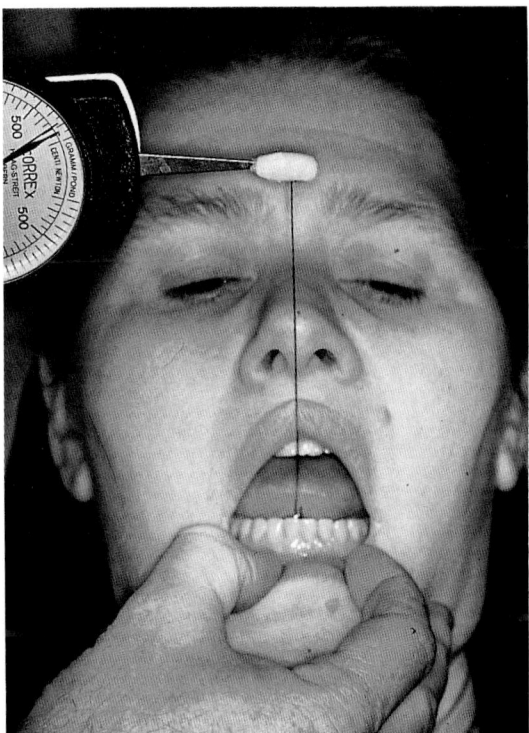

Fig 5 Overdenture retentive force measurements were made by means of a dynamometer. A metal loop was attached to the overdenture, just above the bar to which the wire connecting the dynamometer was fixed.

Patient reactions

At the final examination, the patients' subjective assessment of the denture treatment was solicited. They were also asked to compare the present situation with the original. The assessment was made on a discontinuous analog scale ranging from 1 to 9. Reactions to the overdenture treatment were also related to the amount of jaw resorption. The impact of treatment modality on patient satisfaction was only evaluated for those wearing the overdenture for at least 1 year. The first year was disregarded to avoid the impact of preliminary side effects such as traumatic ulcerations and adaptation.

Statistical analysis

Statistical analysis was performed by means of the statistical analysis system (SAS). Differ-

ences in age, sex, years of edentulism, bone quality and anatomy, antagonistic dental status, implant length, and loading time for both centers were analyzed by means of a t test for equal and unequal variances. To assess the relationship between the number of IME fractures by year and interabutment distances, retentive forces of the overdenture and day and night wearing of the overdenture, Pearson correlation coefficients (r) were computed. The same test was used to reveal any relationship between the objective and subjective measured retention forces of the overdenture and the interabutment distances for both groups combined.

Differences between the systems regarding patient response before and after overdenture therapy, overdenture satisfaction, and differences in overdenture retentive force were as-

Table 3 Overdenture complications (n/total number)

	Brånemark group		IMZ group	
	Max-illa	Man-dible	Max-illa	Man-dible
Overdenture parts				
• Cr-Co fracture	0/2	1/78	—	—
• Corrosion of Jackson magnets	2/2	5/5	—	—
• O-ring box fracture	2/8	—	0/3	—
• Relining	0.6	14/77	0/2	11/69
Opposing complete denture fracture	0/6	7/71	0/2	2/67

sessed by means of the one-way analysis of variance.

For calculation of the interexaminer reproducibility of the overdenture retentive force, all measurements (mean, n = 22) performed by IN and by MQ were examined by means of an analysis of variance with the retentive force as a dependent variable and with the subject and investigator as sources. To estimate the variation between investigators and variation between the three repeated measurements from the same investigator, the $F-$ value was calculated via the mean square of the variations between the investigators over the mean square of the variations between repeated measurements.

Results

Implant loss after loading

During overdenture function in the mandibles for both groups, no implants were lost or showed any mobility or symptoms of pain or infection. In the maxillae the Brånemark group, no implants were lost, while for the IMZ group two implants failed within the same patient after 1 year of loading.

Overdenture failure

All overdentures (86) in the Brånemark group, in maxillae as well as the mandibles, were still in function at the final examination. For overdentures supported by IMZ implants, all prostheses (70) in the mandibles were still in function at the final recall visit; in the maxillae, two of four patients had to revert to complete dentures. In one of these patients, all implants (four) were lost before the abutment connection; in the second patient, all implants (two) failed after 1 year of loading.

Marginal bone loss

At the abutment connection, marginal bone height around the IMZ and Brånemark implants was located at 0.70 and 0.90 mm, respectively, below the implant abutment attachment. For loaded implants, both during the first year of bone healing and remodeling as well as during the following years, the rate of bone loss was found to be significantly higher for the IMZ group. This has also been demonstrated by the estimation of attachment level calculated from the pocket depth and height of the gingival recession.

Complications

For the Brånemark group, complications with maxillary overdentures were related to the attachment systems (Table 3). Previous experience with the Jackson magnets made us abandon their application. Corrosion, rapid loss of retention, and extreme wear were the main reasons for this decision. O-ring box fracture occurred twice in eight O-rings, although they were in function only 5 months.

For the IMZ group, complications were concentrated at the level of the IME. The number of fractures by 1 year was 0.55. For the entire observation period, 0.92 IME per year had been renewed for prophylactic reasons or because of fracture. No correlation could be found between

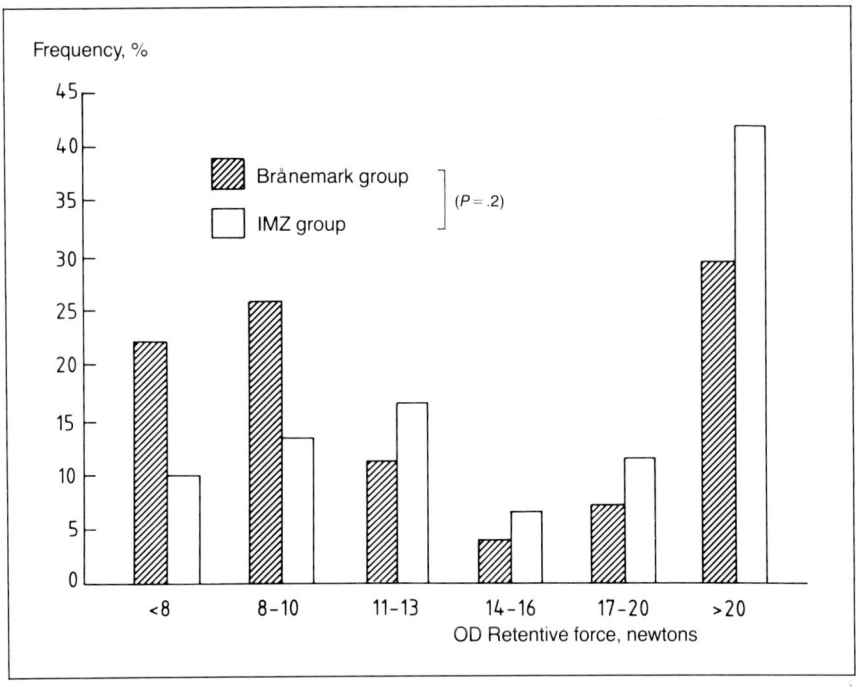

Fig 6 Overdenture retentive force distribution for both groups, mandibles only (*OD* = overdenture).

the number of IME fractures and factors such as the interabutment distance ($r = -.09$, $P = .4$), retentive force of the overdenture ($r = .15$, $P = .2$) or day and night wearing of the prosthesis ($r = -.17$, $P = .1$).

Opposing complete denture fracture occurred in 10% of the Brånemark group and in 3% of the IMZ group. One chrome-cobalt reinforced prosthesis fractured in the Brånemark group, none in the IMZ group. For both study groups, nearly one-fifth of the overdentures had been relined once during the observation period.

Mucositis was noted in 8% and 9% in the mandibles, soreness in 7% and 3%, and ulcer decubitis in 2.7% and 0% for the Brånemark and IMZ groups, respectively. Hyperplasia (defined as any augmentation of the gingiva around the abutments up to a distance of 5 mm) was found around 20% of the Brånemark implants and 14% of the IMZ implants and scored.

However, treatment was only needed in a few patients (5 and 3, respectively).

Overdenture retention

Good interexaminer reproducibility ($P = .6$) was achieved for prosthesis retention force measurements. For repeated measurements performed within the same patient, the inter- and intraexaminer variation was not different ($P = .6$). The 95% confidence interval, calculated from three consecutive scores, was 0.1 N.

Frequency distribution of the retentive force for both systems is graphically depicted in Fig 6. The mean force was 13 N (range 5.5 to 20 N) and 15.3 N (range 4.3 to 20 N) for the Brånemark and IMZ groups, respectively. The difference was not statistically different ($P = .2$). When the data for both systems were pooled, there was no correlation between the retentive

Table 4 Frequency distribution (%) of nonsatisfied patients before and after 1 year of overdenture treatment*

Problem	Before		After	
	Brånemark	IMZ	Brånemark	IMZ
Pain	53.6	53.6	4.9	0
Psychological	46.3	26.8	0	2.4
Retention	92.6	92.6	0	0
Social	51.2	46.3	0	0
Speech	80.4	70.7	0	0

*For the Brånemark and IMZ groups (n = 41).

force and the interabutment distance ($r = .06$, $P = .5$), nor between the subjectively rated retentive force of the overdentures ($r = .03$, $P = .7$).

Stress-breaking effect of the IME

When the old polyoxymethylene IME (n = 62) was replaced by a new polyoxymethylene IME, the mean Periotest value decreased significantly ($P = .001$) from $+3.09$ to $+2.13$, and when the new polyoxymethylene IME was replaced by a titanium IME, a further significant decrease ($P = .001$) could be observed (from $+2.13$ to $+0.65$).

Patients' reactions

The changes in negative subjective experiences before and after prosthesis therapy for patients wearing overdentures for at least 1 year are summarized for both centers in Table 4. The questions posed to the patients were:

- Did you have pain or ulcerations with your old denture?
- Were you obsessed with your old denture?
- Did you have retention problems when chewing with your old denture?
- Were you inhibited in social contacts when talking with your old denture?
- Did you have problems when talking with your old denture?

These questions were repeated concerning the new overdenture. After overdenture treatment, 4.9% of the patients in the Brånemark group revealed pain and 2.4% still had psychological problems with overdentures in the IMZ group.

Patients with limited jaw resorption (resorption anatomy 1 and 2) did not respond differently from those with severe bone loss (resorption anatomy 3, 4, and 5) as noted in both groups (Fig 7).

Patients' reactions to overdenture treatment for both groups were very positive regarding their own satisfaction with function and comfort, with mean values approximately 8.5 (Table 5). There was no difference between the groups except for the retention factor in the IMZ group, in which a significantly better score was obtained ($P = .05$).

More than 96% of the patients answered that their expectations had been fulfilled after overdenture therapy, without any significant differences between the groups ($P = .3$). Prior to treatment, 27.9% never or seldom wore their mandibular dentures in the Brånemark group, while this figure was 22.2% for the IMZ group. After overdenture fabrication, all patients in both groups wore their prostheses during the whole day.

Before overdenture therapy, adhesives were used in the mandibles by 58.6% of the Brånemark group and 46.3% of the IMZ group. No patients used adhesives after implant-supported restorations were in use.

Discussion

A long-term followup over a 10-year period, as internationally recommended, should be the goal.[18] However, it is known that if failures occur with Brånemark implants, these usually occur during the healing or remodeling phase.[18] One could extrapolate the present data to a long-term perspective; however, this was only proven for implants supporting fixed prostheses.[6] Whether the same experience applies to IMZ implants remains undocumented.

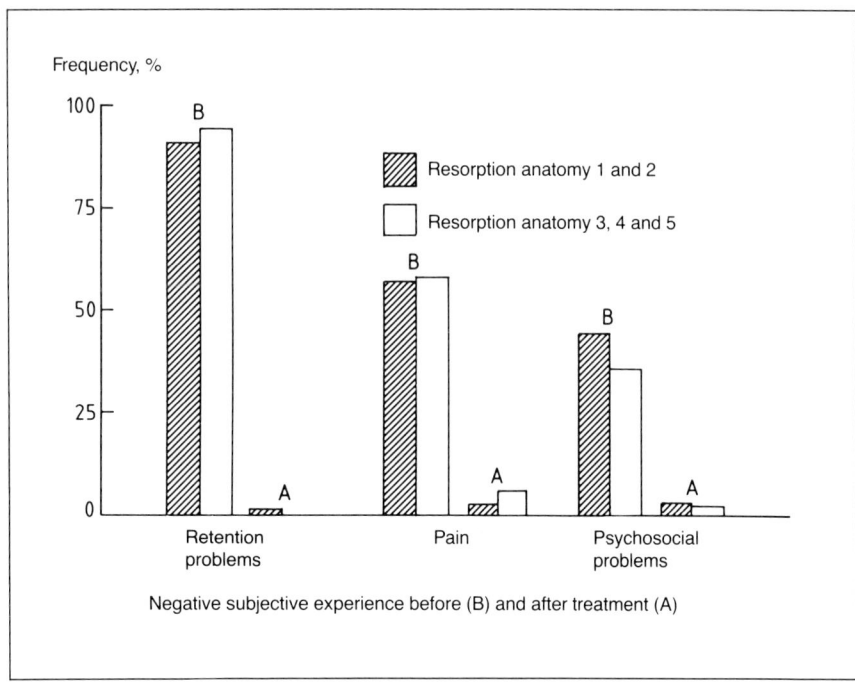

Fig 7 Distribution of patients with negative subjective experience before *(B)* and after *(A)* overdenture treatment according to resorption anatomy.

Table 5 Patient response to overdenture therapy

How do you find your new prosthesis in general?

	1	2	3	4	5	6	7	8	9	
Brånemark	1.4%	—	1.4%	—	5.5%	6.8%	12.3%	16.4%	56.2%	mean: 8.6
IMZ	—	—	—	—	—	1.5%	4.6%	21.5%	72.3%	mean: 8.6

How do you rate the stability of your prosthesis?*

	1	2	3	4	5	6	7	8	9	
Brånemark	1.4%	—	—	1.4%	6.8%	2.7%	9.6%	24.7%	53.4%	mean: 8.3
IMZ	—	—	—	—	1.5%	—	3.1%	13.8%	81.5%	mean: 8.7

How well does your prosthesis function when chewing?

	1	2	3	4	5	6	7	8	9	
Brånemark	1.4%	—	1.4%	1.4%	2.7%	1.4%	13.7%	24.7%	53.4%	mean: 8.4
IMZ	—	—	—	—	—	—	9.2%	18.5%	72.3%	mean: 8.6

How do you find the appearance of your prosthesis?

	1	2	3	4	5	6	7	8	9	
Brånemark	1.4%	—	—	5.5%	4.1%	2.7%	15.1%	19.2%	52.1%	mean: 7.9
IMZ	—	—	1.5%	—	4.6%	—	7.7%	15.4%	70.8%	mean: 8.4

How does your prosthesis function when talking?

	1	2	3	4	5	6	7	8	9	
Brånemark	—	—	1.4%	1.4%	4.1%	2.7%	17.8%	19.2%	53.4%	mean: 8.4
IMZ	—	—	—	—	—	—	7.7%	13.8%	78.5%	mean: 8.7

*Significant difference $P < .05$.

In the mandible, no implants were lost after loading in either group. This is in accordance with the low failure rate (0% to 1%) reported by other centers for the Brånemark[9] and the IMZ[12,13] systems. The range and timing of bone level changes observed around Brånemark implants approaching the zero line after 1 year of loading are similar to those for fixtures supporting fixed prostheses.[21,22] This suggests a favorable prognosis for overdentures in the mandible.

After 2 years, IMZ implants in 20.7% of the patients showed an overall bone loss of 4 mm or more; whereas for the Brånemark implants, such bone loss was not observed in any of the patients.[11,16] Although it seems difficult to establish an exact definition for the rate of bone loss around implants with respect to failure rate, the proportion of "failing" implants for the IMZ implants would increase when extrapolating these data to a long-term perspective. Thus one could question the validity of the assumption that the IME alleviates stress concentrations at the marginal bone level.[14]

In the maxilla category, two IMZ implants failed after 1 year of loading. Bone loss in the maxilla around both implants was considerable. Because of the limited number of maxillary implants involved in the present study, no definite conclusions could be drawn. All overdentures in mandibles for both groups remained in function after a loading time up to 4 years. In the maxillary IMZ group, two patients had to revert to conventional dentures.

The positive results in the mandibles can be explained by the selection of an implant site with optimal bone quality and in which only two fixtures were placed. Moreover, contrary to the Swedish multicenter study,[9] the patient group did not consist of patients in whom prosthesis placement was rendered impossible because not enough abutments remained available. On the contrary, in nearly all but 6% of the patients, a fixed prosthesis on four to six implants was a possible treatment alternative. Financial implications were the primary motivation for overdenture treatment.

Another reason for the success in mandibles may be the prosthesis design itself. By using only two fixtures connected by a bar parallel to the hinge axis, a resilient overdenture design is possible that permits free rotation during occlusal loading and results in a twist-free load transmission to the fixtures in a nearly axial direction.

Although in the Brånemark group all mandibular bar overdentures were reinforced by a chromium-cobalt framework, one fractured because of metal porosity. In the IMZ group, no reinforcement was used and no fractures occurred. The extra financial effort that reinforcement implies may no longer be justified. Fracture of the opposing complete dentures occurred three times as frequently in the Brånemark group as in the IMZ group. However, no conclusions could be drawn because the dentures were fabricated in two different laboratories. The bar concept involves more effort for the practitioner and the technician than the use of magnets, O-rings, or other nonsplinted abutment attachment systems. However, long-term maintenance of the bar design usually involves only activation of the retention clip. Manufacturers of clip attachments should be stimulated to provide a device by which one could objectively quantify retentive force of the clips, thereby preventing overactivation, which could lead to harmful effects on the implant components or the implant/bone interface.

With respect to detrimental effects of anchors on abutment teeth,[23] it has been suggested that these might be influenced by design of the attachment system rather than the retentive force. Damage is more likely to result from overloading caused by the attachments that provide intimate contact of the components during function.[24] Because of the large range in pull-out forces for both systems and the fact that these forces did not correlate with the patients' feelings of overdenture retention, the retentive force for bar overdentures supported by two implants should not exceed 20 N. It is a clinical impression that Ackerman clips could be more precisely activated. The use of Jackson magnets should be discouraged because of corrosion and rapid loss of retention within 1 year. They were not accompanied by adverse tissue reactions in the peri-implant region.

A disturbing complication for the IMZ implant was the frequency of IME (type DH) fracture. Kirsch and Ackerman[12] recommend that the IME be replaced every year. The mean difference in PTV scores obtained from a new polyoxymethylene IME and a titanium IME was 1.48. This difference equals the difference in PTV values between healthy teeth (1.4)[19] or ankylosed oral implants (1)[20] between men and women. Because of this small difference, the use of a polyoxymethylene IME, especially in the bar joint overdenture design, does not appear to offer any major advantage over a titanium IME, and its clinical relevance should be questioned. Hertel,[25] in an in vivo study, and Lill,[26] in an in vitro study, came to the same conclusions.

It has been suggested that IME fractures, especially with overdentures, are the result of patients not paying attention to the removal of their prostheses.[25] A correlation was not found between IME fracture and the retentive force of the overdenture, or the interabutment distance. Retentive forces quantified in this study will be lower than those used by patients to remove their prostheses in a straight vertical direction. The lack of correlation between IME fractures and interabutment distance can be explained by the lack of correlation between retention force and interabutment distance. Longer clips or more clips were not necessarily more activated.

Bite force levels with overdentures are considerable[4] when considering the relatively frequent fracture of the opposing denture. The increased number of conventional maxillary denture midline fractures after fixed prosthetic treatment was reported previously.[27] It is noteworthy that in only one-fifth of the study patients was a reline of the prosthesis base needed. This strengthens the belief that tilting and shifting forces, which are known to be the most detrimental forces for bone resorption, are hardly present in the bar-overdenture concept. Delayed bone resorption can be expected when compared with bone resorption under conventional complete dentures.

After implant treatment in the mandible, more patients complained about lack of retention of their maxillary complete dentures. Improved comfort and bite force with their mandibular prostheses[4] could lead them to unconsciously compare their maxillary dentures with their well-retained mandibular dentures. Regular checkups should be scheduled after overdenture treatment and should include relining when necessary to maintain optimal retention and load distribution.

Whereas no adverse tissue reactions were found when magnets were used, with the use of O-rings, rapid bone loss does occur around the fixtures, at least in the maxillae.[16] Because of the limited series, no conclusions can be drawn in this regard. Followup studies in which fixtures are and are not interconnected, and in which different attachment systems are used, are presently in progress.

Proliferation of the gingiva around abutments supporting overdentures by natural teeth as well as by implants is a well-known fact.[3,9] In the Swedish multicenter study,[9] treatment of hyperplasia was performed in 25% of the patient group. However, in this study very few patients needed treatment and when hyperplasia occurred, it was mostly in the earlier treatment period. In these patients with unattached oral mucosa around the abutments, a gingival grafting procedure was performed. This was only partially successful. Improved plaque control and an atraumatic prosthesis design seem to be essential for the maintenance of healthy soft tissues.

Patient appreciation of the overdenture treatment, as reported in other studies,[9] was very positive in both centers. The IMZ group scored better for the retention factor, which can be explained by the fact that double the number of patients in the Brånemark group had a pull-out force of 10 N or less. Changes in negative subjective experience before and after overdenture treatment were the same for both centers.

Conclusions

Both implant systems can be used with very low failure rates, at least for a medium-term period, for resilient overdenture therapy in the mandible. Not a single failure occurred for bar overdentures retained by two implants in the mandible. However, in the long-term perspective, higher bone loss observed around the IMZ implants may compromise success.

The proposed prosthodontic approach seems to be effective in patients who accept removable dentures but who are handicapped because of instability and lack of retention of their dentures. The overdenture approach is simple, versatile, and relatively inexpensive.

The high rate of polyoxymethylene IME fractures and the small difference in PTV scores between a polyoxymethylene IME and a titanium IME raises questions about the clinical relevance of the device.

Acknowledgments

The authors are very indebted to the advice and encouragement of the late Prof Dr M. De Clercq, former Head of the Prosthetic Department, Catholic University of Leuven, Belgium.

References

1. Bergman B, Carlsson GE. Clinical long-term study of complete denture wearers. J Prosthet Dent 1985; 53:56–61.
2. Blomberg S, Lindquist LW. Psychological reactions to edentulousness and treatment with jawbone-anchored bridges. Acta Psychiatr Scand 1983;68:251–262.
3. Ettinger RL, Taylor TD, Scandrett FR. Treatment needs for overdenture patients in a longitudinal study: Five-year results. J Prosthet Dent 1984;52:532–537.
4. Haraldson T, Jemt T, Stålblad PÅ, Lekholm U. Oral function in subjects with overdentures supported by osseointegrated implants. Scand J Dent Res 1988; 96:235–242.
5. Jemt T, Stålblad PÅ. The effect of chewing movements on changing mandibular complete dentures to osseointegrated overdentures. J Prosthet Dent 1986; 55:357–361.
6. Adell R, Lekholm U, Rockler B, Brånemark P-I. A 15-year study of osseointegrated implants in the treatment of the edentulous jaw. Int J Oral Surg 1981;10: 387–416.
7. van Steenberghe D, Quirynen M, Calberson L, Demanet M. A prospective evaluation of the fate of 697 consecutive intra-oral fixtures ad modum Brånemark in the rehabilitation of edentulism. J Head Neck Pathol 1987;6:53–58.
8. Naert I, De Clercq M, Theuniers G, Schepers E. Overdentures supported by osseointegrated fixtures for the edentulous mandible: A 2.5-year report. Int J Oral Maxillofac Implants 1988;3:191–196.
9. Engquist B, Bergendal T, Kallus T, Linden U. A retrospective multicenter evaluation of osseointegrated implants supporting overdentures. Int J Oral Maxillofac Implants 1988;3:129–134.
10. Naert I, Quirynen M, Theuniers G, van Steenberghe D. Prosthetic aspects of osseointegrated fixtures supporting overdentures: A 4-year report. J Prosthet Dent 1991;65:671–680.
11. Quirynen M, Naert I, van Steenberghe D, Teerlinck J, Dekeyser C, Theuniers G. Periodontal aspects of osseointegrated fixtures supporting an overdenture: A 4-year retrospective study. J Clin Periodontol 1991. In press.
12. Kirsch A, Ackerman KL. The IMZ osteointegrated implant system. Dent Clin North Am 1989;33:733–791.
13. d'Hoedt B, Schulte W. A comparative study of results with various endosseous implant systems. Int J Oral Maxillofac Implants 1989;4:95–105.
14. Fuhrmann G, Kirsch A, Sauer G, Strunz V. Strength and elastic properties of various stress absorbing elements in IMZ implants. German Dent News 1983;38: 123–125.
15. Baier RE, Natiella JR, Meyer AE, Carter JM. Importance of implant surface preparation for biomaterials with different intrinsic properties. pp 13–36 In D. van Steenberghe (ed) Tissue Integration in Oral and Maxillo-facial Reconstruction. Amsterdam: Excerpta Medica, 1986.
16. Quirynen M, Naert I, van Steenberghe D, Deryckere F, De Clercq C, Darius P. Periodontal aspects of Brånemark and IMZ implants supporting overdentures: A comparative study. In Proc 2nd Int Congress on Tissue Integration. Chicago: Quintessence Publ Co, 1992.
17. Lekholm U, Zarb GA. Patient selection and preparation. pp 199–209 In P.-I. Brånemark, G.A. Zarb, T. Albrektsson (eds) Tissue-Integrated Prostheses: Osseointegration in Clinical Dentistry. Chicago: Quintessence Publ Co, 1985.
18. Albrektsson T, Zarb GA, Worthington P, Eriksson AR. The long-term efficacy of currently used dental implants. A review and proposed criteria of success. Int J Oral Maxillofac Implants 1986;1:11–25.
19. d'Hoedt B, Lukas L, Mühlbradt L, Scholz F, Schulte W, Quante F, et al. Das periotestverfahren—Entwicklung und klinische prüfung. Dtsch Zahnärztl Z 1985;40: 113–125.
20. d'Hoedt B, Schramm-Scherer B. Der Periotestwert bei enossalen Implantaten. Z Zahnärztl Implantol 1988; 4:89–95.
21. Adell R, Lekholm U, Rockler B, Brånemark P-I, Lindhe J, Eriksson B, et al. Marginal tissue reactions at osseointegrated titanium fixtures. I. A 3-year longitudinal prospective study. Int J Oral Maxillofac Surg 1986; 1:39–52.
22. Cox JF, Zarb GA. The longitudinal clinical efficacy of osseointegrated dental implants. A 3-year report. Int J Oral Maxillofac Implants 1987;2:91–100.

23. Scholle KV. Ergebnisse der Nachuntersuchungen von Knopfankerprothesen. *Dtsch Zahnärztl Z* 1973;28: 74–79.

24. Stewart BL, Edwards RO. Retention and wear of precision-type attachments. *J Prosthet Dent* 1983;1: 28–34.

25. Hertel RC, Richter EJ. Das intramobile element des IMZ-systems in der klinischen prüfung. *Z Zahnärztl Implantol* 1988;4:43–49.

26. Lill W, Matejka M, Rambousek K, Watzek G. The ability of currently available stress-breaking elements for osseointegrated implants to imitate natural tooth mobility. *Int J Oral Maxillofac Implants* 1988;3:281–286.

27. Lindquist LW, Carlsson GE, Glantz PO. Rehabilitation of the edentulous mandible with a tissue-integrated fixed prosthesis: A six-year longitudinal study. *Quintessence Int* 1987;18:89–96.

The Brånemark Implant Technique: A Standardized Procedure Under Continuous Development*

U. Lekholm

The Brånemark osseointegration procedure has been in clinical practice since 1965. During this period of the system application, improvements and changes have been introduced regarding instrumentation and components. However, according to an earlier publication,[1] most of the alterations took place during the years 1965 to 1971, a time period that consequently has been referred to as the development period of the Brånemark technique.

In 1971 a standardized procedure regarding implant design and surgical handling[2] was introduced that has been utilized, basically unchanged, ever since. The principles thereof can be summarized as follows:

- Commercially pure titanium is used as the material
- The implant design is screw-shaped
- A two-stage surgical procedure is performed
- Atraumatic surgery is essential
- Controlled loading of the implants must be applied.

If these guidelines are followed, it is possible to establish and maintain osseointegration of the implants (fixtures), and thereby create anchorage for various types of prosthetic restorations.[2]

The original standard fixture had a length of 10 mm and a diameter of 3.75 mm, a design that is still used today as the basic unit for implant treatment in many patients. To date, many publications have been presented, demonstrating the outcome of this standard fixture in edentulous and partially edentulous jaws.[1,3–5] According to these reports, the Brånemark procedure has proven to be reliable and predictable, provided the technique has been applied in the correct way. Furthermore, fixture survival rates of 81% and 91% for maxillary and mandibular fixtures, respectively, have been presented in consecutive materials with followup of 5 to 9 years.[1]

Because of expanding application, technical development, and increased clinical experience, new fixtures have been introduced within the system. These are certainly not completely new types of implants but rather are variations of the original design regarding length, diameter, and/or shape. According to the manufacturer (Nobelpharma AB, Göteborg, Sweden), the various Brånemark fixtures are still produced irrespective of design, in accordance with the original principles, thereby giving all of them the same biophysical and biochemical surface characteristics. Regarding implant variability in length and diameter only, they are surgically placed in basically the same way as has been described for the standard 10-mm fixture,[2] utilizing the original biotechnical rationale for surgery as well.

However, those implants that vary in shape (the self-tapping fixtures), have a new cutting tip design, or have a new design of the head (the conical self-tapping fixture), are not placed according to the original protocol. Instead, these fixtures are inserted into the bone site, directly

*Keynote presentation.

following a modified site preparation with stainless steel drills and without any pretapping procedure. Therefore, when using self-tapping implants, it is not just a change in the design, but also a deviation from the surgical protocol that has been introduced. As stated by Albrektsson et al,[6] each change from the original concept should be evaluated per se, and not be presumed a priori to result in the same outcome as for the standard fixture.

The aim of this paper is to report a survey of the literature and to determine what knowledge is available regarding fixture survival in relation to fixture length, diameter, and/or shape.

Materials and methods

According to the Nobelpharma customer price list of January 1990, 19 various fixture types are presently commercially available. These implants can be divided into three subgroups regarding design:

1. Standard fixtures (ϕ = 3.75 mm) of various lengths (7 to 20 mm)
2. Wider fixtures (ϕ = 4.0 mm) of various lengths (7 to 18 mm)
3. Self-tapping fixtures (ϕ = 3.75 mm) of various lengths (10 to 18 mm), with either standard or conical heads

Besides the implants mentioned, other types are also available from the Nobelpharma company, but they are strictly recommended for multicenter studies and/or clinical research projects and have not been included in this investigation. Except for the 10-mm standard fixture that was introduced in 1971,[1] the remaining 18 fixture types have, according to Nobelpharma, been introduced into clinical practice mainly between 1979 to 1984.

When screening the literature for reports of fixture survival related to implant design, no such articles were found. Instead, most of the available data were presented for used fixtures as a group. Sometimes it was not even mentioned in the reports studied that various types of fixtures had been placed. When asking the manufacturer for assistance, it was not possible to obtain any published information regarding this subject based on controlled studies. Because of that, the evaluation of the present report was instead focused upon manuscripts that had recently been accepted and/or submitted for publication. These papers either originated from the Brånemark Clinic in Göteborg (Brånemark Clinic) or had one author based in that clinic. Five such papers were selected[3,7–10] in which the results had been presented in relation to fixture length, diameter, and/or shape. Regarding these data, the followup periods varied in these reports from just after healing,[8] to as much as 10 years of observation.[3,7] However, most of the available results related to success rates of shorter periods, ie, 1 to 3 years.

The parameter studied in the manuscripts was the fixture survival rate presented for the various types of fixtures used. If any specific mention was made regarding complications and/or adverse behavior of the fixtures or the host bone, that information was also collected.

To increase the evaluation base for the present study, specific reference material was also accumulated. All patients selected were those treated between January 1, 1985, and June 30, 1985, at the Department of Oral Surgery, University of Göteborg, Sweden, and followed at the Brånemark Clinic since the start of the clinic in 1986 until now. During the time period mentioned, a total of 85 patients were treated and subsequently subjected to examination. The sample was used to assess fixture survival rates for the various fixture types placed during the period and evaluated at a 5-year followup level (August 1990). It was not possible to reexamine five patients, as three had moved to other centers for followup, one was too ill to come for a checkup, and one had died. The remaining 80 patients (35 males and 45 females), having a mean age of 55 years (range: 15 to 73 years), constituted the specific reference material. In that group, 81 jaws (35 maxillae and 46 mandibles) had been treated,

Table 1 Reference material (Lekholm, 1990) accumulated during treatment at the Department of Oral Surgery, University of Göteborg, Sweden, between January 1, 1985, to June 30, 1985.*

Standard fixtures

7 mm	n = 59	15 mm	n = 68
10 mm	n = 163	18 mm	n = 5
13 mm	n = 69	20 mm	n = 0

Self-tapping fixtures

Standard head		Conical head	
10 mm	n = 17	10 mm	n = 0
13 mm	n = 6	13 mm	n = 2
15 mm	n = 5	15 mm	n = 8
18 mm	n = 0	18 mm	n = 0

*No wider fixtures (ϕ = 4.0 mm) were placed during the period.

Table 2 Survival rates, regarding standard fixtures (ϕ = 3.75 mm)*

	Followup times	
Fixture lengths	5 years	10 years
10-mm fixtures (n = 1004; Routine group I)	88%	85%
7 to 20-mm fixtures (n = 1263; Routine group II)	94%	90%

*Adell et al[3]

and one patient had implants placed in both jaws. A total of 402 fixtures of various designs had been consecutively inserted in these jaws (Table 1). A survival evaluation of these fixtures was done using the journal data available for each patient. Fixtures were regarded as stable and successful if they were still supporting a prosthesis and if radiographically they were not surrounded by any radiolucency at the latest annual checkup. The reference material from these studies in the following text will be referred to as Lekholm (1990).

Results and discussion

The bulk of knowledge regarding fixture survival in long-term followup materials is based mainly on results presented by the Göteborg team.[1,3] When evaluating the outcome of new fixture types, the original data are thus of great importance as a resource reference. In the following text, these figures will also be used when comparing fixture survival to implant length, diameter, and/or shape.

Comparison of fixture survival to implant length

The original 10-mm standard fixture was introduced in 1971, whereas standard fixtures of other lengths (ie, 7 mm, 13 mm, 15 mm, 18 mm, and 20 mm) were produced and first utilized in 1979/1980. From Adell et al,[3] it was found (Table 2) that the original 10-mm fixture had 5- and 10-year survival rates of 88% and 85%, respectively. These figures represented implants placed between July 1, 1971, to June 30, 1976, which were those in routine group I of the study referred to. When looking at the outcome for fixtures of various lengths in the same paper (routine group II; treated July 1, 1976, to June 30, 1981), the corresponding values were 94% and 90% (Table 2). From these results it seems possible to conclude that better stability rates can be established if the fixture length is adapted to the anatomical situation rather than using one implant length in all jaws, irrespective of the jaw shape present.

When looking in more detail at other survival rate data involving various fixture lengths[8,10] (Lekholm, 1990), it was observed (Table 3) that shorter implants (7 mm and 10 mm) seemed to have the least favorable stability rates. For example, as many as 6% of the 7-mm fixtures were reported as failures during the healing phase,[8] and an additional 6% were lost at the end of the first 5 years of function (Lekholm, 1990). Longer fixtures seemed to be more reliable (Table 3), not just after healing but also after longer followup periods. From a review of these figures it could be suggested that 7-mm fixtures should be used with some caution. However, it is also important to observe that all fixture types, independent of length, had stabil-

Table 3 Fixture survival in relation to implant length

Standard fixture lengths (mm)	Friberg et al, 1990 (n = 4641; healing)	van Steenberghe et al, 1990 (n = 522; 1 year)	Lekholm, 1990 (n = 364; 5 years)
7	94% (n = 793)	97% (n = 109)	88% (n = 59)
10		88% (n = 225)	95% (n = 163)
13		94% (n = 85)	96% (n = 69)
15	99% (n = 3848)	100% (n = 74)	91% (n = 68)
18		100% (n = 20)	100% (n = 5)
20		100% (n = 9)	—

Table 4 Fixture survival in relation to implant diameter

	Standard fixtures (ϕ = 3.75 mm)	Wider fixtures (ϕ = 4.0 mm)
van Steenberghe et al, 1990 (n = 558; 1 year)	95% (n = 522)	100% (n = 36)

ity rates exceeding the 85% level, which has been recommended by Albrektsson et al[6] as the minimum level for fixtures in function after 5 years of followup.

The shortest fixtures can also be recommended for clinical use as reliable anchorage units in jaws with advanced resorption. However, it is important to locate them in areas where the bone quality is favorable enough to eventually withstand the load of attached prostheses. From the figures presented in Tables 27-2 to 27-3, it can be concluded that it seems justified to commercially offer all of the various fixture lengths currently available, as they have been clinically used with success in the five manuscripts cited.

Comparison of fixture survival to implant diameter

The original fixture had a diameter of 3.75 mm, a dimension that is still used today for standard fixtures. In 1980, implants with a diameter of 4.0 mm, combined with various lengths, were also introduced. Lately, even wider (ϕ = 5 mm) but also thinner (ϕ = 3 mm) fixtures have become available. However, as these latter types are still only recommended for research purposes in multicenter studies, they are not included in the present review.

When screening the literature for information concerning the outcome of 4.0-mm-wide fixtures, only one report was found.[10] In this work, partially edentulous jaws had been treated and followed as a multicenter project, and the results of the study were presented after 1 year of followup (Table 4). In the reference material (Lekholm, 1990), no wider implants were found and consequently no additional information was available showing the outcome of the 4.0-mm-wide fixtures after 5 years of function.

From the multicenter study it could be seen that wider fixtures, irrespective of length, had a better stability rate (100%) than standard fixtures (95%), at least in the short perspective of 1 year followup. This was a somewhat surprising finding as wider implants normally are used as a kind of "rescue" fixture in situations where standard implants do not have initial stability because of poor jawbone quality or bad surgical technique. The use of a wider fixture in such a situation may improve the fit of the implant into the host site by condensing the bone during the surgical placement of the fixture since the insertion is performed without any pretapping procedure.

Another explanation of the better survival rates observed for the wider fixtures may be the increased titanium surface area that inevitably

Table 5 Fixture survival in relation to implant shape

	Standard fixtures	Self-tapping fixtures	
		Standard head	Conical head
Adell et al[7] (n = 66; 3 y)	—	85% (n = 41)	96% (n = 25)
Jemt et al[9] (n = 23; 3 y)	94% (n = 18)	—	100% (n = 5)
Lekholm, 1990 (n = 402; 5 y)	93% (n = 364)	100% (n = 28)	100% (n = 10)

will be available for contact with the surrounding bone. However, even if the results of the wider fixtures clearly seem to indicate a better survival rate than for standard fixtures, the observation was based on a restricted number of implants (n = 36) being followed only for 1 year. Larger materials and longer observation periods are needed before it can finally be stated that wider fixtures are more successful than standard ones. Furthermore, it must also be remembered that with the use of wider implants follows a need for larger volumes of bone. Unfortunately, that is seldom the case in the clinical situation.

Comparison of fixture survival to implant shape

The most interesting fixtures to evaluate are those that are self-tapping, as they are inserted according to a somewhat changed surgical protocol. Two self-tapping types are available, standard and conical, both having been introduced into clinical practice during 1983/1984. The standard self-tapping fixture is normally used when jawbone density is very low. In such situations there might be only one opportunity to create a threaded canal for the initial stability of the implant, that being with the self-tapping implant itself. Conical fixtures are recommended for use when initial bone remodeling around the neck of the implant is not possible to predict, such as in connection with grafting or fresh extraction sockets. By using a conical fixture in those situations, it is possible to avoid exposed

threads toward the mucosa, even if considerable marginal bone loss takes place during healing or later during function.

From the literature it was observed that results related to self-tapping fixtures were reported in only two papers and in the reference material[7,9] (Lekholm, 1990). That material represented such wide application ranges as grafting, single tooth replacement, and orthodontic treatment. Furthermore, it was found that the number of self-tapping implants reported was low (Table 5). However, the outcome was most interesting, as the presented data corresponded with, or even exceeded, those involving the standard fixtures. The least favorable figures were reported by Adell et al.[7] However, those results can perhaps be explained by the fact that the self-tapping fixtures related to that study were used in conjunction with bone grafts. Consequently, the fixtures had not been placed according to basic principles, and furthermore, they had been inserted into extremely resorbed maxillae jaws. Nevertheless, survival rates varying from 85% to 96% for standard and conical self-tapping fixtures, respectively, after 3 to 5 years of followup, were reported and must be considered as highly acceptable in these difficult cases.

The results presented for self-tapping fixtures used for single tooth replacement and in orthodontic treatment[9] (Lekholm, 1990), were the most favorable. Further indications were thereby obtained that the new type of fixture, regardless of the changed surgical concept, could still result in acceptable and predictable success rates, at least during observation periods of up to 5 years.

A rather interesting side observation was mentioned by Jemt et al[9] regarding the conical self-tapping fixtures. These authors reported that marginal bone remodeling around the neck of the conical implants was more pronounced than around the standard self-tapping fixtures. They found that the bone level had moved down to the first cervical thread of the conical fixtures by the end of a 3-year period, thereby leaving the conical part without any bone contacts. Corresponding amounts of bone loss were not detected around standard implants. The reason for this behavior of conical fixtures is not completely understood, but could be related to the biomechanics of the conical surface. Presumably, axial loading of the surrounding bone may occur in a way other than that of the threaded part of the fixture. However, this observation was based on material involving only five conical fixtures; larger materials are needed to confirm the observation in the future.

Conclusions

In summary it can be stated that few publications are available that report on the outcome of individual fixture types used today. As each new product on the market must be evaluated with regard to its own merits, more studies are certainly needed to demonstrate the potential of each commercially available and individually used implant.

Because many of the new fixture types have been introduced during the latest 5- to 10-year period, no longer-term followup data are available regarding their success rate. Reported values for 15 to 20 years of observation thus refer only to the standard 10-mm fixture.

From the reports reviewed in this article it may be concluded that:

• Shorter fixtures seemed to have a somewhat less favorable stability rate than longer ones.

However, irrespective of length, all types showed acceptable results according to the criteria for success, described by Albrektsson et al.[6]

• Wider fixtures, irrespective of length, have proven to be more stable than standard fixtures, at least during short observation periods.

• Though placed according to a new surgical concept, self-tapping fixtures remained osseointegrated when used on a routine basis.

• All currently available new types of fixtures can be considered reliable and predictable if used appropriately and in the indicated patient situations.

References

1. Adell R, Lekholm U, Rockler B, Brånemark P-I. A 15-year study of osseointegrated implants in the treatment of the edentulous jaw. Int J Oral Surg 1981;10:387–416.
2. Brånemark P-I, Zarb GA, Albrektsson T (eds). Tissue-Integrated Prostheses: Osseointegration in Clinical Dentistry. Chicago: Quintessence Publ Co, 1985.
3. Adell R, Eriksson B, Lekholm U, Brånemark P-I, Jemt T. A long-term follow-up study of osseointegrated implants in the treatment of the totally edentulous jaw. Int J Oral Maxillofac Implants 1990;5:347–359.
4. Albrektsson T, Bergman B, Folmer T, Henry P, Higuchi K, Klineberg I, et al. A multicenter study on osseointegrated oral implants. J Prosthet Dent 1988;60:75–84.
5. Jemt T, Lekholm U, Adell R. Osseointegrated implants in the treatment of partially edentulous patients: A preliminary study on 876 consecutively placed fixtures. Int J Oral Maxillofac Implants 1989;4:211–217.
6. Albrektsson T, Zarb GA, Worthington P, Eriksson AR. The long-term efficacy of currently used dental implants: A review and proposed criteria of success. Int J Oral Maxillofac Implants 1986;1:11–25.
7. Adell R, Lekholm U, Gröndahl K, Brånemark P-I, Lindström J, Jacobsson M. Reconstruction of severely resorbed edentulous maxillae using osseointegrated fixtures in immediate autogenous bone grafts. Int J Oral Maxillofac Implants 1990;5:223–246.
8. Friberg B, Jemt T, Lekholm U. Early failures in 4641 consecutively installed Brånemark dental implants. Int J Oral Maxillofac Implants 1990. In press.
9. Jemt T, Lekholm U, Gröndahl K. A 3-year followup study of early single implant restorations ad modum Brånemark. Int J Periodont Rest Dent 1990;10:341–349.
10. van Steenberghe D, Lekholm U, Bolender C, Folmer T, Henry P, Herrmann I, et al. The applicability of osseointegrated oral implants in the rehabilitation of partial edentulism: A prospective multicenter study on 558 fixtures. Int J Oral Maxillofac Implants 1990;5:272–281.

The Use of Guided Tissue Regeneration for Implants Placed in Immediate Extraction Sockets

W. Becker, B.E. Becker,* C. Ochsenbein, M. Handelsman, T. Albrektsson, and R. Cellete

The purpose of this study was to evaluate bone healing around implants placed into fresh extraction sockets. Three large mongrel dogs were used. There was a total of six test and six control sites, which were randomly chosen. Test sites received 10-mm Brånemark implants (Nobelpharma USA, Chicago, Ill) plus PTFE Augmentation Material (W.L. Gore and Associates, Flagstaff, Ariz), while control sites received only implants (Figs 1 to 5). Standardized probes were used to measure midbuccal implant dehiscences at test and control sites. Three buccolingual measurements were also made at each implant site.

At 18 weeks, second surgeries were performed and measurements of test and control sites were taken (Figs 6 and 7). The animals were sacrificed and specimens were prepared for histologic evaluation.

Test sites had a mean increase in bone height of 2.63 mm and control sites had a mean increase in bone height of 1.0 mm (Figs 8 and 9). Changes in bone height for test sites were significant ($P < .01$). Test sites had a mean increase in buccolingual dimension of 1.5 mm and control sites had an 0.8-mm increase. The differences between these measurements were significant ($P < .01$).

Histologic examination of test and control specimens demonstrated varying degrees of new bone formation as evidenced by bone labeling. Sites receiving augmentation material had the greatest amount of new bone over dehisced implant threads. Implant augmentation material appears to have an application for enhancing bone formation at extraction sites that receive immediate dental implants.

Results of the histologic evaluation will be reported at a later date. We wish to thank Drs Ulf Lekholm and Tomas Albrektsson for their assistance with this project.

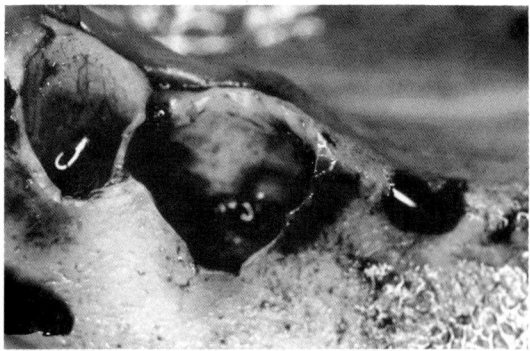

Fig 1 Tooth (P4) has been extracted and the coronal aspect of the extraction socket has been enlarged. A large acrylic resin bur under a constant stream of sterile saline was used to enlarge the socket. An adjacent tooth (P2) was prepared similarly.

*Keynote speaker.

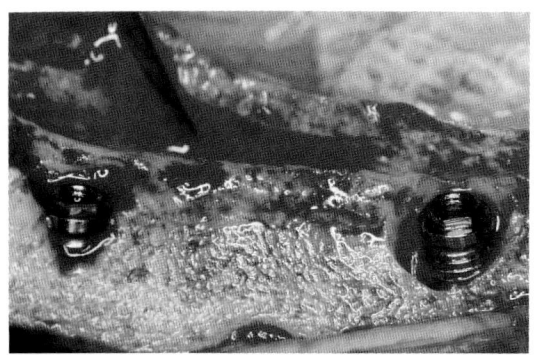

Fig 2 Standard 10-mm Nobelpharma fixtures have been installed into the extraction sockets.

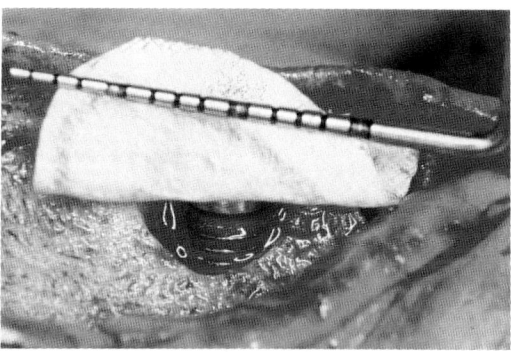

Fig 3 P2 (test) was randomly selected to receive the Gore-Tex augmentation material. The material was appropriately trimmed and fixed to the implant with the cover screw.

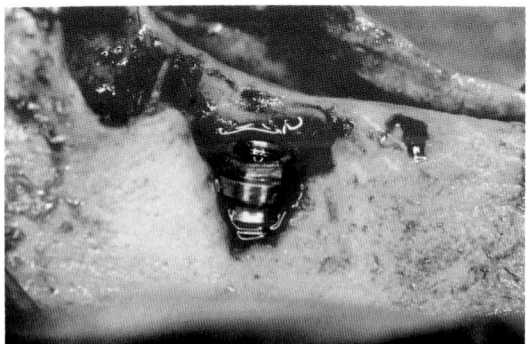

Fig 4 P4 (control) did not receive the augmentation material.

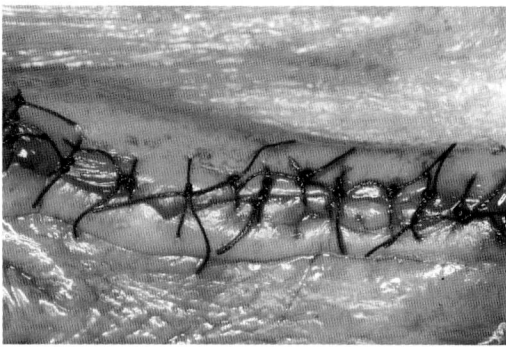

Fig 5 The flap margins were sutured with horizontal and vertical mattress nonresorbable sutures. The sutures were removed at 7 days.

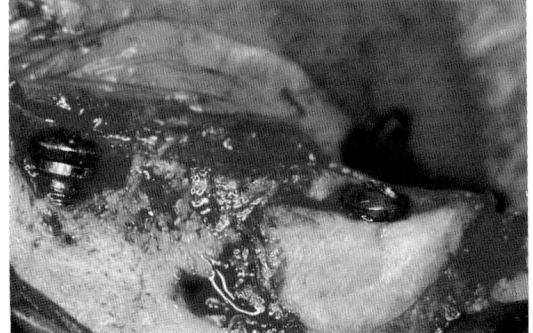

Fig 6 The implant sites were evaluated at 18 weeks post fixture installation. At the control site (P4), two threads remained exposed. At the test site (P2), the augmentation material apparently had bone beneath it. The width of the alveolar ridge appears to have widened when compared with the initial site.

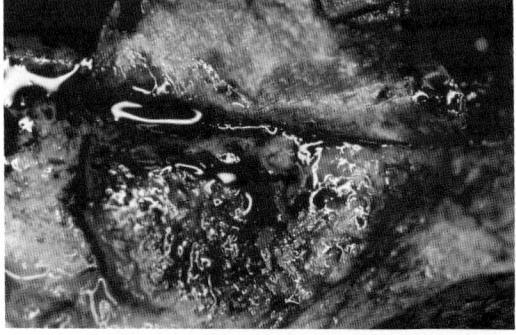

Fig 7 The augmentation material has been dissected from the underlying bone. Bone has formed to the apical aspect of the cover screw (four threads plus the implant rim). There has been a 1.23-mm increase in ridge width.

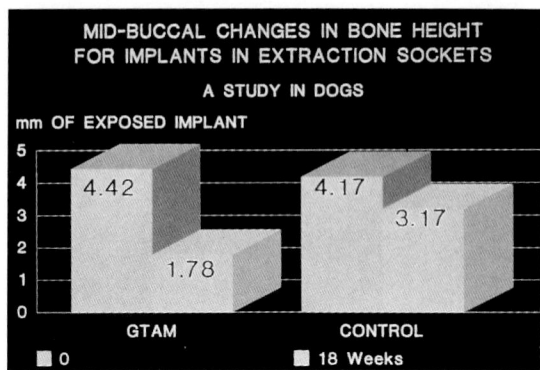

Fig 8 Mean midbuccal changes in bone height for test and control sites.

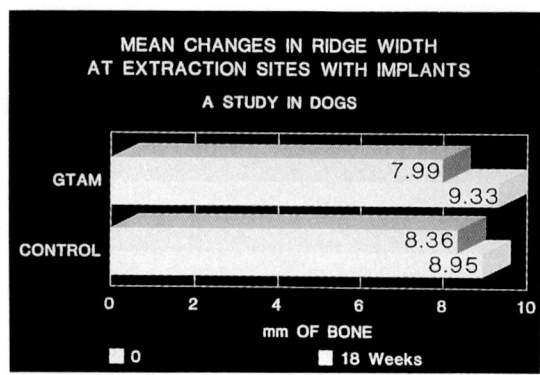

Fig 9 Mean changes in ridge width for test and control sites.

Immediate Implant Placement into Extraction Sites: Surgical and Restorative Advantages

R. J. Lazzara

Since implant dentistry has become a predictable treatment modality, its application has become more widespread in reconstructive dentistry. This paper will discuss a method of preserving vertical bone height as well as locating implants in a more ideal position by placing the implants immediately into extraction sites.

Resorptive patterns of a maxillary alveolar ridge are directed palatally and lingually, as well as apically, following natural tooth extraction. When implants are placed in a matured residual ridge, they are often placed more lingually or are angulated because of the bone topography (Fig 1). As apical resorption of the bone occurs during maturation following extraction, there is less vertical bone height available for implant placement. Therefore, a technique was developed to place implants immediately into extraction sites. Subsequently, a soft tissue covering was provided over the implant and, by epithelial and gingival connective tissue exclusion, bone was regenerated within the extraction socket.

Based on periodontal regeneration procedures using membranes to exclude the epithelium[1-3] and studies on primates whereby implants were placed immediately into extraction sites,[4] a technique was developed to achieve successful bone growth within a socket around an implant. Not only does the membrane exclude the gingival epithelium, but the barrier to gingival connective tissue cells appears to be important.[5] Rather than from the gingival connective tissue or gingival epithelium, it appears that there is a repopulation of the implant surface by cells from surrounding marrow spaces, which promote regeneration of bone adjacent to the implant surface. Furthermore, soft tissue is regenerated over the implant so that the implant remains totally covered with tissue during the integration and regeneration period.

Materials and methods

Following radiographic and clinical diagnosis, tooth extraction is performed, attempting to preserve the integrity of the alveolar walls. Tooth sectioning may be necessary to accomplish an atraumatic extraction and prevent expansion of the alveolus walls during the procedure. Following extraction, thorough degranulation of the tooth alveolus is necessary. Hexed cylindrical implants (Implant Innovations, West Palm Beach, Fla) and pure titanium-threaded implants were utilized in these clinical situations. Preparation of the implant site must extend adequately beyond the alveolus apex to allow thorough stabilization of the implant. Absolute stability of the implant is critical for bone regeneration.

When preparing the implant site, the usual attention should be given to parallelism and ideal prosthetic alignment. If necessary, some modification of the tooth alveolus may be necessary to place the implant in an ideal prosthetic position. This is particularly important in an area that will be visible, such as the maxillary anterior region.

During final placement of the implant in the extraction site, the coronal aspect of the implant

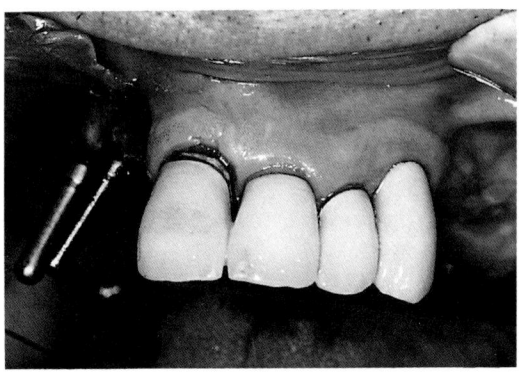

Fig 1 Direction indicators placed at the time of surgery show position and angulation compromise dictated by residual ridge configuration.

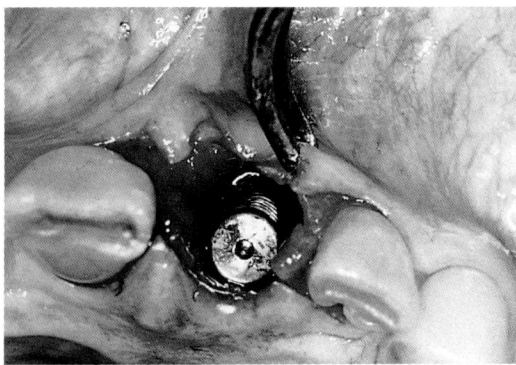

Fig 2 The implant is placed into the extraction site after thorough debridement of the socket walls. Note the voids around the implant and its position apical to the surrounding crest.

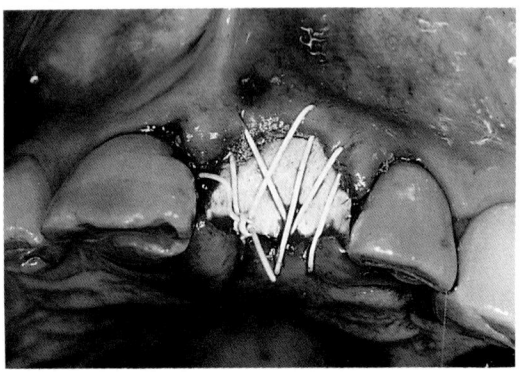

Fig 3 Gore-Tex membrane placed over the extraction site and the flap closed with a crisscross suture technique.

should be a minimum of 2 mm apical to the surrounding alveolus walls. This will permit bone remodeling and osseous regeneration up to the cover screw. In addition, regeneration of the soft tissue over the implant will be promoted for protection and seal during the integration phase. Since the implant is smaller in dimension than the extraction socket, voids will be present around the implant, as seen in Fig 2. To prevent apical migration of the gingival epithelium and repopulation of the implant surface by gingival connective tissue fibers, a membrane technique was developed utilizing Gore-Tex Periodontal Membrane (W.L. Gore and Associates, Flagstaff, Ariz).

Prior to placement of the membrane, the undersurface of the flap in the area adjacent to the tooth should be thoroughly degranulated of any residual epithelium. The membrane material should then be tailored to cover the extraction socket and extend several millimeters beyond the alveolus walls in all directions. The material is laid directly over the bone and the soft tissue is replaced, holding the membrane in position between the replaced flap and the bony surface. The area is sutured utilizing a crisscross pattern, making no attempt to completely coapt the soft tissue at the extraction site (Fig 3). The membrane provides the continuity of closure to protect and seal the implant site.

Postoperative pressure should not be applied to the surgical site since pressure on the membrane will collapse it against the cover screw and could prevent soft tissue regeneration over the coronal aspect of the implant.

The membrane material is left in place for approximately 1 month. When the membrane is removed (Fig 4), immature soft tissue will be noted in the area covering the implant surface. This unepithelialized connective tissue will have regenerated over the implant and has been shown histologically to be immature connective tissue (Fig 5). After removal of the membrane, normal epithelialization of the surgical site will occur in several weeks (Fig 6). A minimum of 6 months is generally considered to be

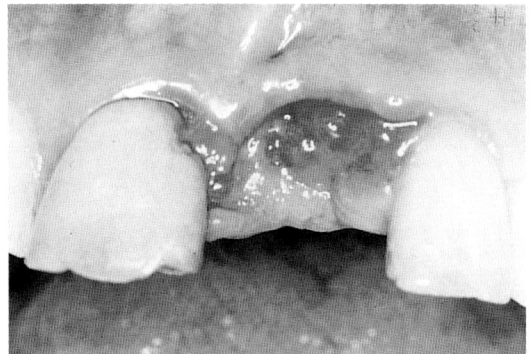

Fig 4 A soft tissue covering has developed over the implant after Gore-Tex removal at 1 month.

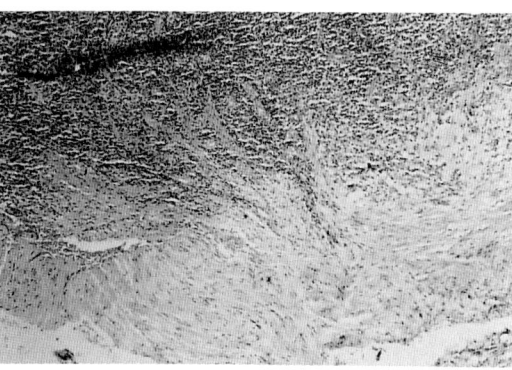

Fig 5 Biopsy specimen of the newly regenerated tissue indicates connective tissue consistent with normal healing of a secondary intention type of wound. Note the absence of epithelial covering associated with the placement of a membrane (hematoxylin-eosin, original magnification × 25).

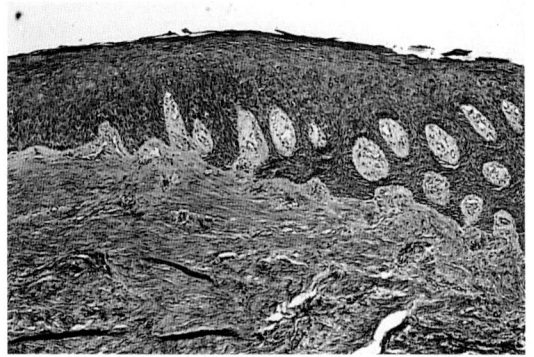

Fig 6 Histologic evaluation of the matured tissue indicates dense collagen formation in the connective tissue layer. The morphology appears to be healthy keratinized gingiva. (Masson trichrome, original magnification × 20).

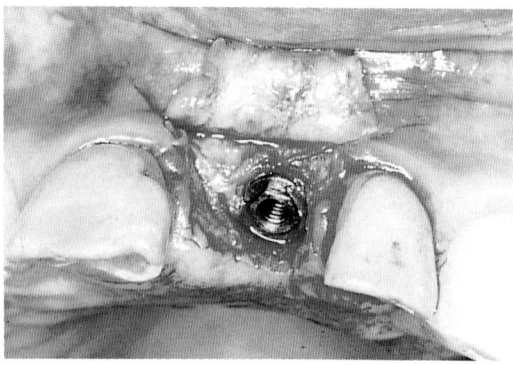

Fig 7 Reentry at 6 months reveals regeneration of bone to the coronal aspect of the implant as well as ridge remodeling.

adequate healing time. Upon reopening the area with the usual secondary surgical procedure, the surgeon will note ridge remodeling and regeneration of bone to the coronal aspect of the implant surface (Fig 7). Following healing, prosthetic reconstruction can be completed using a variety of abutments based on individual prosthetic requirements at the site (Figs 8a and b).

Discussion

Placement of implants into fresh extraction sites allows the surgeon to idealize the position of implants since the implants are placed into a location previously occupied by a tooth rather than an altered ridge position. This should result in a better restorative result, since the screw access opening can be located through the

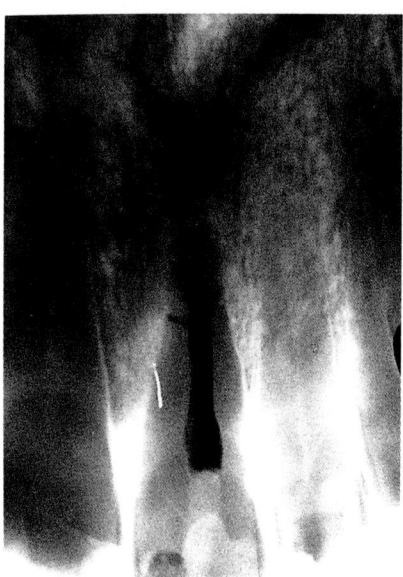

Fig 8a Radiograph of the tooth prior to extraction. Note the bone loss due to root fracture.

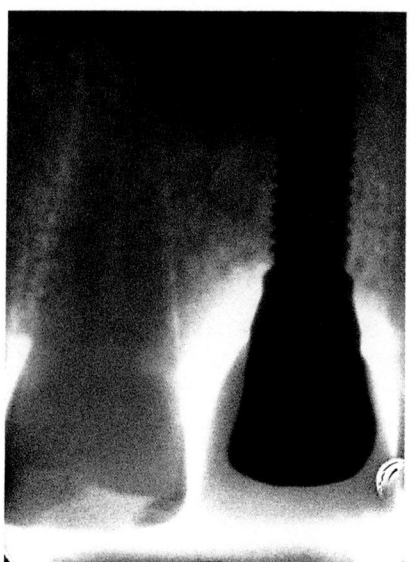

Fig 8b Radiograph of the final restoration at 1 year. Note this single tooth replacement has engaged the hex at the coronal aspect of the implant.

occlusal or cingulum area of the final restoration. In addition, it allows a more normal contour to the facial aspect of the final restoration since the implants can be placed in a more buccal position relative to the adjacent teeth and opposing occlusion.

Since there is regeneration of bone within the extraction socket, this procedure will allow the clinician to place a longer implant. The technique calls for placement of the implant beyond the apex of the extraction site for stabilization, and additional length can be accomplished by regeneration of bone within the socket to provide stronger support. By accomplishing this regeneration, there will be less loss of alveolar height relative to the adjacent dentition; this should result in a more normally sized clinical crown in the final restoration.

In the maxillary posterior region, extraction of the natural dentition oftentimes results in inadequate bone volume for the placement of implants apically without penetrating the maxillary sinus or the use of an inadequately sized implant. Using this immediate placement technique preserves existing bone. Regenerating bone within the alveolus allows the surgeon to place implants in this location that would have been less favorable utilizing the standard technique of extraction, waiting for ridge maturation, and then placement of the implants. In addition, more efficient patient treatment can be accomplished when utilizing this technique. Normally, hopeless teeth are extracted; this is followed by a maturation period of up to 1 year. After ridge maturation, implants are placed and approximately 6 months is permitted for osseointegration. Following the integration period, second-stage surgery is performed and then final prosthesis construction is begun after healing from second-stage surgery.

Utilizing the immediate extraction technique, the period of ridge healing and osseointegration is accomplished concurrently, thereby reducing treatment time for the patient. This can be a major psychological benefit as well as reduce the time that the patient must wear a transitional removable prosthesis.

Conclusion

Placement of implants immediately into an extraction site appears to be a viable technique for preserving bone as well as for regenerating bone at the implant site. It allows the surgeon to maximize the length of implant placed, as well as to ideally place the implant from a prosthetic viewpoint. It helps the restorative dentist create a functional as well as esthetic restoration since implants are placed in a more ideal position rather than a position dictated by a resorbed and altered ridge configuration.

References

1. Gottlow J, Nyman S, Lindhe J, Karring T, Wernstrom J. New attachment formation in the human periodontium by guided tissue regeneration. Case reports. *J Clin Periodontol* 1986;13:604–616.
2. Nyman S, Lindhe J, Karring T, Rylander H. New attachment following surgical treatment of human periodontal disease. *J Clin Periodontol* 1982;9:290–296.
3. Pontoriero R, Nyman S, Lindhe J, Rosenberg E, Sanavi F. Guided tissue regeneration in the treatment of furcation defects in man. *J Clin Periodontol* 1987;14:618–620.
4. Barzilay I, Graser GN, Caton J, Shenkle G. Immediate implantation of pure titanium threaded implants into extraction sockets. *J Dent Res* 1988;67:234.
5. Melcher AH, Dreyer CJ. Protection of the blood clot in healing circumscribed bone defects. *J Bone Surg* 1962; 44B:424–420.

Guided Tissue Regeneration Around Titanium Dental Implants

S. A. Jovanovic, H. Spiekermann, E.-J. Richter, and M. Koseoglu

Long-term clinical studies have demonstrated that osseointegrated implants will successfully support fixed and removable prostheses and that the supporting tissues can be kept in a healthy clinical state for prolonged periods of time.[1-4] Implant therapy is predicated upon the placement of implants into a preoperatively diagnosed bone site, which has a minimum width of approximately 6 mm. Insufficient bone volume will likely result in exposed surface of the implant, less support, and reduced opportunity for implant success. In addition, when an implant is placed into an immediate extraction site, the outcome of the bone response toward the implant is not predictable and can result in an increased initial bone loss. Initial bone loss will result in exposed implant surface, which may create mucosal irritation.

The average marginal bone loss around healthy implants is reported to be approximately 1.5 mm during the first year after implant insertion and 0.1 mm per year in subsequent years.[2] Bone loss exceeding these averages should be viewed with concern, as progressive bone loss is an indication of pending implant failure. The etiology of crestal bone loss adjacent to osseointegrated dental implants in function has varied but falls into two main categories; one relates to the biomechanical factors associated with occlusal overload and the other with bacterial proliferation.[22]

Few studies concerning the success of treatment rendered for failing implants, soft tissue complications, and dehisced implant sites have been reported.[5,6] In several animal experimental studies, the principle of "guided tissue regeneration" (GTR) was used to enhance the formation of bone around dental implants and to exclude the invasion of nonosteogenic extraskeletal soft tissue cells.[7-10]

The accomplishment of bone regeneration was based on the hypothesis that different cellular components in the tissue have varying rates of migration into a wound area around a dental implant. By a membrane technique, the blood clot is protected from the pressure of the overlying tissue so that fibroblasts and other soft connective tissue cells are prevented from entering the bone defect. This technique allows the presumably slower-migrating cells with osteogenic potential to repopulate the bony defect. Recent experimental studies in animals have demonstrated remarkable success with virtually complete bone regeneration and healing of various types of bone defects.[11-13]

Preliminary human clinical applications of this method have shown encouraging results.[14,15] Furthermore, guided tissue regeneration has been used to treat periodontal defects and to regenerate successfully the attachment apparatus in teeth with advanced loss of periodontal tissues.[16-20]

This ongoing study was designed to clinically evaluate the principle of guided tissue regeneration for osteogenesis in three clinical situations (Table 1). Clinical findings of the application of an expanded polytetrafluoroethylene (PTFE) membrane when treating (1) dehisced implant sites, *(2)* implant placement into fresh extraction sites, and *(3)* "peri-implantitis" intraosseous defects are discussed.

Materials and methods

Table 1 Classification of peri-implant bone defects

	Group	No. of implants
Insufficient bone volume	I	17
Extraction sites	II	8
Peri-implantitis defects	III	10

Group I

Ten patients with 17 implants, having a variety of dehisced implant surfaces at the time of placement, were treated by the principle of GTR with a membrane technique. Of the 17 implants, 11 were placed in edentulous maxillae, 3 were placed in edentulous mandibles, and 3 were placed in partially edentulous mandibles.

A remote split- or full-thickness flap design was planned and an incision was made toward the palatal side of the upper ridge crest, or 2 to 4 mm below the mucogingival junction of the lower ridge crest. Vertical releasing incisions were used only when needed. The vertical incision was made one tooth width away from the anticipated placement of the edge of the membrane. Implant placement was performed using the standardized technique described by Adell et al.[2] A varying number of coronal implant threads were exposed after final placement. Measurements were taken to account for the amount of implant surface exposed and the defect location and dimension. These measurements were made from the coronal aspect of the implant head (without the hexagonal part) to the bone crest. Prepackaged sterile Gore-Tex Augmentation Material (GTAM, W.L. Gore and Associates, Flagstaff, Ariz) was trimmed with scissors so that it would overlap the edge of the bone on the periphery of the defect 3 to 4 mm. The membrane was secured with the cover screw and utmost care was used to develop and maintain a space under the membrane. In 2 of the 17 implant sites an intraoral autogenous bone graft was placed between the implant and the membrane to develop and maintain a space for regeneration. The flaps were repositioned over the membrane and sutured to complete coverage with horizontal mattress and interrupted sutures. If indicated, suturing in multiple layers was performed.

Regular postoperative examinations were performed, and reentry operations were carried out after 4.5 to 6 months of healing. All membranes were removed and the implant sites were measured for changes in bone height and width.

Group II

Five patients with eight implants placed into extraction sites were treated with a membrane technique. To ensure complete soft tissue coverage over the extraction site, a modified surgical protocol, which included a tooth extraction and then implant placement a few weeks later, was followed. After all diagnostic procedures were carefully evaluated, an intrasulcular incision was performed. A mucoperiostal flap around the tooth in question was elevated and the tooth was extracted. The flaps were released and soft tissue closure was achieved with vertical mattress sutures. After 4 to 6 weeks the area was evaluated for complete soft tissue coverage of the previous extraction area.

When complete soft tissue coverage had occurred, a "fresh extraction site" flap design was planned. This involved a remote split- or full-thickness incision with elevation of a mucoperiosteal flap. The apex of the alveolus was penetrated for implant placement in the standardized manner. This provided stability after proper alignment of the implant. A varying volume of voids was apparent around the implant.

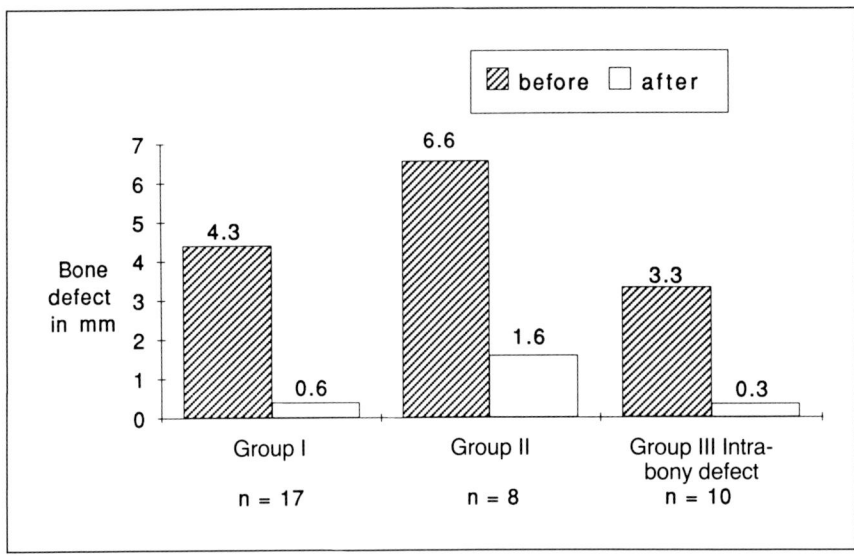

Fig 1 Mean defect height.

Measurements and photographs were taken to account for the amount of implant surface exposed. The GTAM was trimmed and secured by the cover screw. The membrane was placed over the implant and its surrounding osseous defect. The flap was repositioned and sutured to complete coverage. Reentry operations and membrane removal were performed after 6 months of healing. At this stage measurements and photographs were taken to determine osseous tissue gain.

Group III

Seven patients presented with peri-implant disease and radiographically detectable intraosseous defects around ten endosseous implants: six IMZ implants (Friedrichsfeld GmbH, Mannheim, Germany), three Brånemark implants (Nobelpharma AB, Göteborg, Sweden), and one TPS (Friedrichsfeld GmbH) implant. The implants had an average functional phase of 37 months, with a minimum of 11 months and a maximum of 61 months. Documentation included radiographs, gingival index (Löe and

Silness, 1963), plaque index (Silness and Löe, 1964), papilla bleeding index (Saver and Muhleman, 1975), mobility (Schulte, 1986), and probing pocket depth (PD) to the nearest 0.5 mm. After the initial preparation for therapy, the implants were treated to arrest the progressive bone loss and to regenerate bone tissue. The treatment consisted of occlusal adjustment if indicated and surgical intervention.

The surgical therapy included flap management, granulation tissue removal, implant surface cleaning by air powder abrasive,[21] application of detoxifying 1.0% Chloramyne-T solution for 3 minutes (OraTec Corporation, Herndon, Va), saline solution, and e-PTFE membrane placement. The membrane was punctured and placed over the implant to ensure complete coverage of the circumferential intrabony defect and implant surfaces. The flap was repositioned on the outer side of the membrane and readapted with mattress and interrupted sutures to the pergingival implant for complete coverage of the membrane.

The patients were instructed to rinse twice daily for 2 weeks with 0.2% chlorhexidine solution, and an antibiotic regimen was prescribed

Table 2 Filling of bone defects at reentry

Bone defect	No. of implants	Amount of filling			Quality of filling	
		C	P	F	O	Fi
Insufficient bone volume	17	12	3	2	16*	1†
Extraction sites	8	6	2	0	7*	1*
Peri-implantitis defects	10	8	2	0	0	10†

C = complete fill; P = partial fill (> 50%); F = failed fill (< 50%).
O = osseous tissue; Fi = fibrous tissue.
*At 4.5 to 6 months.
†At 5 to 7 weeks.

for 7 days (tetracycline 250 mg four times a day). The sutures were removed after 14 days. The membranes were removed after 5 to 7 weeks as a minor surgical procedure.

Results

Group I

Healing in all surgical sites except three occurred uneventfully, and all 17 implants with surrounding tissues were available for probe measuring and photometric evaluation. After a healing period of 4.5 to 6 months, upon flap reflection the implants were found to be "integrated" and the membranes were retained in proper position under the soft tissue. Considerable force was required to separate the membrane from the surface of the bone.

The mean vertical measurements of the implant dehiscences and bone tissue gain of the 17 test sites at baseline and at reentry are shown in Fig 1. The dehisced implant sites varied between 2.0 and 9.0 mm at baseline, with an average dehiscence of 4.3 mm. Following membrane treatment, an average residual defect of 0.6 mm was measured, resulting in a bone tissue gain varying between 2.0 and 9.0 mm, with an average gain in bone height of 3.7

mm. Alveolar ridge augmentation in a buccolingual direction was also found in several sites.

Table 2 describes the amount and quality of defect filling. Out of 17 test sites, 3 dehisced implant sites showed partial fill (73% to 90%), 2 sites showed less than 50% fill (28% and 42%), and 12 dehisced sites showed complete fill of the defect with bone tissue (Figs 2a to c). Out of 17 test sites, two membranes perforated the soft tissue over an area 3 × 4 mm between the second and fourth week of healing and one membrane site developed a fistula after 8 weeks. In the perforated membrane sites, the removal of the membranes was performed 6 to 9 weeks after placement and a complete fill with a fibrous consistency was noted. At reentry this fibrous tissue had partially resorbed and a defect fill of 28% and 42% with bone was seen (Table 3). The mean percentage of bone tissue gain of the 17 dehisced sites was 89.4%, varying from 28% to 100%.

Group II

Healing in all surgical sites except two occurred uneventfully and all eight implant sites could be measured for bone changes. At second-stage surgery, 6 months after placement, the membranes were found to be retained in proper position under the soft tissue.

The mean vertical measurements of the implant dehiscences and the mean residual defect of the eight implants at baseline and at reentry

Table 3 Membrane position versus defect fill

Group	Membrane coverage	Fill	Membrane exposure	Fill	Fistula to membrane	Fill
I	14	11C/3P	2	2F	1	1C
II	5	5C	2	2P	1	1C
III	7	7C	3	2P/1C	0	0

C = complete fill; P = partial fill (>50%); F = failed fill (<50%).

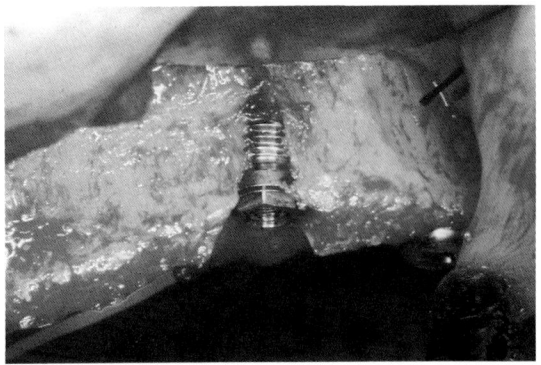

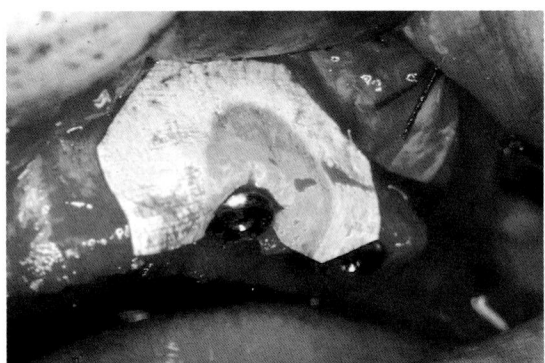

Fig 2a One of the treated patients in group I. Buccal view following reflection of mucoperiosteal flaps and placement of a Brånemark implant. Note exposed implant threads.

Fig 2b Following placement of the membrane secured to the implant with a cover screw. Note development of space under membrane.

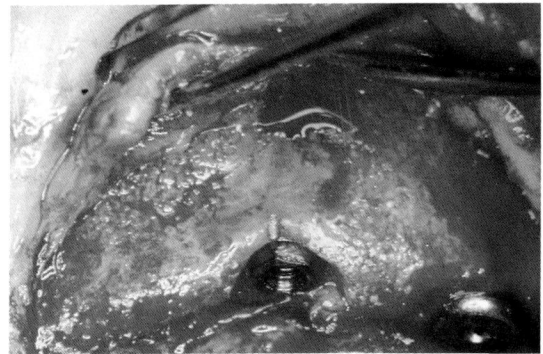

Fig 2c Membrane has been removed 6 months postoperatively and new bone formation is seen over previously exposed implant threads.

are shown in Fig 1. The mean defect was measured as 6.6 mm. At reentry 6 months later, there was a mean residual bone defect of 1.6 mm. Out of eight implants placed into a fresh extraction site six test sites showed a complete fill of the defect with hard bonelike tissue (Figs 3a and b). Alveolar ridge augmentation in a buccolingual direction was an additional finding in several sites.

Two test sites treated with a membrane perforated the soft tissue during the 3rd and 12th weeks of healing, respectively. The exposed material was kept in place for 5 and 6 weeks, respectively. At the 8-week removal time,

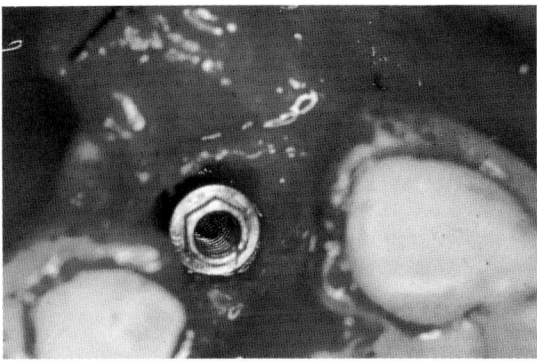

Fig 3a One of the treated patients in group II. Peri-implant voids after placement of implant into extraction site.

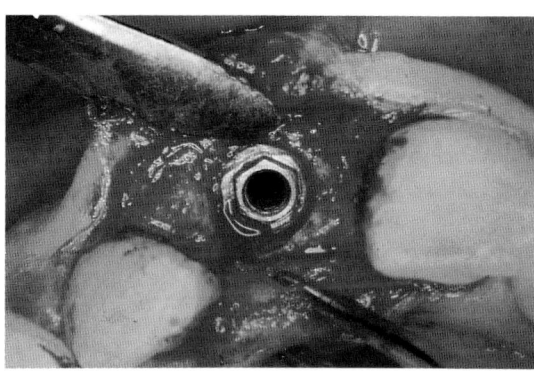

Fig 3b Reentry and membrane removal 6 months later reveals complete regeneration of bone up to the implant surface.

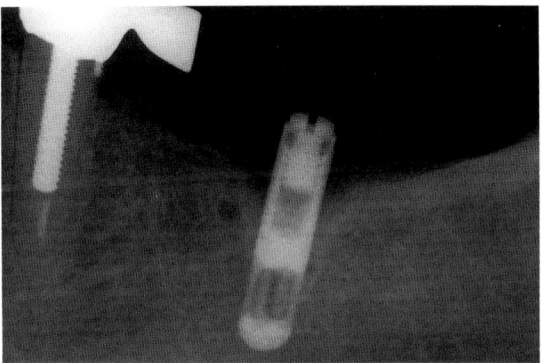

Fig 4a One of the treated patients in group III. Initial radiograph of peri-implant intrabony defect at the time of treatment and membrane placement.

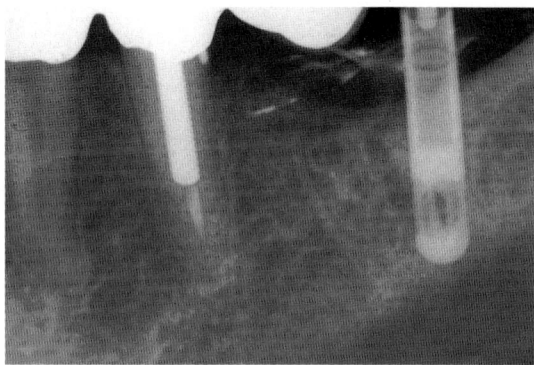

Fig 4b Six months postoperative radiographic appearance. Note the regeneration of bone within the intrabony defect.

regenerated tissue was noted with a fibrous consistency, and at the 18-week removal time regenerated tissue was noted with a combination of osseous and fibrous consistency. At the 6-month reentry time both test sites showed a partial fill of the defect with bone tissue (Table 3).

Group III

Premature exposure of the membrane was seen in three of the ten implant sites. The initial mean plaque score was 1.7, while at the final 6-month postoperative examination it was 0.6.

The initial mean gingival score was 2.1, while the final score was 0.3. The mean papilla bleeding index at the initial examination was 2.5, while at the final examination it was 0.5. The average initial probing depth was 6.8 mm and 6 months later it was 4.1 mm. Following surgical therapy and the initiation of a carefully supervised plaque control regimen, the gingival condition at all sites improved significantly. Implant mobility was not seen during the course of the study.

The topography of the ten peri-implant bone defects involved a moderate to advanced circumferential horizontal bone loss and a circumferential narrow to wide intrabony defect. The membranes were removed after 5 to 7 weeks.

Out of ten treated peri-implant defects, seven bone defects were filled with soft fibrous tissue and three defects were filled with dense fibrous tissue at the time of membrane removal. The mean initial dimension of the intrabony aspect of the total defect was 3.3 mm and a significant amount of defect fill occurred on an average of 3.0 mm at the time of membrane removal.

Comparison of the ten treated implants between baseline and final radiographs 6 months postoperative appeared to demonstrate radiographic evidence of excellent repair with bone regenerative capacity of this membrane technique in seven intrabony defects (Figs 4a and b). Three intrabony defects remained apparent during the course of the study and did not demonstrate any defect fill. Two of the failed regenerated defects had premature membrane exposure (see Table 3). No radiographic evidence was seen for regeneration of bone tissue coronal to the intrabony component of the peri-implant defect.

Discussion

This clinical study was performed to test the principle of guided tissue regeneration in a variety of indications for the repair of implant defects. An expanded PTFE membrane was used to isolate the implant surface from soft tissue cells, thereby allowing bone cells to repopulate the bony defect around the implant.

Most of the treated implants in groups I and II presented practically complete bone coverage of the exposed threads. The treated peri-implant bony defects in group III showed, to a lesser extent, a bone regenerative capacity. This incomplete bone regeneration may be related to a contaminated implant surface. In addition, the treatment methodology for group III included placement of the membrane around a pergingival implant. Since an intraoral communication through the implant sulcus was present, the time of membrane removal was decreased

to 5 to 7 weeks after placement. This was in contrast to the test sites in groups I and II, where the membrane removal was performed between 18 to 24 weeks.

Although the results of the present study indicate that the GTR technique is conducive to bone tissue regeneration, caution should be exercised in estimating prognosis. The amount of new bone formation will depend on the variation of the space volume between the membrane and the surface of the implant. Another aspect of great importance is the appropriate management of surgical flaps and the need to keep the membranes submerged during a healing time of at least 4.5 to 6 months. If flap separation occurs and a membrane becomes exposed, a maintenance problem develops and a higher risk for a decreased gain in bone tissue is seen. An exposed membrane should not be kept in place for much longer than 6 weeks.

Conclusion

When evaluating regenerated tissue as seen in this study, it can be noted that three different qualities of tissue were seen: (1) bone tissue, (2) a combination of bone and soft tissue, and (3) thick fibrous soft tissue. This surgical application of an e-PTFE membrane provided a clinical method to enhance bone formation around dehisced dental implants and implants in fresh extraction sites. Implants with "peri-implantitis" bone defects demonstrated radiographic bone fill in the intrabony component of the defect, but no gain in bone tissue coronal to the intrabony component of the defect. Further long-term clinical investigations are needed.

References

1. Brånemark P-I, Hansson BO, Adell R, Breine U, Lindström J, Hallen O, et al. Osseointegrated implants in the treatment of the edentulous jaw. Experience from a 10-year period. *Scand J Plast Reconstr Surg* 1977; 11(suppl 16).

2. Adell R, Lekholm U, Rockler B, Brånemark P-I. A 15-year study of osseointegrated dental implants in the treatment of the edentulous jaw. *Int J Oral Maxillofac Surg* 1981;10:87.

3. Albrektsson T, Dahl E, Enbon L, Engevall S, Engquist B, Eriksson AR, et al. Osseointegrated oral implants. A Swedish multicenter study of 8139 consecutively inserted Nobelpharma implants. *J Periodontol* 1988;59:287–296.

4. Albrektsson T. A multicenter report on osseointegrated oral implants. *J Prosthet Dent* 1988;60:75–84.

5. Adell R, Lekholm U, Rockler B, et al. Marginal tissue reactions at osseointegrated titanium fixtures. A three-year longitudinal prospective study. *Int J Oral Maxillofac Surg* 1986;15:39–52.

6. Gammage DD, Parham JR, Charles M, et al. Clinical management of failing implants: Four case reports. *J Oral Implant* 1989;15:24.

7. Choi P, Oyen O, Bissada N. Guided tissue regeneration and bone formation around endosseous dental implants. *J Dent Res* 1989;68:264.

8. Zablotsky MH, Meffert RM. Guided tissue regeneration on dehisced HA-coated and titanium endosseous implants. *J Dent Res* 1990;69:347.

9. Becker W, Becker BE, Handelsman M, Celletti R, et al. Bone formation at dehisced dental implant sites treated with implant augmentation material: A pilot study in dogs. *Int J Periodont Rest Dent* 1990;10:93.

10. Dahlin C, Sennerby L, Lekholm U, Linde A, et al. Generation of new bone around titanium implants using a membrane technique: An experimental study in rabbits. *Int J Oral Maxillofac Implants* 1989;4:19.

11. Dahlin C, Linde A, Gottlow J, Nyman S. Healing of bone defects by guided tissue regeneration. *Plast Reconstr Surg* 1989;5:672.

12. Dahlin C, Gottlow J, Linde A, Nyman S. Healing of maxillary and mandibular bone defects using a membrane technique. *J Dent Res* 1989;68:914.

13. Seibert J, Nyman S. Localized ridge augmentation in dogs incorporating the principle of guided tissue regeneration. *J Periodontol* 1990;61:157.

14. Lazzara R. Immediate implant placement into extraction sites: Surgical and restorative advantages. *Int J Periodont Rest Dent* 1989;9:333.

15. Nyman S, Lang N, Buser D, Bragger U. Bone regeneration adjacent to titanium dental implants using guided tissue regeneration: A report of two cases. *Int J Oral Maxillofac Implants* 1990;5:9.

16. Nyman S, Lindhe J, Karring T, Rylander H. New attachment following surgical treatment of human periodontal disease. *J Clin Periodontol* 1982;9:290.

17. Gottlow J, Nyman S, Lindhe J, Karring T, Wennstrom J. New attachment formation in the human periodontium by guided tissue regeneration: Case reports. *J Periodontol* 1986;13:604.

18. Becker W, Becker B, Berg L, Prichard J, Caffesse R, et al. New attachment after treatment with root isolation procedures: Report for treated class III and class II furcations and vertical osseous defects. *Int J Periodont Rest Dent* 1988;3:2.

19. Pontoriero R, Lindhe J, Nyman S, Karring T, et al. Guided tissue regeneration in degree II furcation-involved mandibular molars. *J Clin Periodontol* 1988;15:247.

20. Cortellini P, Pini Prato G, Baldi C, Clauser C. Guided tissue regeneration with different materials. *Int J Periodont Rest Dent* 1990;10:137.

21. Philip L, Parham JR, Charles M, et al. Effects of an air-powder abrasive system on plasma-sprayed titanium implant surfaces: An in-vitro evaluation. *J Oral Implant* 1989;15:78.

22. Newman MG, Flemmig TF. Periodontal considerations of implants and implant-associated microbiota. *J Dent Educ* 1988;52:737.

Session III Discussion

Question to D. Lundgren (Jönköping, Sweden): How much time elapsed from the primary surgery (implant placement) to the connection of the implant to the prosthesis?

D. Lundgren: Three to 5 months.

Question to D. Lundgren: How did you connect the type-2 cases to the prosthesis?

D. Lundgren: A gold beam was cast and screwed to the framework of the prosthesis and to the fixture abutment via the gold cylinder.

Question to D. Lundgren: Do you think that the tooth hypermobility is reversible, ie, will the mobility of the tooth-supported prosthesis increase again if it is released from the implant?

D. Lundgren: Perhaps. The screw-coupled prostheses had very reduced periodontal support. Tooth mobility might therefore increase again if the implant support is removed. However, if the connection is unscrewed the passive support might be enough to prevent recurrence of the tooth hypermobility.

Question to D. Lundgren: Is this a special way of treating advanced periodontal disease?

D. Lundgren: By no means! The periodontal disease had previously been cured. The presented measures were undertaken only to prevent or reverse a progressive hypermobility of the abutment teeth.

Question to B. Becker (Tucson, Arizona): Did you try any of the resorbable membranes with this technique?

B. Becker: We have not used any other membranes in conjunction with the placement of immediate implants in our studies. It has been well documented that the polytetrafluoroethylene (PTFE) membrane can be successfully used for guided tissue regeneration in periodontal therapy, and it has been documented that PTFE can be used to treat fenestration defects over implants at the time of placement in dogs and in rabbits. There have been no long-term studies published showing the efficacy of using resorbable membranes for periodontal regeneration or with implants. Therefore, at the present time all of our research has been with the PTFE membranes.

Question to S. Jovanovic (Aachen, Germany): Do you think that the treatment of failing implants is predictable and that regeneration of hard tissue can be achieved?

S. Jovanovic: The treatment of progressive peri-implant bone loss is related to a compromised implant site. Most probably, a peri-implant infection has been established and the surface of the implant is contaminated with pathogenic bacteria. Treatment should eliminate all possible etiological factors such as bacterial infection and occlusal overload. Up to 3-year results demonstrate an excellent response of the peri-implant tissues after resective "peri-implant surgery," with the establishment of a healthy peri-implant seal. However, the outcome of regenerative surgery is more complex and dependent on an aseptic implant surface, an intraosseous defect, and bone repair. The short-term results of our treatment procedures show good regeneration of the vertical defects, but further investigation on implant surface detoxification and regeneration techniques is necessary.

Question to S. Jovanovic: Do you feel that the membrane should stay submerged during the healing period of the implant, and what happens if the membrane perforates the flap?

S. Jovanovic: The minimum time for healing to regenerate osseous tissue is unknown and will most probably vary with patient and site selection. Although animal experiments demonstrated that after 6 weeks the regeneration of osseous tissue occurred, our data show compromised bone regeneration with early retrieved membranes. Therefore, we feel that the membrane should be kept in place during the entire submerged healing of the implant for at least 6 months. To achieve and maintain this submerged healing, modified flap designs are needed. If a membrane becomes exposed due to flap separation or pressure from a prosthetic appliance, a maintenance problem develops. To eliminate the risk of compromising the regeneration site, exposed membranes should not be kept in place for longer than 4 to 6 weeks.

Question to S. Jovanovic: Why did you wait for soft tissue closure after the extraction of hopeless teeth?

S. Jovanovic: In our early results with immediate implant and membrane placement, we saw a high degree of membrane exposure and the development of fistulae. We then changed our surgical protocol to a delayed implant placement. This allowed us to achieve a more predictable soft tissue closure over the surgical sites. Although the callus formation is disturbed during the placement of the implant, we feel that full coverage with soft tissue is detrimental to the protection of the blood clot and the success of regeneration.

Implant Component Compatibility

P. Binon, D. Weir, L. Watanabe, and L. Walker

Following the introduction of the Swedish Biotes System (Nobelpharma AB, Göteborg, Sweden) into North America, several alternative systems with fixtures and components that closely emulate the original design and treatment protocol became available. Claims of equivalency and compatibility soon followed.[1,2] These products offer an attractive alternative because they are less expensive, offer more prosthetic flexibility, and are easier to obtain. Physically, the replicates are similar in shape, size, and thread design. These "Brånemark" clones are often grouped together without distinction and it is possible and even likely that components from different manufacturers are used interchangeably in restorations using this type of implant.

The coupling of imprecisely matched components can influence long-term implant prognosis. The clinical implications of poor component fit and compatibility are: frequent loose screws, chronic screw fracture, high bacterial plaque retention, adverse soft tissue response, and ultimately, the loss of integration.[3–9] The purpose of this study was to evaluate machining accuracy and consistency and the compatibility of four different systems' component parts.

Materials and methods

Implant components from Nobelpharma USA, Chicago (Biotes); Collagen Corp, Palo Alto, Calif (Osseodent); Core-Vent Corp, Encino, Calif (Swede-Vent); and Implant Innovations, West Palm Beach, Fla (SID Threaded) were evaluated for compatibility within and between systems. Three of the systems consisted of an implant, abutment cylinder with retaining screw, and a gold cylinder and screw. The fourth system (Swede-Vent) varied in having one-piece abutments. The different components are identified throughout the study by the following letters:

Nobelpharma = N, NP; Swede-Vent = S, SV; Osseodent = O, OD; Implant Innovations = I, III.

The accuracy and consistency of machining is based on the direct measurement of five randomly selected implants and abutments from each system with a digital micrometer and a micrometer microscope, accurate to one micrometer. Measurements from selected locations that reflect easy and difficult machining tasks are reported in this preliminary report. The difference between the high and low values measured at each location was used as an indicator of accuracy and precision. Large differences reflect greater machining tolerances and variations in component dimensions. The respective components were then assembled into as many different combinations as possible and measured for interface fit at the fixture/abutment (F/A) level and the abutment/gold cylinder (A/C) level. Assembly of the components was standardized by using a Nobelpharma torque wrench. High-magnification 35 mm transparencies for each interface were obtained using a Nikon F3/T with a 105 mm lens (Nikon,

Table 1 Implants: Accuracy and consistency of matching

Implant	OD* Head (μm)	OD Hex (μm)	Length (μm)	Composite (μm)
Nobelpharma	4	14	10	28
Implant innovations	11	13	15	39
Swede-Vent	12	61	15	88
Osseodent	9	39	54	102

*OD = outside diameter.

Table 2 Implant abutments: Accuracy and consistency of matching two-piece abutments

Implant	Collar		Screw			Composite value (μm)
	Width (μm)	Length (μm)	Hex width (μm)	Length (μm)	Hex length (μm)	
Implant Innovations	9	25	94	92	46	266
Nobelpharma	14	34	92	80	90	310
Osseodent	8	143	320	71	50	592

Tokyo, Japan) mounted on a bellows incorporating a 1,000 watt strobe and using Ecktachrome 100HC film (Kodak, Rochester, NY). The slides were projected and direct interface and abutment width measurements were made. The discrepancy was then calculated using the following equation:

$$\frac{X \text{ (interface gap in μm)}}{\text{Known abutment width}} = \frac{\text{Measured interface error (mm)}}{\text{Measured abutment width (mm)}}$$

Representative scanning electron microscopic (SEM) views for each of the matings were also obtained. A cross section of each system's assembled component was also evaluated.

Results

Comparing the implants on the basis of outside diameter of the head, outside diameter of the hex, and full length of the fixture resulted in composite values ranging from 28 to 102 μm (Table 1). The best machining tolerances were demonstrated by NP and III fixtures.

Comparing the two-piece abutments made by NP, OD, and III implant components on the basis of collar length and width, and screw length and hex length and width, the resulting composite values ranged from 266 to 592 μm (Table 2). The least variation and the best machining tolerances were demonstrated by III and NP. Core-Vent one-piece abutments (TTA-5 and TSA-4) were also evaluated. Three points were measured on each and the composite scores reflected tight machining tolerances (Table 3).

Summary data for unmated fixtures and abutments (Table 4) ranged from 315 to 694 μm, with III and NP demonstrating the tightest machining tolerances.

Component fit within the same system was then evaluated. The fixture/abutment interface

Table 3 Implant abutment: Accuracy and consistency of machining one-piece Core-Vent

Abutment	1-Width (μm)	2-Length (μm)	Full length (μm)	Composite (μm)
TSA-4	15	6	10	31
TTA-5	34	24	38	96

Table 4 Summary data for fixture and abutment: Accuracy and consistency of machining conventional and one-piece abutments

Conventional	Fixture (μm)	Abutment (μm)	Composite (μm)
Implant Innovations	39	266	315
Nobelpharma	28	310	338
Osseodent	102	592	694
One-piece abutments			
TSA-4	88	31	119
TTA-5	88	96	184

was measured (N = 30) and the calculated interface error was recorded at 20 μm (III), 23 μm (OD), and 49 μm (NP). High magnification slides and corresponding SEMs illustrating typical matings are shown in Figs 1a to f. The higher values recorded for the NP interface are the result of the typically rounded edge found on all NP abutments (Fig 1f). This appears to be a limited surface phenomenon and not indicative of an open penetrable interface.

The SV fixtures were mated with Core-Vent one-piece abutments (TTA-5 and TSA-4). Fixture/abutment discrepancy was measured at 15 μm for the SV/TSA-4 (range, 7 to 21 μm, N = 10) and 18 μm for the SV/TTA-5 (range 14 to 28 μm, N = 10). Typical interface adaptation is shown in Figs 2a and b.

Component fit for mixed systems (mixed manufacturers) was then evaluated at the fixture/abutment interface. The results are shown in Table 5. The smallest mean discrepancy (21 μm) recorded at this interface was obtained between Swede-Vent fixtures and Implant Innovation abutments (Fig 3).

The abutment/gold cylinder interface was evaluated next (Fig 4). Typical matings of components from the same system are illustrated in Figs 5a to f. The results are shown in Table 6. The interface discrepancy noted for III was 32 μm (range, 21 to 49 μm) and 35 μm for NP. The OD average discrepancy was 62 μm with a range of 28 to 119 μm.

Component mating from mixed systems (manufacturers) was subsequently evaluated. Results of the different combinations are shown in Table 6. When III and NP abutments are fitted with their own and competing gold cylinders, the values range from 32 to 41 μm. When OD abutments were mated with their own, III, and NP gold cylinders, discrepancies of 56 to 62 μm (range, 21 to 161 μm) resulted. These matings were often skewed to the side (Figs 6a and b), with one side open more than the other. The ×200 SEM of the NP/III abutment to gold cylinder illustrates a representative good fit (Fig 7). A typical poor fit is exemplified by the OD/NP mating in Fig 8.

A representative stack of each system components was embedded in resin, sectioned, polished, and examined with SEM. The resultant cross sections support the surface measurement data. All three samples (III, NP, OD) demonstrated tight fixture/abutment interface fit. The NP section verified a sealed interface and the typical rounded abutment edge. The TSA-4 abutment/Swede-Vent fixture mating confirmed the previously noted tight interface fit.

The abutment/gold cylinder interface for III, NP, OD is visualized in Figs 9a, b and c. The fit of the internal bevel for III and NP is crisp and tight. The OD internal bevel shows skewed seating between components. A higher magnification of the abutment/gold cylinder interface demonstrates complete and incomplete seating of the components (Figs 10a and b).

Discussion

Variation in machining tolerances was noted between the four different systems evaluated.

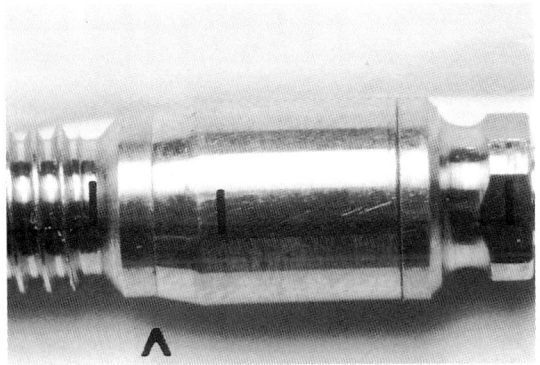

1a

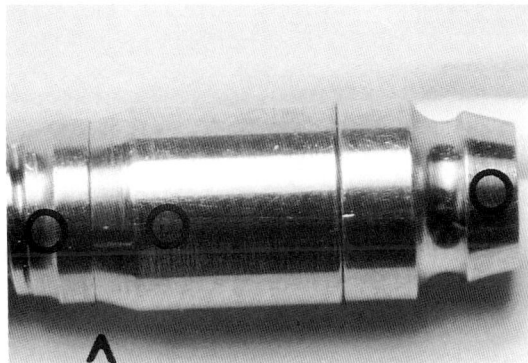

1b

Figs 1a to c High-magnification slides of assembled component parts. Letters designate system and the arrow points to the fixture/abutment interface being evaluated.

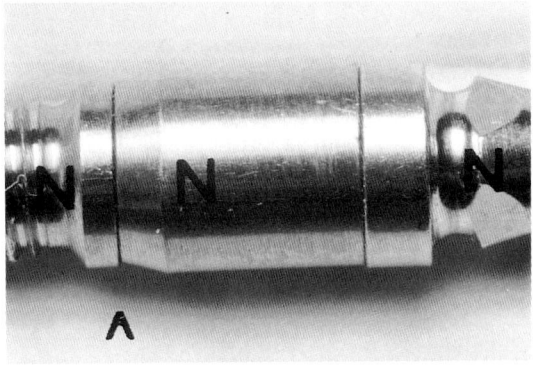

1c

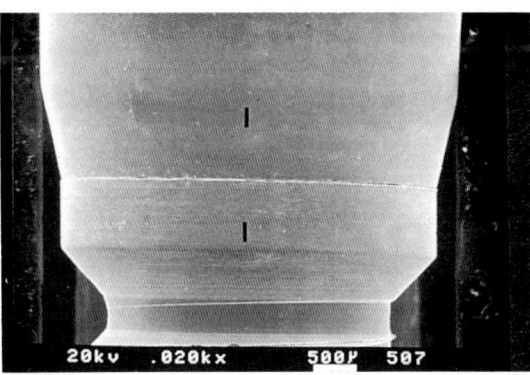

1d

Figs 1d and e SEM views (×20) of the fixture/abutment interface.

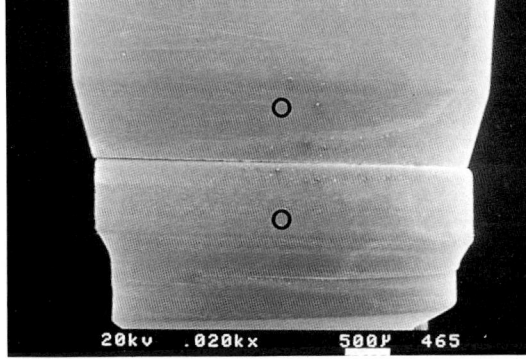

1e

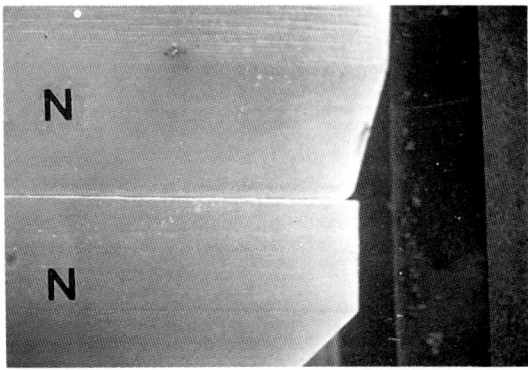

Fig 1f The typical rounded outside edge of the NP abutment collar. The interface is, however, sealed.

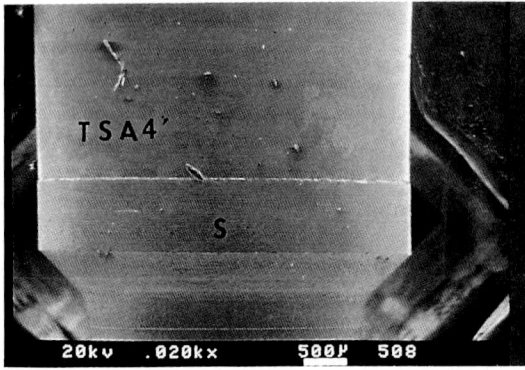

Fig 2a An SEM (×20) of the one-piece TSA-4 abutment mating with the SV fixture.

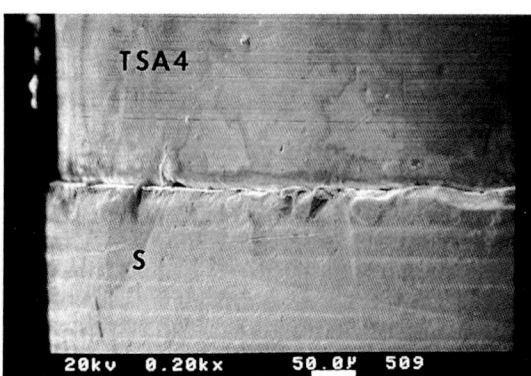

Fig 2b An SEM (×200) of the same interface, demonstrating excellent fit.

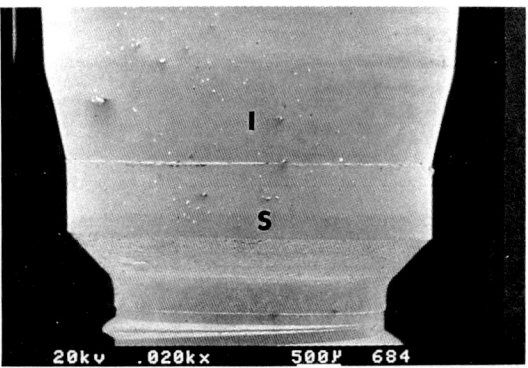

Fig 3 An SEM (×20) of the fixture/abutment interface between SV and III components. An example of an excellent fit of components of different systems.

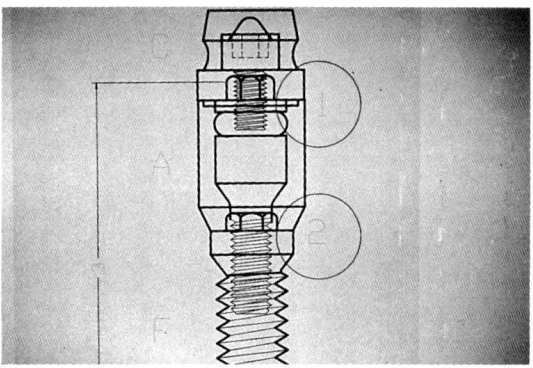

Fig 4 Schematic showing component assembly. Interface 1 (abutment/cylinder) and 2 (fixture/abutment) are marked as reference.

Table 5 Mixed system components fixture/abutment (F/A) interface*

F/A interface	Mean discrepancy (μm)
III/III	20
III/OD	24
III/NP	65
OD/OD	23
OD/III	37
OD/NP	66
NP/NP	49
NP/III	27
NP/OD	27
SV/III	21
SV/OD	25
SV/NP	45

*III = Implant Innovations; OD = Osseodent; NP = Nobelpharma; SV = Swede-Vent.

Table 6 Mixed system components abutment/gold cylinder (A/C) interface*

A/C interface	Mean discrepancy (μm)	Range (μm)
NP/NP	35	14–63
NP/III	32	21–49
NP/OD	39	21–56
III/III	32	21–49
III/NP	37	14–70
III/OD	41	21–63
OD/OD	62	28–119
OD/NP	56	21–126
OD/III	61	28–161

*III = Implant Innovations; OD = Osseodent; NP = Nobelpharma; SV = Swede-Vent.

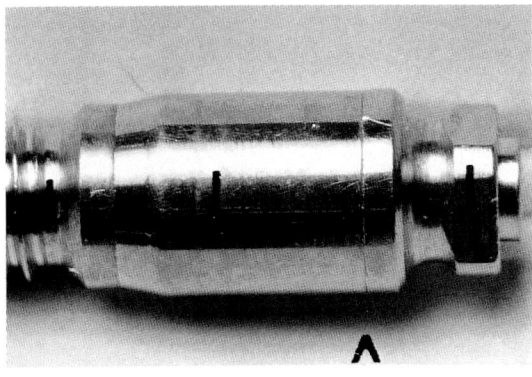

5a

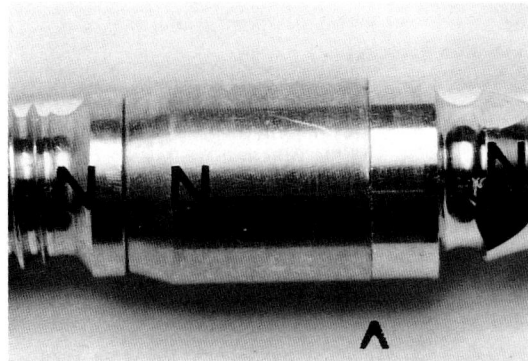

5b

Figs 5a to c High-magnification slides of assembled component parts. The arrow indicates the interface being examined (abutment/cylinder). In Fig 5c, the interface demonstrates an interface discrepancy clearly visible with the naked eye.

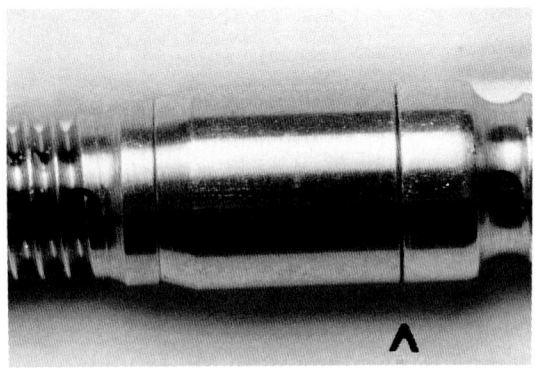

5c

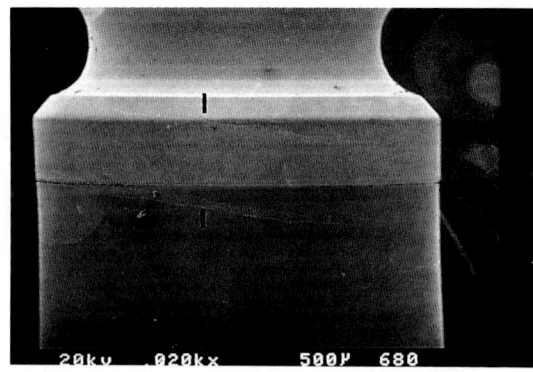

5d

Figs 5d to f SEM views of the abutment/cylinder interface. Figure 5e is a high magnification (× 200) of the excellent fit achieved with the NP components.

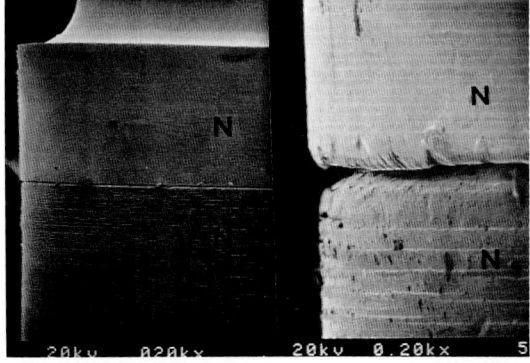

5e

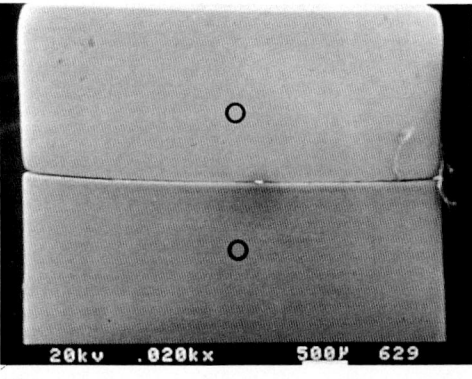

5f

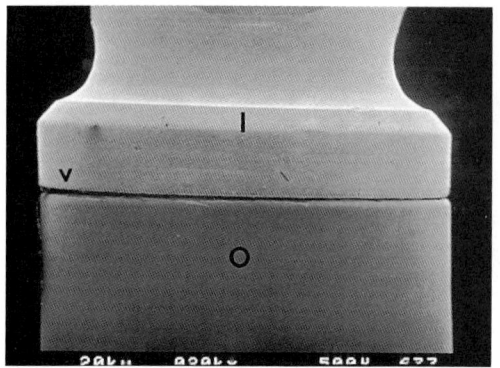

Fig 6a SEM view of the abutment/cylinder mating of OD and III components. The gold cylinder is skewed off center, resulting in an open margin of 85 μm.

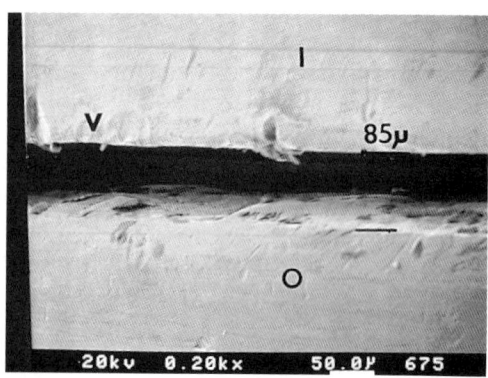

Fig 6b Higher magnification of the location marked with an arrow in Fig 6a.

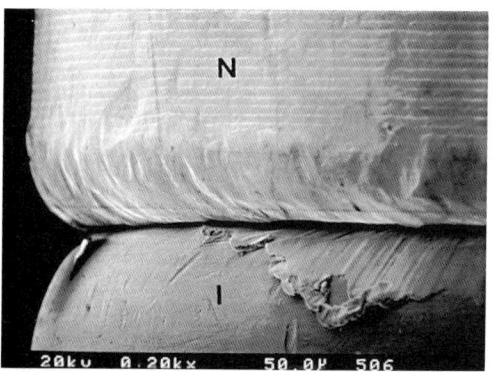

Fig 7 SEM view (×200) of an excellent abutment/cylinder interface fit between III and NP components.

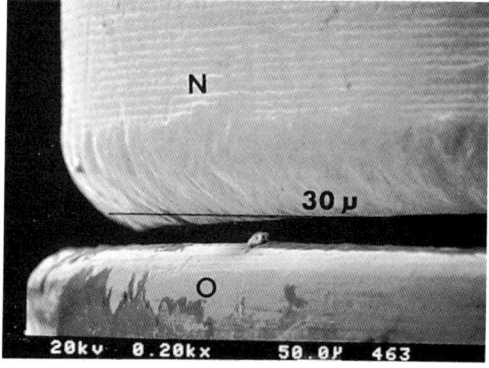

8a

Figs 8a to c SEM view of an abutment/cylinder interface between OD and NP components. Notice the skewed seating in Fig 8b. This results in an open margin of 30 μm on the right and 90 μm on the left. The material seen in the interface is conducting liquid that moved via capillary attraction up from the SEM mount.

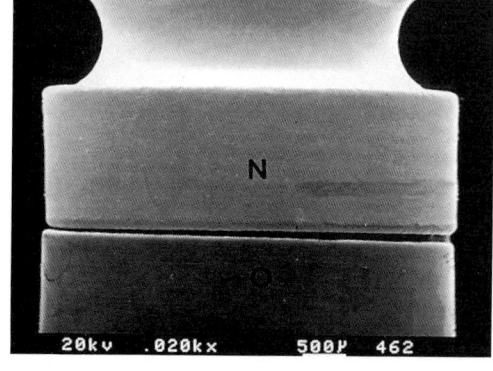

8b

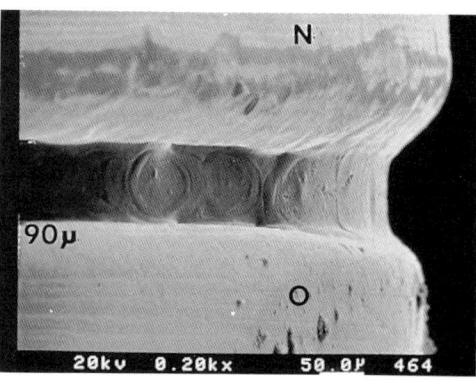

8c

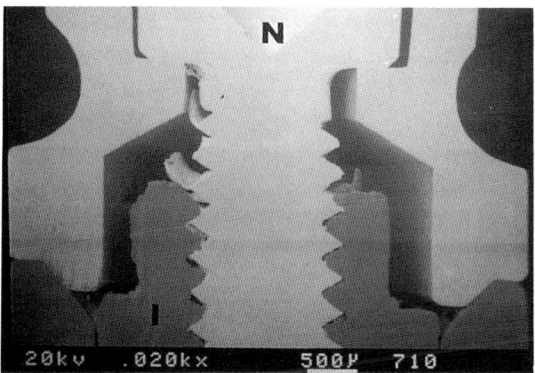

9a

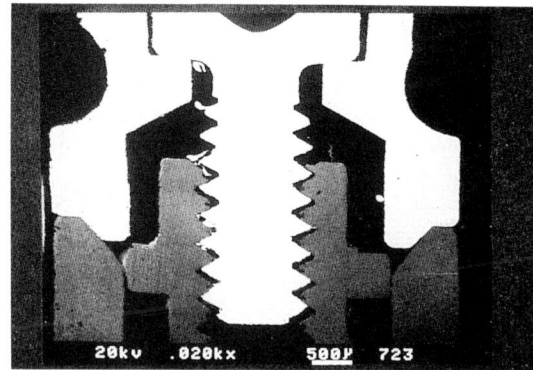

9b

Figs 9a to c SEM view of cross sections at the abutment/cylinder interface of III, NP, and OD components. The abutment/cylinder bevel of the III and NP components fit together and seal the interface. The OD interface does not seal completely.

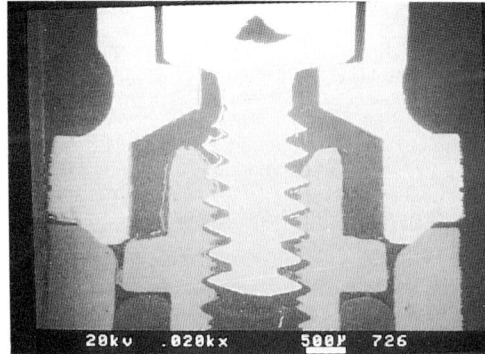

9c

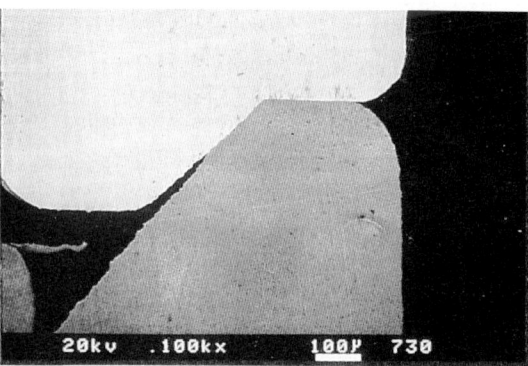

Fig 10a High-magnification SEM view of the III interface.

Fig 10b *(right)* High-magnification SEM view of the OD interface. Figure illustrates thickness of the abutment's internal bevel, which is responsible for the poor seating identified in some of the components.

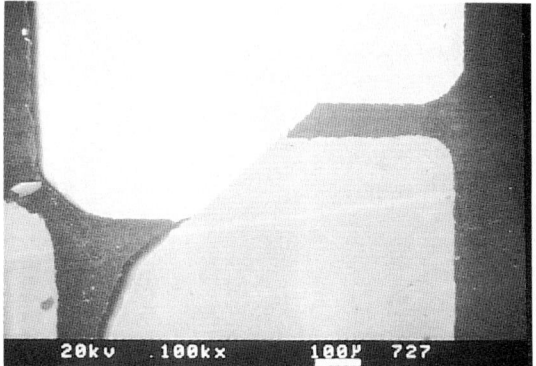

Inconsistencies in machining component parts can have a profound effect on interface fit. Preliminary results indicate that the NP and III system component parts evaluated demonstrate excellent accuracy and machining consistency. The SV one-piece abutment system also demonstrated excellent and consistent fixture/abutment interface fit. From a clinical perspective, component fit within and between the four systems evaluated can be considered acceptable, the only exception being the OD abutment/gold cylinder interface. The one variable that consistently resulted in a poor abutment/cylinder interface, both within its own system and when mated with the other systems, was the OD abutment. The SEM photos document a skewed seating of the gold cylinders. The SEM cross section of an OD mating shows that the gold cylinder cannot seat completely because the bevels are mismatched. A noticeable difference in angularity of the inside bevel of the OD abutment collar is present. It is logical to conclude that inconsistencies in the machining of this bevel have resulted in an unacceptable interface fit.

Conclusions

The preliminary results suggest that there are two systems available (III/two-piece abutment and SV/one piece abutment) that meet or exceed the machining and design criteria set by the original Swedish system. Components from these two systems can be mated with each other and those of the Swedish system to achieve an acceptable level of compatibility. It is prudent however to carefully inspect the fit of all components on a clean implant before use.

Although these systems meet high machining standards, long-term biological efficacy must still be documented in clinical trials.

Acknowledgments

We would like to acknowledge and thank the Nobelpharma (Göteborg, Sweden), Core-Vent (Encino, Calif), and Implant Innovations (Irvine, Calif) Corporations for providing the components used in this study.

References

1. Orcon Sciences. Brochure no. 8028-01-1187. Osseodent implants meet or exceed the strict design criteria of the Swedish system. Brochure no. 8049-01-0788. Compatible with several different abutment types, both fixed and removable. Palo Alto, Calif: Collagen Corp.
2. Core-Vent Corp. Brochure no. 4 NOBEL 2. Encino, Calif: Core-Vent Corp.
3. Sones A. Advanced problem solving: Complications with osseointegrated implants. 53rd Annual Scientific Meeting, Pacific Coast Society of Prosthodontists, Sun River, Ore, 1988.
4. Lekholm U, Adell R, Brånemark P-I. Possible complications. p 237 In P.-I. Brånemark, G.A. Zarb, T. Albrektsson (eds) *Tissue-Integrated Prostheses: Osseointegration in Clinical Dentistry*. Chicago: Quintessence Publ Co, 1985.
5. Adell R, Lekholm U, Rockler B, Brånemark P-I. A 15-year study of osseointegrated implants in treatment of the edentulous jaw. *Int J Oral Surg* 1981;6:387–416.
6. Worthington P, Bolender CL, Taylor TD. The Swedish system of osseointegrated implants: Problems and complications encountered during a 4-year trial period. *Int J Oral Maxillofac Implants* 1987;2:77–84.
7. Balshi T. Preventing and resolving complications with osseointegrated implants. *Dent Clin North Am* 1989; 33:821.
8. Beumer J, Lewis S. p 239 In *The Brånemark Implant System—Clinical and Laboratory Procedures*. St Louis: Ishiyaku EuroAmerica Inc, 1989.
9. Hobo S, Ichida E, Garcia L. p 239 In *Osseointegration and Occlusal Rehabilitation*. Tokyo: Quintessence Publ Co, 1989.

Removal Torques of Commercially Pure Titanium and Vitallium Implants in Rabbit Bone

C.B. Johansson and T. Albrektsson

Commercially pure (CP) titanium and the cobalt-chrome alloy Vitallium represent two generally used implant materials in oral and orthopedic surgery.

Tissue reactions to CP titanium implants have frequently been reported in the literature, whereas reports on tissue-Vitallium reactions have been rare. The aim of this study is to compare the two materials with respect to removal torque and histomorphometry after insertion in rabbit bone.

Materials and methods

Two screw-shaped implants (diameter 3.5 mm, length 10 mm) of each metal to be tested were inserted in each proximal tibial methaphysis of seven adult New Zealand white rabbits. Three months later, the animals were sacrificed and seven implants of each metal were removed with a 6 BTG-N Tohnichi Gauge Instrument (Tohnichi Mfg Co, Ltd, Tokyo, Japan). The remaining 14 implants (7 of each metal) with surrounding bone were fixed and further processed for cutting and grinding and finally analyzed histomorphometrically using databased Leitz Microvid equipment (Leitz, Inc, Wetzlar, Germany).

Results

The average removal torque for the CP titanium implants was 24.9 N/cm (range 18 to 30 N/cm), SD 5.0. Vitallium implants had an average of 11.7 N/cm (range 7 to 19.5 N/cm), SD 4.5. The results from the histomorphometrical part of the study will be completed during the first half of 1990.[1]

Conclusion

The present study has demonstrated a clear significant difference in removal torque between the two materials. Screw-shaped CP titanium implants presented a higher removal torque than Vitallium implants 3 months after insertion in rabbit bone.

Reference

1. Johansson CB, Sennerby L, Albrektsson T. A removal torque and histomorphometric study of bone tissue reactions to commercially pure (CP) titanium and Vitallium® implants. *Int J Oral Maxillofac Implants* 1991; 6:437–441.

Removal Torques for Titanium Implants Following Irradiation

Å. Hansson, K. Johnsson, M. Jacobsson,* and I. Turesson

The effect of irradiation on osteogenesis has been studied by several authors. Jacobsson and co-workers[1] have earlier demonstrated that the regenerative capacity of bone is much retarded after administration of 15 Gy of cobalt 60 irradiation. From a clinical point of view, the disturbed bone healing pattern may be a serious drawback. For instance, after tumor resection in the craniofacial area and therapeutic irradiation, there is often a need for bone reconstruction with grafts and/or implants.

Bone grafts in many craniofacial locations often result in failure, particularly when the host bone has been irradiated. In one study, O'Brien et al[2] reported 24 cases of mandibular reconstruction using autologous bone with successful overall treatment (patient alive, disease free, with viable graft) in 42% of the cases. The complication rate was 65%. Thirty-eight percent of the patients were dead at the time of followup (6 months to 3.5 years). In that material it was not possible to evaluate whether the patients actually benefitted from reconstruction. Albert et al[3] presented a study of ten patients with malignant tumors in whom mandibular reconstruction was undertaken using a Dacron mesh tray and cancellous bone. Eight of the reconstructions were stable for an average of 21 months (6 months to 3 years), but 40% of the patients were dead within an average of 12.5 months (6 months to 2.5 years).

The attitude toward implant insertion in irradiated bone at many clinics is very conservative, if at all recommended. The newly irradiated bone

is not the ideal host site for either a bone transplant or an implant. It has been suggested[4] that a delay of the bone surgical intervention may be advantageous compared to surgery in fairly recently irradiated tissue. If delayed surgery is combined with an extremely gentle surgical technique, to disturb as little as possible the potentially reduced healing capacity of the bone, clinically more favorable results are deemed possible in restorative surgery after irradiation.[5]

The aim of the present study was to evaluate how irradiation affects the degree of bone tissue integration for commercially pure titanium implants, as measured with the torque necessary for removal of implants, ie, simulating a clinically applicable situation.

Materials and methods

Animals

A total of ten adult New Zealand white rabbits of both sexes were used in the study. Closure of the epiphyseal plates was confirmed by radiography.

Implants

The implant consisted of a screw of commercially pure titanium with an exactly known composition. The implant had been manually

*Keynote speaker.

graded, cleaned in n-Butylalcohol (Merck) and absolute alcohol in ultrasonic baths and then autoclaved. The screw had an outer diameter of 3.6 mm and the bottom represented a perfect cylinder without pores or cuts and with a square top that fitted to a specially constructed connector (Fig 1).

Anesthetic procedure

During irradiation and the surgical sessions, the animals were anesthetized with intramuscular injections of a combination of fentanyl and fluanison (Hypnorm, Mekos) at a dose of 0.5 mL/kg body weight and intraperitoneal injections of diazepam (Valium, Roche) at a dose of 2.5 mg. Postoperatively intramuscular injections of buprenorphine (Temgesic, Reckitt & Colman) were given in doses of 0.1 mg.

Irradiation procedure

The rabbits were irradiated at a temperature of 22°C. During irradiation the femur and tibia were placed on a 10-cm-thick polystyrene phantom. Gamma irradiation (Co60) was used to minimize the difference in the absorbed dose in soft tissue and bone. Source skin distance (SSD) was 60 cm. The dose rate was approximately 2 Gy per minute. A 5-mm bolus was applied to ensure full buildup. A single dose of 15 Gy was given to the right hind limb.

Surgical procedure

After irradiation, the animals were divided into two groups with five animals in each. Group A had implants inserted directly after irradiation had been completed, whereas group B had implants inserted 12 weeks after irradiation. The implants were inserted under aseptic conditions using a very gentle surgical technique with sharp drills and low drill speeds. Ample cooling with saline solution was performed when preparing the implant sites by drilling as well as when the implants were carefully

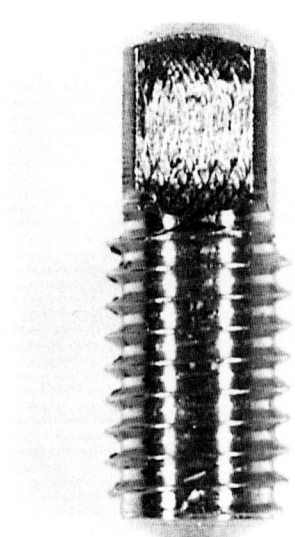

Fig 1 The implant consists of a screw made up of commercially pure titanium. The outer diameter of the implant is 3.6 mm and the bottom represents a perfect cylinder without pores or cuts. The top is square and fits to a specially constructed connector.

screwed into the tibial and femoral cortical bone sites. The fasciae were sutured in separate layers and the skin closed. The animals were allowed to be fully weight-bearing after surgery.

Removal torque measurements

Eight weeks after implant insertion the animals were again anesthetized according to the method described earlier. The skin and fasciae were opened and the implants unscrewed using a torque gauge instrument (Tohnichi 15 BTG-N; Tohnichi Mfg Co, Ltd, Tokyo, Japan), which gave direct readings of the torque (in N/cm) necessary for loosening of the implant.

Statistical methods

Comparison between the irradiated and the nonirradiated side was performed with the Wilcoxon test for pair comparison with respect to the sum of the forces required for loosening

Table 1   Removal torques for group A*

Animal no.	Right tibia	Left tibia (control)	Right femur	Left femur (control)
1	15	29	17	24.5
2	9	21.5	17	22
3	10	11.5	11.5	37
4	4	23	17	18
5	11.5	15	17	17

*Measurements for removal torques are given in N/cm.

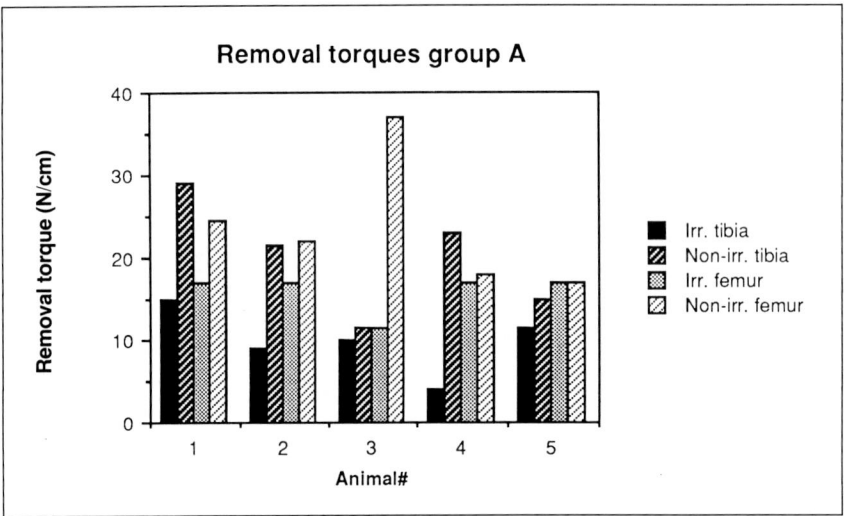

Fig 2   Graph illustrating removal torques for the animals in group A.

the implant in the upper and lower limbs. Two-sided tests were used. To elucidate the effect of a delay in implanting the screws, a 95% confidence interval for the difference between the two groups with respect to the difference, the sum of forces at the irradiated side minus the sum of forces at the nonirradiated side was determined. Also within each group a confidence interval was determined for the last mentioned difference.

Results

The mean removal torque for the tibial test implants of group A ranged from 4 to 15 N/cm as compared to 11.5 to 29 N/cm for the corresponding control implants. The corresponding results for the femoral implants were 11.5 to 17 N/cm for the tests and 17 to 37 N/cm for the controls (Table 1 and Fig 2).

For group B the torque necessary to remove the tibial test implants varied from 9 to 19 N/cm and 17 to 23.5 for the controls. For the femoral test implants the removal torque varied from 12 to 24 N/cm as compared to the control implants with a range of 19 to 25 N/cm (Table 2 and Fig 3). The difference between the sum (upper and lower limb) of forces at the nonirradiated side and the irradiated side is summarized in Table 3.

When applying the Wilcoxon test for pair comparison on the difference between the nonirradiated and the irradiated side for the whole

Table 2 Removal torques for group B*

Animal no.	Right tibia	Left tibia (control)	Right femur	Left femur (control)
1	10.5	23.5	24	25
2	19	17	17	20
3	8.5	19	18	24
4	9	21.5	12.5	19
5	8.5	22	12	22.5

*Measurements for removal torques are given in N/cm.

Table 3 Statistical evaluation

	Group A	Group B
Number of animals	5	5
Mean	− 17.9	− 14.9
SD	8.8	8.6
95% confidence interval	− 28.8 to − 7.0	− 25.6 to − 4.2

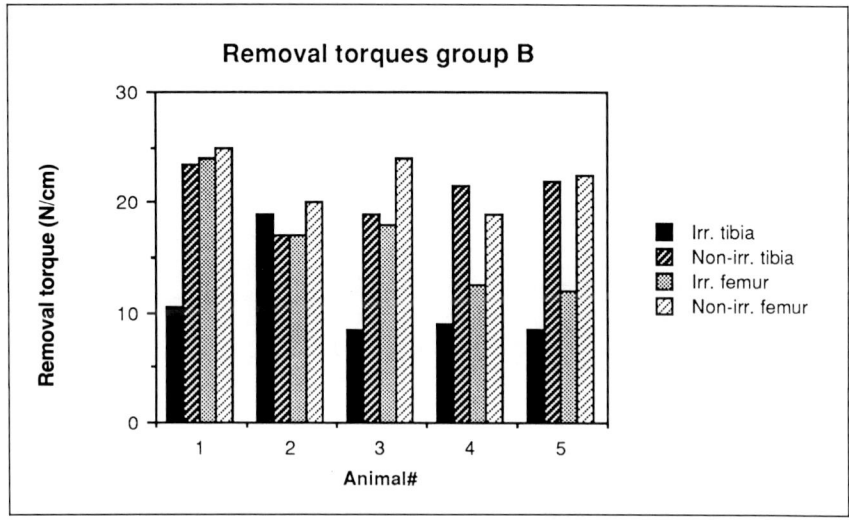

Fig 3 Graph illustrating removal torques for the animals in group B.

material (groups A and B), a significant reduction of required removal torque as a result of irradiation ($P<.01$) was found. The confidence interval for the difference between groups A and B was − 15.7 to 9.7, which contains zero. Thus no effect of a delay of 12 weeks could be demonstrated.

Discussion

It is well known that irradiation inhibits bone healing for extended periods of time after irradiation trauma.[4] The methods previously used measured, qualitatively and quantitatively, bone tissue formed within implants, such as the Bone Growth Chamber or the Bone Harvest Chamber, after irradiation.[6] These studies have provided important data and methods to accurately measure the healing capacity of bone tissue, but not its ability to incorporate an implant. What is studied in this investigation is a more complex situation in which other factors beside bone healing are involved. It can be said to be a reflection of the status of the bone-to-implant interface.

The present method, initially devised by Johansson et al,[7] provides an opportunity to mimic a clinical situation with an implant in situ in living bone tissue. From the study by Johansson et al,[7] it is apparent that the amount of bone formed around a similar titanium implant design will increase with time. After 21 days Johansson could show microscopic evidence of mostly soft tissue in the interface; at 30 days, more bone was observed in the implant threads, and at 90 days there was good contact between implant and mature bone tissue.

When the implant and tissue are brought into contact, different types of interaction will start. The implant may induce changes in the biological system, that in turn, via surface reactions, will induce changes in the implant material. The interface zone is the region where such changes occur.[8]

Upon insertion of an implant, the first reaction that will occur is diffusion of proteins and lipids to the implant surface. The proteins not irreversibly adsorbed can be exchanged for others. Structural and conformational changes occur in the adsorbed protein layer. After these initial reactions of up to a few minutes' duration, diffusion into the implant surface may also take place.[9] Then cells will start to interact with the surface and its protein layer. This will take place when the protein layer reaches a thickness of more than 1 nm.[10] Eventually, new bone may be formed.

The present results clearly show that the incorporation of a titanium implant is adversely affected by irradiation of a single dose of 15 Gy. The study did not show any significant difference in torque removal force between group A and group B animals, which is in contrast to the improvement in bone healing after an initial depression following irradiation demonstrated in another study.[4] This fact may have several explanations. One is that the presently used method may be more insensitive to small changes in bone behavior. Another explanation may be that the process of implant incorporation involves many other facets than the amount of bone formed close to the implant. These include the adhesion of biomolecules to the implant oxide layer and the capability of the bone tissue to affect the implant surface, secondarily influencing the adhesion between bone and implant. It is not unreasonable to assume that the osteoblasts and their precursors may form bone tissue that, while reduced in amount and functional capacity because of the irradiation

trauma, may still provide such a high adhesive capacity that the difference in affinity directly after and 12 weeks after irradiation is not discernible with the presently used method.

Conclusion

To the knowledge of the present authors, this is the first study to measure the torque necessary to remove a titanium implant from its implant site after irradiation. The findings of the reduced capacity of the irradiated bone tissue to incorporate implants as measured directly and 3 months after irradiation prompt a conservative approach in the clinical situation. Thus it is probably better to let the irradiated bone tissue recover from the irradiation trauma if possible, so as to encourage a better incorporation of the implants.

References

1. Jacobsson M, Jönsson K, Albrektsson T, Turesson I. Dose-response for bone regeneration after single doses of 60Co irradiation. *Int J Radiat Oncol Biol Phys* 1985;11:1963–1969.
2. O'Brien CJ, Archer DJ, Breach NM, Shaw HJ. Reconstruction of the mandible with autogenous bone following treatment for squamous carcinoma. *Aust NZ J Surg* 1986;56:707–711.
3. Albert TW, Smith JD, Everts EC, Cook TA. Dacron mesh tray and cancellous bone in reconstruction of mandibular defects. *Arch Otolaryngol Head Neck Surg* 1986;112:53–60.
4. Jacobsson M, Jönsson K, Albrektsson T, Turesson I. Short- and long-term effects of irradiation on bone regeneration. *Plast Reconstr Surg* 1985:76:841–848.
5. Jacobsson M, Tjellström A, Thomsen P, Albrektsson T, Turesson I. Integration of titanium implants in irradiated bone. Histologic and clinical study. *Ann Otol Rhinol Laryngol* 1988;97:337–340.
6. Albrektsson T, Eriksson AR, Jacobsson M, Kälebo P, Strid KG, Tjellström A. Bone repair in implant models: A review with emphasis on the Harvest Chamber for bone regeneration studies. *Int J Oral Maxillofac Implants* 1989;4:45–54.
7. Johansson C, Jacobsson M, Albrektsson T. Removal forces for osseointegrated titanium implants. In *Implant Materials in Biofunction,* C. de Putter, G.L. de Lange, K. de Groot, A.J.C. Lee (eds), *Advances in Biomaterials.*

Amsterdam: Elsevier Science Publishers BV, 1988; 8:87–92.

8. Kasemo B, Lausmaa J. Surface science aspects on inorganic biomaterials. *CRC Crit Rev Biocompat* 1986; 2:335–380.

9. Albrektsson T, Brånemark P-I, Hansson HA, Kasemo B, Larsson K, Lundström I. The interface zone of inorganic implants in vivo: Titanium implants in bone. *Ann Biomed Eng* 1983;11:1–27.

10. Kasemo B, Lausmaa J. Metal selection and surface characteristics. pp 99–116 In P.-I. Brånemark, G.A. Zarb, T. Albrektsson (eds) *Tissue-Integrated Prostheses: Osseointegration in Clinical Dentistry.* Chicago: Quintessence Publ Co, 1985.

The Effect of Radiation at the Titanium/Bone Interface

S.A. Hum and P.E. Larsen

Cancer is the second most frequent cause of death in the adult population.[1] In 1990, it is estimated that 30,500 new oral cancers will occur, representing 4% of all new cancer cases.[1] The relative 5-year survival rates for oral cancer is estimated to be 54%. Surgery, radiation therapy, or a combination of both is utilized in the treatment of malignant tumors of the head and neck region. The use of combined modalities is typically reserved for Stage 3 and 4 tumors with 5-year survival rates of <30% by either modality alone.[2] The approach to advanced disease has produced a population of patients who have significant functional and cosmetic defects that are further compounded by radiation injury of host tissues.

Radiation therapy causes bone tissue to experience a marked decrease in cellularity and hemopoietic activity, dilation of sinusoids, and endosteal fibrosis.[3] The principle factor in bone damage is radiation injury to the bone vasculature.[4–6] Bone that has been exposed to radiation does not tolerate traumatic insult, healing very slowly or even progressing to osteoradionecrosis.[6]

Osseointegrated implants would serve as an excellent foundation for the fabrication of an oral or maxillofacial prosthesis. However, potential morbidity subsequent to surgical manipulation of irradiated bone has created appropriate concern for the placement of implants in head and neck cancer patients. Implant placement is generally considered to be contraindicated in irradiated bone. This contraindication represents an empiric rather than a scientific judgment. This study was undertaken to evaluate the effect of radiation at the tissue interface of actively integrating titanium implants.

Materials and methods

New Zealand white rabbits were selected for use in this study since rapid bone turnover in this species allows evaluation of integration at 6 weeks.[7,8] The proximal tibia was selected as the surgical site because of the ease of access and its successful use in previous implant studies.[7,9–11] Adult rabbits (at least 6 months old), were used to ensure complete fusion of the proximal tibia epiphyseal center.[8] Implants were placed in both proximal tibiae of ten New Zealand white rabbits. The left tibia received external beam radiation while the right tibia served as an internal control. One rabbit experienced a longitudinal fracture of the tibia during placement of the implant and was removed, leaving nine experimental animals to complete the study.

General anesthesia was induced with a ketamine (50 mg/kg) and xylazine (5 mg/kg) intramuscular injection and were maintained under anesthesia with Halothane. A 3.3 × 8 mm plasma-sprayed titanium implant cylinder (IMZ, Interpore, Irvine, Calif) was placed bilaterally in the proximal tibia (Fig 1).[12] External saline irrigation was utilized to prevent thermal bone trauma.[11] A two-layer dissection was performed to ensure adequate soft tissue coverage of the

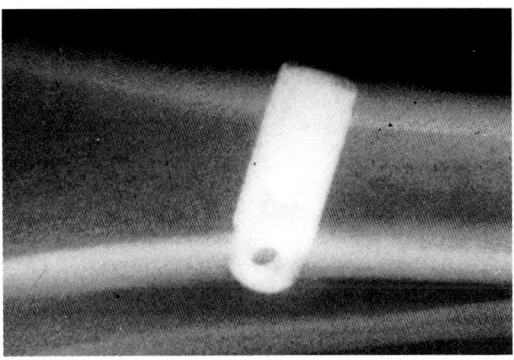

Fig 1 Postsurgical radiograph of titanium cylinder implant placed in the rabbit proximal tibia.

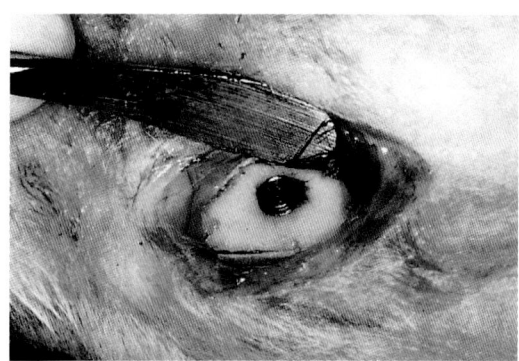

Fig 2 Medial approach to rabbit proximal tibia. A two-layer dissection was performed to allow muscle to cover the implant and prevent skin dehiscence.

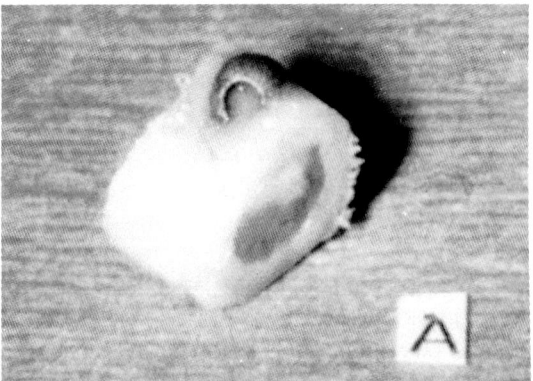

Fig 3 Postsacrifice tibia implant specimen. All implants were clinically integrated and without mobility.

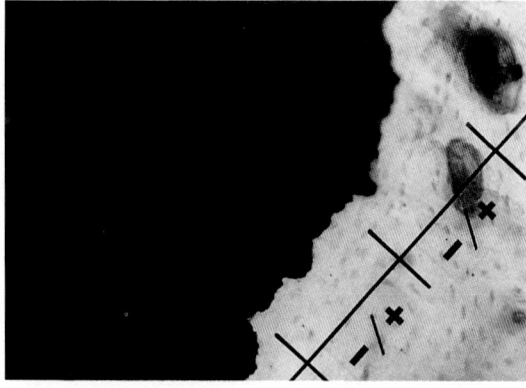

Fig 4 Representation of ocular grid adapted to the light microscope. At ×10 magnification, each grid represents 100 μm.

implant heads (Fig 2). A 2-week healing phase followed to ensure wound closure prior to radiation.

At week 2, a course of radiation delivered from a Cesium 137 source (0.66 MV) was begun on the experimental tibia. The radiation was delivered in nine fractions of 450 rads over 19 days for a total of 4,050 rads. This is a radiation equivalent dosage of 1,728 Rets. Intramuscular ketamine/xylazine was used during the radiation. Fluoroscopy was used as an aid in localization of the implant and the radiation was delivered parallel to the longitudinal axis of the

implant. During radiation the control tibia was retracted from the surgical field and secured with sandbags.

The rabbits were sacrificed 8 weeks postimplantation with an intravenous euthanizing solution (T-61), administered through an ear vein. The evaluation of the implants was accomplished by clinical, radiographic, and histologic examination.[13] Standardized radiographs were exposed utilizing a portable dental x-ray unit and dental periapical film. The implants were harvested with an oscillating saw, and an evaluation of clinical integration and mobility was

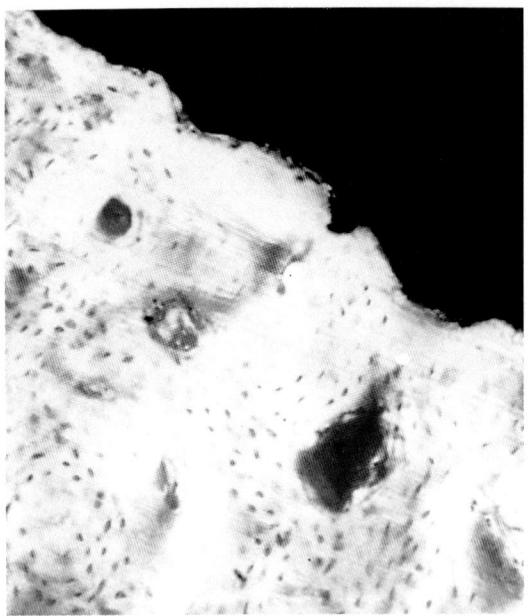

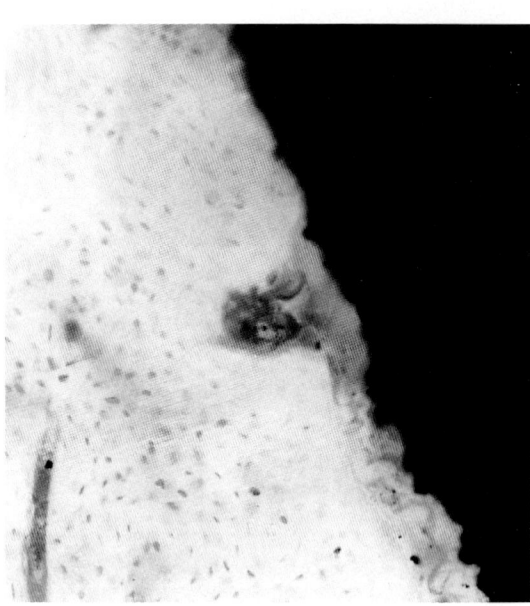

Fig 5 Photomicrograph ($\times$10) of bone/implant interface. This section represents an area of successful osseointegration in an irradiated implant.

Fig 6 Photomicrograph ($\times$10) of bone/implant interface with soft tissue interposed between the implant and bone. This section represents an area of failure in a control implant.

accomplished by a blinded evaluator using a dissecting probe to palpate the implant (Fig 3). The bone-implant specimens were fixed in a 5% glutaraldehyde solution. Specimens were embedded in a methyl methacrylate embedding medium. One 300-μm-thick longitudinal section was produced for each implant specimen with a diamond circular saw. These sections were evaluated unstained with light microscopy ($\times$10). An ocular grid was adapted to the light microscope to divide the bone implant interface into 100-μm intervals (Fig 4). Only the cortical bone-to-implant interface was evaluated, as the central hemapoietic marrow portion of the tibia cannot osseointegrate because of its largely cellular/vascular composition. Each interval was then judged by a blinded evaluator as having either successfully achieved or failed osseointegration. Successful osseointegration was defined as a close, intimate approximation of bone to metal without any interposed fibrous connective tissue (Fig 5).[9] If any portion of a grid

was judged not to be a success by the above criteria, the entire grid was counted as a failure (Fig 6). An average of 68 grids were evaluated for each implant.

Results

There was no gross mobility noted in either the experimental or control groups and all implants appeared grossly integrated. Postsacrifice radiographs were examined for any evidence of peri-implant radiolucency (Fig 7). There was no evidence of any radiographically detectable bony changes on standardized radiographs in either the control or irradiated implant groups.

Evaluation by light microscopy of nondecalcified histologic specimens revealed successfully osseointegrated surfaces in 94.8% of the 647 grids evaluated in the control group (Table 1). The experimental group displayed 76.2% of 589 grids possessing successful osseointegration (Table 1 and Fig 8). This difference is statistically significant by Mann-Whitney-Wilcoxon nonparametric evaluation of means at the $P<.05$ significance level.

Discussion

It is generally accepted that a history of exposure to radiation therapy for head and neck malignancies is a contraindication to the placement of osseointegrated implants. Brånemark even suggests the exposure to standard dental and panoramic radiographs should not be allowed during the integration phase of these implants.[14] These contraindications have recently been challenged.[15] Some surgeons place implants in irradiated bone and their early data supports this technique.[16] Concern regarding potential long-term morbidity of titanium implants in irradiated bone prompted this study. Although implants are usually placed during the postradiation time period, in this study, implants were placed prior to irradiation in an attempt to simulate implant placement at the time of cancer resection.

The ability to deliver equivalent radiation dosage to an experimental model is essential in the study of radiation effects. Radiation courses of different fractions, dosages, and protraction schedules may be related by the equation:

$$RD = D \times F^{(-0.24)} \times T^{(-0.11)}$$

where RD is the radiation equivalent dosage expressed as Rets (rad-days), D is the total dosage in rads, F is the number of fractions, and T is the time of treatment in days.[17] The typical radiation course for human head and neck radiation therapy is 6,000 rads delivered in 30 fractions of 200 rads each over a 6-week time period. This represents 1,758 Rets. The radiation equivalent dosage in this study was 1,728 Rets. This should produce a tissue dose and injury in the rabbit model similar to that seen in humans undergoing radiation therapy for head and neck cancer.

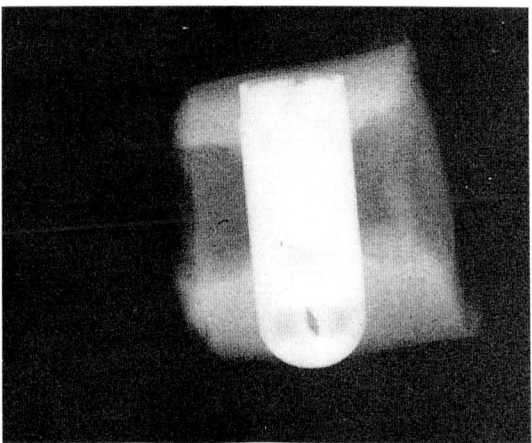

Fig 7 Postsacrifice radiograph. No evidence of peri-implant radiolucency occurred in any of the specimens. Only the cortical interface was evaluated in this study.

Table 1 Total grids evaluated for each tibia and the percentage of grids with osseointegration*

Rabbit	Grids	Control	Grids	Experimental
A	85/87	97.7	76/99	76.7
B	55/71	77.4	75/85	88.2
C	62/64	96.8	34/41	82.9
D	75/80	93.7	43/68	63.0
E	74/74	100.0	54/66	81.8
F	67/70	95.7	59/71	83.0
G	34/38	89.4	34/61	55.7
H	96/96	100.0	51/59	86.4
I	65/67	97.0	23/39	58.9
Total	613/647	94.8	449/589	76.2

*Nonparametric evaluation confirms a statistically significant difference between the control and experimental tibiae. There was no statistically significant difference in the number of grids evaluated for each group.

The clinical evaluation of short-term implant success is accomplished by examination of the exposed implant for evidence of gross mobility. Implant mobility is a definite indicator of integration failure.[13,18,19] Radiographs of the implant at the time of exposure are evaluated for any evidence of peri-implant radiolucency. Radiolucent zones are an indicator that the implant is anchored by fibrous connective tissue and not bone.[13,20] These clinical indicators are only

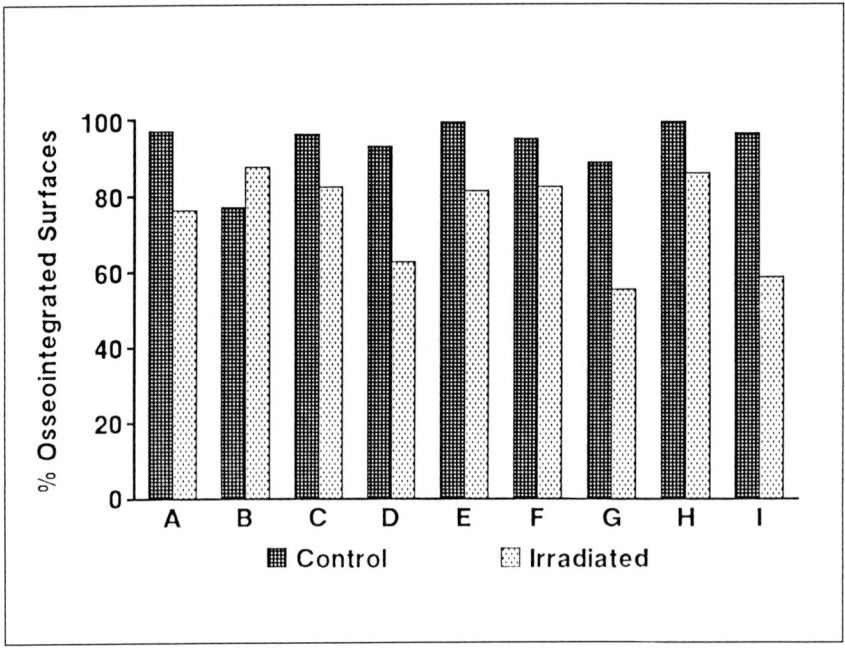

Fig 8 Bar graph representation of percentage of osseointegrated surfaces for both control and irradiated implants.

rough estimates of the actual quality of the bone/metal interface.

Histologic examination is not feasible in human patients. Albrektsson defines osseointegration as a direct contact between bone and implant at the light microscopic level.[9] Histologic success is defined as an implant possessing greater than 95% osseointegrated surface area.[9] Histologically demonstrable osseointegration was seen in over 94.8% of the implant surface area in the control group. This supports the validity of the rabbit tibia model. The decrease in successfully integrated surface area (76.2%) in the irradiated tibia is statistically significant and is of potential clinical significance. The potential failure of an implant with diminished osseointegration is associated with an unacceptable morbidity in irradiated bone. The lack of absolute failure and apparent success of the implants in irradiated bone by clinical parameters is encouraging. Further study is necessary to clearly establish the short- and long-

term effects of radiation on both the hard and soft tissue/implant interface. Hyperbaric oxygen is successfully utilized in bone grafting and osseous healing of irradiated bone to increase host tissue oxygen tension.[6] Hyperbaric oxygen could be applied to irradiated host bone prior to implant placement or utilized as salvage therapy for implants that fail or progress to osteoradionecrosis. Long-term success of irradiated implants after exposure and prosthetic loading was not addressed in this study.

Conclusion

The exposure of actively integrating titanium implants in a rabbit model produced a statistically significant decrease in the percentage of successfully osseointegrated surfaces from 94.8% in controls to 76.2% in the irradiated group. Application of clinical success parameters—implant mobility and peri-implant radiolucency—demonstrated no differences between control and irradiated implants.

References

1. Silverberg E, Lubera JA. Cancer Statistics, 1990. *Cancer* 1990;39:1.
2. DeVita VJ. *Principles and Practice of Oncology.* 2nd ed. Philadelphia: JB Lippincott Co, 1985.
3. Knospe WH, et al. Regeneration of locally irradiated bone marrow. *Blood* 1966;28:3,398–415.
4. King MA, et al. A study of irradiated bone. *J Nucl Med* 1979;20:1142–1149.
5. Cutright DE, Brady JM. Long term effects of radiation on the vascularity of rat bone. *Radiat Res* 1971; 48:402–408.
6. Marx RE. Osteoradionecrosis: A new concept of its' pathophysiology. *J Oral Maxillofac Surg* 1983;41:283–288.
7. Roberts WE, et al. Osseous adaptation to continuous loading of rigid endosseous implants. *Am J Orthod* 1984;86:95–111.
8. Crary DD, Swain PB. Genetic differences in growth rate and maturation of rabbits. *Growth* 1960;24:111–130.
9. Albrektsson T, Jacobsson M. Bone-metal interface in osseointegration. *J Prosthet Dent* 1987;57:597–606.
10. Roberts WE. Bone tissue interface. *J Oral Implant* 1988;14:217–222.
11. Eriksson AR, Albrektsson T. Temperature threshold levels for heat-induced bone tissue injury. *J Prosthet Dent* 1983;50:101–107.
12. Kirsch A, Mentag P. The IMZ endosseous two phase implant system. *Oral Implant* 1986;12:4,416.
13. Albrektsson T, Zarb GA, Worthington P, Eriksson AR. The long-term efficacy of currently used dental implants: A review and proposed criteria of success. *Int J Oral Maxillofac Implants* 1986;1:11–25.
14. Brånemark P-I. Osseointegration and its experimental background. *J Prosthet Dent* 1983;50:399–410.
15. Jacobsson M, et al. Dose response for bone regeneration after single doses of Cobalt 60 irradiation. *Int J Radiat Oncol Biol Phys* 1985;11:1963–1969.
16. Marx RE. Implants for the rehabilitation of cancer patients. Presented at the AAOMS Clinical Congress, San Diego, Calif, 1990.
17. Vaeth J. Frontiers of Radiation Therapy and Oncology. vol 6. Baltimore: University Park Press, 1972.
18. Brånemark P-I, et al. Osseointegrated implants in the treatment of the edentulous jaw. Experience from a 10-year period. *Scand J Plast Reconstr Surg* 1977; 11(suppl 16).
19. Adell R, et al. A 15-year study of osseointegrated implants in the treatment of the edentulous jaw. *Int J Oral Surg* 1981;10:387.
20. Niznick G. A probing look at dental implants. Presented at the 12th Annual USC Periodontal Symposium, Los Angeles, 1986.

Implant Surface Physics and Chemistry: Improvements and Impediments to Bioadhesion

R.E. Baier, A.E. Meyer, and J.R. Natiella

The organizers of the Second International Congress on Tissue Integration requested that "pertinent, current, provocative" information on implant surface properties critical to improving oral, orthopedic, and maxillofacial reconstruction be provided. The key issue in this regard is how to make an implant become part of a patient's body—a part that will, with its adjacent natural tissues, be able to reheal repetitively at the implant/tissue interface just as severed or fractured natural tissue would. That is, in the face of lifetime use and inevitable trauma, the implants or the prostheses they support must demonstrate continuous stability. Successful "integrated" implants are those that regain stability after unanticipated trauma; that is, they have a large range of "physiologic forgiveness."

For osseointegrated implants, this means that once they are funtionally immobile and traumatically (even by cumulative micromotions during normal prosthetic usage) rendered mobile, they will spontaneously return to their desired immobile condition. Failure to reheal in this way will lead to less desirable secondary stabilization by interposed connective tissues, which may, nevertheless, be sufficient for sustenance of function. Truly integrated biomaterial/tissue interfaces will be (1) initially stable, (2) repeatedly stable (after trauma), and (3) self-stabilizing.

What is the Current Situation?

Almost all implant/bone histologic illustrations that have been published over the years, particularly of screw-type implants longitudinally sectioned and pushed out, show the thread pattern perfectly replicated in the adjacent bone. This is mute but convincing testimony to the lack of true adhesion at the implant/bone interface. Otherwise, the pushout tests would have fractured the bones to leave much less esthetic reproductions of the implant surface features. The current situation is not much different from that illustrated in the pioneering studies of Predecki and coworkers.[1]

Professor Brånemark illustrates the current state of the art with a picture of clenched hands, where interdigitated fingers show that it is mechanical interlocking—not actual integration in the adhesive scientists' sense—that is responsible for early mechanical strength of emplaced screw-type, root-form implants. The quantity of interdigitation is most important, considering that adhesive debonding occurs in yet unmineralized, corticalizing osteoid, which always represents the weakest (cohesively) common site for failure of bony tissues. Intrinsically high–surface-energy materials include commercially pure titanium, titanium alloys, cobalt-chromium alloys, alumina and other inert ceramics, calcium-phosphate ceramics, and various glasses. These can all establish at least initial physical-chemical binding to wound site substances and through that binding stimulate cellular growth and repair processes. Some of these biomaterials, such as CP titanium, glow-discharge treated or not, may actually engage in local chemical modifications of the wound healing events per local peroxide generation. Calcium oxide layers that represent the most superficial aspects of most hydroxyapatite-coated implants may also chemically interact. These surface oxides become "slaked lime" pastes that can form implant/tissue interfaces that will immobilize more or less quickly than uncoated implants. In either situation, the participation of a "bioactive" implant in the healing process generally seems to beneficially suppress local immunologic events, blunt "foreign-body" responses, and allow more prompt integration with tissue while also possibly inhibiting the initiation of biomaterials-centered infections.

From the perspective of the implant and biomaterials science communities, the first few minutes to about the first hour of interaction of materials in the host sites are the most critical. The actual surface condition of the implant dictates the host response, as subsequently manifested in secondary macrophage activity and tissue maturation at the implant sites.

The host/material "interlock" occurs through formation of a host-deposited "conditioning" film, maturation of that film by dynamic interchanges with newly arriving substances, and continuing host changes in response. This dynamic equilibrium certainly continues over very long periods. The current state of the art with conventional "osseointegrating" implants is best illustrated in the recently completed graduate thesis work of Dr I. Barzilay (University of Rochester/Eastman Dental Center). Figure 1 illustrates, in a macroscopic section, the excellence of bony approximation to a Brånemark fixture in the primate jaw. Actual quantitation of the degree of bone/metal adaptation was done to assess the meaning of this functional integration by inspection of cross and longitudinal sections of decalcified and undecalcified tissues.

Mandibular implants sectioned with a diamond disc and then ground to 30 μm (thinner than most prior studies) before multiple staining with modified trichrome preparations revealed resorptive phenomena at the implant neck region, with crests of bone adjacent to this critical area and intervening approximated soft tissue. Even after 6 months there was a variation in

response along the implant contour, but generally very little soft tissue was found deeper than the first screw thread, which is in agreement with the findings of Albrektsson and Sennerby.[2] As evidence of the amazing "biocompatibility" of the implant material, Fig 2 shows an actual haversian system forming within a single screw-thread undulation. Compare this with Fig 3, a ground section of normal primate bone. At lower magnification (Fig 4) open spaces exist both above and below each screw thread, which (although in part the result of sectioning-induced trauma/artifact) also represent the labile nature of the bone/metal interface when mechanically challenged. It would have been easy to photograph selected regions of these sections and suggest direct contact of bone throughout.[2] In our experience, if sections are ground thinly enough there will always be spaces illustrating the delamination of the bone from the metallic surface. A great deal of prior work, photographing only 75- to 100-μm sections, overlooks this evidence of easy separation.

Having invested the laborious preparation and inspection resources required, it is now clear from the very thin ground sections of well-integrated dental implants that actual bone bonding does not frequently occur. Thus, the previous work by scanning electron microscopy showing essentially bone-free implants pushed or twisted from well-functioning implant sites, and the parallel representations of bony screw-thread impressions in decalcifying mating tissues, is confirmed: Functional tissue integration, at least in bone, does not in fact correlate with actual adhesion across the bone/metal interface.

Can This Situation Be Improved?

In our experience, the actual bonding of metallic, ceramic, and glassy implants to tissues—both hard and soft—can be obtained by first treating the implants by the process of radiofrequency glow discharge. This treatment assures their cleanliness (at least), increasing their surface energies to more bondable values, and perhaps

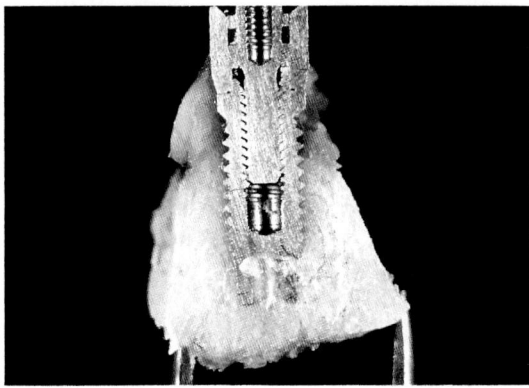

Fig 1 Longitudinal section through well-integrated titanium implant in primate jaw.

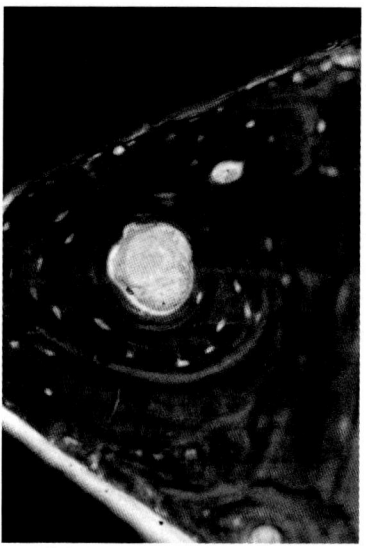

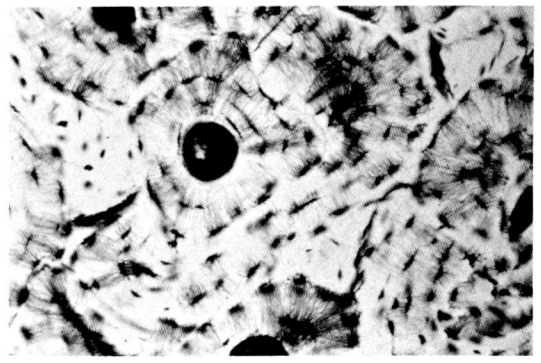

Fig 2 Modified trichrome-stained, high-magnification view of a complete haversian system within a section of thinly ground primate bone adjacent to the screw thread. Note that in spite of the generally circular nature of the bone lamella, bone layers adjacent to the implant are locally parallel to the metal. This illustrates how the maximum strength of this system in shear is limited by the weakest layers of parallel-oriented, unmineralized osteoid.

Fig 3 Histologic appearance of normal, thinly ground primate bone with interlocking, multidirectional bone lamella. This multioriented, strength-enhancing feature is eliminated as bone healing approximates implant surfaces of all types.

mitigating the circumstances that otherwise allow biomaterials-centered infections. Use of hydrogen peroxide rather than argon or air as the low-pressure gas phase, in which the cool "glow" is generated around the implants, can also lead to their absolute sterilization while greatly increasing their passive surface oxide thicknesses. In peroxide vapors, glow-discharge processes move from the level of disinfection, scrupulous cleaning, and improved passivation against corrosion to the level of complete sterilization required for general acceptance of this technique in the clinic. Combined glow-discharge and peroxide vapor devices allow dry, noncorroding sterilization of materials inside their final packages, all accomplished at ambient room temperatures. Bioactive ceramic and so-called "HA" implants, even though self-cleaning by partial surface dissolution, are also further activatable by glow-discharge treatment. Our preliminary evidence suggests this to be a potential major improvement in the manufacturing-to-implantation cycle for plasma-sprayed materials.

The importance of glow-discharge treatment for obtaining the high surface energies needed for spontaneous flow and filling of porous and textured implants is obvious. Glow-discharge treatment prompts rapid filling of voids, eliminating pockets of microbial debris and removing stress-concentrating vacancies. Even when sterilized by this process inside their final packages, certain traditional advantages of glow-discharge processing persist: improved passivation against corrosion, as compared with acid passivation; cleaner implant surfaces, as compared with autoclaving or other conventional sterilizing techniques; and maintenance of the edges of sharp tools and the integrity of heat-sensitive materials, since the process is carried out at room temperature. Availability of small glow-discharge treatment devices in the clinic will have the additional benefit of being able to rapidly overcome worries about possible lack of sterility resulting from accidental contamination of tools or prostheses during procedures. Further, since superficial exogenous factors (such as dead bacteria or other debris) can stimulate antibody-producing cells and result in implant complications, prophylactic or clinical glow-discharge treatment of appliances can also be a good precautionary step.

With "osseointegrated" tooth root replacements now entering the domain of the general dentist, there is an increasing need for protection against failures caused by interfacial debris and/or the possible re-use of components (such as healing caps). Small, inexpensive, user-friendly radiofrequency glow-discharge treatment devices could fulfill these requirements.

Benefits of radiofrequency glow-discharge treatment will not be demonstrable in simple mechanical tests—after short-term healing (less than 90 days)—because of the universal failure of bone-surrounded implants in their weaker osteoid layers. However, clear differences that persist in the arrangement of the tissue at the variously prepared implant interfaces suggest that longer-term healing or rehealing properties may be positively influenced. The basic problem with obtaining greater strengths is the habit of bone to heal around implants by the process of corticalization, even to glow-discharge–sterilized hydroxyapatite implants.

It has already been mentioned that with many implants in bone, and specifically dental implants, there is "cornering" of the healing cortical bone that results in the loss of bone contact

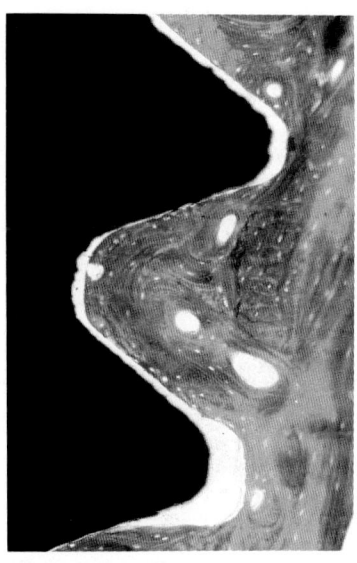

Fig 4 Thinly ground section of titanium/bone interfacial zone from a functionally well-integrated implant in a primate jaw. Note the locally parallel bone lamellar orientations at all aspects. If separations of the distances shown occur during implant function in vivo, the initial surface qualities present at the tissue/implant interface may be critical to the subsequent rehealing by bone growth or, less desirably, fibrous tissue intrusion into the spaces created or, worse, bone resorption.

at least down to the first fret in cases of even well-integrated specimens. It thus becomes clear that, since all bone-emplaced biomaterials are healed by corticalization, there is a need for attention to gross surface geometric features of implant designs as well as to their specific surface energies and surface textures at the level of cellular detail. Recent work in our laboratories separated these variables, revealing unambiguously the influence of the surface energy term for the first time. Equally smooth commercially pure titanium specimens were given specific surface modifications to high–, medium–, and low–surface-energy states. They were placed into rabbit femoral cortical defects drilled at low speed to diameters 1% smaller than those of the specimens. Figure 5 shows the resultant histologic view of a near-cortical region of such

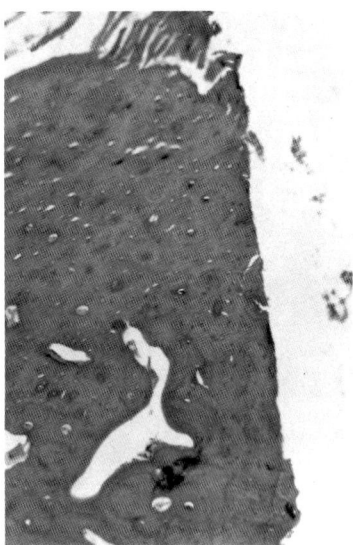

Fig 5 H & E stained thin section of rabbit femoral bone after pushout, from bottom to top (medullary to cortical), of a smooth cylinder of CP titanium. Note that the midspecimen bone lamellae are oriented predominantly perpendicular to the axis of the implant space, as were the splintered cortical spicules seen at the top of this section. The implant was in place for less than 1 hour before its pushout test. No bone resorption or healing phase occurred.

an instrumented defect immediately after the titanium specimen had been placed, the bone had been excised and stabilized in an epoxy resin, and the implant had been pushed out from its medullary portion through the cortical surface. Since no bone healing process occurred in this case, it is clear from inspection of Fig 5 that the bone architecture was predominantly normal (perpendicular) to the axis of the implant, and that because of the interference fit, the pushout test actually lifted and fractured the exterior lamellar cortical zone.

Figure 6 shows the resultant site histology after pushout of a deliberately organic-contaminated titanium specimen, healed into place for 8 weeks with the animal fully mobile immediately after surgery. Note the presence of a downwelling, thick, implant-paralleling cortical

zone. This zone is marked by the darker-stained reversal line, where bone regrowth began after the initial pressure-induced necrosis was resolved. Also note that the low–surface-energy coated titanium specimen was expressed from the healed site by failure in an interfacial osteoid zone. Inspection of the implants of these types, after pushout from many similar sites, revealed only a small amount of soft organic debris on their surfaces. Figure 7 is a hematoxylin-eosin–stained section of the failure site for an implant that carried with it a bit more adherent healed tissue. Energy-dispersive x-ray analyses of the lower–surface-energy implants showed no evidence of organic materials clinging to them.

In contrast, implants that were simply glow-discharge treated before placement (and stored under cool, boiled distilled water until the implant site was ready) left mainly fractured new bone at their failed sites after pushout tests. These findings are typified by the histologic view in Fig 8. Note that almost the entire zone of newly corticalized bone that formed adjacent to the implant and parallel to it was transferred with the implant as it was sheared from the site. Again, however, the failure "cylinder" was in a zone of unmineralized osteoid. Thus, even though the pushout strengths for the glow-discharge–treated implants were statistically superior to the strengths for organic-coated or simply detergent-washed specimens, this was a small gain in comparison to the tenfold greater strength of the adjacent, intact bone. Inspections of the high–surface-energy (glow-discharge–treated) implants retrieved after 8-week healing periods, using scanning electron microscopy, energy-dispersive x-ray analysis, and electron spectroscopy for chemical analysis (ESCA), clearly showed a considerable thickness of calcium- and phosphate-rich matter still attached. The main benefit, therefore, of glow-discharge treatment of implants is that re-healing of such a fracture would occur wholly in bone tissue, without requiring recolonization of the initially foreign interface.

As well-noted by Hobkirk,[3] new bone forms first at the defect walls, not adjacent to the implants. Bone grows toward the implants, ori-

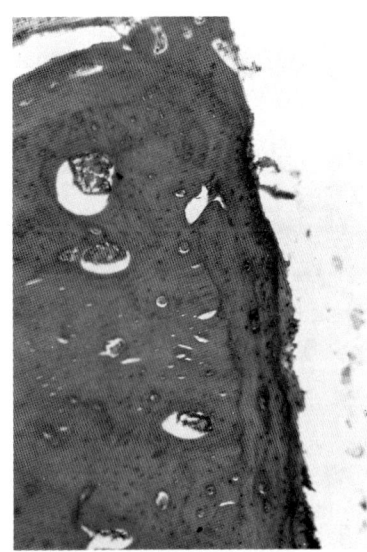

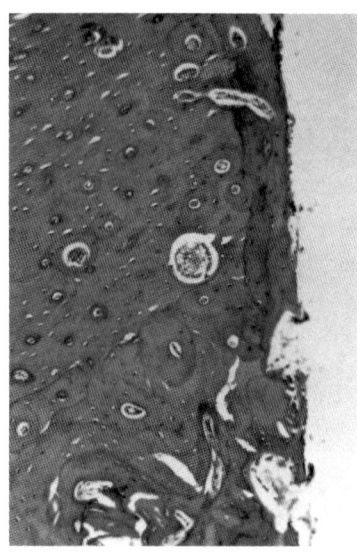

Fig 6 H & E stained thin section of a rabbit femoral implant site following pushout of a low–surface-energy (organic-coated) CP titanium cylinder after 8 weeks of healing. Note the thick, rounded, down-welling zone of new cortical bone left behind as the implant exited from the site.

Fig 7 H & E stained thin section of a deeper zone of the failed implant/bone interface in a rabbit femoral implant site from which an organic-contaminated titanium cylinder was pushed out after 8 weeks of healing.

enting parallel as it goes. When the implants are of high–surface-energy types, there is also generally a "cortical bulge" adjacent to them that often resorbs during function. If, as with healed bone, other tissues are also always locally oriented horizontally and parallel to adjacent implant surfaces, additional attention must be directed to this type of cellular differentiation as a major determinant of integration.

Our research efforts have revealed obvious differences in this regard in the degrees of flattening of interfacially localized cells and in the overall cellular and extracellular matrix densities. Zonal differences in cell abundance and orientation vary as a function of distance from the implanted material surfaces and the nature (surface energy, at least) of each biomaterial. It is lamentable that surface energy and surface geometry (texture as well as gross contour) terms were not well separated in most prior implant trials. Especially at the portions of implants that emerge from one tissue type to an-

other (bone to connective tissue or connective tissue to epidermal tissue) or from tissue into colloidal biofluids (such as permucosal posts from the integrated implant into the oral cavity), the "edge" effects might be substantial. Indeed, the implant surface physics and chemistry, as defined through the phenomenon of the "critical contact angle" (θ c) of Gibbs' inequality condition may be the controlling factor. This is, perhaps, the previously missing clue to why there always is "cornering," leading to corticalization and possibly inevitably to "craterization" or "saucerization" for implants emerging from bone.

Simply put, discontinuities of the slopes of implant surfaces can lead to situations in which excess unhealed volumes near edges can be very large even when precautions are taken to assure that the equilibrium contact angles are very small.[4,5] For example, the Gibbs equation (θ c = [180° – ϕ] + θ e, where θ e is the equilibrium advancing contact angle of fluid

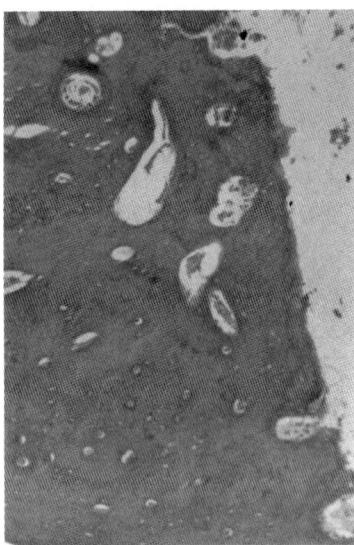

Fig 8 H & E stained thin section of failure zone in 8-week healed rabbit femoral bone surrounding a glow-discharge–treated, smooth titanium cylinder. Note that most of the interfacial new bone was transferred with the implant as it was pushed out from the site.

[cells, tissues] phases on a flat specimen, ϕ is the solid (implant) edge angle where spreading or cellular contact and growth is desired, and θc is the critical value of the fluid [tissue] contact angle required for the advancing tissue contact line to cross the edge and maintain coverage) still applies even when the equilibrium contact angle for a tissue phase (or fluid) is zero and when transition zones are made less abrupt (eg, by chamfering the edges). The fluid (tissue) will not spontaneously "wet" across certain shape changes, even though perfect wetting and spreading is already established nearby.

An increase of a material's surface free energy, eg, by glow-discharge treatment, to produce tissue/material contact angles of zero (normally prompting complete spreading and rapid cell growth) unfortunately cannot guarantee movement (growth, coverage, etc) over discontinuities in surface slope. Therefore, there may always be tendencies for peri-implant sul-

cus or "cupping" regions or poorly integrated sites that can entrap microorganisms and make implant maintenance and hygiene problematic.

What Can Be Done About This New Challenge?

Because prompt and complete tissue integration provides a potential theoretical barrier to control of biomaterials-centered infection, the answer may be to reverse the bioadhesive potential of exposed, at-risk implant segments entirely. Conveniently, this can be done with implant abutments in the same glow-discharge treatment devices that surface energize (while passivating against corrosion) the portions of the devices that will be buried. The required modification is simply to admit volatile precursor vapors of medical-grade silicones while the glow-discharge process is active. These vapors are added at such a concentration that the "glow" acts mainly to polymerize and crosslink a thin silicone layer on the implants at a more rapid rate that it removes it. The depositing film forms a completely conformal, microscopically thin protective envelope. The benefits of glow-discharge disinfection and surface cleaning of adventitious debris are preserved in this micro-coating process. The final device carries an invisible veneer of fouling-release silicone, with the same apparent self-cleansing qualities as intraoral mucosa.

Technical characterization of these low-adhesion, medically safe coatings has already generated several hundred pages of summary data tables, plots, and spectroscopic records, which, together with the material safety data sheets for the preferred starting material, hexa-methyldisiloxane (HMSDS), document their safety and effectiveness. Heptafluoropropoxy-silane (3-HEPT) and tetrafluoroethylene (TFE) vapors also give good results.

For testing coating effectiveness and persistence, three types of test plates were utilized in various saltwater exposure series: *(1)* Uncoated controls, *(2)* 3-HEPT–coated test plates, and *(3)*

HMDS-coated test plates. The uncoated controls were cleaned and then treated by radiofrequency-induced gas plasma before immersion in strong salt solution (artificial seawater) at three different temperatures. The contact angles of distilled water droplets were measured on all uncoated control plates prior to immersion; all angles were less than 10 degrees. The 3-HEPT–coated test plates were prepared by a chemical immersion technique that produced fluorinated coatings of the maximum possible durability, exceeding even the usual quality produced by the US Navy's process for coating periscope head windows; the contact angles of water droplets on these surfaces all were greater than 90 degrees. The HMDS (methyl silicone) coating was applied to the test plates by an experimental gas plasma polymerization process that was empirically selected. This coating process will require optimization before its routine use. The water contact angles on the HMDS-coated test plates prior to immersion in saltwater also averaged 90 degrees or more, and their desired critical surface tension values between 20 and 30 mN/m were independently validated on some specimens. Spectroscopic transmission qualities (UV, visible, infrared) measured prior to immersion showed the HMDS-coated test plates as well as the 3-HEPT–coated test plates to have the essential transparency of nonreactive, very thin films. Subsequent postexposure spectral analyses demonstrated that the coatings did not at all degrade the properties of their substrata plates during the 8-week exposure in saltwater.

The average water contact angles on postexposure samples (after excess salts were removed) remained relatively constant for both the uncoated controls and the 3-HEPT–coated samples. The initial complete water wettability of glow-discharge–treated pre-exposure controls (<10 degrees) was not maintained, since retention of the very high surface free energy produced by gas plasma treatment cannot be accomplished, even by storage in a vacuum chamber. After contamination with oil, detergent cleaning, and, finally, gas plasma treatment (8-week samples), all test plates again displayed water contact angles less than 10 degrees; these data demonstrate that the surfaces (control, 3-HEPT–coated, and HMDS-coated) can be repetitively cleaned and brought to their initial precoating state without difficulty.

The average water contact angles on postexposure HMDS-coated samples indicated that the coating as currently applied is increasingly degraded by immersion in saltwater as a function of exposure time and temperature. Test plates kept at 4°C throughout the test period experienced an average decrease in water contact angle of only 10 to 15 degrees. Those maintained at higher temperatures showed further time- and temperature-related average decreases of 45 to 60 degrees, with the most severe and rapid decrease observed for specimens immersed in 40°C saltwater. It should be emphasized that optimization of the gas plasma polymerization and coating procedures can overcome this durability problem if further short-term testing indicates the value of the coating in resisting microbial plaque retention. Loss of the HMDS coating from the surface does not degrade the properties of the test plates in any way, in that the coating failure seems to be by partial lifting and detachment rather than by chemical reaction.

Exposure of 4-week saltwater-immersed test plates (all types) for an additional 4 weeks in air at varying temperatures did not further degrade the properties of the samples. Likewise, exposure of 6-week saltwater-immersed test plates to intense UV/visible light for an additional week did not cause changes in the properties of the samples.

No significant differences in water shed times or shed droplet sizes were noted among the various sample types, exposure times, or temperatures. On average, only a 50 to 60 μL water droplet size was required before spontaneous shedding (by gravity flow) within a 1-second timeframe for all specimens.

Previous results have demonstrated the HMDS coating to be superior to all other materials with regard to safety and handling. It is now necessary to optimize coating application techniques to extend the coating lifetimes and im-

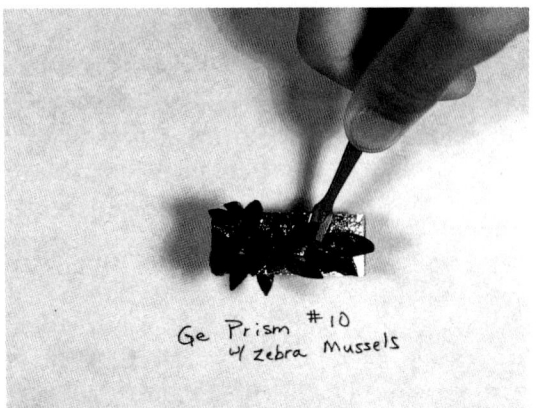

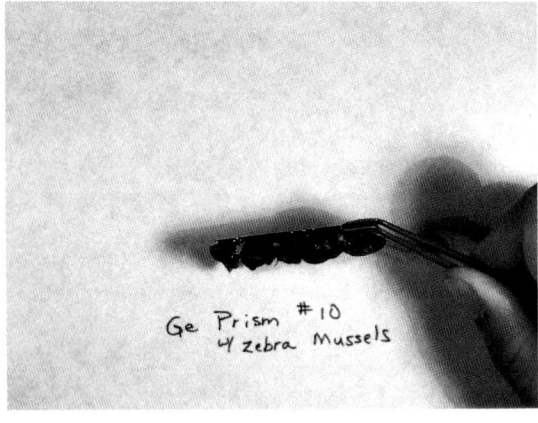

Fig 9 Face view of zebra mussels *(Dreissena poly-morpha)* from Lake Erie water spontaneously adherent to a germanium internal reflection prism.

Fig 10 Edge view of a 1-mm-thick plate of germanium with tenaciously adherent zebra mussels, established and retained by a DOPA-rich glycoproteinaceous cement at the tiny bases of spiderweb-like byssus strands.

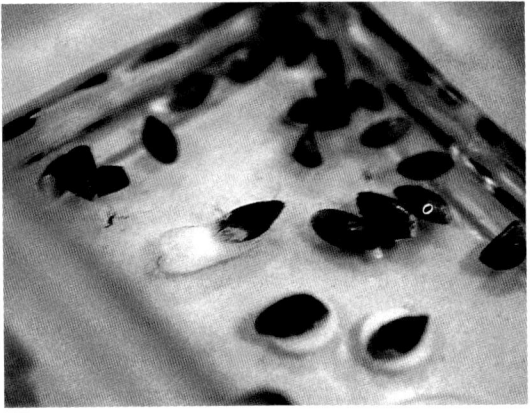

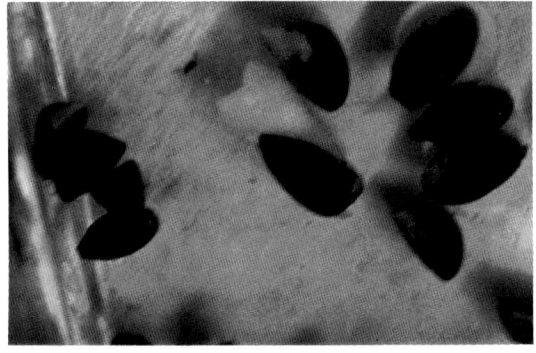

Fig 11 In a dish of Lake Erie water containing numerous young-adult zebra mussels, spontaneous and tenacious adhesion is established by the mollusks to a tooth and to two circular discs of Synamel (dense hydroxyapatite from Calcitek).

Fig 12 Close-up view of zebra mussel attachment to tooth and hydroxyapatite illustrating that tooth drying, etching, and instrumenting in any fashion may all be unnecessary to adhesive bonding when the principles of bioadhesion are adequately understood.

prove their durabilities, assuming that spontaneous shedding or release of microbial deposits from coated specimens is observed to be as easy with these coatings as has been shown in the past.

In fact, it is only low–surface-energy coatings of the quality just described that will resist the amazing underwater adhesion capabilities of barnacles, tube worms, algae, and now the zebra mussels that have been proliferating explosively in the waters of the Great Lakes and nearby freshwater systems. Figures 9 and 10 show, respectively, face and edge views of flat plates to which zebra mussels spontaneously adhered in abundance from natural Lake Erie water. The plates were, in fact, internal reflection prisms allowing analyses of the adhesive cement of these animals while they were still alive (the cement is a DOPA-rich glycoprotein, by these analyses).

Figures 11 and 12 illustrate that prompt and strong attachment occurs directly to harvested human teeth and to discs of dense hydroxyapatite (Synamel, from Calcitek). The attachment is so strong that one must break the tendon-like byssus threads of these animals to detach them, rather than having failure at the bond. With such examples from nature, it is not too optimistic to conclude that both promotion of biological adhesion and its prevention, where that is desired, will become possible for tissue-integration specialists before the year 2000. With sufficient understanding of the interfacial details of these events, adverse findings (such as "bone" formation in artificial hearts and heart valves) may become the harbingers of entirely new ways to integrate prostheses. In the jaw, for example, one may use the same elastomeric coatings as used in artificial hearts, spontaneously mineralized in vivo, to serve as implantable replacements for bone-attached periodontal ligaments.

Summary and Forecast

It is now possible to ensure that mechanical failure of an implant system will either be, or not be, at the interface. The tasks of the prosthodontist, the implant manufacturer, and the surgeon are to select and provide device and host-site features that can guarantee the "plane of parting" during intended physiologic function to be sufficiently and repeatedly distant (or near) the material interface to maintain an implant's intended function indefinitely. The challenge has been passed from biomaterials selection to biomaterials engineering.

There is a specific need for increased attention to surface geometries and textures of the finally fabricated devices. There is also a need for more data on dynamic remodeling of initially deposited layers, such as might transpire through periosteum-like cells observed at some implant/bone interfaces. More information is also required on the relationships of tissue factors to materials factors in relation to (1) "biocompatibility," to carry prognosis from initial responses to involvement of fluids and cellular exudates; (2) growth factors, to modification of the initial responses by corrosion events; and (3) biodegradation.

Future test rationale must assume initial implant instability and must monitor the rate of first attainment of stability and subsequent rates of reattainment of stability after mechanical challenge. First attainment of stability (attainment of stability once) is an insufficient demonstration of suitability for long-term function. Integrated implants must be able to heal repeatedly. This implies a process of dynamic stability at minimally functional levels. It is clear that more complete knowledge and control of implant surface physical and chemical features will be critical in this continuing effort.

Acknowledgments

We are grateful to the organizers of the Second International Congress on Tissue Integration for inviting our participation, to Dr I. Barzilay for experimental specimens, to J. Earle for histotechnology support, to M. Stachowski for rabbit femoral pushout specimens, to Dr L. Carter for histopathology of the rabbit implant sites, and to L. Lankes for professional preparation of the manuscript.

References

1. Predecki P, Auslaender BA, Stephan JE, Mooney VL, Stanitski C. Attachment of bone to threaded implants by ingrowth and mechanical interlocking. J Biomed Mater Res 1972;6:401–412.
2. Albrektsson T, Sennerby L. Direct bone anchorage of oral implants: Clinical and experimental considerations of the concept of osseointegration. Int J Prosthodont 1990;3:30–41.
3. Hobkirk JA. Patterns of cortical bone growth around alumina implants. J Oral Rehabil 1981;8:143–154.
4. Oliver JF, Huh C, Mason SG. Resistance to spreading of liquids by sharp edges. J Colloid Interface Sci 1977;568–581.
5. Bayramli E, Mason SG. Liquid spreading: Edge effect for zero contact angle. J Colloid Interface Sci 1978;66:200–202.

A Clinical Trial of a Partially Porous-Coated, Endosseous Dental Implant in Humans: Protocol and 6-Month Results

D.A. Deporter, P.A. Watson, R.M. Pilliar, M. Pharoah, M. Chipman, and D.C. Smith

Dental implantology has become a rapidly developing field of research and clinical application since Brånemark and co-workers[1] reported their results of a 15-year followup in humans treated with a threaded implant design of pure titanium. The Brånemark system, however, is considered by some to be expensive, complicated to place, and technique-sensitive. There is, therefore, a need for simpler, less invasive, and biologically more compliant dental implant systems that could be used reliably by a wider group of practitioners.

We have previously reported on the design and testing in dogs of a new partially porous-coated endosseous dental implant system that appears to have several advantages over threaded implant designs.[2] The implant root component is fabricated from Ti-6Al-4V, has a tapered, truncated cone shape to facilitate implant placement and optimize stress transfer at the bone/implant interface, and utilizes a powder-sintered, porous surface topography to promote integration by means of bone ingrowth over selected regions of the implant. In a comparative study in beagle dogs, this implant performed as well as a threaded implant system of pure titanium over an 18-month functional period. However, the results indicated that porous-coated implants could be shorter than threaded implants because of the increased surface area per unit length of implant available for bone ingrowth with the porous design.[2]

This report is concerned with an experimental protocol and 6-month results from the first human trial in which this partially porous-coated implant system has been used to treat completely edentulous patients, the majority of whom had severe mandibular alveolar ridge resorption. In keeping with our objective of developing simple treatment approaches that would be relatively inexpensive and applicable by a large group of practitioners, these patients were managed using three implants in the anterior mandible and a removable overdenture.

Materials and methods

Patient selection

Fifty-two otherwise healthy edentulous adults (17 male, 35 female), age 34 to 69 years (mean, 56.0 ± 9.0), were accepted from a group of referred patients using the following criteria.[3,4] To be included in the study each patient had to show one or more of the following: (1) severe bone loss in the mandibular denture-supporting areas that seriously limit denture retention, (2) poor oral muscular coordination impairing denture control, (3) low tolerance of mucosal tissues to contact with denture materials making patient comfort a problem, and (4) parafunctional habits leading to recurrent soreness and denture instability. The details of the procedure, of alternative treatments available, and of the anticipated benefits and risks were carefully explained to each patient verbally and in writing, and each patient was required to sign an in-

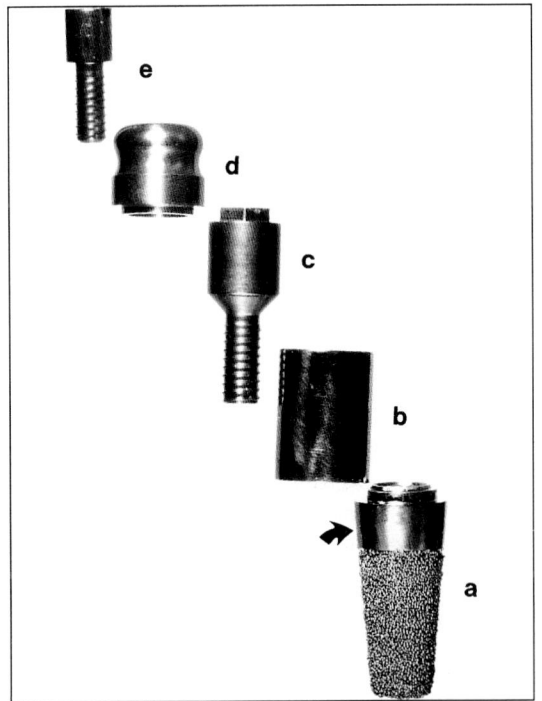

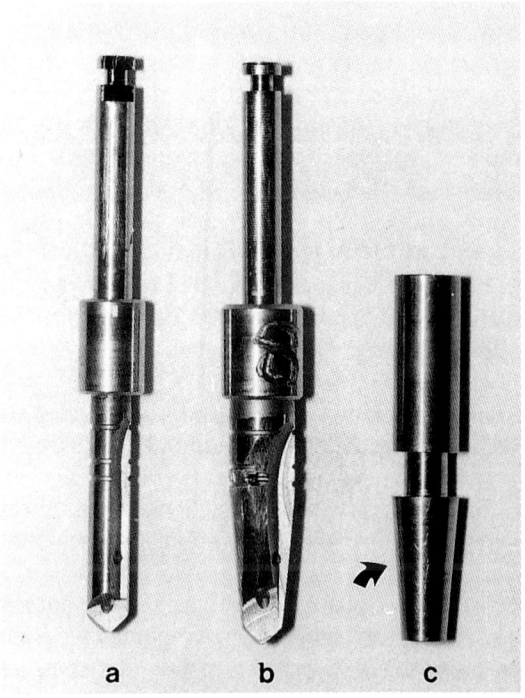

Fig 1 The components of the implant system included the implant root component (a), the transgingival collar (b), the collar-retaining screw (c), the prosthodontic cylinder (d), and the cylinder retaining screw (e). The coronal 2-mm segment of the implant root component has a machined surface (arrow), whereas the remainder of this component is porous-coated. (Original magnification × 4.)

Fig 2 The specialized surgical burs and trial-fit gauge used to place the implants. The pilot bur (a) is used first and is followed by one or both of the implant burs (b). There are two implant burs available (only one is shown), one being 0.1-mm larger in diameter than the other. The trial fit gauge (c) is used to check the size and direction of the implant channel. The end of this gauge to be inserted into the implant channel (arrow) is the same diameter as the implant root component but is not porous-coated. (Original magnification × 2.75.)

formed consent form previously approved by peer review.

Patient records

The following records were collected:

1. A medical questionnaire and written evidence of a recent medical examination
2. A clinical examination including intraoral and extraoral color photographs
3. A radiographic examination including panoramic and lateral and posterior skull views
4. A blood sample to determine baseline blood levels of titanium, aluminum, and vanadium
5. A quality of life questionnaire to provide an objective assessment of the patient's satisfaction with his/her existing dentures
6. A self-administered questionnaire to assess psychiatric health

The implant system and instrumentation

The components of the implant system were larger in dimension but similar in overall design to those used in our animal experiments with few exceptions (Fig 1). Thus, the implant root component was a truncated cone with a maximum (coronal) diameter of 4.0 mm, a 5-degree taper angle, and a flattened apex. The coronal 2 mm had a machined surface whereas the remainder of the implant root component was coated with beads of Ti-6Al-4V so as to create a three-dimensional porosity with a pore size in the range of 50 to 200 μm. Implants of 7-, 8-, 9-, and 10-mm lengths were available for use. A button-shaped prosthodontic cylinder and retaining screw (Fig 1) were used to support and engage the undersurface of the overdenture. The components were cleaned and sterilized using a standardized procedure as used earlier in our animal work.[5]

To conduct implantation, very few specialized instruments were required and these included:

1. Three special surgical burs (Fig 2) including a pilot bur and two implant burs, one being 0.1-mm smaller in diameter than the other
2. A slot-head screwdriver for removal of the temporary cover screw and healing cap at the reentry procedure, and for attaching the prosthodontic cylinder and its retaining screw
3. A hexagon-head screwdriver for placing the transgingival collar and collar-retaining screw
4. A trial-fit gauge (Fig 2) (the same diameter as the implant, but without porous coat) for checking the size of the prepared implant site just prior to implantation and for checking mutual alignment between sites

The implantation procedure

In this investigation implants were placed only in the anterior mandible for the following reasons. Firstly, the mandible is most often the jaw selected for treatment in completely edentulous patients,[6] as the majority of such patients are satisfied with the service provided by a complete maxillary denture. Secondly, the anterior mandible is the most predictable site for placing

dental implants,[7] and it was reasoned that any new system should first be tested in such a site. Thirdly, in keeping with our original objective of developing a simpler approach, it was desirable to place the implants in a site that would not involve the need and extra experience and skill required to expose and reflect the mental neurovascular bundles. Therefore, only three implants were placed so as to avoid completely any impingement on the mental foramina while still providing more than adequate support for an overdenture.

The location of each mental foramen was determined from a panoramic radiograph, whereas the appropriate implant length(s) was chosen after measuring the available bone height from the lateral and posterior skull views (measurement error ± 1 mm). In selecting the implant length for each patient, the objective was to use the longest implant possible, while being certain not to risk perforating the inferior cortex. In many patients, the inferior cortex was not involved in stabilizing the implant.

The preoperative preparation of the patient and surgical procedure were generally similar to the protocol suggested by Adell et al.[8] Thus, the labial mucoperiosteum was incised horizontally in the depth of the vestibule, and a lingually based, full-thickness flap was raised sufficiently to expose the underlying alveolar ridge. The three implant sites were prepared using a speed-reducing handpiece driven by an electric motor that was coupled to a control box equipped with variable speed control, and using external saline irrigation only.

One implant was placed close to the midline and one to either side of it with a minimum interimplant distance of 4 mm. To prepare each site, a preliminary channel was cut to an appropriate depth with the pilot drill (Fig 2). This was subsequently enlarged with the smaller of the two implant burs, checked for size and orientation with the trial fit gauge (Fig 2), and if necessary, enlarged slightly by using the larger implant bur. This final bur was still 0.05-mm smaller in diameter than the corresponding implant and this, together with the tapered implant shape, ensured a tight initial fit of implant to bone. Following thorough irrigation of the site with saline, the implant (already containing a healing cap and cover screw) was carefully placed in the site by holding it with forceps touching only the coronal machined (ie, nonporous) segment and then fully seated with three to four firm taps delivered with a small surgical mallet and a Teflon-tipped punch. The flap was then repositioned and sutured, and the patient was asked to maintain pressure on the flap for several hours by biting gently on gauze.

The patients were prevented from using their existing mandibular dentures for the first 10 to 14 days, at which time they returned for suture removal. At this time the base of the patient's existing denture was relieved and lined with tissue conditioner (Visco-gel, Dentsply Ltd, Surrey, England) to minimize pressure on the healing implant sites. With few exceptions, the reentry procedure was scheduled for 10 weeks following implantation.

The reentry procedure

Our earlier work in dogs had indicated that the porous design had become fixed by bone ingrowth and would be ready for function by 4 weeks of initial healing.[5,9] Therefore, it was decided that the implant would be stable after a shorter initial healing period than the usually recommended 4 to 6 months. Ten weeks was arbitrarily selected and this has worked well, but at this point, it is not possible to say whether a shorter interval of 8 weeks (twice that needed in dogs), for example, may suffice.

At reentry, an incision was made along the crest of the ridge overlying each implant, and the mucosa was raised minimally around each implant to facilitate removal of the screw and healing cap and placement of the collar and collar-retaining screw. The mucosa was then repositioned and sutured tightly around each collar. The denture was modified again and further relined with Visco-gel to act as a temporary overdenture, and the patient was appointed to begin new denture fabrication approximately 2 weeks later.

The prosthetic phase

The removable overdenture was selected as the restoration of choice in this trial for the following reasons:

1. It is substantially less expensive than a fixed restoration and therefore more accessible to patients in routine clinical practice.
2. It is a technique easily managed by a general dental practitioner as it utilizes conventional denture therapy procedures.
3. Modifications and repairs of the prosthesis are more easily and less expensively managed than with a fixed prosthesis.
4. It often gives a better esthetic result as it provides superior facial soft tissue support.
5. It permits easier daily cleaning of the implants by the patient, and simpler periodic professional assessment and maintenance of the implants and prosthesis.
6. It is more forgiving than a fixed restoration with regard to imperfections in interimplant alignment.
7. The loss of one or more implants is less critical to the continued success of the existing prosthesis.

Conventional procedures were utilized for the prosthodontic therapy, including the use of transfer copings to locate implant analogues within the mandibular cast. Maxillary and mandibular complete dentures with acrylic resin teeth were fabricated for each patient. A silver palladium (Maestro; J.F. Jelenko Co, Armonk, NY) metal bar was incorporated into the lingual flange of the mandibular denture to minimize the risk of fatigue fracture, especially in the regions of the undercut receptacles (Figs 3a and b) created in the denture base to house the prosthodontic cylinder component of each implant assembly. At the time of denture insertion, these receptacles were lined with President (medium or heavy viscosity depending upon the degree of retention desired) silicone impression material (Coltene AG, Allslatten, Switzerland) such that a minimum of 1.5 mm of this material surrounded each prosthodontic cylinder. This material provides excellent retention but is suf-

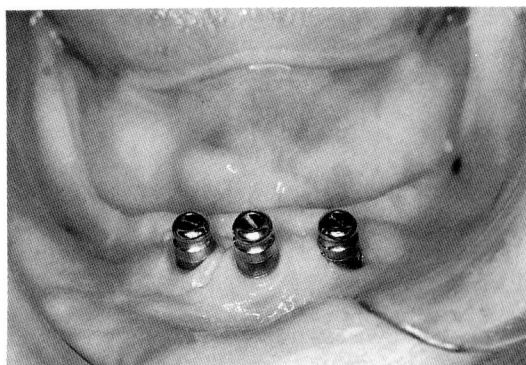

Fig 3a An example of a patient who has passed the 1-year function point.

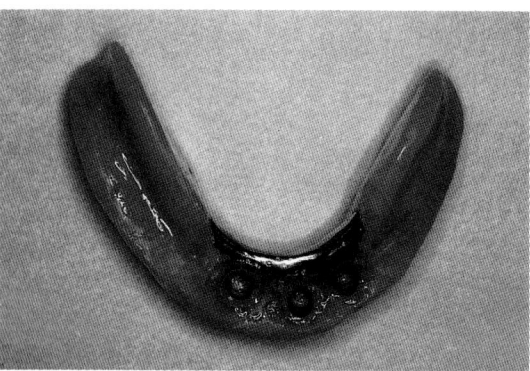

Fig 3b The overdenture design used has a metal bar incorporated into the lingual flange for added strength. The undercut receptacles used to house the prosthodontic cylinders of the implant system are lined with silicone impression material.

ficiently resilient to cushion the occlusal forces being delivered to the implants. Experience by one of the investigators with another implant system has shown that the silicone needs to be changed annually, a procedure that can be done chairside in 10 minutes.

Radiographic examinations

Standardized periapical radiographs of each implanted site in each patient were obtained just prior to insertion of the prosthesis to provide baseline data and to ensure that the collar was fully seated on the implant. The experimental protocol then provided for sequential radiographs at 3, 6, and 12 months of function and at yearly intervals thereafter. All films (Ultraspeed DF-57, size no. 1, Kodak, Rochester, NY) were exposed while being held in a specialized film holder, similar to that described by Cox and Pharoah.[10] This holder attaches directly to each implant, thereby ensuring that the plane of the film is always parallel to the long axis of the implant and that the image geometry in sequential radiographs is constant. Exposure of all films was done at 70 KVp, 10 mA, and 38 impulses with a constant focal-film distance (49.2 cm) using an S.S. White (Spacemaker)

x-ray machine routinely tested for consistency of output and timer accuracy. All films were processed in an identical fashion using a manual method with freshly mixed Kodak 6BX developer and fixer (no. 190-1859) to minimize variation in film density.

Analysis of the radiographs

The primary objective of the radiographic assessment was to verify that there were no peri-implant radiolucencies and to determine the extent and progress, if any, of alveolar bone resorption adjacent to the implants. With threaded implant systems, specifically the Brånemark implant, successful implants are reported to show a maximum loss of crestal bone of 1 mm in the first year and 0.1 mm per year thereafter,[1] although more recent work[11] suggests that the majority of Brånemark implants show stable bone levels after 2 to 3 years of function. Our animal work with the porous implant design used here[12] revealed that once initial bone remodeling occurred down to the region of the machined surface/porous coat junction, the crestal bone level became stable. This was demonstrated at least to the end of the 18-month period studied, presumably because of adequate stress transfer from implant to bone by the porous surface topography. It was anticipated that progressive bone loss with time would not occur with the porous-coated implant once initial remodeling was complete. The experimental protocol called for radiographs to be examined in three ways. Firstly, they were analyzed visually under ×6 magnification by an experienced radiologist (MP) who checked for peri-implant radiolucencies and determined the crestal bone height in relation to the machined surface/porous coat junction on each of the mesial and distal aspects of each implant. As well, they were analyzed by a technician using computer-assisted technique. The films were transverse-illuminated and projected onto a monitor using a video camera (DAGE-MTI Ine, model N70, Michigan City, Ind). The image was digitized using a two-image digitizing board (Matrox Corp, Dorval, Quebec) and mounted in a graphics-oriented computer (Silicon Graphics Inc, model IRIS 3120, Mountainview, Calif). A customized program was created to measure the crestal bone height in relation to the machined surface/porous coat junction on the mesial and distal aspect of each implant. The program was also designed to account for variations in film density and to provide a continuous measurement of bone density immediately adjacent to the mesial and distal aspects of each implant. The details of these analyses will be published in a separate report.

Clinical examinations

The clinical parameters (other than radiographs) that were used to assess implant status included implant mobility and absence/presence of pain to luxation and percussion. Implants were examined manually for visible buccolingual and mesiodistal mobility by applying alternating force with two hand instruments. Healthy implants display no mobility or associated pain.

Other clinical parameters such as a gingival index or periodontal probing depth have not been included in the protocol (although gingival index is recorded to satisfy FDA requirements)

as these are recognized as having minimal value in assessing dental implant status.[13]

Metal iron release studies

Recently, Black et al[14] reported on studies of titanium, aluminum, and vanadium concentrations in serum and urine taken from patients with titanium alloy orthopedic implants. The results of the atomic absorption analyses indicated no significant increase in aluminum levels and a very slight increase in titanium. Vanadium levels could not be determined with sufficient sensitivity. Further studies of metal ion uptake in blood samples drawn from our dental implant patients have been undertaken. Blood samples are being collected before implantation; at 3, 6, and 12 months after implantation; and at yearly intervals thereafter for 5 years. All blood samples will be analyzed using atomic absorption spectrophotometry methods developed in our group.[15,16]

Results

This trial was begun in January 1989 and the final initial surgery was completed in July 1990. All of the surgery was performed by one operator (DAD). One hundred fifty-six implants have been placed in 52 patients. At the time of this report (August 1990), 28 patients had passed the 6-month functional period and 15 patients had been functioning with their implant-supported overdentures for more than 1 year. One patient died shortly after the 3-month functional period. To date, a total of 123 implants have been exposed to the oral cavity (the remaining 33 implants will be re-exposed shortly) and of these, 4 implants (3%) failed to osseointegrate and were removed before being placed into function. Three of these implants were in one patient (patient number 10) and their failure to osseointegrate cannot be explained except to say that there was minimal resistance to drilling and virtually no bleeding from the prepared

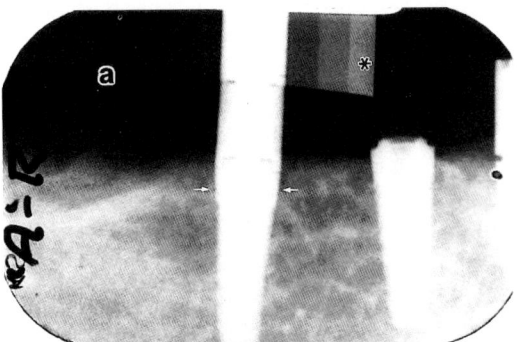

Fig 4a Sample radiograph of an implant at the time of prosthesis insertion.

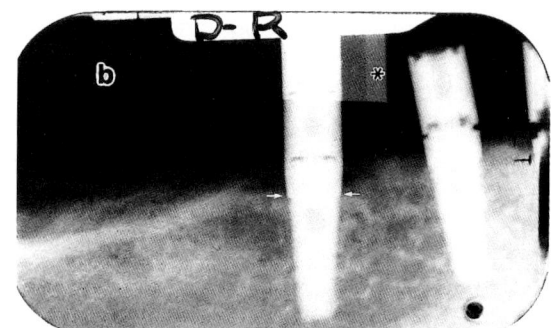

Fig 4b Sample radiograph of implant after 1 year of function. The crestal bone can be seen to have resorbed down to the region of the machined surface/porous coat junction *(arrows)*. Any apparent differences in implant length are the result of differences in photographic reproduction. The image of the hydroxyapatite stepwedge(*) incorporated into the specialized filmholder as a density reference can be seen in both a and b.

sites, suggesting poor bone quality and insufficient osteoprogenitor cells to permit fixation by bone ingrowth in the 10-week healing period allowed. The other implant was lost because of wound infection following early loss of sutures. This patient is functioning satisfactorily using two implants to support his overdenture and has passed the 1-year function point without further problems. Only one other implant has been lost, and while this occurred at 6 months, the patient reported having had physical trauma to the implant within 2 weeks after the reentry surgery. She is functioning satisfactorily using the two remaining implants and has passed the 1-year function point without further problems.

As indicated, radiographs of each implant site are scheduled to be obtained just prior to insertion of the associated prosthesis and then sequentially at 3, 6, and 12 months of function and at yearly intervals thereafter. Bone levels will be assessed both visually and using computer-assisted methods, and will be reported in relation to the machined surface/porous coat junction. This data will be reported when the whole group of 52 patients has passed the 1-year function point. Qualitative evaluation of the 15

patients who have already passed 1 year of function indicates a pattern of bone remodeling similar to that seen in our earlier animal work (Figs 4a and b).[2,12]

Discussion

This is an interim report on our first prospective study to evaluate in humans a new partially porous-coated, endosseous dental implant system. The study involves 52 edentulous patients and 156 consecutively placed implants, three per patient, which were all placed in the anterior mandible and in each case used to support an overdenture. While it is intended that these patients will be followed for a minimum of 5 years and success rates reported at appropriate intervals, it was the purpose of this report to describe the experimental design and to reveal our experience to date.

Of the 156 implants placed, 123 have already been uncovered while the 33 remaining implants are still undergoing initial healing. Of these 123 exposed implants, 4 failed to integrate while 1 was lost at 6 months, probably because of facial trauma that occurred shortly after reentry. Since it is still very early in the study and since it is our intention always to report cumulative failure rates, it seems premature to make any comments on overall success and failure rates at this time. Rather, we prefer to wait until all of the implants have passed the 1-year function point, and to limit discussion here to the implants that have failed to integrate to date.

Only one other published prospective study in which implants were used to support a mandibular overdenture was found. In this study by Naert and co-workers,[17] 44 patients were treated each with two or three Brånemark implants in the anterior mandible. Of these, one implant of the 88 uncovered (ie, 1.1%) failed to integrate. By comparison, in a retrospective study by Engquist et al[18] in which data from 11 Swedish centers were reported, of the 148 Brånemark implants placed in the anterior mandible and intended for use with an overdenture, eight implants (5%) failed to integrate. In the much quoted report by Adell et al,[1] the number of Brånemark implants placed in the mandible that failed to integrate ranged from 2% to 15%, the highest failure rate occurring in their random group I. Zarb and Symington,[6] in their first replication study with the Brånemark implant, reported that 7 of 69 implants (10%) placed in the anterior mandible failed to integrate; in a subsequent report on this same replication study, this initial failure rate escalated to 13.6%.[19] In another study of a different group of patients, Symington et al[20] reported that 10.9% of implants in the anterior mandible failed to integrate. While the reasons for these divergent failure rates (1.1% to 15%) are not clear at this time, these data support the conclusion that our figure of 3% failing to integrate is quite acceptable, especially given the fact that this is the first group of patients treated with this new, porous-coated implant.

The pattern of bone remodeling observed in radiographs obtained to date in the present study has been as predicted from earlier animal work.[2,12] Thus, once the implant is loaded, the crestal bone at the implant surface resorbs down to the region of the machined surface/porous coat junction and appears stable thereafter. This initial remodeling ("loss") occurs, it is assumed, because the coronal 2 mm of the implant has a machined surface that, unlike the porous coat, is ineffective in allowing force transfer from implant to bone, resulting in disuse atrophy. In the dog, it took up to 12 months for this initial bone remodeling to occur; it is too soon to comment on how long this process will take in the human. However, once bone remodeling approximates the machined surface/porous coat junction, it is expected to remain stable thereafter, if the animal work is truly predictive. Bone levels in relation to the machined surface/porous coat junction will be reported regularly.

The pattern of bone remodeling around Brånemark implants in humans has recently been elucidated by Bower et al.[11] They reported that there was a large range of crestal bone loss up to 18 months following insertion of an implant-supported prosthesis and that this was due to initial remodeling. Thereafter, a steady state was reached and for the majority of implants (84% at year 3) no further bone loss occurred. These observations are supported by our findings in the dog with a threaded implant design,[12] and lend support to the notion that bone loss around implants need not be progressive, once initial remodeling has occurred.

Acknowledgments

The authors wish to thank the Innova Corporation, Downsview, Ontario, Canada, for supporting this trial and the Medical Research Council of Canada for supporting the earlier extensive animal research. The technical assistance of Mr D. Abdulla, Ms Denise Booker, Mrs Susan Carter, Mrs Judy Davis, Mrs Monical Mills, and Mrs Nancy Valiquette are also acknowledged with much appreciation. Dr Bunnai Ogiso, Nihon University, Toyko, Japan, provided excellent surgical assistance. Mrs Caroline Chu kindly prepared this manuscript and Mrs Rita Bauer took numerous clinical photographs. Finally, the patients were wonderful and most appreciative.

References

1. Adell R, Lekholm U, Rockler B, Brånemark P-I. A 15-year study of osseointegrated implants in the treatment of the edentulous jaw. *Int J Oral Surg* 1981;6:387–416.

2. Deporter DA, Watson PA, Pilliar RM, Chipman ML, Valiquette N. A histological comparison in the dog of porous-coated vs. threaded dental implants. *J Dent Res* 1990;69:1138–1145.

3. Lekholm U, Zarb GA. Patient selection and preparation. pp 199–209 In *Tissue-Integrated Prostheses: Osseointegration in Clinical Dentistry*. Chicago: Quintessence Publ Co, 1985.

4. Laney WR. Selecting edentulous patients for tissue-integrated prostheses. *Int J Oral Maxillofac Implants* 1986;1:129–138.

5. Deporter DA, Watson PA, Pilliar RM, Melcher AH, Winslow J, Howley TP, et al. A histological assessment of the initial healing response adjacent to porous-surfaced, titanium alloy dental implants in dogs. *J Dent Res* 1986;65:1064–1070.

6. Zarb GA, Symington JM. Osseointegrated dental implants: Preliminary report on a replication study. *J Prosthet Dent* 1983;50:271–276.

7. Schnitman PA, Rubenstein JE, Woehrle PS, Da Silva JD, Koch GG. Implants for Partial Edentulism: Proceedings of NIH Consensus Development Conference on Dental Implants, NIDR, Office of Medical Applications of Research, NIH and FDA, 1988, pp 53–56.

8. Adell R, Lekholm U, Brånemark P-I. Surgical procedures. pp 211–232 In *Tissue-Integrated Prostheses: Osseointegration in Clinical Dentistry*. Chicago: Quintessence Publ Co, 1985.

9. Deporter DA, Watson PA, Pilliar RM, Howley TP, Winslow J. A histological evaluation of a functional endosseous, porous-surfaced, titanium alloy dental implant system in the dog. *J Dent Res* 1988;67:1190–1195.

10. Cox JF, Pharoah M. An alternative holder for radiographic evaluation of tissue-integrated prostheses. *J Prosthet Dent* 1986;56:338–341.

11. Bower RC, Radny NR, Wall CD, Henry PJ. Clinical and microscopic findings in edentulous patients 3 years after incorporation of osseointegrated implant-support bridgework. *J Clin Periodontol* 1989;16:580–587.

12. Pilliar RM, Deporter DA, Watson PA, Valiquette N. Dental implant design-effect on bone remodelling. *J Biomed Mat Res* 1991;25:467–483.

13. Smith DE, Zarb GA. Criteria for success of osseointegrated endosseous implants. *J Prosthet Dent* 1989;62:567–572.

14. Black J, Skipor A, Jacobs J, Urban RM, Galante JD. Release of metal ions from titanium-base alloy total hip replacement prosthesis. Abstract, p 501. 35th Annual Meeting, Orthop Res Soc, Las Vegas, Feb 6–9, 1989.

15. Lugowski S, Smith DC, van Loon JC. The determination of Al, Cr, Co, Fe and Ni in whole blood by electrothermal atomic absorption spectrophotometry. *J Biomed Mater Res* 1987;21:657–674.

16. Lugowski S, Smith DC, van Loon JC. The determination of titanium and vanadium in whole blood. *Trace Elements in Med* 1987;4:28–34.

17. Naert I, De Clercq M, Theuniers G, Schepers E. Overdentures supported by osseointegrated fixtures for the edentulous mandible: A 2.5-year report. *Int J Oral Maxillofac Implants* 1988;3:191–196.

18. Engquist B, Bergendal T, Kallus T, Linden U. A retrospective multicenter evaluation of osseointegrated implants supporting overdentures. *Int J Oral Maxillofac Implants* 1988;3:129–134.

19. Cox JF, Zarb GA. The longitudinal clinical efficacy of osseointegrated dental implants: A 3-year report. *Int J Oral Maxillofac Implants* 1987;2:91–100.

20. Symington JM, Listrom RD, Watson PA, Brown A, Copp PE. Applications of osseointegrated implants. A preliminary report on 35 cases. *Can Dent Assoc J* 1986;52:139–142.

In Vitro Performance of a Fixation System for Free-Vascularized Bone Graft in Staged Operation

E.Y.S. Chao, F.M. Schultz, L.L. Berge, and Y.N. Li

Massive autogenous grafts required to bridge skeletal defects caused by wide resections are usually obtained from the iliac crest, ribs, or fibulae.[3–6,9,16] Using a portion of the distal femur or proximal tibia to fuse the knee joint has been successful, but not without complications.[13,14,17] When the region of resection is more extensive (> 6 to 8 cm), this method of reconstruction becomes less effective since the mechanical strength of the graft and the fixation devices cannot withstand the repetitive load applied, while progressive weakening of the autogenous graft caused by resorption and remodeling further reduces the strength of the reconstruction. In addition, if the fixation at the graft ends is not rigid, nonunion between the graft and host may occur. If the fixation device is too rigid, the graft may become atrophic, especially when nonvascularized grafts are used in patients aged 40 years and older. Although free-vascularized grafts of the proximal fibula have been advocated to enhance union and graft hypertrophy, complications including graft fracture, resorption, or infection persist.[8,12,19,20] The preparation of screw holes and application of screws and a plate can cause significant vascular damage to the graft and host, which may adversely affect bone union.[11,15,18] Better fixation that provides initial stability to enhance bony union while allowing subsequent graft modeling and hypertrophy is needed.

Fixation of a free-vascularized bone graft using screws alone does not provide adequate stability because screw insertion creates a layer of necrotic bone near the screw threads, which may become fibrous tissue and eventually lead to loss of fixation under repetitive load. Osseointegration provides a better screw/bone interface, and improved anchorage may allow the use of a less rigid metallic device for staged operation to enhance tissue vascularity and graft hypertrophy. Direct bone/metal interface without fibrous tissue lining is defined as osseointegration. If successfully achieved, such a biologic condition permits direct and secure load transmission with diminished incidence of late failure.[1,2]

The objectives of this study were to develop special titanium fixtures and the corresponding plate and fixation screw system for vascularized fibular graft transplantation, and to compare the in vitro fixation between the titanium graft fixation system and the conventional stainless steel ASIF (Association for Study of Internal Fixation) compression screw and plate system strength in an orthotopic bone graft transplantation model. The results of this study could provide information concerning the need for weight-bearing protection when staged fibular transplantation is to be utilized. If the essential fixation rigidity and strength could not be accomplished by the experimental devices, new design and development must be pursued before the concept of osseointegration and staged transplantation of vascularized fibular grafts can be safely tested.

Materials and methods

Two fixture screw/plate fixation systems were

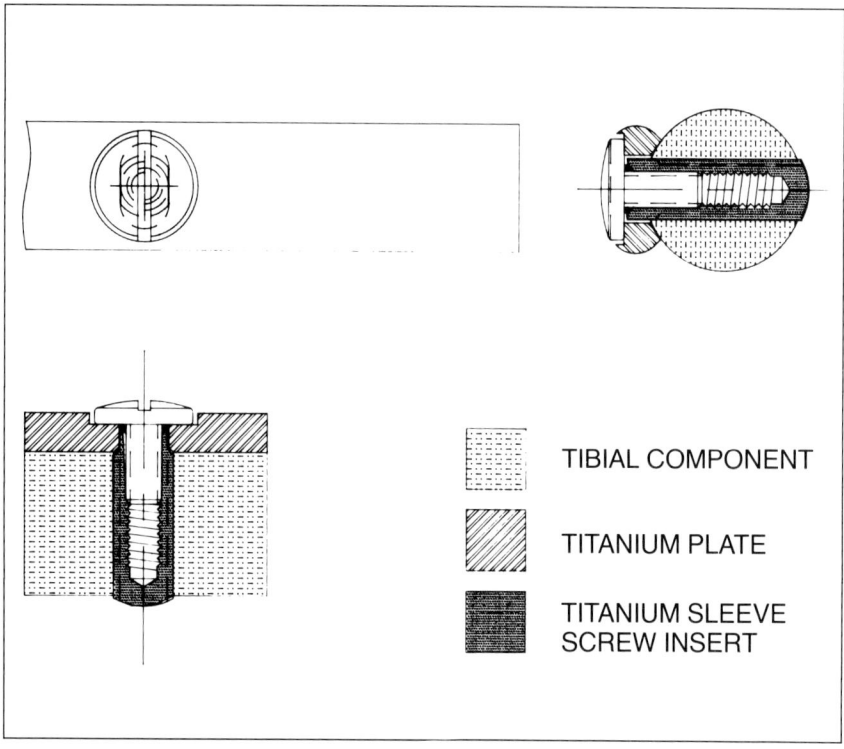

Fig 1 The sleeve titanium fixture screw design with cap screw and plate for segmental bone graft fixation to the host following a staged implantation procedure.

developed and tested for their adequacy in fixing segmental bone graft transplantation. The first system involved a hollow sleeve screw with both internal and external threads (Fig 1). The external threads allow initial fixation of the screw fixture in bone for osseointegration during the first stage of the graft transplantation procedure. The internal threads permit plate fixation using tightening cap screws, which will be used in the second stage of graft transfer and fixation.

The second fixation system used a solid screw fixture with external threads only. Plate fixation was later accomplished by using cap nuts over the screw heads engaged within the screw holes of the plate (Figs 2a and b). The fixture screws, cap screws, and cap nuts were made of commercially pure titanium (surgical grade) and the fixation plate was made of Ti-6Al-4V alloy. For comparison, conventional ASIF compression screws made of stainless

steel and the same titanium plate in the screw fixture system were used.

Two bone models were used in the experiment. The first model was a solid circular rod made of self-curing polyurethane material, "RF-100" foam (Daro Products, Inc, Milwaukee, Wisc), 1 inch in diameter (Fig 3). This material has been carefully studied for its adequate mechanical properties to simulate the human humerus.[7] The foam bone model measured 210 mm in length, with the middle section 48 mm in length and osteotomized to simulate the bone graft for orthotopic transplantation and fixation.

The second bone model used was the canine tibia sectioned and fixed identically to that performed for the foam bone model. After sectioning and fixation, the bone models were carefully embedded in Wood's metal (Cerrobend Alloy, Satterlee Company, Minneapolis, Minn), with a melting temperature of 78°C, maintaining con-

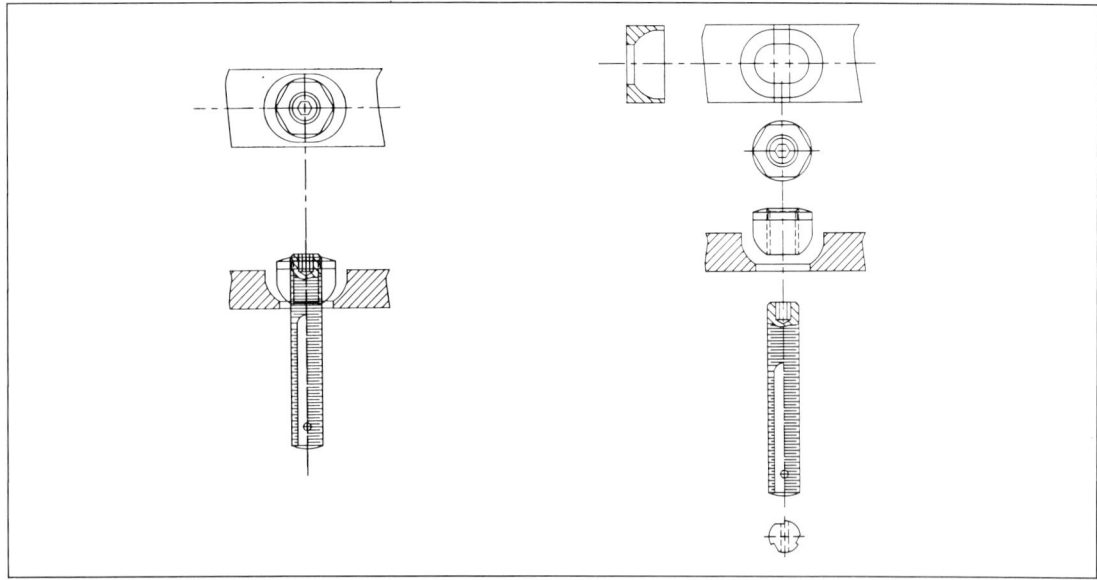

2a

Figs 2a and b The solid titanium fixture screws with cap nuts and Ti-6Al-4V plate for segmental bone graft fixation to the host following staged implantation procedure in order to achieve osseointegration of the screw fixtures with bone. (2a) Schematic diagrams of the fixture screw, cap nut, and plate design and assembly illustration. (2b) Finished solid screw fixtures, cap nuts, and fixation plate.

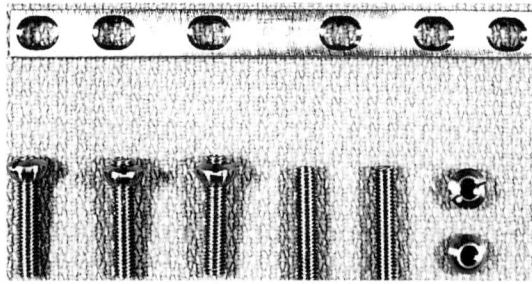

2b

sistent orientation and placement using a special mounting guide (Figs 4a and b). All screws applied to either the foam bone model or the canine tibia were tightened consistently using an instrumented torque wrench (Fig 5).

Torsion and 4-point bending tests were used to study fixation stiffness properties, and a failure test was performed only under torsion for fixation strength determination (Figs 6a and b). In the 4-point bending test, two plate locations were used; one with the plate placed on the tension side (anteroposterior bending) and the other with the plate positioned laterally to the direction of bending (mediolateral bending). Stiffness values, ultimate torque, total rotation, and energy required at failure were determined from the force-deformation curves in each test

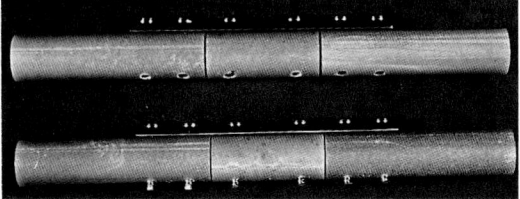

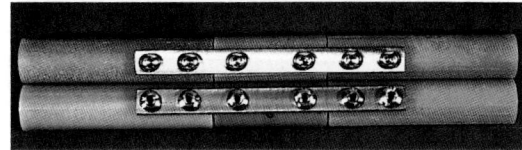

Fig 3 The titanium screw fixture and the ASIF screws used to fix the simulated graft transplantation using the foam bone model. The same titanium plates were used in each fixation method to minimize the plate rigidity effect.

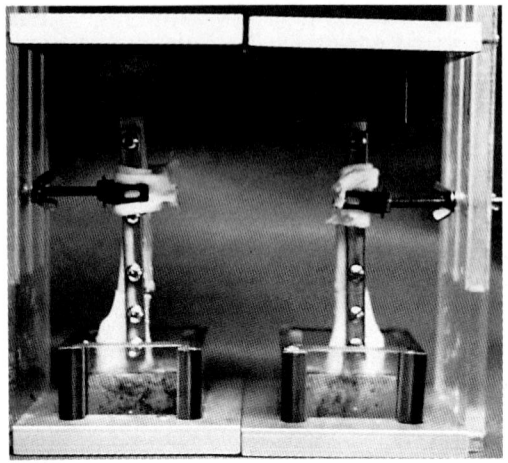

4a

Figs 4a and b The canine tibia model used to compare the sleeve screw fixtures and cap screw fixation strength and rigidity with that stabilized by ASIF screws using the same titanium plate. (4a) The mounting guide used to embed the test specimen in Wood's metal to ensure consistent placement and orientation of each pair of canine tibiae. (4b) The securely mounted tibiae with their mid-diaphyseal section fixed by two methods for stiffness and strength comparison.

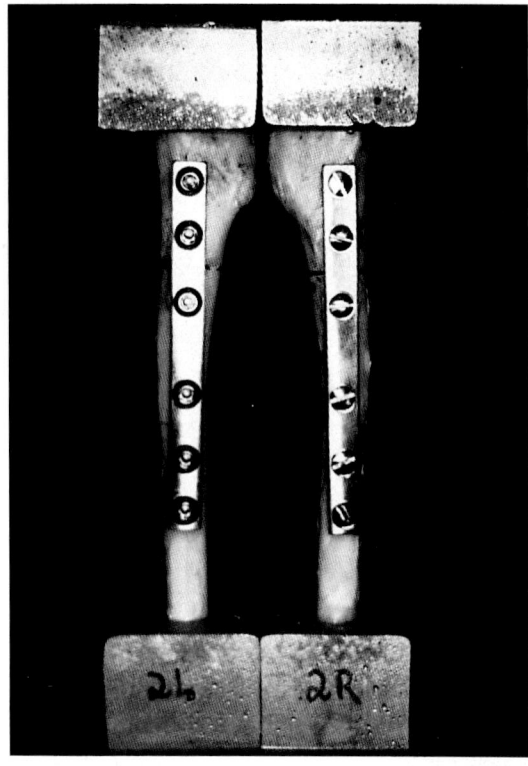

4b

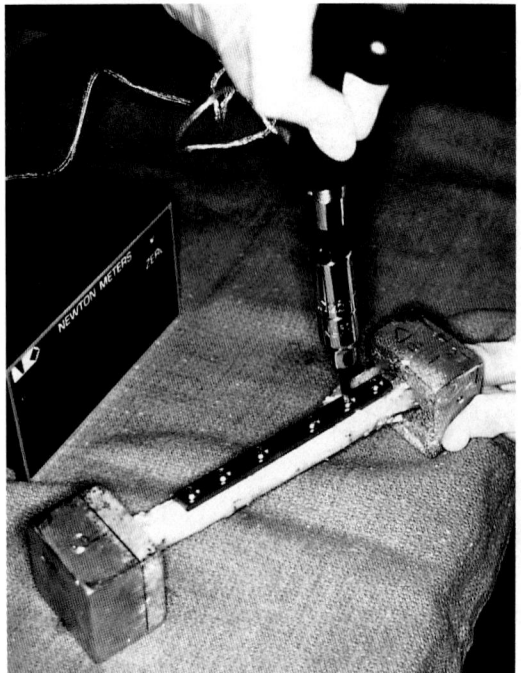

Fig 5 The instrumented torque wrench used to standardize the tightening torque for each screw fixture, cap screw, cap nut, or ASIF screw before mechanical testing.

sequence. To save testing time and the number of required specimens for the experiment, the first fixture sleeve screw system (hollow with cap screws) was tested against the ASIF screws using the canine tibiae. The solid fixture screws fixed to the plate with cap nuts were tested against the ASIF screws using the foam bone model. All results were expressed as the percentage of the intact specimens so as to minimize the variation in model dimension and mechanical property. A Student's *t* test was used to detect the difference in experimental fixture systems with that obtained by using the conventional ASIF screws. After torsional failure the modes of failure were examined and compared.

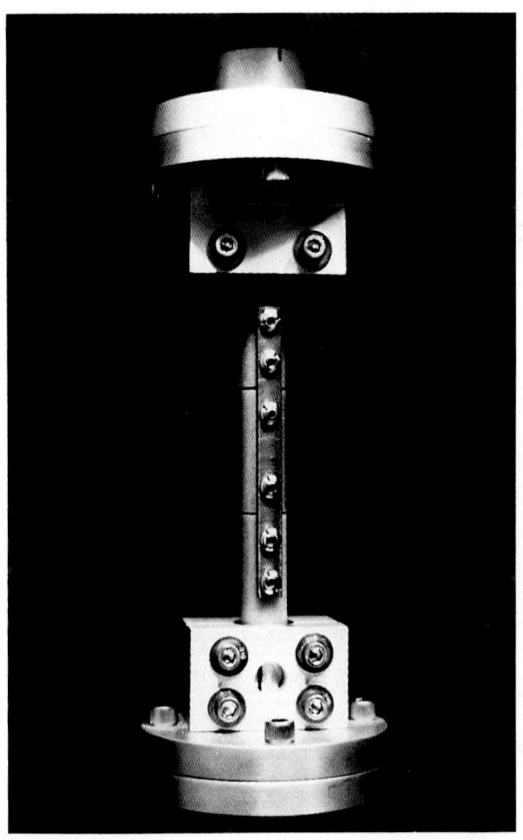

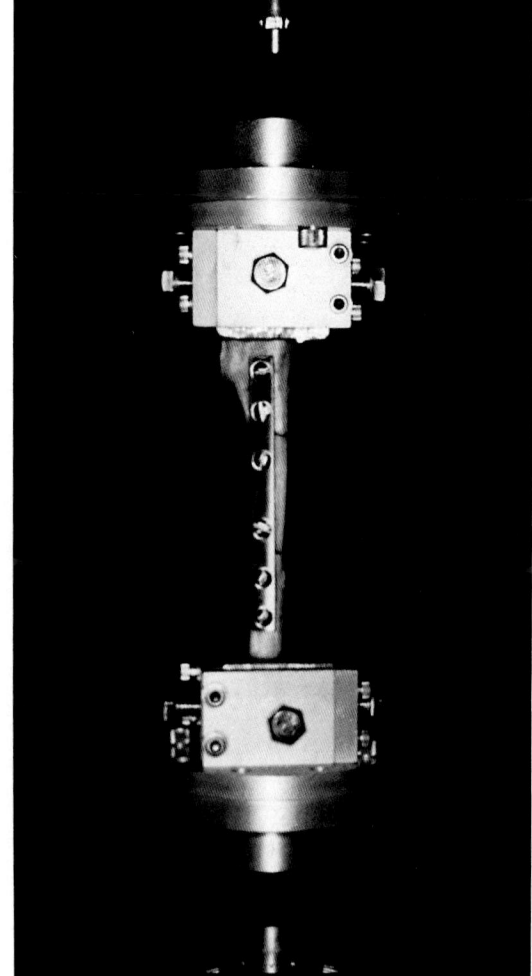

Figs 6a and b Specimen testing under different loading conditions. (6a) Torsional test for stiffness and strength determination. (6b) 4-point bending test in anteroposterior direction.

Results

The hollow fixture screw system with cap screws compared favorably with the ASIF screws in bending stiffness property, but the torsional stiffness was significantly lower ($P <$ .05) in the titanium system (Table 1). The torsional strength was less in the titanium fixture screw group; however, the difference was not statistically significant (P = .13). When compared to the intact bone data, the stiffness and strength values were less than 50% of the intact value. The ASIF screw fixed model can provide close to 60% of the intact model's torsional strength. The most common failure mechanism in the ASIF screw fixed group was the fracture

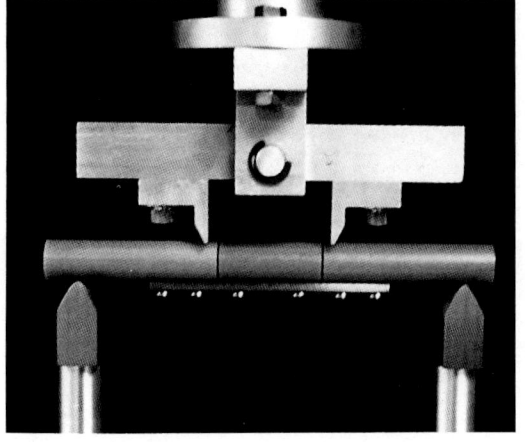

6b

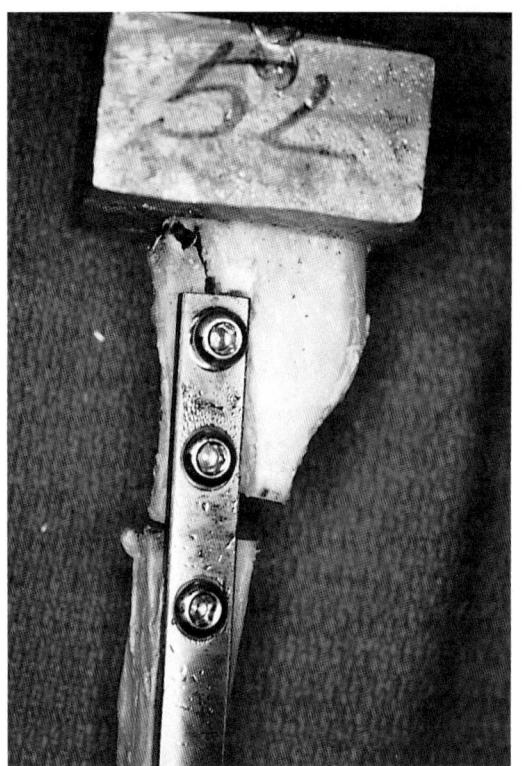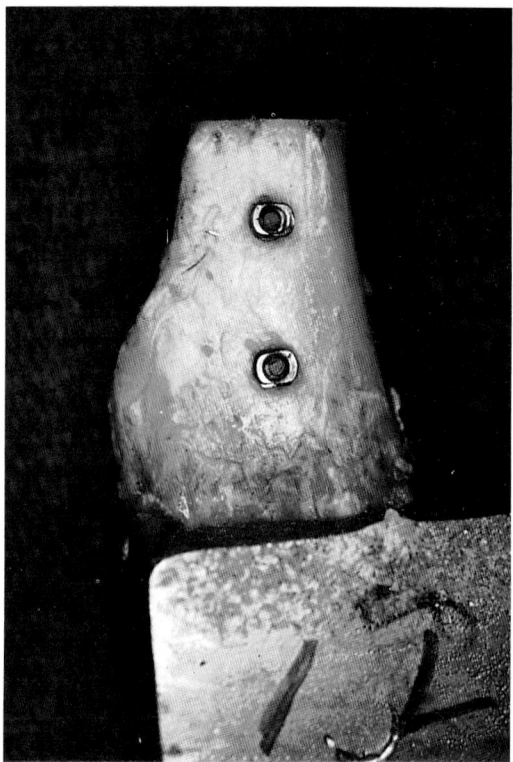

Figs 7a and b The failure mechanisms involved in different fixation methods using a canine tibial model. (7a) Bone fracture and screw bending in ASIF screw and titanium plate fixation group. (7b) Failure through cap screw fracture with bone and screw fixture intact.

Table 1 Comparison of fixation stiffness and strength between a titanium screw fixture/plate system with cap screws and the conventional ASIF screws in a canine tibial model

Specimens	Fixation stiffness			Maximum torque to failure (N-m)
	AP bending (N-cm/deg)	ML bending (N-cm/deg)	Torsion (N-cm/deg)	
Intact canine tibia (n = 6)	2945 ± 605 (100%)*	2569 ± 568 (100%)	238 ± 92 (100%)	29 ± 8 (100%)
ASIF screws and Ti plate (n = 6)	1066 ± 166 (36%)	342 ± 64 (13%)	53 ± 5† (19%)	17 ± 5 (59%)
Ti fixture with cap screws (n = 6)	1074 ± 144 (36%)	411 ± 130 (20%)	39 ± 8† (14%)	14 ± 2 (47%)

AP = anteroposterior; ML = mediolateral.
*All percentage values in parentheses are expressed in reference to intact canine tibia value.
†Significantly different between the ASIF and Ti system ($P < .05$).

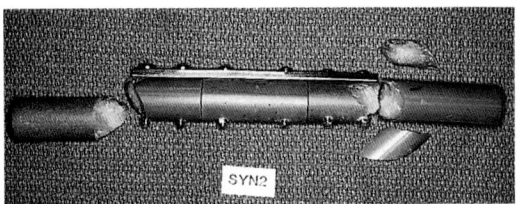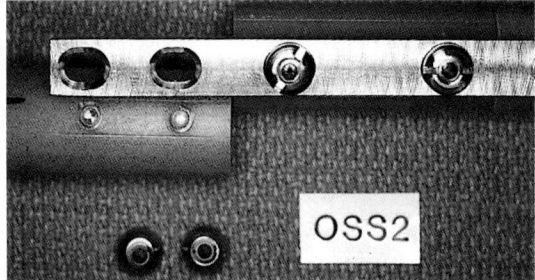

Figs 8a and b The failure mechanisms involved in different fixation methods using synthetic foam bone model. (8a) Fracture of the bone model at the end of the plate in ASIF screw fixed side. (8b) Fracture of the head of the solid screw fixture at the base of the hexagonal socket used for tightening of the cap nut.

Table 2 Comparison of fixation stiffness and strength between a titanium screw fixture/plate system with cap nuts and the conventional ASIF screw fixation in a foam bone model

Specimens	Fixation stiffness			Maximum torque to failure (N-m)
	AP bending (N-cm/deg)	ML bending (N-cm/deg)	Torsion (N-cm/deg)	
Intact foam bone model (n = 4)	414 ± 36 (100%)	414 ± 36 (100%)	81 ± 8 (100%)	32 ± 3 (100%)
ASIF screws and Ti plate (n = 4)	732 ± 22 (177%)	318 ± 26* (77%)	59 ± 5 (73%)	25 ± 2* (78%)
Ti fixture screw with cap nuts (n = 4)	609 ± 43 (147%)	263 ± 10* (64%)	52 ± 4 (64%)	18 ± 1* (56%)

AP = anteroposterior; ML = mediolateral.
*Significantly different between the ASIF and Ti system ($P < .05$).

at the bone end with screw bending (Figs 7a and b). On the titanium fixture screw side, cap screws on the bone-end section were frequently sheared off in addition to bone fracture.

The solid titanium fixture screw with cap nut did not improve its graft fixation stiffness and strength when compared to the ASIF screw system (Table 2). The bending stiffness and torsional strength were significantly lower on the titanium side ($P < .05$). The artificial foam bone model was adequate for fixation strength and stiffness test except in anteroposterior bending, which was too flexible when compared to the metallic fixation systems as reflected by the increase in bending stiffness value after fixation. Failure associated with the ASIF screw

system mainly involved model fracture while failure in the titanium fixture system occurred through fracture of the fixture screw at the seat of the hexagonal socket (Figs 8a and b). This was related primarily to the poor design where the end of the hexagonal socket coincided with the maximum stress area resulting in a compounded effect of stress concentration and structural weakness. Thus, the modified design change utilizing cap nuts for plate fixation to screw fixtures did not provide any improvement.

Other biomechanical testing parameters did not offer any new information. The failure mechanisms involved in each model and fixation method were consistent. Under microscopic examination of the thread surfaces, there was less osseous damage and closer screw/bone interface on the titanium fixture screw side. However, all screw/bone interfaces showed significant microfractures and abrasive tears caused by mechanical tapping and screw insertion.

Discussion

Rigid and strong fixation of the intercalary bone segment of substantial length is difficult to achieve. Using only cortical screws would not be sufficient to provide the necessary strength needed to achieve graft/host union. Failure of fixation may occur even with weight-bearing protection. Using either one long plate to cross both osteotomy sites or two short plates bridging the gaps at either end seems to provide inadequate fixation stability and strength, which was mainly limited by the weak screw/bone interface and the number of screws placed in the bone segment. The multiple osteotomy sites plus bone end mismatch both in size and geometry will further reduce the fixation strength. Application of long plates in two planes will no doubt increase both the fixation strength and stiffness, but such rigid fixation may predispose the graft to severe atrophy. Therefore, an optimal fixation method allowing the graft to unite with the host and achieve hypertrophy through remodeling is a challenging problem in vascularized fibular graft transplantation.

In the preliminary in vivo study using canine tibia, osseointegration was demonstrated by positive bone remodeling and hypertrophy around the implanted screw fixture.[10] This study further demonstrated bone resorption at the screw thread interface during the initial time period of 2 to 4 weeks after implantation. Hence, a two-stage operation utilizing the screw fixture and fixation plate system presented here may be beneficial for successful graft union and hypertrophy. Bone remodeling within the screw thread space and new bone formation around the screw will provide increased fixation strength when the bone plate is applied in the second stage of operation and graft transplantation.

Unfortunately, the present fixation system designs did not provide sufficient stiffness and strength to allow safe and effective graft immobilization. Although improved design for the cap screw or nut and fixation plate could be developed, proper balance between fixation rigidity and the potential graft atrophy must be weighed in order to achieve optimal results. The current models used do not provide a realistic situation because of the dimension and geometric mismatch between the fibular graft and the host bone. This mismatch of graft/host site will further weaken the fixation strength. Finally, the fibula is a comparatively weak long bone with a rather small cross section. Implanting a sizable screw fixture with the fibular cortex will further weaken its load-carrying ability unless significant graft hypertrophy was achieved before transplantation. Therefore, weight-bearing protection may be inevitable in most fibular graft transplantation cases.

The significance of the improved microscopic appearance of bone thread surface after low speed drilling and tapping adopted in titanium fixture screw insertion cannot be ascertained in the present in vitro study. The main advantage of the present concept is to enhance the vascular status of the graft at the time of transplantation without violating the established microvascular network around and within the fibular graft. This advantage, along with other potential benefits, including ease of graft fixation and avoidance of local irradiation effect before or after fibular graft transplantation, should provide sufficient justification to pursue the current concept further. The same principle, when perfected, can be effectively applied to different bone graft transplantation sites other than the major long bones.

Acknowledgment

This study was supported in part by a Public Health Service grant, number CA40583, awarded by the National Cancer Institute, Department of Health and Human Services. We wish to thank Larry Berglund for his assistance in performing the specimen testing and data reduction.

References

1. Brånemark P-I. Osseointegration and its experimental background. *J Prosthet Dent* 1983;50:399–410.
2. Brånemark P-I, Zarb GA, Albrektsson T. *Tissue-Integrated Prostheses: Osseointegration in Clinical Dentistry.* Chicago: Quintessence Publ Co, 1985.
3. d'Aubigne MR, Meary R, Thomine JM. La resection dans le traitement des tumerus des os. *Rev Chir Orthop* 1966;52:305–324.
4. Enneking WF, Burchardt H, Puhl JJ, Thornby J. Temporal and spatial activity in mirror segments of mature dog fibula. *Calcif Tissue Res* 1972;9:283–295.
5. Enneking WF, Shirley PD. Resection-arthrodesis for malignant and potentially malignant lesions about the knee using an intramedullary rod and local bone grafts. *J Bone Joint Surg* 1977;59A:223.
6. Enneking WF, Edy J, Burchardt H. Autogenous cortical bone grafts in the reconstruction of segmental skeletal defects. *J Bone Joint Surg* 1980;62A:1027.
7. Hein TJ, Perissinotto A, Hotchkiss R, Chao Edmund YS. Analysis of bone model material for external fracture fixation experiments. Biomedical sciences instrumentation. Paper presented at 24th Annual Rocky Mountain Bioengineering Symposium, North Dakota State University, Fargo, North Dakota, 27–28 April 1987. *ISA* 1987;23:43–48.
8. Hsu RWW, Wood MB, Chao EYS, Sim FH. Free vascularized fibular graft in the skeletal defect reconstruction after tumor resection. *J Bone Joint Surg* 1990;submitted for publication.
9. Langlais F, Aubriot JH, Postel M, Tomeno B, Vielpeau C. Prosthese de reconstruction de l'extremite superieure du femur. Resultat a moyen terme de 20 resection pour tumeurs. *Rev Chir Orthop* 1986;72:415–425.
10. Li YN, Bishop AT, Chao EYS. Titanium fixture screws in canine tibial diaphysis following osseointegration principles. In W.R. Laney, D.E. Tolman (eds) *Tissue Integration in Oral, Orthopedic, and Maxillofacial Reconstruction: Proceedings of the 2nd Int Congress.* 23–27 September 1990. Mayo Medical Center, Rochester, Minn, Chicago: Quintessence Publ Co, 1992.
11. O'Sullivan ME, Chao EYS, Kelly PJ. Current concepts review. The effects of fixation on fracture healing. *J Bone Joint Surg* 1989;71A:306–310.
12. Pho RWH. Free vascularized fibular transplant for replacement of the lower radius. *J Bone Joint Surg* 1979;61B:362–365.
13. Sim FH, Beauchamp CP, Chao EYS. Joint arthrodesis: With particular reference to knee arthrodesis using a porous-coated intercalary prosthesis. pp 102–113 In R. Coombs, G. Friedlaender (eds) *Bone Tumour Management.* London: Butterworth and Co, Ltd, 1987.
14. Sim FH, Beauchamp CP, Chao EYS. Reconstruction of musculoskeletal defects about the knee for tumor. *Clin Orthop* 1987;221:188–201.
15. Smith SR, Bronk JT, Kelly PJ. Effects of fixation on fracture blood flow. *Orthop Trans* 1987;11:294–295.
16. Springfield DS. Massive autogenous bone grafts. *Orthop Clin North Am* 1987;18:249–256.
17. Tomeno B, Languepin A. Resection arthrodesis of the knee using "Juvara-Merle d'Aubigne" procedure. Analysis of forty-five cases. pp 39–45 In E.Y. Chao, J.C. Ivins (eds) *Tumor Prostheses for Bone and Joint Reconstruction: The Design and Application.* Chicago: Thieme-Stratton, Inc, 1983.
18. Uhthoff HK, Finnegan M. The effects of metal plates on post-traumatic remodelling and bone mass. *J Bone Joint Surg* 1983;65B:66–71.
19. Weiland AJ, Moore JR, Daniel RK. Vascularized bone autografts: Experience with 41 cases. *Clin Orthop* 1983;174:87–95.
20. Wood MB, Cooney WP III, Irons GB Jr. Free vascularized fibula graft transplantation: Skeletal indications and results. *Mayo Clin Proc* 1985;60:729–734.

Titanium Fixture Screws in Canine Tibial Diaphysis Following Osseointegration Principles

Y.N. Li, A.T. Bishop, and E.Y.S. Chao

Increased utilization of limb sparing procedures for malignant bone and soft tissue tumors in the extremities frequently results in the creation of large bony defects. Reconstruction of these extremities may require the use of a free-vascularized bone graft, either alone or in combination with conventional grafts. Using screws alone to fix the graft to the host cannot provide the necessary stability and strength because screw insertion causes a layer of necrotic bone near the screw threads, which turns to fibrous tissue and may eventually cause loss of fixation. Among the complications reported in the use of free bone transfer, nonunion requiring reoperation is the most common.[6,7] Furthermore, overly rigid fixation may cause severe stress shielding osteopenia to the graft, leading to resorption. Osseointegration may provide a better screw/bone interface to improve screw anchorage to bone and thus prevent graft fracture, nonunion, or resorption. Direct bone-to-screw osseointegration has not been widely studied apart from the dental implant application. If this principle can be repeatedly demonstrated, it should be considered in joint arthroplasty design, fracture fixation, limb lengthening procedures, as well as anchorage of tendon and ligament.

A novel form of skeletal fixation, initially developed by Brånemark and co-workers in Sweden, enables direct bone-to-screw contact resulting in improved long-term fixation subjected to repetitive loading.[1-3] The technique has been widely utilized for fixation of dental implants but has not been employed in orthopedic surgery except for experimental implantation of meta-

carpophalangeal arthroplasty.[5] This form of fixation has potential application in staged skeletal reconstruction for infection or tumor when segmental defect reconstruction by vascularized bone transfer is planned. A two-staged procedure with initial implantation of titanium fixtures into the donor bone (eg, fibula) followed by free-vascularized transfer once direct bone-to-implant osseointegration is assured may enable plate and screw fixation to the anchored fixtures with greater initial and long-term strength.

Further, minimal fixation is frequently used because of concern for disruption of donor bone vascularity. Staged transfer will likely allow recovery of intramedullary circulation and even result in a hyperemic state of bone blood flow, as well as the accompanying bone hypertrophy. Improved rigidity and intraosseous circulation should both enhance bone healing. Finally, optimal fixation rigidity can avoid overly stiff mobilization using massive implants, which may cause graft resorption caused by stress-shielding osteopenia.

The extensive research of Brånemark and his colleagues and others has elucidated the parameters needed for successful osseointegration.[4] The implant must be made of tissue-tolerant material. Its configuration and surface characteristics should allow an exact fit with adjoining bone and provide adequate initial mechanical stability. A rough finish may improve biomechanical parameters. Integration will occur in either a cortical or cancellous bed; thus, bone type is less important than other parameters. Of critical importance is gentle surgical

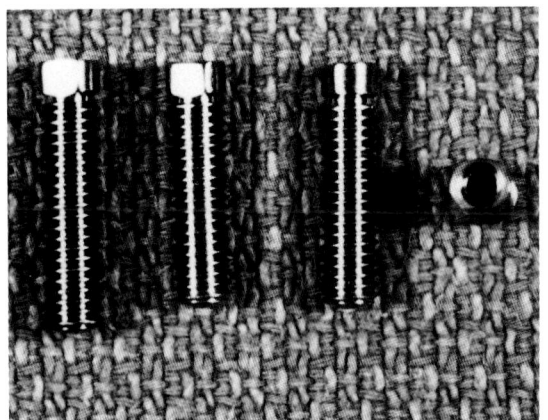

Fig 1a Special screw fixtures (sleeve screws) used to achieve osseointegration with canine tibia. Close-up view of the titanium screw fixtures.

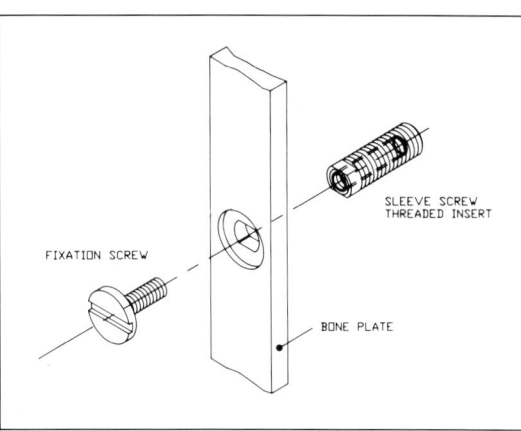

Fig 1b Schematic diagram illustrating the plate fixation to the sleeve screws in the staged operation involving graft transplantation.

technique to prevent osteocyte death resulting from excessive heat generation or mechanical damage, as well as protection from loading and resultant micromotion until osteogenesis and integration have occurred.[2–4]

The long-term goal of this investigation is to examine in depth the feasibility of osseointegration for fixation of free-vascularized bone transfers. The expertise gained in the techniques utilized for this study will likely serve as a basis for future investigations of a broad range of potential applications of osseointegration principles in orthopedics. The specific objective of the present investigation was to examine roentgenographic, histomorphological, and biomechanical characteristics of osseointegrated screws/fixtures in a canine tibia.

Materials and methods

Special screw fixtures (sleeve screws) were designed and fabricated using surgical grade pure titanium. The screw threads had fine pitch (10 ~ 32 machine screw thread) to ensure proper engagement with canine tibial cortex. Two screw lengths were available to allow full bone penetration in cortices of varying width.

The screw contained a hollow sleeve with internal threads for fixation screw application so as to fasten a rigid titanium plate for graft fixation in staged operation (Figs 1a and b). Screw placement jigs and drill guides were used to allow accurate placement of the fixture sleeve screws. Different sized drills (1.57 to 4.0 mm) were incrementally stepped in the drilling procedure to allow careful and atraumatic preparation of the screw bed. A sharp tap was used for final bone thread preparation. A slow-speed drill (20 rpm) was used for drilling, whereas the final tapping was performed by hand. To avoid contamination of the screw surface, a titanium forcep was used to handle all screws. These instruments were placed in a special rack to facilitate surgical implantation (Fig 2).

Five adult, mixed-breed dogs weighing 22 to 30 kg were used. Maturity was confirmed radiographically by physeal plate closure. After intravenous induction of general anesthesia (pentobarbital, 30 mg/kg) and aseptic draping, the tibia of one of the hind limbs was exposed. Six custom-made osseointegration titanium fixture screws were inserted transversely to the mid-diaphysis of the tibia. A template was used to obtain the precise location of these screws and to avoid damaging the nutrient vessels. An instrumented wrench was used to standardize

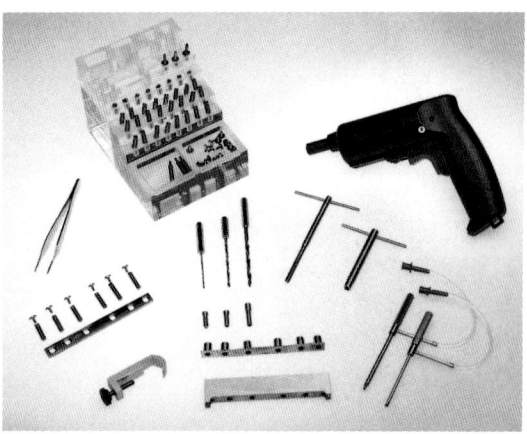

Fig 2 Titanium fixture screws and insertion instruments including drill bits, drill guides, bone holding jig, screw holding forcep, instrument with irrigation tube, and the slow-speed drill.

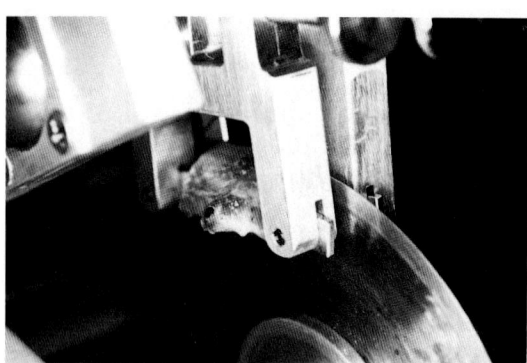

Fig 3 A section of tibial cortex containing the titanium screw fixture mounted on the Isomet diamond saw to be cut into halves in the longitudinal direction, bisecting the sleeve screw.

the final tightening torque. During bone thread preparation and screw insertion, abundant saline irrigation was used to minimize bone temperature. The periosteum was repaired and soft tissue closed in layers. The procedure was then repeated on the contralateral tibia during the same anesthetization period.

All animals were allowed to bear weight immediately. Continuous fluorochrome labeling (25 mg/kg tetracycline) was given orally once daily throughout the experimental period. Anteroposterior and mediolateral radiographs of the tibiae of each animal were taken just before surgery and every 2 weeks until euthanasia. One dog each was euthanized at 2, 4, 6, 8, and 10 weeks.

After euthanasia, both tibiae were harvested with all soft tissue stripped. Both bone and surrounding soft tissue samples were sent for infection testing. All screw fixtures and equal amounts of adjacent tibial cortex were cut transversely using an Isomet low-speed diamond circular saw (Buehler, Ltd, Lake Bluff, Ill) at low speed and under saline irrigation. Each segment of tibial cortex containing the titanium screw fixture was then cut longitudinally, bisecting the screw using the same cutting technique (Fig 3). Half of each screw specimen was randomly selected and used for histomorphologic analysis and the other half for a biomechanical push-out test.

For histological analysis, the specimens were fixed immediately in alcohol and subsequently embedded in methyl methacrylate resin. Longitudinal slices of 200 μm in thickness of the screw/bone interface were obtained using the Isomet low-speed saw with diamond blade. These slides were then ground 54 to 70 μm thick for quantitative histologic analysis using contact microradiograph, ultraviolet light, and polarized light microscopy before and after paragon stain. A semiautomated counting method was used for old bone, new bone, and porosity determination. The bone/thread contact length within each thread space was also measured for comparison.

The remaining half of each specimen was embedded in Wood's metal (Ceffo Bend Alloy) using a special fixation jig for the push-out test (Figs 4a and b). The push-out strength of the osseointegration screws was compared with those implanted in fresh cadaveric canine tibiae (simulating a 0-week specimen). The force/displacement curve of the push-out test was used to determine ultimate push-out force, shear stiffness (slope of the linear position of the load/deformation curve), and energy to failure. These values were normalized based

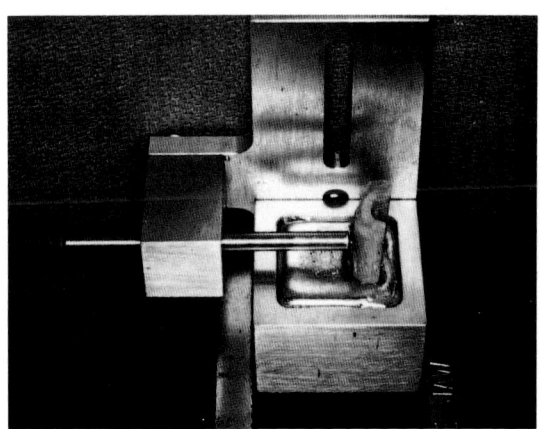

Fig 4a Canine tibial cortex with osseointegrated screw fixture prepared for the biomechanical push-out test. One end of the bone/fixture composite is being fixed in the Wood's metal, guided by a precision jig and a holding pin screwed into the sleeve screw. When the Wood's metal hardens, the jig will be turned over to embed the opposite side in the same manner.

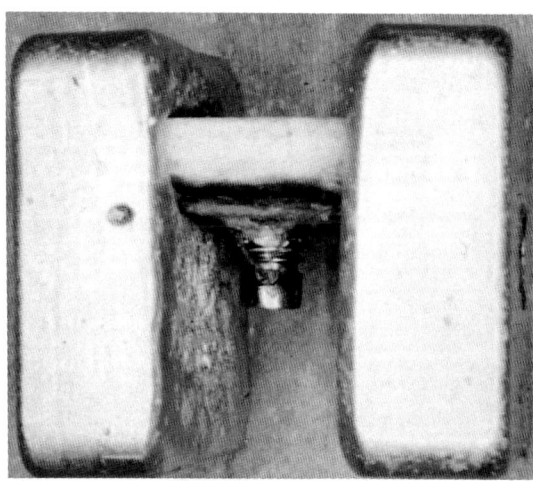

Fig 4b The fixed bone/fixture composite with the fixture screw pushed out after the test. Note the direction of push-out is always from endosteum to periosteum.

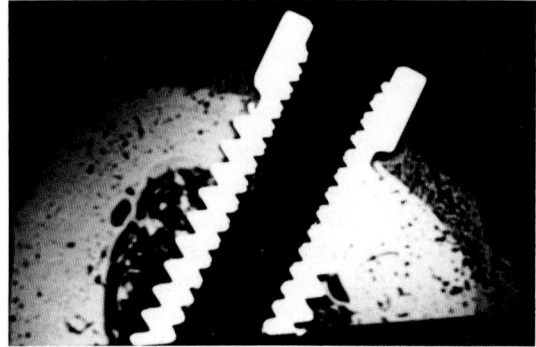

Fig 5a Microradiographs of the osseointegrated titanium screw fixture in canine tibial cortex after 10 weeks. New bone formation at the entry cortex. Note that a significant amount of new bone had to be removed in order to expose the screw fixture head.

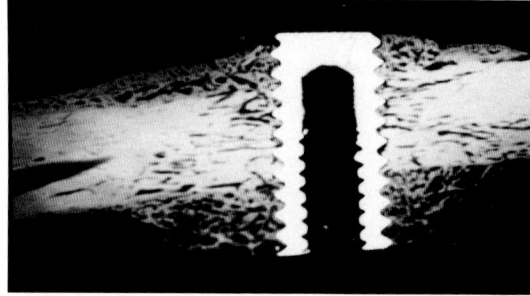

Fig 5b New bone formation at the exit cortex with both endosteal and periosteal thread coverage.

on the thickness of the bone cortices. ANOVA and paired Student's *t* tests were used for comparison.

Results

All five dogs survived the experimental periods without complications. The tissues examined

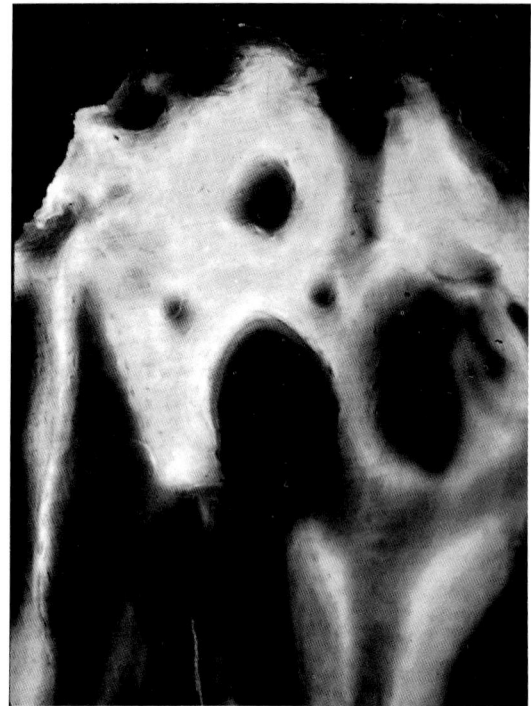

Fig 6a Histologic section of bone within the screw fixture's threads viewed using ultraviolet light microscopy. The brighter color indicates the tetracycline labeled new bone. Bone 4 weeks after implantation.

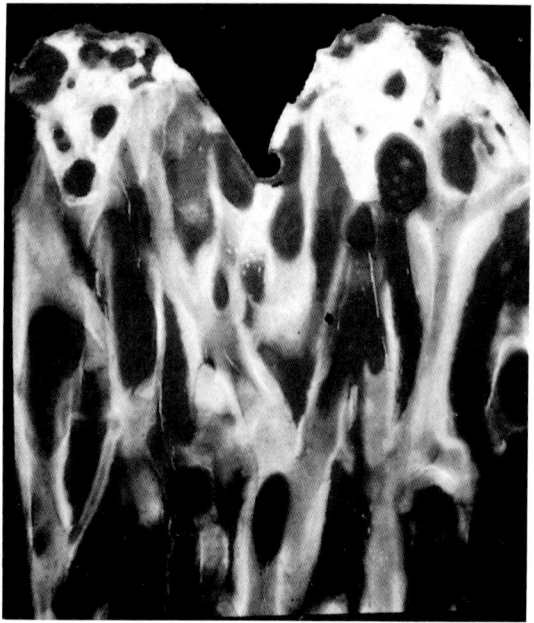

Fig 6b   Bone 6 weeks after implantation.

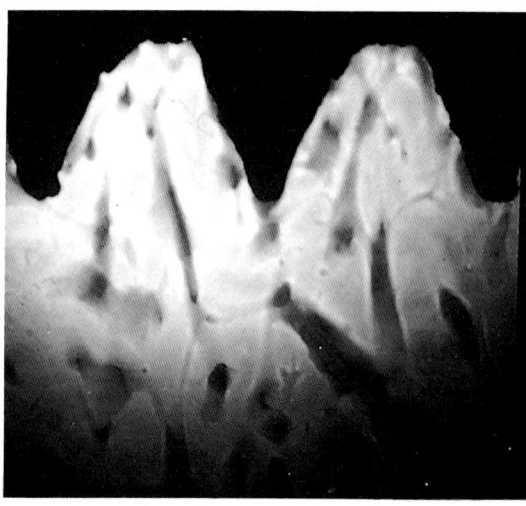

Fig 6c   Bone 10 weeks after implantation.

showed no sign of infection. At 2 weeks there was an area of radiolucency around each screw regardless of location. By 6 to 8 weeks there were halos with increasing radiodensity surrounding the implants. At 10 weeks the halo signs were more defined and there were no radiolucent lines around the implant. In addition, new bone formation was evident around the screw in the medullary canal.

The microradiographs showed bone apposition throughout the screw threads with both endosteal and periosteal new bone formation. This new bone formation occurred at both the entry and exit cortices (Figs 5a and b). Under ultraviolet light microscopy, the histologic slides showed clear progress of new bone formation within the threads with time (Fig 6a to c). Using new bone contact length with thread surface expressed as percentage of available threads engaged in each cortex, there was a statistically significant

Table 1 Bone/screw thread contact length expressed in percentage of available thread length in each cortex

Followup time (weeks)	Sample size	Bone/screw thread contact length (% of available thread length)	
		Entry cortex (%)	Exit cortex (%)
2	12	27 ± 9*	4 ± 4*
4	12	40 ± 14*	47 ± 19*
6	12	73 ± 37*	70 ± 35*
8	12	77 ± 16	80 ± 15
10	11	74 ± 20	89 ± 4

*Significant increase of bone/screw thread contact with increasing time ($P < .05$).

Table 2 Normalized maximum push-out strength (force/cortex thickness)

Specimen location	Normalized maximum push-out strength (Nmm)					
	0 Weeks (n = 72)	2 Weeks (n = 12)	4 Weeks (n = 12)	6 Weeks (n = 12)	8 Weeks (n = 12)	10 Weeks (n = 12)
Entry cortex	433 ± 156	392 ± 49	379 ± 42†	481 ± 99†	568 ± 214*†	343 ± 79*
Exit cortex	367 ± 105*	253 ± 48*†	419 ± 59†	392 ± 149†	536 ± 89*†	432 ± 76*

*There were significant decreases in push-out strength between the two adjacent time periods ($P < .05$).
†There were significant increases in push-out strength between the two adjacent time periods ($P < .05$).

increase of bone contact with time (Table 1). There was no difference in bone/thread contact between the entry and exit cortices.

In the biomechanical push-out test, 72 specimens (12 tibiae with six screws in each) were prepared from canine cadaveric tibiae to standardize the push-out strength for the zero time group. There were no statistical differences in normalized push-out strength between any two screw positions on the tibial cortex ($P > .05$). Using the normalized maximum push-out strength (total force in Newtons divided by cortex thickness), there was a significant decrease in push-out strength with time from 0 to 2 weeks and from 8 to 10 weeks (Table 2). From 2 to 8 weeks there was a steady increase in normalized push-out strength. Although there is a trend toward higher entry cortex screw push-out, the difference was not statistically significant. Other biomechanical push-out strength parameters such as stiffness and energy absorption at push-out did not offer any new information. However, when bone/thread contact length was correlated with push-out strength, there were significant correlations between entry cortex bone contact length and push-out strength ($P < .003$) and between exit cortex bone contact length and push-out strength ($P < .002$).

Discussion

The present results seem to show the potential for better screw fixation in long bone following the osseointegration principle. In early time periods, the interface osseous tissue adjacent to screw thread surface appeared to become avascular and went through a resorption process as

273

reflected from the radiographic and histologic results. Such biologic change seems to have occurred regardless of the meticulous surgical preparation of bone threads through low-speed multiple drilling and tapping, along with copious irrigation. Close bone/titanium contact was accomplished using pure titanium material without special surface treatment as previously advocated in the dental implant fabrication process.[2–4] It is postulated, therefore, that the most important factor in orthopedic application may be the crucial unloading period, which allows undisturbed bone resorption and formation.

It was difficult to obtain ultrathin histologic slides to study the tissue/metal interface for evidence of the type of biologic bonding. Our specimens could only provide qualitative observation because of the large thickness of the tissue slices and the routine light microscopy techniques used. The true significance of direct cell bonding with the implant in orthopedic application has not been well demonstrated and this could only be studied using implants under in vivo loading conditions.

The increased push-out strength with time seems to correlate closely with the amount of new bone formed within the thread space. This finding was not surprising under the type of testing load adopted for the present study. Direct push- or pull-out load may not occur under realistic conditions, and such limitations must be carefully considered in interpreting the present results. However, since screw push-out strength can increase beyond, the time zero value must reflect some sort of surface bonding with the implant. Whether such bonding will occur using other types of implant materials remains to be elucidated. Finally, the lack of continuous strength increase at 8 to 10 weeks is difficult to explain. Newly formed bone may undergo remodeling and rapid turnover because of vascular invasion, which may be responsible for such change. Longer followup would be necessary to validate such a finding and provide a more convincing explanation.

The present experiment used only one animal per time period, although multiple screws were used in both tibiae. The lack of sufficient sample size would certainly diminish the significance of the data reported here. However, during the data analysis process, all screw results were pooled together and subjected to ANOVA, which should justify the statistical findings reported herein. It is clear that osseointegration principles can provide certain beneficial effects in orthopedic application, such as the staged free-vascularized fibular graft transplantation proposed herein. Extensive investigations are needed before practical application of such a concept can be realized. The present study, implants, and experimental procedure utilized should provide sufficient incentive to further pursue this idea.

Acknowledgments

This study was supported by the National Institutes of Health grant CA40583, awarded by the National Institutes of Health, Public Health Service, Department of Health, Education, and Welfare. We would especially like to acknowledge the most significant contribution made by Linda Berge and Fred Schultz in implant design and instrument fabrication.

References

1. Adell R. Clinical results of osseointegrated implants supporting fixed prosthesis in edentulous jaws. *J Prosthet Dent* 1983;50:251–254.
2. Adell R, Lekholm U, Rockler B, Brånemark PE. A 15-year study of osseointegrated implants in the treatment of the edentulous jaw. *Int J Oral Surg* 1981;10:387–416.
3. Albrektsson T, Brånemark P-I, Hansson HA, Lindström J. Osseointegrated titanium implants: Requirements for ensuring a long-lasting, direct bone-to-implant anchorage in man. *Acta Orthop Scand* 1981;52:155–170.
4. Brånemark P-I, Breine U, Adell R, Hansson BO, Lindström J, Ohlsson A. Intraosseous anchorage of dental prostheses. *Scand J Plast Reconstr Surg Hand Surg* 1969;3:81–100.
5. Hagert CG, Sollerman C, Brånemark P-I, Albrektsson T. Directly bone-anchored metacarpophalangeal joint implants. Transactions of the 8th Meeting of the Society for Biomaterials and the 14th International Biomaterials Symposium 1982;5:33.
6. Weiland AJ, Moore JR, Daniel RK. Vascularized bone autografts: Experience with 41 cases. *Clin Orthop* 1983;174:87–95.
7. Wood MB. Free vascularized bone transfers for nonunions, segmental gaps, and following tumor resection. *Orthopedics* 1986;9:810–816.

Bone Modeling and Remodeling Around Control and Axially Loaded Fixtures in Canine Tibiae

S.J. Hoshaw, J.B. Brunski, G.V.B. Cochran, and K.W. Higuchi

Scientists have long been interested in how bone grows and responds to the challenges of both excess and reduced mechanical usage. Meade[1] and Carter[2] provided reviews of the vast literature of studies examining the relationship of bone to its mechanical environment. In attempts to gain additional information, many other researchers have studied the biomechanics of implants and stress transfer to surrounding bone; this is especially true for both orthopedic and dental implants.[3–6] However, few studies[7–9] have examined implant experimental results in light of theories and mechanisms of bone modeling and remodeling. Therefore, this study attempts to evaluate a bone-implant model in terms of a theory developed by Frost,[10] which proposes a relationship between strains in bone and bone modeling and remodeling activities.

In years past, the term "bone remodeling" has been used to describe almost all types of bone growth and turnover. To avoid confusion, and in accordance with recent publications,[10–12] the following definitions for bone modeling and remodeling will be used throughout the paper. The deposition or removal of bone from existing bone surfaces is defined as modeling. Modeling results in an overall change in the size or shape of the bone. Bone remodeling involves the sequence of events that result in the formation of secondary osteons within the existing bone tissue. A remodeling cycle does not alter gross bone architecture or size.

According to current theory, most activities underlying skeletal physiology and disease, including modeling and remodeling, take place through actions of a collection of multicellular units with properties that the individual cells of the unit lack. This organ-level organization of skeletal tissue has been referred to as the intermediary organization of the skeleton.[13] It is well established that bone remodeling, via the formation of secondary osteons, is a result of the activity of basic multicellular units (BMU), each of which include osteoclasts, osteoblasts, and appropriate precursor cells. BMU-based bone remodeling begins with an activation stimulus (A), followed by osteoclastic resorption (R) and bone formation (F) by osteoblasts. Often a quiescent period (Q) follows the active resorption phase. In the case of modeling, activation is followed directly by either bone resorption (A-R) or bone formation (A-F). In modeling, resorption and formation are uncoupled, while in remodeling they are coupled. An increase in the number of active modeling and remodeling sites, over and above the ambient, often occurs as a result of surgery, trauma, or some other stimuli. Frost has labeled this behavior a regional acceleratory phenomenon (RAP).[14]

The existence of a limiting strain range or minimum effective strain (MES) has also been postulated by Frost[10] as a controlling factor in bone response to mechanical usage (Table 1). Strains above the MES act to turn the adaptive mechanism(s) "on," and strains below this threshold leave the system in the "off" state. According to the theory, bone strains above the MES bring about an increased modeling response on bone surfaces and decreased re-

Table 1 Summary of Frost's theory of bone response to mechanical usage*

According to Frost's Theory	
Modeling (MES ~ 1500–3000 $\mu\epsilon$):	↑ MU $\Rightarrow$ ↑ Modeling response
Remodeling (MES ~ 100–300 $\mu\epsilon$):	↑ MU $\Rightarrow$ ↓ Remodeling response

*MES = minimum effective strain, MU = mechanical usage.

modeling activity in the cortex. Consequently, increased mechanical usage tends to conserve existing cortical bone because of decreased remodeling activity and increase bone mass as a result of the increased modeling.

Frost's theory of bone modeling and remodeling in response to mechanical usage was developed for skeletal bone without the complicating presence of an implant; however, he has suggested its application to bone around orthopedic and dental implants through some proposed design criteria.[15,16] For example, if the placement and subsequent use of an implant in bone generated strains in the host bone that were greater than the MES for that tissue, changes in the modeling and remodeling behavior for that bone would be theoretically expected. Observation of those changes could be made histomorphometrically and the data compared to appropriate experimental controls. This study represents an in vivo model that should allow tests of the theory at a bone/implant interface.

Materials and methods

Two 7-mm-long screw-shaped titanium Brånemark fixtures were placed 25 mm apart in medial, mid-diaphyseal sites in the tibiae of six coonhounds. After a healing period of 12 months, the fixtures in the left tibias were accessed through small skin incisions; each implant was connected to a servohydraulic test system via a titanium connecting pin screwed into the internal thread in the implant. Implants were loaded in axial tension with a sawtooth waveform, 330 N/s, 300 N maximum, 10 N minimum for 500 cycles per day for 5 consecutive days. Implants in the right tibias were undisturbed.

Four fluorochrome bone labels, each fluorescing a different color when excited by light of the proper wavelength, were given to mark calcifying tissue; these labels act as a time marker for bone modeling and remodeling events at the interface. In this study, labels were given intravenously at 3 months postimplantation, 3 weeks preloading, and at 4 and 8 weeks postloading. Two dogs were sacrificed at 6 weeks postloading, while the remaining four dogs were sacrificed at 12 weeks postloading.

Tibial segments, each containing one implant, were sectioned mediolaterally, bisecting the implant with a slow-speed diamond saw. These 25-mm-long segments, each containing an implant half, were embedded in polymethyl methacrylate resin (PMMA). Block sections were metallographically polished to 0.3 μm and examined in reflected and fluorescent light microscopy.

Results and Discussion

For ease of discussion of the histological results, the bone/implant interface is divided into four regions of interest: *(1)* the periosteal surface, *(2)* the endosteal surface, *(3)* the cortex within 1 mm of the implant, and *(4)* the proximal and distal cortices (Fig 1).

In regions 1 and 2, the periosteal and endosteal surfaces, the modeling response was visible to the naked eye in both loaded and control interfaces (Figs 2a and b). There was bone growth over the shoulder and around the apex of the implant. Area measurements of the modeled bone were used to compare loaded and control samples; the extent of the modeling response was significantly greater ($P < .025$) in

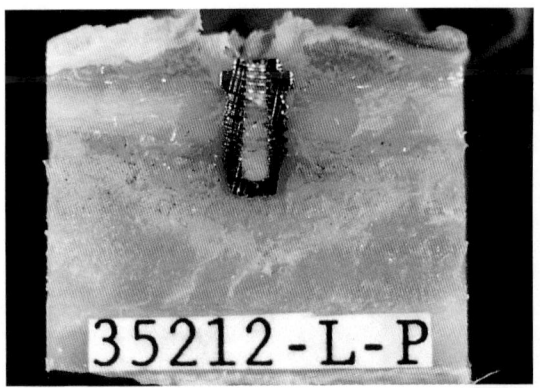

Fig 1 Schematic diagram of a typical histological section showing four regions of interest: *(1)* periosteal surface, *(2)* endosteal surface, *(3)* cortex within 1 mm of the implant, and *(4)* proximal and distal cortices.

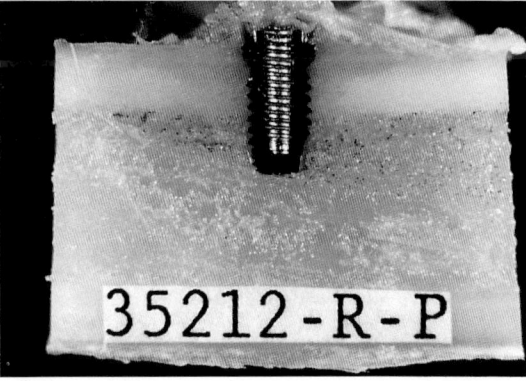

Figs 2a and b Macrophotographs of (a) a loaded and (b) a control bone/implant interface pair. Note extent of periosteal and endosteal modeling in loaded versus control interface.

the loaded samples. This result is consistent with predictions based on Frost's theory of bone modeling in response to mechanical usage. Assuming that the applied load on the implant created bone strains above the MES for modeling, the expected response would include increased postloading modeling on bone surfaces near the implant, as was observed. The preloading modeling, ie, that which occurred in both the loaded and control interfaces before loading began, is probably the result of the RAP brought on by the surgical placement of the implants. Notably in all cases, the modeling activity was localized to the implant region; the bone on the lateral aspect of the tibia, directly opposite the implant, did not show any visible modeling response.

Also, in these bone surface regions 1 and 2,

there was evidence of the fluorochrome bone labels given 3 weeks preloading and the two labels given 4 and 8 weeks postloading (Figs 3a and b). The label appeared both in diffuse bands and well-defined stripes, which may indicate lamellar bone formation. In some cases, the fluorochrome label given 8 weeks postloading suggested that the bone deposited early in the modeling phase was being remodeled by secondary osteons. However, presence of the label given 3 months postimplantation was not detected.

In the cortical region within 1 mm of the implant, region 3, secondary osteons were observed whose Haversian canals were perpendicular to the plane of the longitudinal section (Figs 4a and b). This orientation is rotated 90° from the usual orientation of osteons in the tibial

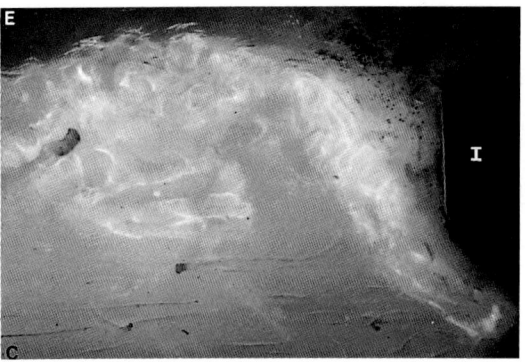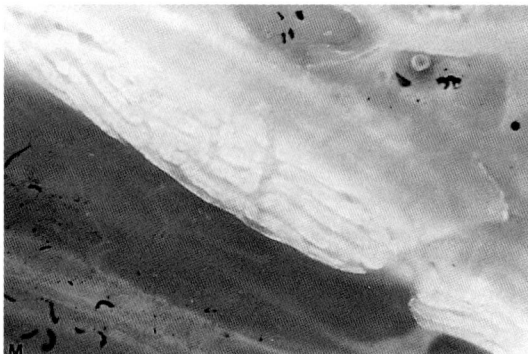

Figs 3a and b Fluorescent light photomicrographs of typical (a) periosteal and (b) endosteal modeling for loaded implants. (C = cortex, I = implant, E = embedding medium, M = marrow space.)

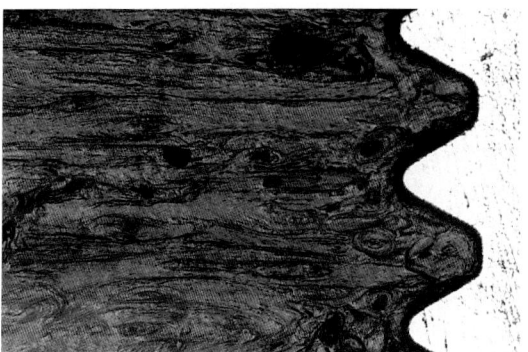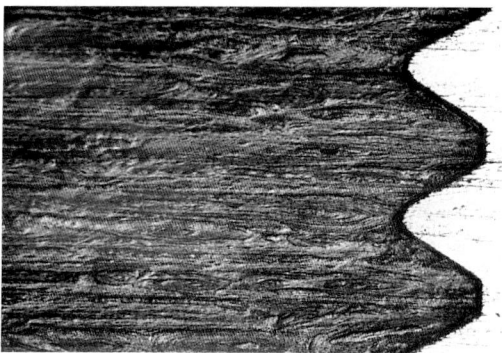

Figs 4a and b Reflected light photomicrographs of (a) in vivo and (b) freshly inserted bone/implant interfaces. Note change in osteon orientation near the implant in (a).

cortex, which is parallel to the long axis of the bone (see Fig 4b of a freshly inserted implant in cortical bone). These observations, seen in both loaded and control samples, indicate that the bone within about 1 mm of the implant has been completely remodeled; this is consistent with the virtual absence in this region of the fluorochrome label, which was given 3 months postimplantation. The mechanism(s) by which osteons develop this orientation is undetermined.

For both loaded and control implants, there was little evidence of the 3-week preloading label in the cortical region within 1 mm of the implant. This may indicate that bone in this location has resumed a state of remodeling activity that is characteristic of the ambient found elsewhere in the tibial cortex. Also, this region contained few deposits of the label given 4 weeks postloading. This result may be caused by three possibilities: (1) technical difficulty in exciting and viewing the label, (2) the label was given during the A-R(Q) portion of the remodeling cycle, ie, before the F phase began, and (3) the A phase was depressed so that there was no subsequent F phase to take up the label. The label given 8 weeks postloading did mark secondary osteons forming within 1 mm of the implant (Fig 5); however, significant differences between loaded and control interfaces were not observed.

As a consequence of the possibilities discussed here, the remodeling results near the

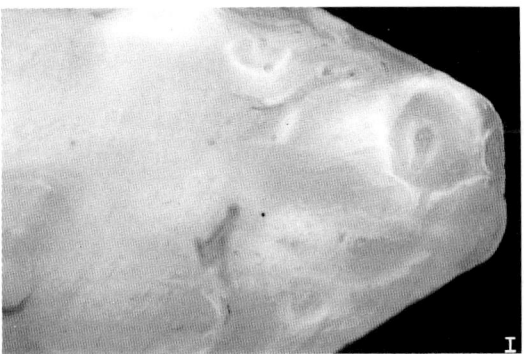

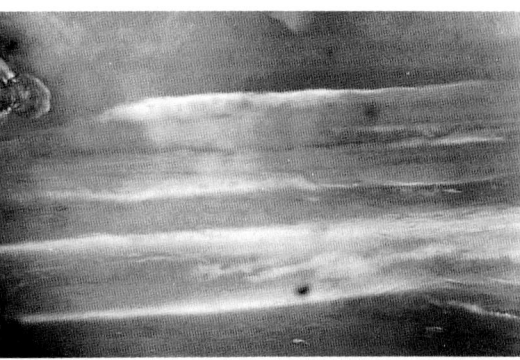

Fig 5 Fluorescent light photomicrograph of bone within control implant thread. Note osteons labeled with 8-week postloading label.

Fig 6 Fluorescent light photomicrograph of two longitudinal forming secondary osteons in the distal cortex of a control implant.

implant are inconclusive with regard to Frost's theory of bone response to mechanical usage, which predicts different remodeling responses depending on the strain magnitude in the region. If the generated strains in the bone had been greater than the MES for remodeling, which Frost identifies as 100 to 300 $\mu\epsilon$,[10] there should have been fewer new BMUs in the loaded interfaces. Alternatively, if the strains had been large enough, about 3,000 $\mu\epsilon$,[16] to initiate a damage response through the formation of microfractures, then the number of new BMUs should have been greater in the loaded interfaces. However, to date in this experiment, the number of new BMUs, as determined by an analysis of the two labels given postloading, does not indicate a difference between loaded and control interfaces in the amount of remodeling, either increased or decreased. Therefore, neither one of the two scenarios can be confirmed.

In region 4 (the proximal and distal cortices 3 to 5 mm away from the implant), numerous forming osteons were marked by the fluorochrome label given 3 months postimplantation (Fig 6). These osteons were oriented parallel to the long axis of the tibia and were equally apparent in both the loaded and control samples. However, few of these osteons were observed in the lateral cortex opposite to the implant. It is suggested that these osteons, formed 3 months

postimplantation several millimeters away from the implant, are good evidence of an RAP triggered by the implant placement surgery. Similar findings were reported by Martin,[7] but no explicit evidence exists that these labeled osteons are a direct consequence of a surgical RAP.

Conclusion

This in vivo model did provide a limited experimental investigation of Frost's theory of bone modeling and remodeling in relation to a loaded bone/implant interface (Table 2). The increased modeling response near the implant, especially in the loaded samples, was an expected result given the predictions of the theory. However, the remodeling activity near control and loaded implant threads was inconclusive. It remains to be seen if a more quantitative histomorphological analysis of these bone/implant interfaces will reveal statistically significant differences between loaded and control samples. In addition, knowledge of the strains generated in the bone adjacent to these loaded and control implants is necessary for a complete analysis. Data from finite element and strain gauge studies of bone/implant interfaces of this type should provide useful quantitative strain information in this context.

Table 2 Summary of experimental results

Region	Results summary	Agreement with Frost's theory
1 & 2	• Modeling observed on bone surfaces • Significantly greater at loaded interfaces • 3 weeks preload, 4 and 8 weeks postload labels	Consistent
3	• Change in osteon direction • No significant difference between loaded and control • 4 and 8 weeks postload labels	Inconclusive
4	• Numerous forming osteons • 3 months postimplanation label • Similar finding for both loaded and control	RAP (?)

Acknowledgments

This study was supported by the National Institute of Dental Research grant T32 DE 07054-12, Veterans Administration Rehabilitation Research & Development Project no. 160.

References

1. Meade JB. The adaptation of bone to mechanical stress: Experimentation and current concepts. pp 211–251 In S.C. Cowin (ed) *Bone Mechanics*. Boca Raton, Fla: CRC Press, 1989.
2. Carter DR. The relationship between in vivo strains and cortical bone remodeling. *CRC Crit Rev Biomed Eng* 1982;8:1–28.
3. Brunski JB. Biomaterials and biomechanics in dental implant design. *J Oral Maxillofac Implants* 1988;3:85–97.
4. Fitzgerald RH, ed. *Non-cemented Total Hip Arthroplasty.* New York: Raven Press, 1988.
5. Meroueh KA, Watanabe F, Mentag PJ. Finite element analysis of partially edentulous mandible rehabilitated with an osteointegrated cylindrical implant. *Oral Implant* 1987;13:215–238.
6. Soltész U, Siegele D. Principal characteristics of the stress distributions in the jaw caused by dental implants. pp 439–444 In R. Huiskes, D. VanCampen, J. DeWijn (eds) *Biomechanics: Principles and Applications.* The Hague, The Netherlands: Martinus Nijhoff Publ, 1982.
7. Martin RB. Osteonal remodeling in response to screw implantation in canine femora. *J Orthop Res* 1987;5:445–452.
8. Roberts WE. Bone tissue interface. *J Dent Educ* 1988;52:804–809.
9. Roberts WE, Smith RK, Zilberman Y, Mozsary PG, Smith RK. Osseous adaptation to continuous loading of rigid endosseous implants. *Am J Orthod* 1984;86:95–111.
10. Frost HM. Vital biomechanics: Proposed general concepts for skeletal adaptations to mechanical usage. *Calcif Tiss Int* 1988;42:145–156.
11. Martin RB, Burr DB. *Structure, Function and Adaptation of Compact Bone.* New York: Raven Press, 1989, pp 143–144.
12. Parfitt AM. The physiologic and clinical significance of bone histomorphometric data. pp 143–223 In R.R. Recker (ed) *Bone Histomorphometry: Techniques and Interpretation.* Boca Raton, Fla: CRC Press, 1983.
13. Frost HM. The skeletal intermediary organization. *Metab Bone Dis Rel Res* 1983;4:281–290.
14. Frost HM. The regional acceleratory phenomenon: A review. *Henry Ford Hospital Med J* 1983;31:3–9.
15. Frost HM. Suggested vital biomechanical design criteria for load-bearing bone, dental and joint endoprostheses. Unpublished document.
16. Frost HM. Skeletal structural adaptations to mechanical usage (SATMU):2. Redefining Wolff's law: The remodeling problem. *Anat Rec* 1990;226:414–422.

Session IV Discussion

A. Broner (New York University, New York): Dr Baier, it appears that the high energy level surface of the glow-discharge implant plays an important role. How long does the energy level last? As a corollary to that, should we be glow-discharging just prior to placement regardless of any manufacturer claim?

R. Baier: This high surface energy lasts a very short period of time. The ideal circumstance would be to glow-discharge, treat, and place it immediately into the prepared site. We have found adequate storage means to simply glow-discharge, treat, and place the implant from the glow-discharge chamber into boiled, distilled water. This will hold the high implant surface energy for as long a period of time as 5 years, as demonstrated in tests that we completed with glass specimens.

A. Broner: Dr Baier, in light of your new feelings about implant surface texture without compromising chemistry, what comments can you offer about the acid-etched surface of the Swede-Vent implant?

R. Baier: I cannot offer any specific comments about the acid-etched surface of the Swede-Vent implant. However, I can comment that acid etching is not itself a cleaning technique. I have been amazed that one can go through standard acid passivation according to the American Society for Testing and Materials and still have a greasy, waxy overcoat on the surface in spite of thickening of the oxide. It passivates in the sense of thickening the oxide and making it slightly more resistant to corrosion. However, it does that by thickening the oxide underneath a contaminating layer of organic material so it is still a lower-energy, although more oxidized, surface. One side benefit has been found with the glow-discharge treatment, as noted when we have been examining whether or not the "cure was worse than the disease" (maybe we were glow-discharging away the oxide and making the implant more subject to corrosion). Glow-discharge treatment can uniformly thin and energize the implant so that immediately upon exposure either to air or preferably to liquid systems, reoxidation is strongly favored. A good, thick, dense oxide layer is produced that diminishes further corrosion, as contrasted with standard autoclaved and acid-passivated samples.

G. Niznick: Dr Baier, while glow-discharge treatment removes organic material left on the surface, it does nothing to remove the inorganic contamination from machining that you have pointed out is so important to remove. Don't you think that once the implant comes off the machine with all the tungsten carbide grinding bits on it, that something should be used aggressively to remove the inorganic material and glow-discharge to remove the organic material?

R. Baier: I would agree with the general principle. Certainly one must be concerned with polishing grits, alumina grits, investments, things that are sapphirelike, aluminum-oxide–like because they are very difficult to eliminate. I do have one caution with regard to hydrofluoric acid-treated materials, however. Fluoride, whether from hydrogen fluoride or any other source that fluoridates the surface, will diminish its surface energy. You have probably checked the existing surface energies, but there is a potential disadvantage of using hydrogen fluoride.

G. Niznick: You need to neutralize it so further treatment is needed once the surface has been etched.

G. Niznick: Dr Deporter, the Weiss implant that was marketed in the 1980s also had a bead-type surface and was quite extensively clinically tested in a number of centers. Unlike your implant, which has a straight collar, it had a narrow neck that left a defect at the top, yet when the bone reached the porous surface it became a plaque collector and bone loss seemed to be quite progressive at that point. Do you see any difference in what you are doing and why the results should be any different than what was already experienced with the Weiss implant?

D. Deporter (Toronto, Ontario, Canada): The Weiss implant had a wire mesh that was added to its surface. We do have a different surface configuration here, perhaps more facility for bone ingrowth.

We have done extensive animal testing and found that bone remodels down to the region of the machined-surface–porous-coat junction; but even where bone loss has occurred so that a little bit of the porous coat is exposed, it is filled with an oriented connective tissue. There are no signs of any bacterial plaque penetration into the porous coat. We have been concerned about this from the beginning and, in fact, we have even carried the experiment a step further and added a small hydroxyapatite collar to the machined surface and found that the hydroxyapatite will keep bone even higher and further away from the porous coat. We are conducting a clinical trial in a limited group of humans in the hope of replicating our animal findings. I can only say that obviously time will tell whether or not our experience is better, the same, or worse

than that of Dr Weiss and his co-workers.

S. Sachs (Lake Success, New York): Dr Jacobsson, did you suggest that one can wait 1 year following full therapeutic radiation and place fixtures into the mandible? I am aware of some of your work with temporal bone and maxilla, but are you making that as a suggestion or speculation, or do you have some clinical or laboratory evidence to support that?

M. Jacobsson (Göteborg, Sweden): I have no intraoral results to back that up. No, that is what we have recommended for the extraoral applications with which I am mainly concerned.

There are scattered reports from different places but none as to the amount of radiation or time after radiation before proceeding. We know very little in this field, unfortunately.

B. d'Hoedt (Tübingen, Germany): Dr Deporter, in your abstract you mentioned that your implant requires a shorter healing period than others. On what measurements is this based?

D. Deporter: In dogs, this particular implant was fully osseointegrated and ready to function within 4 weeks. We have been using 10 weeks as our standard initial healing period in this human trial. In all except for two patients in whom the four implants were located, this was perfectly satisfactory. Even though we are using the shortest healing period that has been reported, we probably can use an even shorter period.

T. West: Dr Baier, does that glycoprotein primer coat you describe vary in width? What factors of cleanliness and surface energy make it vary in width? Can we see it in a microscope and might that primer coat be the unmineralized portion that may or may not be artifact against implant materials?

R. Baier: The glycoprotein primer coat is almost always in the range of 200-Å thick. That material differs in organization on different implants, but not in composition. It is the material that has the greatest deposition potential from the wound healing fluid. The absorbed or deposited configuration that these molecules assume is based upon whether there are anchoring points, "hot spots" if you will, on the solid surface. Microscopic evidence of interfacial translucency, nonmineralized areas, or greater thicknesses where there is not frank bone adjacent to an implant almost always reflects a circumstance where the glycoproteinaceous film has not been well anchored. It is then able to engage in a lot of "turnover" events and keep the interface in flux, preventing adhesion.

T. West: Can you see it in the scope and in the transmission electron micrograph?

R. Baier: You could certainly see it in the transmission electron microscope. It is there every time in every circumstance.

H. Staffileno (Evanston, Illinois): My comment is directed to Dr Larson and possibly a couple others. The rabbit is a frequent animal model and possibly because of the propensity for osseous response in the rabbit, it is very exuberant. However, it may be more prudent to use dogs and baboons as we have seen and particularly to extend our studies over longer periods of time.

G. Huré (Paris, France): Dr Baier, can a special machine called Picotron, which is a decontaminating machine with argon gas, be used in our daily practice in order not to discard contaminated implants?

R. Baier: I routinely use three Picotron units in my own laboratory for that general purpose. When this was first being developed and sold, the devices that were first shown were, in fact, inadequate. I asked Park Dental not to put them on the market until I fully tested them in my own laboratory to my own satisfaction for over 1 year. The unit that they now have built is a device that can adequately clean, surface prepare, and maintain preexisting sterility. One of the problems with the Picotron is that you cannot fill it

with hydrogen peroxide gas to get absolute sterility of packaged products and deep porous materials because it contains indwelling commercially pure titanium electrodes. The electrodes are directly in the vapor space and the peroxide so beautifully thickens the oxide and passivates the titanium that you can no longer get the glow to start and these titanium electrodes no longer function. They become so passive that the device cannot run. As a routine laboratory or even a clinical tool to give yourself assurance of surface cleanliness, the answer is yes. If the material is washed to get rid of obvious debris that you see with your eye, glow-discharge treatment in that device is capable of removing all the rest in my experience.

G. Huré: Dr Baier, is there any chance of getting contamination with the oil pump, vacuum pump?

R. Baier: Yes, there is a chance that there will be backstreaming of the silicone oil vapor from the pump, again diminishing the surface energy on the treated device. One of the improvements that was made during the year of testing was to put a solenoid between the pump and the device so that when it is off, the solenoid closes off the vacuum pump to the chamber so that it cannot refill in any way with any contaminating vapor. The device should not be run without the solenoid.

C. Berman: Dr Baier, the last question dealt with contaminated implants and whether one could recycle them through an argon glow-discharge machine. Now, specifically what does the term "contaminated implant" mean? Are we talking about a failed implant removed from a patient that, after being cleaned in a glow-discharge machine, can be reimplanted in another person? Or was the question about an implant that fell on the floor and picked up some inorganic material? Certainly a glow-discharge machine can decontaminate that.

R. Baier: With regard to clinical advice, clinical handling is dependent upon the scruples and standards of individual practitioners. We have found acceptable decontamination routinely in our laboratories using germanium prisms, by simply scrubbing with a soft brush and detergent, rinsing, and then glow-discharge treating for 2 minutes. The prisms are put into fixtures in our own mouths and we study the natural history of dental plaque formation from human to human within our own laboratory group without any problem of infection. We have that confidence in the glow-discharge process, if practiced properly.

C. Berman: I have been doing glow-discharge work since 1984. I have found no difference in the clinical results using glow-discharged Brånemark implants and using Brånemark implants taken directly from the package. Have you any evidence to support the fact that glow-discharge treatment of clean, sterile implants from the manufacturer improves the clinical result of the treatment?

R. Baier: The answer to that is clearly no.

C. Berman: It surely delays the surgery as you are aware, because you have to wait for the thing "to cook."

R. Baier: A couple of minutes. But having no benefit beyond 95%, that certainly then has to be your choice. As a general tool, however, considering a system that has 60% or 75% success, or might diminish resting time before loading from a period of 6 months to 3 to 10 weeks, or whatever, as we learn more of how to control surface energy together with surface texture, it is one of the tools in the armamentarium.

C. Berman: As an implant is screwed in, is the body perhaps cleaning it as it is put into place? You talked about that little thin layer; as you torque an implant into place, is it possible that those surface cells at the top of the osteotomy are cleaning the implant? And as the implant goes in, is it then cleaned of that layer and in effect the glow-discharge therapy that you just did was null and voided?

R. Baier: I would disagree entirely with that. It would be macroscopically cleaner but on a microscopic level, basically you would be squeezing the local cells like sponges and they would be expressing their tissue juice. This procedure is never totally atraumatic and so what has been made available at the site will be sufficient macromolecular- and lipid-type material to adsorb to the surface. If the surface to receive these components is a nonstick surface, in essence one has a failed implant going in unless the implant can somehow recover as a result of dynamic transfer at the interface. If, on the other hand, that implant surface is extraordinarily receptive to binding to whatever is put down, I think you are in a much more secure situation in terms of subsequent colonization and remodeling.

H. Amstutz (Los Angeles, California): Dr Baier, you noticed that radiation, for example, can change the physical and mechanical properties of ultrahigh molecular weight polyethylene. Most of the evidence, at least in friction and wear, suggests that it takes five or more resterilizations to produce change. Do you have any evidence that glow-discharge treatment does not change the properties of the material, specifically with respect to friction and wear, and is there any potential danger in using more than one method of radiation if it came out initially that way, and then resterilize with glow-discharge treatment?

R. Baier: I do not have good evidence on friction and wear. I have some cell culture results and contact angle-based surface studies. Our evidence is that glow-discharge treatment can provide quick and adequate sterilization with no disadvantage, whether it is previously radiation-sterilized or is being done the first time. The one clear difference is that the material starts out nonadhesive to cellular growth. One cannot do cell cultures on ultrahigh molecular weight polyethylene. They will round up and bead off and there will be no propagation. Glow-discharge–treated polyethylene is equal in cell culture experiments to tissue-culture polystyrene.

E. McGlumphy (Columbus, Ohio): Could Dr Johansson or Dr Jacobsson comment on how the magnitude of torque removal from rabbit bone might contrast with what might be expected from human bone?

M. Jacobsson (Göteborg, Sweden): We have done some studies in humans and for different periods of time after insertion. Removal torques are greater in the human skull bone than those in rabbits. I do not have the figures here for those experiments, but they are greater and increase with time reaching a peak at about 1 to 1$^1/_2$ years after insertion in the temporal bone.

J. Brunski: Dr Baier, I want to return to the push-out tests of the titanium cylinders that were prepared with the three different surface energies, zones 1, 2, and 3. You suggested that the mode of failure in zones 1 and 2 type materials, with the lower surface energy materials, seems to be some "weak plane" relatively close to the surface of the titanium, whereas in the glow-discharge/higher energy surface there was a failure region out in the bone.

R. Baier: That is not correct; I probably stated it wrong. The failure planes all seemed to be in an osteoid layer, whether it was closer to the implant or further from the implant, so that we were never deep enough into the bone in any failure to be encountering true bulk bone properties. I was very much concerned that surface property changes were not providing different problems of bone adhesion.

M. Block: Dr Baier, concerning the line of site of the glow-discharge, how would that apply to abutment heads or gingival collars etc, that we may want to put into the glow-discharge and energize the surface?

R. Baier: Up until the recent introduction of hydrogen peroxide, glow-discharge treatment could not be used with confidence for anything with any sulci. With hydrogen peroxide gas being used, one can actually get sterilization of fiberoptics, deep porous implants, and in fact, if you are not worried about the persistence of the

high surface energy, you can actually put an implant in a standard plastic paper pouch and get sterilization by glow-discharge treatment inside the pouch better with complete sterilization, without persistence of high surface energy. You do get some of the benefits of the ambient temperature cool sterilization without the packaging, where it is not necessary to put the thing into boiled distilled water unless one is really fanatic about surface energy.

D. Altobelli (Boston, Massachusetts): Dr Baier, have you done any work to introduce to that high energy glow-discharged surface an initial controlled coating that could enhance the healing at that site, ie, some specific glycoprotein, mucopolysaccharide, or even growth factor?

R. Baier: I think that is an excellent suggestion and I presume studies like that are in progress elsewhere. We are not doing any such study. A member of our faculty prefers, during his normal implantation trials, to preimmerse the implant in the patient's blood. He takes the implant that we have glow-discharge treated for him and stored in boiled, distilled water, and pours off almost all the water, keeping the implant covered. Then he actually syringes some of the patient's blood from the site and puts it into the bottle and does the precoating there. He says that this gives him greater freedom to fit and back out and make small modifications. It is his clinical impression of the results in a few cases thus far, that the procedure is just as good as placing it immediately in the site. In essence the site is brought to the implant rather than the implant to the site, to get that first coating.

R. Yanase (Torrance, California): Dr Baier, is there any indication that there could be a greater amount of bone-to-surface contact established to explain possible accelerated healing?

R. Baier: Not any evidence that I have. Our basis for suggesting that healing is occurring quicker is that if we take equal materials and glow-discharge—treat one set and conventionally sterilize the other set (by autoclave, for example) and just put cells of any type on them, the glow-discharge–treated surface leads to rapid cell growth and proliferation. Cells cover the glow-discharge–treated materials in a very short period of time, perhaps 3 days, while the same cells on untreated materials kind of bead around the microcluster and just ignore the surface.

G. Sandor (Toronto, Ontario, Canada): Dr Hoshaw, do you think that Frost's theory was the microscopic correlate for Wolff's theory, and if so, wouldn't it have been interesting to try and correlate your study with a radiographic analysis as well?

S. Hoshaw (Troy, New York): Frost's theory is certainly not the only one in which you can look at a bone/implant interface in this kind of a study. It does have similar sorts of implications. However, as to Wolff's law, I think it takes into account some of the bone physiology principles that some of the other theories do not directly take into account. In terms of a radiographic study, I am not sure how much refined and detailed information can be obtained from a single radiograph. We have planned on looking at these specimens and using some backscattered scanning electron microscopy, which may provide such information as you are suggesting.

Osseointegrated Joint Prosthesis in the Hand

G. Lundborg, C. Sollerman, and P.-I. Brånemark

Osteoarthrosis of the small joints of the hand remains a major clinical problem. The etiology may vary. Rheumatoid arthritis constitutes an enormous problem wherein involvement of the wrist, metacarpophalangeal (MCP) joints, and proximal interphalangeal (PIP) joints may cause instability, subluxation, impaired range of motion and chronic pain. Other common causes are infectious arthritis and intra-articular fractures. Primary osteoarthrosis of the PIP joints is a frequent problem, especially among postmenopausal women.

Various techniques have been described for treatment of small joint destruction in the hand. Perichondrial transplantation has proved successful in selected cases,[1,2] but has no place in the large average patient groups. Although having the advantage of not introducing foreign material, soft tissue interposition techniques[3,4] ultimately result in progressive stiffening of the joints. Arthrodesis is always a possible salvage procedure to achieve stability and pain relief, but the loss of mobility is a definite disadvantage.

The dominating approach to this problem is the use of some kind of endoprosthetic replacement.[5] The most common technique is based on interposition of a silicone spacer.[6] According to this principle, the spacer is not rigidly fixed to adjacent bone structures. On the contrary, the stems extending from the middle part move longitudinally in the bone marrow cavities with movements of the fingers, thereby helping to distribute the bending forces within the whole spacer material. Although this technique is well accepted for treatment of vast patient groups,

unfavorable tissue reactions in the bone as well as in the surrounding soft tissues may ultimately lead to progressive stiffening of the joints.[7–13] Other techniques based on rigid fixation of a joint mechanism with cement[14] have not proven to give satisfying long-term results.

In 1986 a report was published describing the first application of the osseointegration principle for fixation of an endoprosthesis replacing MCP joints in six patients.[15] At followup, which was extended to 3 years, osseointegration seemed to persist as assessed by radiological techniques, but the joint mechanism did not work adequately. Because of bad functional outcome the technique was temporarily abandoned.

Three years ago a new generation of clinical trials was initiated, aimed at application of the osseointegration principle to approach MCP and PIP joint problems of the hand. The aim was to combine many years of experience with osseointegration of titanium fixtures in other parts of the body[16–19] and a noncomplicated and replaceable joint mechanism. In the present article our experiences involving the use of such prostheses in 63 cases of small joint destruction in the hand in 39 patients are described.

Concept of joint replacement

The purpose was to develop an endoprosthesis based on a replaceable joint mechanism anchored to osseointegrated fixation elements with titanium screws, designed in principle according to previous experience in the oral region[17,20–22] where the screws were used as anchorage components. After individual measurements were made in each case, the screws were made at the Institute for Applied Biotechnology, Göteborg. The diseased joint was resected to leave adequate space between adjacent bone resection sites. Following a gentle preparation of the marrow cavities, the titanium screws were carefully introduced longitudinally into the bones adjacent to the resected joint. A silicone joint mechanism of the hinge type (Atos Medical AB, Hörby, Sweden) was used as a spacer replacing the resected joint. In the central axis of each titanium screw there was an extended cylindrical space fitting exactly to short titanium stems fixed to the joint mechanism via titanium plates incorporated in the polymer material (Figs 1a and b).

The titanium stems of the joint mechanism were introduced into the cylindrical space in each titanium screw (Fig 1). Because of a slight incongruency between the stems and the corresponding spaces, rotation stability was achieved. By a simple maneuver, the joint mechanism could be easily released from the titanium screws and replaced if needed.

Surgical procedure

For replacement of the MCP joints, dorso-ulnar longitudinal skin incisions were used. The extensor hood was incised laterally and after retraction of the extensor tendon the joint could be explored. The collateral ligaments were saved as far as possible. The joint was resected to leave sufficient space between the resection sites. The titanium screws and joint mechanism were introduced as described previously. Following suture of the hood, skin dressings were applied and the hand was immobilized in a functional position.

For the PIP joints a dorsal curved skin incision was used. The central slip of the extensor mechanism was incised longitudinally, each component being retracted laterally. The procedure was then carried out in accordance with that previously described.

The hand was mobilized after 1 week according to a meticulous rehabilitation program. During the first 3 weeks, careful passive mobilization was applied two to three times per day under supervision of an occupational therapist. With time, active exercises were progressively introduced. Full loading was first allowed after 3 months.

Clinical material

Forty-five MCP joints in 24 patients and 18 PIP joints in 15 patients have been operated on since 1988, ie, a total of 63 joints. The main indications for treatment have been rheumatoid arthritis, primary osteoarthrosis or arthrosis of post-traumatic or postinfectious etiology. In five cases of postinfectious arthrosis involving MCP joints, the joint destruction was combined with necrosis of the extensor tendon. In these cases the joint replacement had to be combined with reconstruction of the tendon, carried out as a two-stage grafting procedure. Five MCP joints in 4 patients have been followed for more than 2 years, and 21 MCP joints have been followed in 14 patients for more than 1 year. Two PIP joints in two patients have been followed for more than 2 years, and 12 PIP joints have been followed in 12 patients for more than 1 year. Clinical and radiological assessment was made in all cases at 3 months, 6 months, and at 1-year intervals following surgery.

Results

MCP joints

There were two initial failures because of early postoperative infections requiring removal of screws and the mechanism. In a second stage

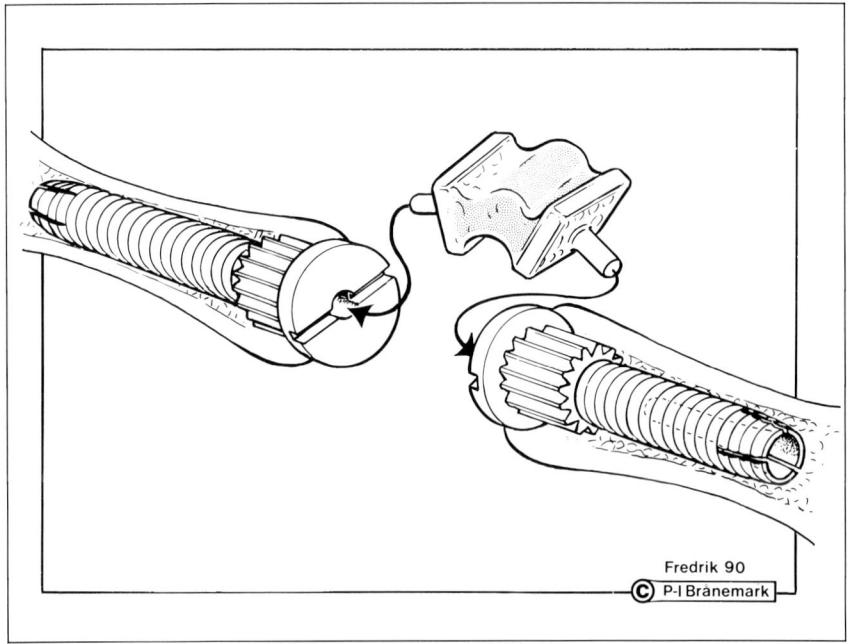

1a

Figs 1a and b Schematic drawing of the joint mechanism and titanium fixtures before application (a) and after surgery (b).

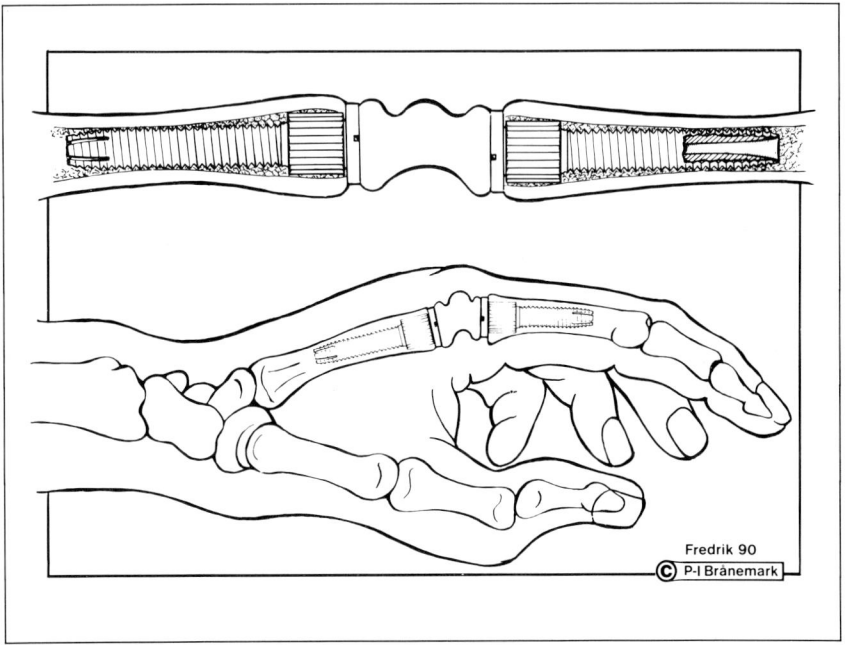

1b

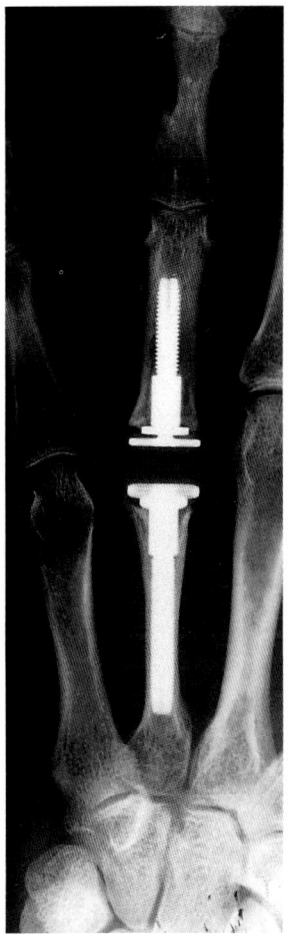

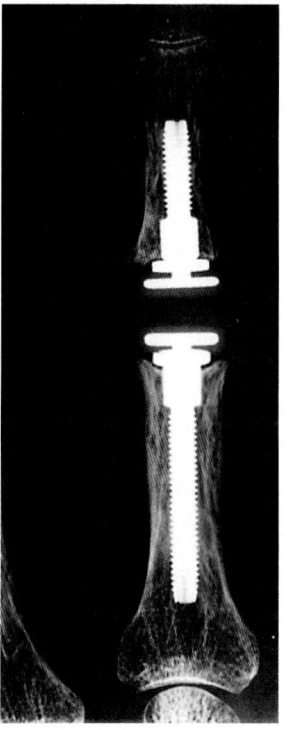

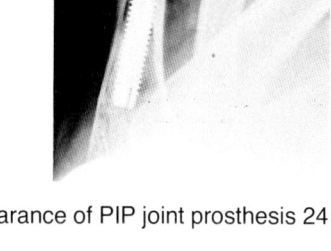

Fig 2 Radiological appearance of MCP joint prosthesis 18 months after surgery.

Figs 3a and b Radiological appearance of PIP joint prosthesis 24 months after surgery.

these patients were treated with soft tissue interposition plasty. In all the remaining 43 cases, osseointegration as judged by radiological examination has been achieved and maintained (Figs 2 and 3).

The clinical results varied with indications and preoperative status. A consistent observation was that the patients described early pain relief. In rheumatoid cases without complicating tendon or other soft tissue problems, the range of motion at followup was consistently satisfying with a range of motion of 40° to 65°.

The cases of postinfectious osteoarthrosis

were often complicated by extensor tendon destruction, requiring a two-stage extensor tendon reconstruction. Such cases usually showed an active extension defect of 20° to 30°, but in favorable situations full extension was achieved (Figs 4a and b).

In one patient fracture of the silicone material occurred at about 1 year following surgery. A reason for this may be the use of a small "PIP joint model" for the MCP joint in this special case, because of the extremely small size of the bone structures. The spacer was successfully replaced, with the osseointegrated fixtures

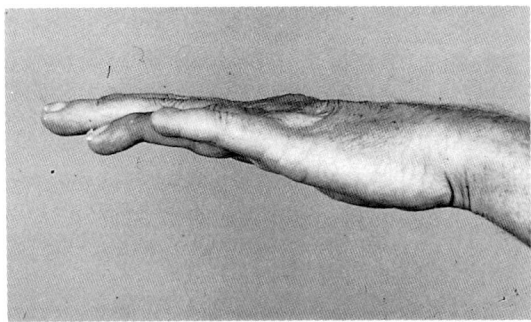 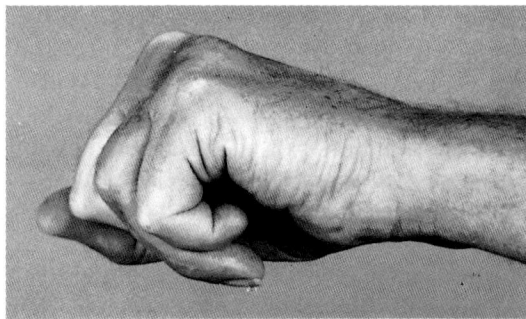

Figs 4a and b Clinical result following replacement of the fourth metacarpophalangeal joint (the case illustrated in Fig 2). In this patient, joint destruction was combined with necrosis of the corresponding extensor tendon. The joint replacement procedure was combined with a two-stage reconstruction of the extensor tendon.

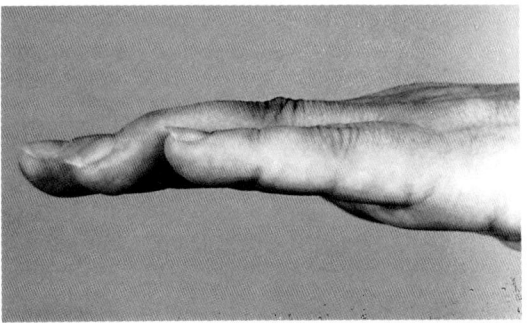 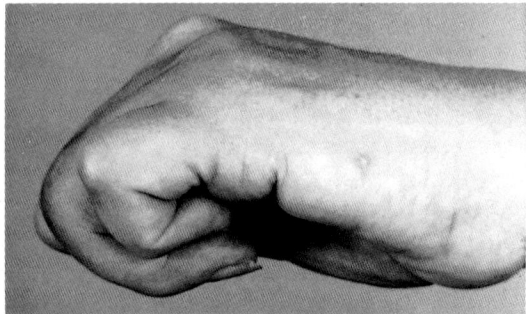

Figs 5a and b Range of motion in the patient illustrated in Fig 3.

working as adequate anchorage points for the new joint mechanism.

PIP joints

Osseointegration occurred in all patients (Figs 3a and b). In cases of primary osteoarthrosis without complicating tendon or other soft tissue problems, the range of motion was sometimes extremely good and approached 90° (Figs 5a and b). In patients with previous intra-articular fractures, often operated on one to two times before joint replacement, the results vary depending on the preoperative status of periarticular soft tissue structures.

Discussion

The principle for joint replacement is based on two concepts: (1) the utilization of osseointegrated fixation components for an endoprosthesis and (2) the use of a noncomplicated and replaceable joint mechanism. In this way the patient is offered immediate pain relief and satisfying function, but the joint mechanism can still be replaced if it fails or if an improved mechanism has been developed. Screw fixation is based on well-documented corresponding principles in the oral and maxillofacial region, showing permanent and successful osseointegration of titanium to bone in 80,000 patients, some of them followed for more than 25 years.[18] With this clinical base the authors feel well motivated to also use the same principle for joint replacement in young patients. An especially interesting group in this respect includes patients with juvenile rheumatoid arthritis, a disease for which the possibilities for joint replacement in the hand so far have been very limited.

With respect to healing and rehabilitation, the hand is much different from other regions of the body where the osseointegration principle has been applied. Nonloading of the fixtures has been regarded as a critical issue in the initial postoperative period for achieving osseointegration in the oral region. Such nonloading is not possible in the hand, since extended immobilization of the hand would lead to permanent joint stiffness. Consequently, mobilization is initiated early at 1 week following surgery, although with extreme care and under the supervision of an occupational therapist. The rehabilitation program represents a balance act between successful osseointegration and acceptable functional restitution of the hand. Thus far early mobilization has not resulted in loosening of any fixtures. A factor of interest is the direction of load applied to the screws in the hand, as compared to the jaws; with movement of fingers, load is applied sidewise in an angulated direction rather than in a longitudinal axial direction.

Complicated joint mechanisms, designed to imitate a normal joint, do not always result in satisfactory function.[15,23] The joint, mechanism used in the present study is of simple design. The long-term mechanical properties of the material remains to be evaluated. So far the joint mechanism should be regarded as a spacer, apparently with adequate mechanical properties. Improved joint mechanisms are under development. In an extended time perspective, improved endoprostheses can even be utilized in previous surgical patients since the construction allows replacement of the joint component even when the titanium fixtures are permanently integrated into the bone.

References

1. Engkvist O, Johansson SH. Perichondrial arthroplasty: A clinical study in twenty-six patients. Scand J Plast Reconstr Surg 1980;14:71.
2. Millesi H. Arthroplasty of the finger joints following posttraumatic conditions (with the exception of the saddle joint). Hefte Unfallheilkde 1980;141:229.
3. Weilby A. Resection arthroplasty of the metacarpophalangeal joint a.m. Tupper using interposition of the volar plate. Scand J Plast Reconstr Surg 1977;11:239.
4. Vainio K, Reiman IU, Pulkki T. Results of arthroplasty of the metacarpophalangeal joints in rheumatoid arthritis. Reconstr Surg Traumatol 1967;9:1.
5. Eiken O, Hagert CG. Finger joint replacement. Recent Adv Plast Surg 1981;2:101.
6. Swanson AB. Flexible implant resection arthroplasty in the hand and extremities. St Louis: CV Mosby Co, 1973.
7. Hagert CG, Eiken O, Ohlsson NM, Aschan W, Movin A. Metacarpophalangeal joint implants. I. Roentgenographic study of the silastic finger joint implant. Swanson design. Scand J Plast Reconstr Surg 1975;9:147.
8. Klems H. The Swanson-joint in traumatic stiffness of finger joint. Z Orthop 1975;113:495.
9. Brace DW, Millender LH. Failure of silicone rubber wrist arthroplasty in rheumatoid arthritis. J Hand Surg 1986;11A:175.
10. Fatti JF, Palmer AK, Mosher JF. The long-term result of Swanson silicone rubber interposition wrist arthroplasty. J Hand Surg 1986;11A:166.
11. Peimer CA, Medige J, Eckert BS, Wright JR, Howard CS. Reactive synovitis after silicone arthroplasty. J Hand Surg 1986;11A:624.
12. Vahnanen V, Viljakka T. Silicone rubber implant arthroplasty of the metacarpophalangeal joint in rheumatoid arthritis. J Hand Surg 1986;11A:333.
13. Paplamus SG, Payne CM. Axillary lymphadenopathy 17 years after digital silicone implants: Study with x-ray microanalysis. J Hand Surg 1988;13A:411.
14. Helbig B, BuckGramcko D. Ergebnisse nach Alloarthroplastik traumatisch geschädigter Fingergelenke. Handchir Mikrochir Plast Chir 1977;9:213.
15. Hagert CG, Brånemark P-I, Albrektsson T, Strid KG, Irstam L. Metacarpophalangeal joint replacement with osseointegrated endoprostheses. Scand J Plast Reconstr Surg 1986;20:207.
16. Brånemark P-I, Breine U, Lindström J, Adell R, Hansson BO, Ohlsson Å. Intra-osseus anchorage of dental prostheses. I. Experimental studies. Scand J Plast Reconstr Surg 1969;3:81.
17. Brånemark P-I, Hansson BO, Adell R, Breine U, Lindström J, Hallén O, et al. Osseointegrated implants in the treatment of the edentulous jaw: Experience from a 10-year period. Scand J Plast Reconstr Surg 1977;suppl 16.
18. Brånemark P-I. Introduction to osseointegration. p 11 In P.-I. Brånemark, G.A. Zarb, T. Albrektsson (eds) Tissue-Integrated Prostheses: Osseointegration in Clinical Dentistry. Chicago: Quintessence Publ Co, 1985.
19. Tjellström A, Rosenhall U, Lindström J, Hallén O, Albrektsson T, Brånemark P-I. Five-year experience with skin-penetrating bone-anchored implants in the temporal bone. Acta Otolaryngol 1983;95:568.
20. Adell R, Lekholm U, Rockler B, Brånemark P-I. A 15-year study of osseointegrated implants in the treatment of the edentulous jaw. Int J Oral Surg

1981;10:387.

21. Albrektsson T. The response of bone to titanium implants. *Crit Rev Biocompat* 1985;1:53.

22. Albrektsson T, Brånemark P-I, Hansson H-A, Lindström J. Osseointegrated titanium implants: Requirements for ensuring a long-lasting direct bone-to-implant anchorage in man. *Acta Orthop Scand* 1981;52:55.

23. Hagert CG. Anatomical aspects on the design of metacarpophalangeal implants. *Reconstr Surg Traumatol* 1981;18:92.

Avoiding Complications With Craniofacial Implants

A.M.S. Brown, D.W. Proops, and M.J.C. Wake

The pioneering work of P.-I. Brånemark has brought a revolution of respectability to intraoral implants, making some other forms of prepros- thetic surgery obsolete. Extraoral implantology will have a similar effect on the treatment of craniofacial defects but is presently in its in- fancy. The exchange of information between users is inadequate, and this inevitably leads to the duplication of avoidable problems and com- plications. Our experiences with the use of the Nobelpharma system (Nobelpharma AB, Göte- borg, Sweden) during 3 years have been highly favorable, and serious complications have been unexpectedly few. What few complications there have been are identified by an ongoing audit process as largely avoidable, and most of these occurred during the early phase of our program.

Bone problems

Primary failure of osseointegration

Osseointegration with craniofacial implants is so reliable that it may almost be considered routine. Occasionally, however, nonintegration does occur and may often be associated with previous irradiation.[1] It remains to be seen what effect the use of hyperbaric oxygen may have on the incidence of nonintegration in these cases. Nonintegration is far less likely to occur in the temporal region than in the facial skele- ton.[1,2] This may be partly the result of a gener- ous thickness of compact bone in the cranium and the favorable architecture of the diploic bone. An audit of our first 110 fixtures inserted revealed that only two have failed to integrate (1.8%) and that both were in facial bone that had undergone radical radiotherapy.

Case one: Orbital prosthesis

A boy 11 years old had lost both eyes through retinoblastoma in early infancy. Radical external beam radiotherapy followed enucleation of the left eye. Based on the impression that the eye- brow had been little affected by the radiotherapy (Fig 1), it was assumed that the underlying supraorbital bone similarly had been little af- fected. Three fixtures were placed (Fig 2), but only 14 weeks elapsed between first- and second-stage surgery. The most lateral fixture loosened upon gentle tightening of the abut- ment, and the fixture was later removed.

Case two: Nasal prosthesis

This patient represents our only complete fail- ure. A male patient had suffered subtotal nasal amputation for squamous cell carcinoma of the nasal tip that had recurred after radical radio- therapy some years earlier. At first-stage sur- gery, radical nasal septal resection was per- formed and the pyriform aperture and nasal floor were exposed. Three fixtures were placed in the nasal floor, but only minimal cortical bone was found, with open textured cancellous bone.

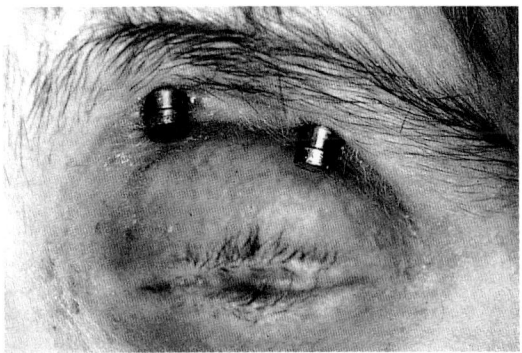

Fig 1 Orbital defect showing the survival of relatively normal eyebrow hair and excellent periabutment skin condition. That the abutments emerge through a full-thickness skin graft cannot be seen in this view. Long abutments keep the magnet/abutment interface well away from the skin surface.

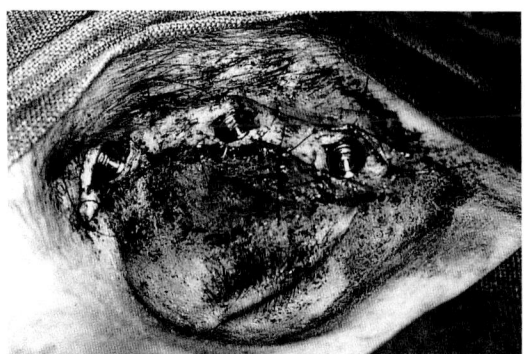

Fig 2 The same case as in Fig 1. Three abutments emerge through a full-thickness graft. The most lateral abutment loosened on gentle abutment tightening and was removed.

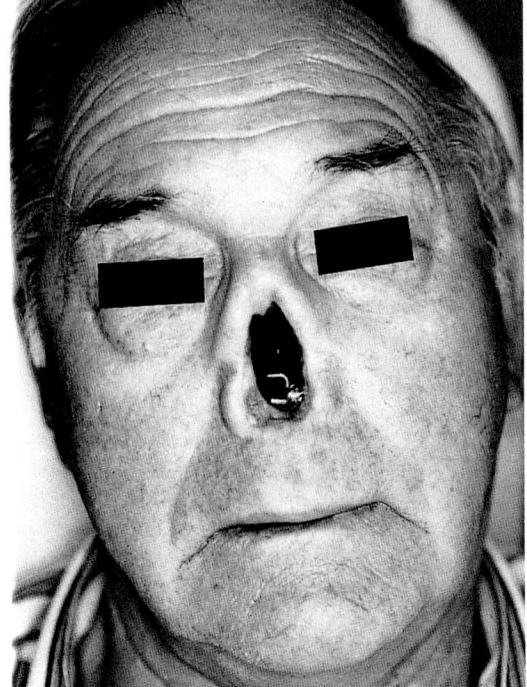

Fig 3 Supporting framework in place on the last surviving abutment.

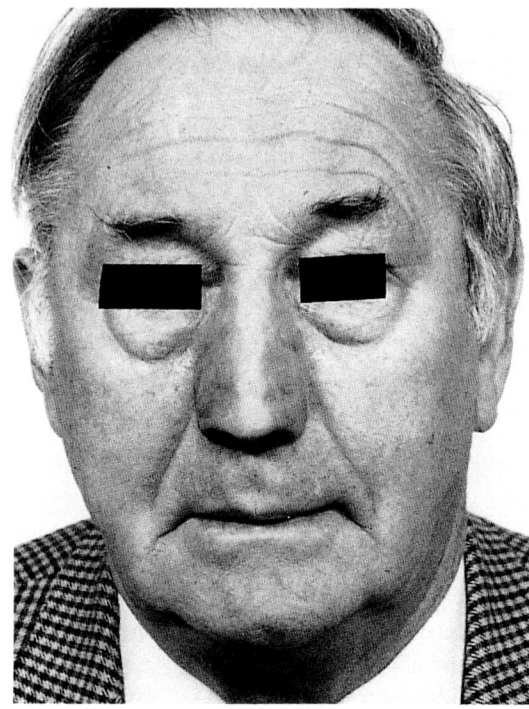

Fig 4 Completed nasal prosthesis for the patient in Fig 3, three months before loss of integration.

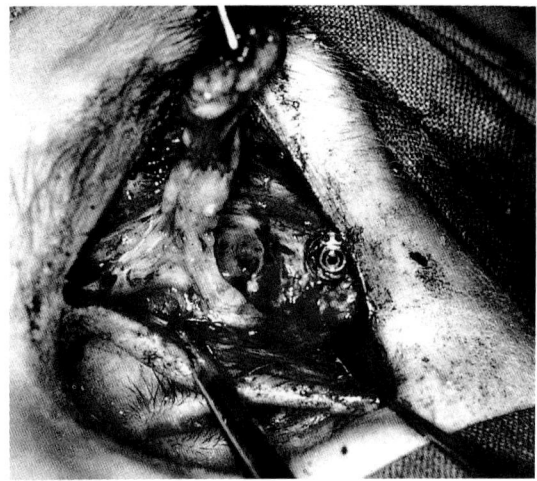

Fig 5 Extensive subcutaneous resection of periorbital tissues in the case of Fig 1.

At second-stage surgery only 17 weeks later (the nasal floor was said not to have been within the radiation field), one fixture was found to be nonintegrated and was removed.

It is highly likely that the inappropriately short healing period between first- and second-stage surgery was at least partly responsible for the nonintegration in these two cases. In both it had been thought that the radiation field had spared the implanted bone.

Secondary loss of integration

Of the first 110 fixtures placed, two have been removed as a result of loss of osseointegration, both in the same nasal case previously described. One was lost early, before it was loaded, and the other was lost after having been loaded for 3 months. Figure 3 shows the abutment and supporting framework in place, and Fig 4 shows the finished prosthesis with which the patient was delighted until it failed. This degree of loading on a single fixture, in all directions including rotation, was clearly unsustainable. It should be noted that the soft tissues in both instances responded normally.

What might have rendered this case successful?

1. A longer interval should have occurred between first- and second-stage surgery.[1]
2. The use of longer intraoral type fixtures might have been possible.
3. Hyperbaric oxygen therapy may have been used adjunctively.
4. Bone grafting of the nasal floor and lateral walls would likely have provided better quality bone in positions where functional stresses could be better shared.

Thin cranial bone

In some cases, for example auricular replacement in congenital disorders such as first arch syndrome, the temporal bone may be so thin that dura mater is exposed by initial drilling to a depth of less than 3 mm. This may result in the placement of fixtures in locations incompatible with a satisfactory prosthesis, and in any case, thicker bone may not be available and may indeed be unnecessary. All that is required is to widen the hole enough to enable a flat blunt instrument (such as the smallest dental "flat plastic") to be used to gently separate the dura mater from the deep surface of the bone. The spiral drill and tap can then be used just short of the full depth, and the fixture itself used to self-tap the deepest part. It is likely that new bone will form around the fixture in the extradural space.

Soft tissue problems

Unexplained recurrent periabutment skin infections

Occasionally a patient will suffer intermittent suppuration around an abutment for no apparent reason, despite all the recommended measures having been taken to optimize the soft tissue response.

The orbital case already described serves as an example. At second-stage surgery, radical

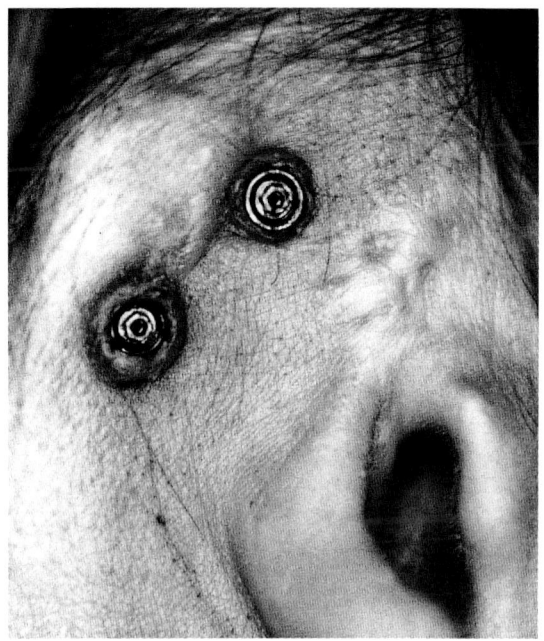

Fig 6a Intractable periabutment infection caused by loose abutments.

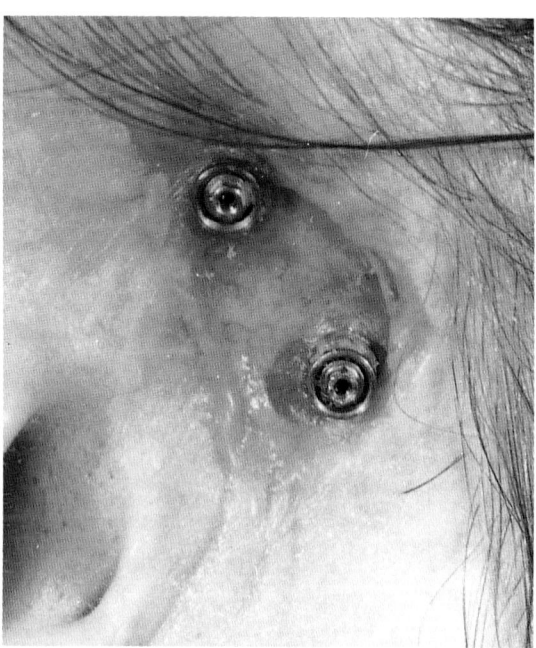

Fig 6b Three months after excision and split skin grafting of affected skin. Graft contraction of at least 30% has taken place.

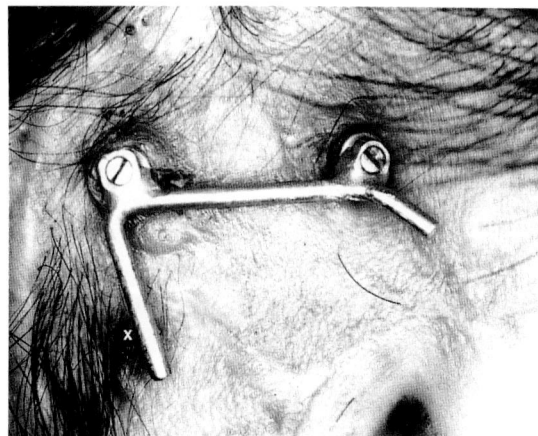

Fig 7a The results of failure to observe basic principles (see text). The abutment at X emerged through hairy skin and was removed because of infection. Above that, the periabutment skin is infected, and the anterior abutment has also suffered infection.

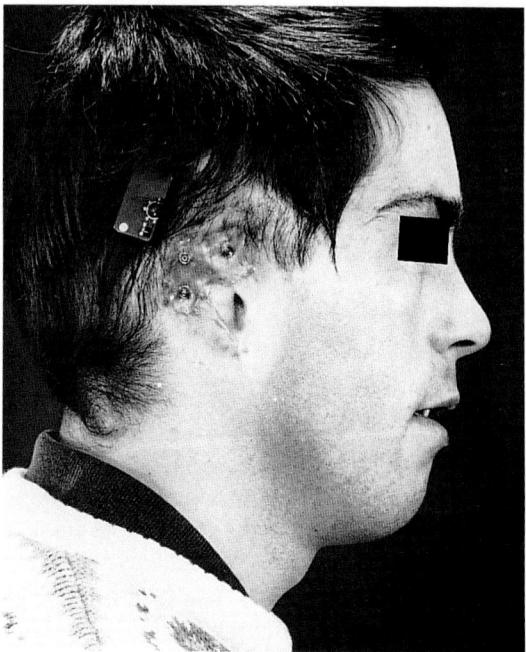

Fig 7b The whole area has been excised and split skin grafted. Some temporalis and sternocleidomastoid muscle had to be resected. The inferior fixture has once again received an abutment.

soft tissue thinning was performed (Fig 5) and in addition, to avoid hairy skin and distortion of the eyebrow position, a postauricular full-thickness skin graft was placed (Fig 2). The skin has been healthy with excellent hygiene, but on three occasions in the past 18 months, acute suppuration has occurred around the medial abutment, normally resistant to local measures and antibiotics, and normally lasting about 6 days. No explanation is offered for this behavior.

Explanation of periabutment skin infections

Abutment loosening

Loosening of an abutment invariably leads to intractable periabutment infection. This is an uncommon occurrence but has been encountered in two situations. In two patients, intraoral abutments were attached rather than extraoral ones. These are superficially identical, but as the retaining screw is longer in the intraoral abutment, the abutment will not seat fully.

In two other patients, abutment loosening has been a recurrent problem. Damage to the hexagonal seating of the abutment may have occurred when they were originally fitted. Figure 6a illustrates the reaction around the problem abutments, and Fig 6b shows the same patient after replacement of the abutments, excision of the auricular remnant, and excision and split skin grafting of the affected skin.

Inadequate soft tissue preparation

This is the most common cause of adverse skin reactions, which is surprising because the requirements for success are well defined.[2] Fastidious adherence to these principles, at least in the temporal region, will almost always guarantee a favorable skin reaction, but contravention of them will almost as surely result in an unfavorable reaction.

The important principles are the provision of periabutment skin that is thin, nonmobile, and nonhairbearing. Figure 7a illustrates the results

of failure to observe these principles. This patient, who was accepted for the provision of bilateral auricular prostheses and a bone-anchored hearing aid, received inadequate soft tissue preparation including inadequate periabutment skin flap thinning, failure to resect muscle overlying the fixtures, and failure to provide nonhairy periabutment skin. All three abutments were plagued by periabutment skin infection, and the most inferior abutment, which emerged through hairy skin, was removed early, and is absent in Fig 7a. Eventually, the whole area was excised and grafted with split-thickness skin taken from the upper arm, with the inferior abutment being resurrected, following which there have been no problems (Fig 7b).

Unfavorable soft tissues

Patients having congenital microtia and those in whom scalp flaps have been used in reconstruction pose particular soft tissue problems. Figure 8a illustrates a patient with a congenital defect who will require a new hairline, both to enable satisfactory positioning of the prosthetic ear and to supply nonhairy periabutment skin. The use of an acrylic resin template (Fig 8b) is useful in such cases. It permits the maxillofacial technologist to determine the ideal position for the fixtures, defines the amount of shaving required preoperatively, makes locating the fixtures easier at second-stage surgery, and indicates the area of skin excision and grafting that will be required.

Problems with the use of magnets

Particularly in the orbital region, magnets designed to couple with Nobelpharma abutments can provide considerable flexibility in fixture positioning and angulation, can enable the use of implants where there would otherwise be insufficient orbital size, and make periabutment cleaning easier.

Caution should be exercised in this regard, however, until it is known that the lack of mutual

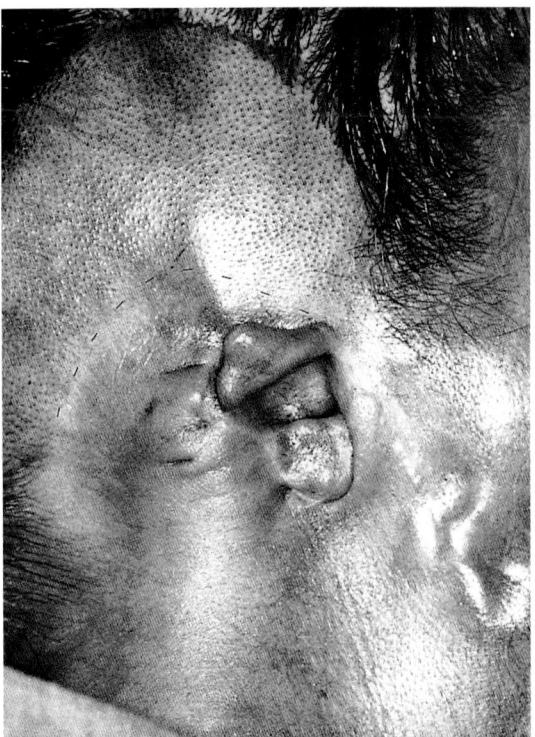

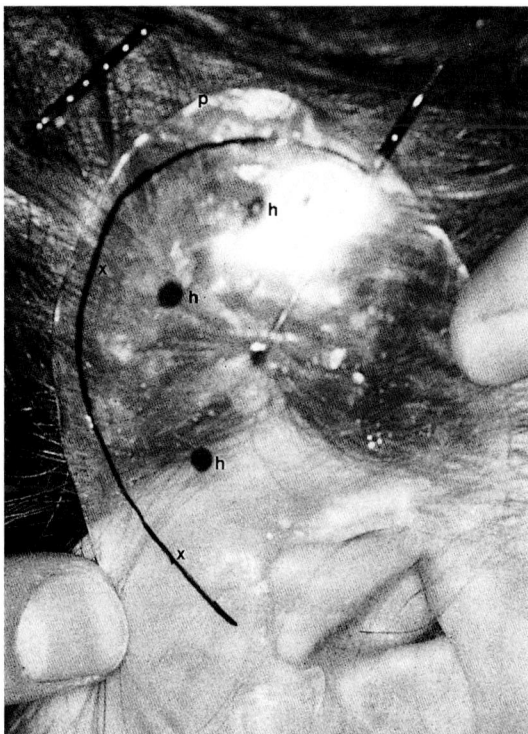

Fig 8a A case of first arch syndrome being prepared for a prosthetic ear. The hair has been shaved to just beyond the location of the desired new hairline. The natural hairline is marked by the dashed line. Extensive excision and grafting are necessary.

Fig 8b An acrylic resin template to aid in planning the surgery. The periphery *(p)* is used to delimit preoperative shaving, the line *x-x* encloses the area that must eventually be denuded of hair to facilitate an optimal prosthesis, and holes *(h)* enable percutaneous ink marking of the bone at the ideal sites for fixtures.

linkage does not adversely affect success rates, especially since there is a small but significant fixture failure rate in the orbital region.[1,2]

Magnets (Inovadent Techniques, Leeds, UK) have been used in only four patients and a significant problem was encountered in one instance that led to the removal of an abutment. In this case, corrosion occurred at the magnet/abutment interface, leading to skin inflammation and pain that could only be resolved by removal of the abutment. The length of the abutment was only marginally adequate, allowing the corrosion to encroach on the skin. Longer abutments will obviate this problem, as in Fig 1.

Skin graft behavior and management

Periabutment skin reaction in patients who have received grafts with full- or split-thickness skin is generally not a problem. Figure 9 illustrates a patient who had received split-thickness grafting to one-half of the head following severe burns. There has never been a hint of periabutment inflammation in this situation. The most superior abutment was removed only because it was poorly placed for prosthetic purposes.

Two technical points are worthy of mention. In a case such as that illustrated in Fig 9, viability of the skin depends almost entirely upon the

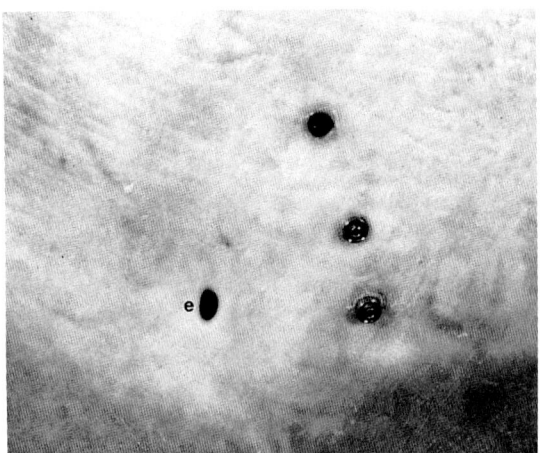

Fig 9 Extensive postburn skin grafting of the side of the head. The external auditory meatus is marked *e*. The most superior abutment has just been removed, but only because it is not ideally positioned. The skin response is excellent.

periosteal blood supply. Any attempt to raise separate cutaneous and periosteal flaps at first-stage surgery will lead to skin necrosis. Dissection should be exclusively subperiosteal.

The successful "take" of any skin graft depends on its capacity to incorporate a blood supply from the recipient vascular bed. For extensive grafts, this necessitates the attainment of absolute hemostasis and the use of a conforming pressure dressing. Figures 10a to c illustrate the consequences of failure to fulfill these conditions. While this patient did not actually receive a graft, the skin flap has been thinned at dermal level so that it effectively behaves as a full-thickness graft. Postoperative reactionary hemorrhage was compounded by the loss of a pressure dressing only a few hours postoperatively and the failure to replace it. The formation of hematomas beneath the skin led to widespread necrosis.

One insoluble problem is the inability to predict how much graft contraction will occur. Full-thickness grafts usually contract very little, but split-thickness skin (or more accurately, the

scar tissue that forms beneath it) can contract considerably, up to 50% by area especially when cut thinly,[3] with most contraction completed by 6 months. It is advisable to err on the side of generosity when split-thickness skin grafts are used, even though the grafted area may look far too extensive at operation. This is demonstrated in Fig 6b where the clearance around the abutments is only adequate 3 months after grafting, although immediately postoperatively the patient thought that excision had been excessive.

Prosthetic difficulties

The retention of auricular vestiges

A large proportion of patients presenting for auricular prostheses will still possess auricular tissue in the form of postexcision or posttraumatic remnants, or microtic vestiges. Earlier efforts were conservative and as much tissue as possible was retained. However, experience has demonstrated that this decision was almost always wrong. Although a prosthesis could be fabricated that was perfectly satisfactory on a plaster model, living tissues in the region of the lobe are closely related to the mandibular ramus and thus move during jaw movements. It may be desirable to remove all microtic or other remnants in the auricular area before prosthesis fabrication so as to obtain a stable soft tissue base for the restoration.

Conclusions

The benefits of implant retention for prostheses are numerous. Serious complications have been remarkably few. Those few problems that have been encountered are primarily the result of failure to observe well-established principles.

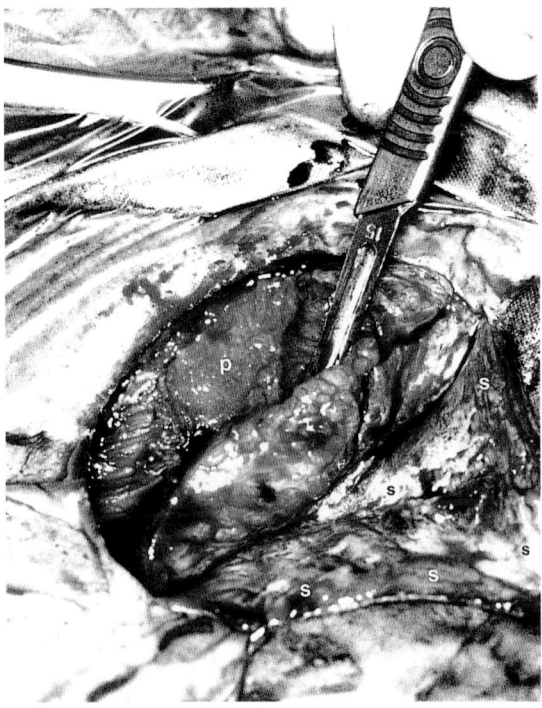

Fig 10a Second-stage surgery for an auricular prosthesis. Subcutaneous tissue is radically excised between the periosteum *(p)* and the dermis of the skin flap *(s)*.

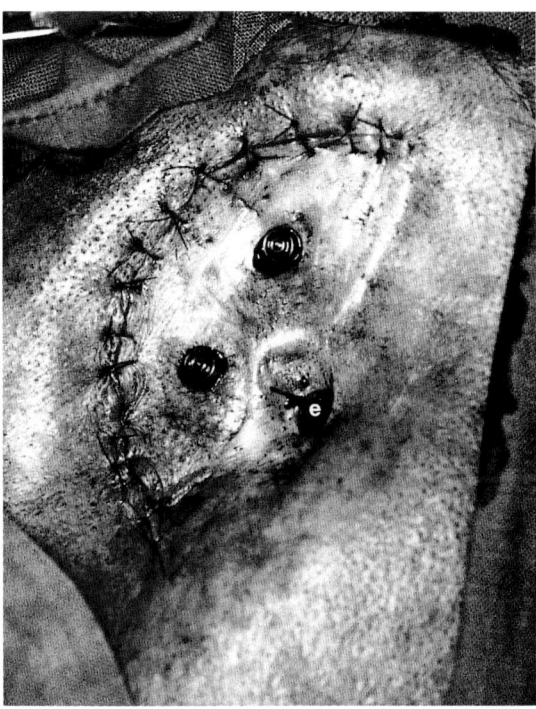

Fig 10b The radically thinned skin is sutured back into place and perforated to accept the abutments. *(e)* External auditory meatus.

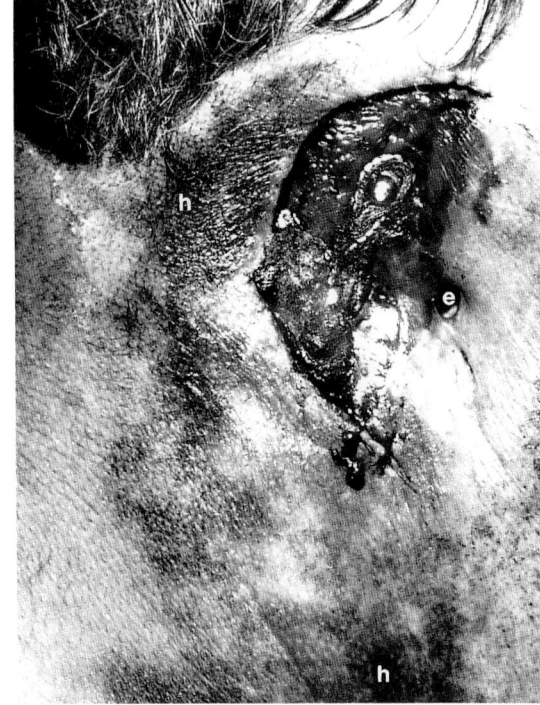

Fig 10c Almost complete skin necrosis caused by loss of the pressure dressing and reactionary hemorrhage. *(e)* External auditory meatus; *(h)* subcutaneous hematoma spreading into the neck.

Acknowledgments

We would like to express our sincere thanks to our maxillofacial technologist colleagues Martin Deadman and Steve Worrollo. Were it not for their skills, we would be wasting our time. All of these implants have been provided at no cost to the patients, and have not been funded by the National Health Service. We owe a debt of gratitude to all those who have worked so selflessly to raise the charitable money that has enabled this work to proceed.

References

1. Jacobsson M, Tjellström A, Thomsen P, et al. Integration of titanium implants in irradiated bone: A histological and clinical study. *Ann Otol Rhinol* 1988;97:337–340.
2. Tjellström A. Osseointegrated systems and their applications in the head & neck. *Adv Otolaryngol Head Neck Surg* 1989;3:39–70.
3. Grabb WC, Smith JW. *Plastic Surgery: A Concise Guide to Clinical Practice.* 2nd ed. Boston: Little, Brown & Co, 1973, pp 49, 50.

The Use of Titanium Fixtures for Intraoral Anchorage to Facilitate Orthodontic Tooth Movement

K. Higuchi and J.M. Slack

Proffitt et al[1] have defined anchorage as "the resistance to unwanted tooth movement," or "the resistance to reaction forces that is provided by other teeth, or by structures outside the mouth." Orthodontic tooth movement has always been limited to action-reaction reciprocal force mechanics because of the absence of a fixed anchorage point in the mouth. Extraoral headgear retraction of maxillary molars is currently the most effective way of obtaining anchorage for the orthodontic movement of teeth.

Roberts et al[2] have stated that inadequate anchorage is one of the most limiting aspects of orthodontic therapy, and that biomechanical horizons would be considerably advanced by an effective means of attaining direct osseous loading. Since 1965, when Brånemark and associates[3] introduced the concept of osseointegration, pure titanium threaded implants have been successfully utilized in the clinical treatment of edentulism.

Brånemark[3] has defined osseointegration as a direct structural and functional connection between living bone and the surface of a load-carrying implant. Osseointegrated titanium implants (fixtures) have been repeatedly observed to be rigidly anchored in bone, so that removal is dependent on the ultimate failure strength of the supporting bone, rather than separation at the implant/bone interface. Adell et al[4] have cited unpublished data from 1970 indicating that osseointegrated implants in dogs could not be moved by conventional orthodontic forces.

The purpose of this prospective study was to evaluate the efficacy of using osseointegrated titanium implants as anchorage units in a series of adult patients, to achieve orthodontic tooth movement. The assessment of protraction and retraction forces of varying magnitudes on the osseointegrated titanium implants was planned. The movement of full arches, not just single teeth, was to be attempted.

Materials and methods

Seven adult patients, five females and two males, with an age range of 22 to 41 years, were selected. Table 1 summarizes the pretreatment clinical data and length of treatment.

Ten-millimeter Brånemark (Nobelpharma USA, Inc, Chicago, Ill) implants were placed bilaterally in the third molar region of the mandible for six patients and in the first molar region for one patient (JS) with missing mandibular molars. The surgical procedures were performed according to the principles established by Brånemark.[3]

During the period of healing, standard orthodontic aligning and levelling was accomplished. Four to 6 months later, the implants were uncovered and a single Nobelpharma abutment cylinder was placed. The abutment height was reduced to avoid contact with the opposing maxillary dentition and to accommodate the mucosal tissue level when necessary. A customized composite resin crown was placed over the abutment and an edgewise bracket was secured. After orthodontic arch alignment, a

Table 1 Summary of pretreatment clinical data and length of treatment

Patient	Age	Sex	Occlusion type	Orthodontic time (mo)	Total treatment time (mo)
JV	22	F	Class II retruded	25	31
LE	36	F	Class II	27	32
RH	34	M	Class II	35	39
JZ	27	F	Class II retruded	17	21
JS	40	M	Missing molars; Class III mutilated	26	30
TB	32	F	Class II	28	32
SE	41	F	Class II retruded	18	22

rectangular wire (.018 × .025 inch) was connected to the implant-abutment unit and orthodontic forces were applied from the implant to the orthodontic appliances.

In the single case of retraction, the same osseointegration principles were used except placement of the implants was farther forward in the mandible so that they could be used for prosthetic restoration later. The mandible was bilaterally edentulous.

After orthodontic arch alignment, a rectangular wire (.018 × .025 inch) was connected to the implant-abutment unit and orthodontic forces were applied from the implant to the orthodontic appliances. Initially, forces of 150 to 200 g were applied to each abutment. Later, after it became apparent that the implant abutments were accepting the load, forces were increased to 400 g to each abutment unit. This group of seven patients was under active orthodontic treatment for a period of 18 to 30 months, with average treatment time being 26 months. The abutments were engaged after the arches had been orthodontically aligned and leveled. At this point, protraction or retraction were instituted, with the abutments used as anchorage.

All patients were evaluated using standardized pretreatment and posttreatment cephalometric head films obtained with the same radiologic equipment. The head films were traced using conventional anatomic landmarks. Specifically, maxillary incisor inclination to sella-

nasion (SN) and mandibular plane (MP) were measured. In addition, the change in distance in millimeters in the incisal edge, from pretreatment to posttreatment, was recorded as well as bodily movement (mm) of the mandibular second molars (Tables 2 and 3).

Results

In the seven patients, all 14 of the implants placed remained clinically stable during the entire treatment period. Two fixtures have since been used for prosthetic restorations, which serve as single-tooth first molar replacements. No paresthesia was reported by any of the patients, and no complaints were registered regarding pain or discomfort from the area of the abutment/implant units. There was an absence of hyperplasia, or inflammation, from the tissue adjacent to the abutment/mucosa interface. The only technical problem experienced was the loosening of abutment screws, which occurred several times. Retightening of this screw reestablished the rigid connection to the osseointegrated fixture. Following completion of orthodontic treatment, the abutment connectors were removed and cover screws were placed on the fixtures. The tissue was then surgically closed over the buried fixtures.

Overall treatment time for patients in this

Table 2 Clinical change with respect to incisor axial inclination

Patient	Pretreatment 1 to SN	Posttreatment 1 to SN	Degree of maxillary incisor tipping	Pretreatment 1̄ to MP	Posttreatment 1̄ to MP	Degree of mandibular incisor tipping
JV	86°	99°	13°	73°	90°	17°
LE	90°	90°	0°	75°	89°	14°
RH	95°	95°	0°	75°	89°	14°
JZ	84°	104°	20°	79°	96°	17°
SE	95°	104°	9°	80°	91°	11°
JS	102°	108°	4°	95°	84°	−9°
TB	76°	97°	21°	83°	107°	24°

Table 3 Clinical change with respect to incisor-molar movement

Patient	Anterior movement of 1̄ forward incisal edge to incisal edge (mm)	Anterior movement (molar) 7̄ (mm)
JV	5	3
LE	3	6
RH	4	2
JZ	5	2
SE	3	2
JS	−5	No molars present
TB	4	1

study was comparable to, or slightly longer than, that required for typical adult orthodontic treatment. The length of treatment involved 4 to 6 months of healing prior to abutment connection, while the actual orthodontic phase of treatment ranged from 17 to 35 months, with a mean treatment time of 25 months. Six Class II patients were treated with protraction orthodontic mechanics, and one patient (JS) had correction of a Class III anterior crossbite with retraction forces on the fixture-abutment unit. A notable correction of a Class II malocclusion was seen in one patient (LE), in whom a 6-mm Class II incisal discrepancy was corrected with protraction of the entire dentition.

Tables 2 and 3 summarize the clinical changes with respect to change in incisor axial inclination, incisor movement, and bodily movement of the mandibular second molars. In each of the seven patients treated, the fixture-abutment unit did serve as effective rigid anchorage, enabling occlusal correction. The fixture-abutment units did not show any movement when pretreatment and posttreatment head films were evaluated. The axial tooth inclinations of patients with retruded dentition were corrected to more favorable alignment with the mandibular incisor axial inclination change ranging from 9° to 24° (Table 2).

Maxillary incisor changes were similar and occurred concurrently with maxillary tooth movement (Table 2). The mean change in maxillary incisal movement in the seven patients was 4.1 mm (Table 3). Bodily movement of the mandibular second molars was also recorded. The mandibular molars averaged 2.3 mm of anterior protraction with a range of 2 to 6 mm (Table 3). The range of anterior mandibular incisor movement was between 1 and 6 mm (Table 3). All spaces were closed at the completion of treatment.

Discussion

The concept of rigid intraoral anchorage had not been predictably achieved prior to the use of osseointegrated implants. The use of titanium fixtures has provided a modality to permit unidirectional tooth movement without reciprocal action. If it is possible to create a point of rigid anchorage, then theoretically, by placing rigid connectors such as heavy rectangular arch wires to that point, the transfer of that rigidity can be moved anteriorly or to other strategic locations in the dental arch. These new points of rigid anchorage can then be used to implement conventional orthodontic mechanics such as protraction, retraction, leveling, and transverse changes to correct various malocclusions.

Four patients were treated (JV, LE, JZ, SE) using protraction mechanics to advance the entire dentition. They were selected because of dissatisfaction with their retruded facial and dental appearance. All had had four first premolars extracted from previous orthodontic treatment, and all extraction spaces were closed. In all four patients, after the incisors had been protracted, lip and facial profile was improved. Alternative options included a reverse pull type of headgear or anterior protraction with the creation of an edentulous space in the premolar area.

The surgical placement of implants in the ramus and third molar region was difficult in some patients, primarily because of access limitations. Mandibular opening capability, opposing maxillary dentition, and soft tissue anatomy all affected the final fixture position. Overall efficiency of both surgical and orthodontic phases of treatment improved with experience. Total length of treatment time undoubtedly was extended somewhat because of early minimal force loads.

The technical mechanics of connecting the abutment unit to the orthodontic arch wire initially proved to be a challenge. Initially, the abutment connection was brought out on the buccal side of the composite resin crown to the double buccal tube of the second molar. Tissue impingement by the abutment, crown, and arch wire connecting the abutment to the molar proved to be a problem. Placing a bracket on the lingual side of the molar eliminated this difficulty. Connecting the attachment to the molar initially proved to be a challenge until experience was gained.

Conclusion

This report is believed to be the first prospective study utilizing standardized rigid anchorage in a series of patients treated with osseointegrated titanium fixtures.

Brånemark osseointegrated titanium implants were placed in the posterior mandible and used to protract the entire dentition in the maxilla and mandible. They also have been used effectively for retraction and correction of a Class III anterior crossbite malocclusion with missing molar teeth. All of the implant-abutment units remained stable throughout treatment with no observed mobility. Orthodontic forces ranging from 150 to 400 g were applied during the clinical course of treatment. Based on this initial series of patients, it seems that the achievement of fixed anchorage intraorally is possible utilizing the process of osseointegration.

References

1. Proffitt WR, et al. *Contemporary Orthodontics*. St Louis, Mo: CV Mosby Co, 1986, p 260.
2. Roberts WE, Smith RK, Silberman Y, et al. Osseous adaptation to continuous loading of rigid endosseous implants. *Am J Orthod* 1984;86:95–110.
3. Brånemark P-I. Introduction to osseointegration. pp 11–76 In P.-I. Brånemark, G.A. Zarb, T. Albrektsson (eds) *Tissue Integrated Prostheses: Osseointegration In Clinical Dentistry*. Chicago: Quintessence Publ Co, 1985.
4. Adell R, Lekholm U, Rockler B, Brånemark P-I. A 15-year study of osseointegrated implants in the treatment of the edentulous jaw. *Int J Oral Surg* 1981;6:387–416.

Future Challenges for Craniofacial Implantation

G. R. Holt

In the United States, the greatest challenge currently is in obtaining FDA approval for craniofacial applications of osseointegrated implants. That includes the hearing aid application. This does not detract from the efforts that have been made thus far, but it is frustrating to investigators to have this opportunity and not be able to share it with so many more colleagues around the country.

Dr Brown has indicated that deleterious effects can result, and he discussed how we might prevent some of them as potential complications for craniofacial applications. (see pages 294 to 302). There are no clear-cut solutions for many of these problems. They deserve not only the attention to detail but research in the future concerning how we may positively affect some of the adverse or relative patient problems.

What are some of the future challenges? It is easy to bring ideas forward, but the hard part is to decide how to address the proposals and to develop some very basic principles and protocols to look at these. We can see problems that occur at the tissue/implant interface and understand them from a biomaterials point of view as well as from a molecular and biochemical point of view; it is important to look at these in-depth and understand what is happening at the interface. However, one must also not lose sight of the fact that the clinical applications must also be looked at in-depth.

One area under investigation at the University of Texas Health Science Center at San Antonio concerns the possibility of being able to positively influence the osseointegration procedure by inducing or facilitating bone formation, particularly in those areas where bone formation may be retarded or may be a problem. Synthetic transforming growth factor beta, some of which is proprietary but some of which will be available in the very near future, can be utilized inside the fixture. Our own analytical bone implant uses it within a large chamber to facilitate bone growth for computerized cystomorphometry. It seems conceivable that one could also apply it outside the fixture as an integral part of the coating or even as a filler within a larger cavity to increase the osteogenic potential of a particular site.

What is the best implant surface coating? Obviously, with commercially pure titanium, the surface is titanium oxide—acquired upon exposure to air. Is an alloy of titanium just as good as commercially pure titanium? If so, what does the surface coating then form, and is it as acceptable for tissue integration as the commercially pure form? Can hydroxyapatite as an osseoconductive material be important in the integration of some of these fixtures? That certainly is important and is now being reported in the orthopedic literature, but the topic should also be studied by researchers.

There are many bone inductive factors. Some have been mentioned and some are yet to be discovered. Solutions are needed to encourage the integration of implants in patients with deleterious factors such as radiation or poor health. A local factor may be of benefit, or perhaps a systemic bone inductive factor can be developed, which taken orally or parenterally could help particular sites.

What is the best surface pore and ridge contour? What is the depth or height of the irregular surface? Is sputtering a good way to externally coat it?

Can hollow fixtures be used? Many of us are using hollow screws as part of a plating or fixation device for craniofacial fractures and reconstruction. They work very well. Does the fixture now used need to be solid with the exception of the central portion that is fluted, or can it be hollow? Can one actually have a fixture within a fixture to increase the total surface area of the osseointegrated process? Can one have a fixture that is perforated and yet have a central cylinder for the abutment attachment? These possibilities need to be considered as far as expanding the design of the implants themselves.

Where can implants be placed? Certainly the zygoma and the pterygoid plate; these are potential sites that could receive longer fixtures than the standard 3- to 4-mm craniofacial fixtures now being utilized. For thin bone, can an expanding fixture be utilized, such as inserting a screw into a hollow wall that expands once it penetrates the wall? Could this approach be used in areas such as the maxillary sinus or the frontal sinus to gain additional area for retention? Is it possible to fill the sinus with bone-inducting material which will solidify that sinus and permit screw fixation?

The temporomandibular joint should be a very exciting site for further investigation into the use of implants in the replacement of that particular structure. Other areas for consideration include the orbit, the base of the skull, and the cranium. We have seen that it is possible to move teeth. Soviet studies have shown that long bones can be moved with a distraction technique. Compressive techniques have been used in treating bone fractures. Could fixtures that are osseointegrated be used to expand any area of the face or the skull that is desired? Synostosis, hemifacial atrophies—many of these defects have been treated by onlay grafting or expansion with osteotomies in the past. These could be potential sites for expansion.

Access to the intracranial contents seems very appropriate for this sort of technique. Fixtures that are now available can certainly be solid. They can be stable and have longevity that would allow for the transmission of electrodes intracranially. Such electrodes could go to the cochlea, to the eighth nerve, to the cochlear nuclei themselves, or to various areas of the brain for electrical stimulation or retardation. In addition, with the ability to project electrical images upon the occipital cortex for vision, this could be an exciting area for the transmission of those particular electrodes in that disability.

Currently under consideration is the question of bone expansion in areas that are very thin or not conducive to healing. The nasal bones, the orbit, and postmaxillary defects could potentially be grafted. What are the best graft materials? We think that probably calvarial bone may be better than iliac crest bone as far as resorption properties are concerned. When one uses a bone graft in the orbit, for example, is it secured with a titanium fixture? Is a titanium screw used? Should it be a temporary fixture or should it be permanent? These are ideas that need to be considered.

The idea of augmentation with grafting is important. Is it possible to actually induce further bone growth in a subperiosteal area by placing bone-conductive and bone-inductive materials between the bone and the periosteum? Will it allow for thickening of the bone without having to graft it?

One of the best opportunities for bioengineers is to develop the capacity to have a consensual gaze eyeball in an orbital prosthesis. Current procedure utilizes an eyeball that is fixed and does not track. But a 20-year-old woman who has lost her orbit contents because of some malignant process and appears to be free of disease could certainly be better rehabilitated having an eye that tracks with the other eye and somehow takes its signal from electromyograms of the occular muscles on the opposite side.

A real problem exists currently with hearing aid applications. Hearing aids are too big, too bulky, and are very unsightly. Unfortunately the emphasis in developing hearing aids has not kept up with modern technology. Microchips and microelectronic circuits are available that permit these hearing amplification devices to be housed in a very small area. The challenge to those involved in this field ought to be the miniaturization of the hearing device to make it as small and inconspicuous as possible so that it is not always necessary to place the fixture for this device back behind the hairline and perhaps have to graft. Is it also possible to incorporate this vibration device within an auricular epithesis or prosthesis itself? Additionally, the whole idea of anchoring mechanical and electrical vibrators and stimulators in the middle ear, the ear canal, and on the promontory is within our grasp.

Cranioplasty has long been accomplished typically with biomaterials that fall in the polymer range. It would seem possible to utilize tissue-integrated fixtures to anchor much more cleverly designed and developed cranioplasty repair materials than ever before. The understanding and technology are available to develop and machine an exact-sized prosthesis for a defect utilizing reconstructive three-dimensional and computer-generated robotic-type production. It should also be possible to anchor them with the latest technology in a very unobtrusive manner that will not be visible under a very thin scalp defect.

Orthopedic surgeons have considerable insight into the utilization of these materials and fixture techniques for the cervical spine. Should clinicians delve further and deeper into base-of-skull surgery, it would not be long before the base-of-skull approach for tumors at the foramen magnum could be used. An integrative fixture technique could be utilized to secure fixation devices whether they be bone grafts or other biomaterials at the base of the skull.

Reconstruction of the Compromised Patient Using Titanium Two-Stage Osseointegrated Implants and Three-Dimensional Computed Tomography Scanning

C.A. Babbush

When an individual is missing some or all natural teeth and wishes to have them reconstructed with dental implants, certain procedures must be carried out as part of the presurgical evaluation of the implant candidates.[1] This evaluation includes a clinical examination that involves an evaluation of the hard and soft tissues of the jaw. In addition, a dental and medical history, as well as selected laboratory procedures, are necessary. Until recently, the various radiographic techniques performed for evaluation of potential implant receptor sites were achieved through the use of panoramic, occlusal, lateral cephalometric, and perhaps tomographic films. These rather routine radiographic procedures do not allow one to accurately examine the potential receptor site in a three-dimensional manner; furthermore, they do not disclose sufficiently accurate anatomical information to define bone dimensions and configurations. The desired information should include the configuration of bone in a dynamically accurate three-dimensional image.

The development of computer tomography (CT) has provided additional information that can ultimately create horizontal images.[2,3] In addition, more recent technological developments have made possible sagittal as well as coronal images by reformation through a sophisticated software package called Dentascan (General Electric, CT Division, Milwaukee, Wisc). These reformatted images have provided more accurate and essential information for the creation of three-dimensional examinations. With the development of Dentascan, it

has become possible to reconstruct successive cross-sectional images of the maxilla and mandible that are perpendicular to the maxillary and mandibular curvatures with a reformatting computer program (Figs 1a to c).[4–6]

To further interpret this information for treatment planning purposes, an analysis that has previously been published, provides precise anatomic information concerning the edentulous areas of the maxilla and mandible.[7] The successive numbering of the cross-sectional images is initiated from the right side of the ridge and progresses to the left side. The height and width of each successive cross-sectional image at a specified level is measured. These measurements of the height and width of cross-sectional slices are plotted geographically according to the number image. This technique of graphically displaying the cross-sectional dimensions has been termed maxillary-mandibular shape pattern analysis (MSPA) (Fig 2). The MSPA technique creates a profile of a patient's maxilla and mandible. This profile results in an accurate presurgical assessment that includes the selection of appropriate implant sizes as well as the location for implant placement. In addition, MSPA enables the clinician to determine the deficiencies and anatomic structures that either contraindicate implant placement or require alternative treatment modalities. Alternative treatment modalities may include maxillary antroplasty with augmentation bone grafting, mandibular and mental nerve transposition, and vestibuloplasty procedures. A series of moderately to severely compromised individuals have

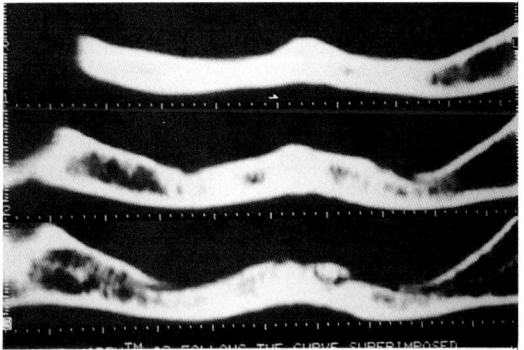

Fig 1a CT-Dentascan examination demonstrates three-dimensional evaluation of implant receptor sites. Panoramic serial views.

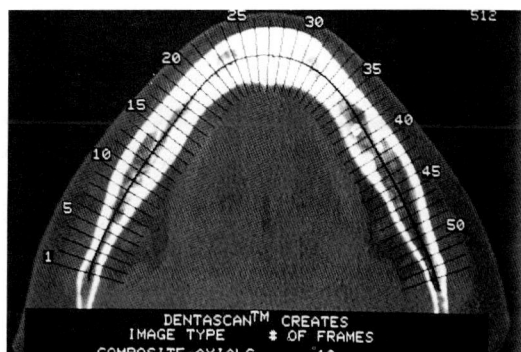

Fig 1b Occlusal view of residual arch.

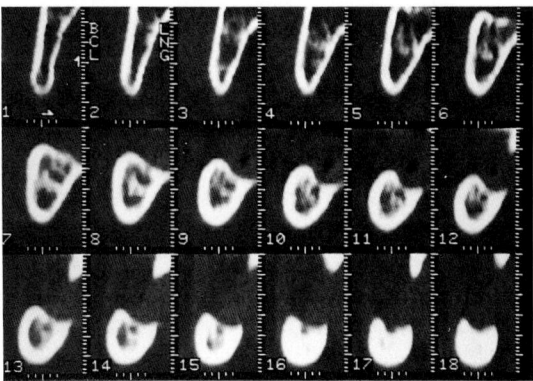

Fig 1c Cross-sectional views.

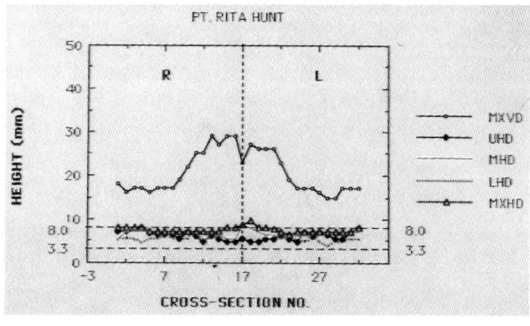

Fig 2 Graphic MSPA display from Dentascan examination.

been reconstructed over the past 2 years, requiring secondary reconstruction following tumor, trauma, or advanced atrophic presentation. Such treatment would not have been possible without the combined advanced technology of Dentascan and the two-stage osseointegration procedure. Representative patient treatment is illustrated by the following case histories.

Case I

Patient number one was a 75-year-old healthy man with more than a 20-year history of wear-

ing complete maxillary and partial mandibular removable prostheses. Two remaining mandibular canines were removed several months prior to the implant evaluation because of periodontal disease (Figs 3a and b). Clinical and panoramic radiographic evaluation revealed a knife-edge ridge configuration in both the maxilla and mandible. CT-Dentascan was carried out for both the maxilla and mandible. MSPA was performed and confirmed the knife-edged configuration (Fig 4). The treatment planned for this patient involved an aggressive alveoloplasty for the occlusal or superior third of each arch to reduce the severe knife-edged ridge and create a broad base so that two-stage osseointegrated IMZ Implants (Interpore International,

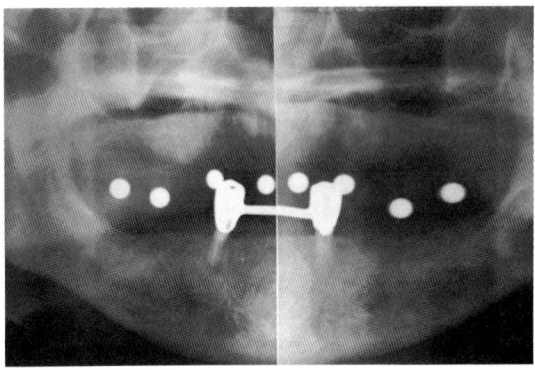

Fig 3a Original panoramic radiograph.

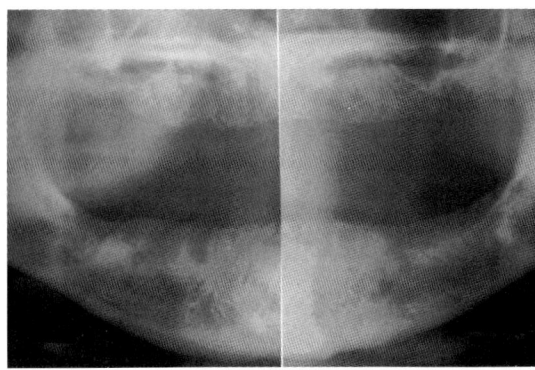

Fig 3b Postextraction panoramic radiograph.

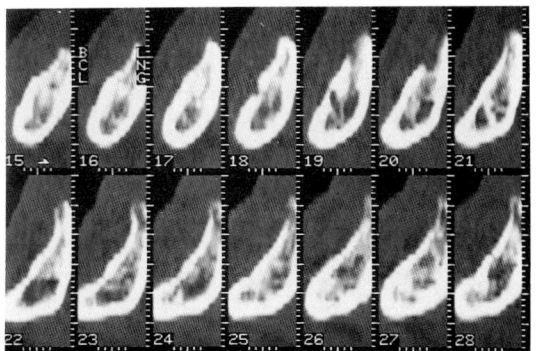

Fig 4 Dentascan demonstration of severe knife-edge configuration.

complete maxillary prosthesis for more than 10 years is the second patient example. The maxillary removable prosthesis had compromised stability and function. This patient had a minimal amount of residual maxillary bone; however, CT-Dentascan demonstrated the potential for the placement of four 4.0 × 8.0 mm IMZ implants, which were ultimately placed (Figs 6a to e). This patient declined maxillary antroplasty procedures with augmentation graftings and would only undergo a straightforward implant reconstruction. Prosthetic reconstruction was completed using a connector bar with an overdenture and internal clip fixation (Fig 7).

Irvine, Calif) could be placed (Fig 5a).[8] Ultimately, a series of eight IMZ implants was placed in the mandible and seven in the maxilla in addition to augmentation of the labial aspect of the left maxilla with porous hydroxyapatite granules (Fig 5b). The patient's teeth were ultimately reconstructed with a screw-on implant-supported prosthesis, both in the maxilla and the mandible (Fig 5c).

Case II

A 60-year-old woman who had severely advanced atrophy of the maxilla and had worn a

Case III

Patient number three was a 26-year-old woman who had undergone mandibular resection to remove a benign tumor. She was secondarily reconstructed with an autogenous rib graft that had been placed 2 years prior to implant consultation (Fig 8). To analyze the possibility of implant reconstruction, a CT-Dentascan was obtained for the residual mandible and the reformatted program was instituted (Figs 9a to d). The horizontal plane image, the reconstructive vertical image, and the cross-sectional views were assessed. The bone graft portion of the jaw was seen from cross sections num-

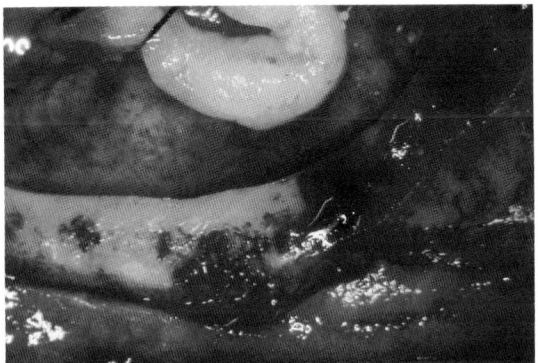

Fig 5a Alveoloplasty was carried out to achieve favorable implant receptor sites.

bered 34 to 59 on the reconstructive panoramic image. The region between cross-section numbers 10 and 60 was selected and plotted on the MSPA graph. The location for the implant placement could only be carried out in the right mandible. The patient's teeth were ultimately reconstructed with four IMZ implants and a screw-on long cantilevered implant-supported prosthesis (Fig 10).

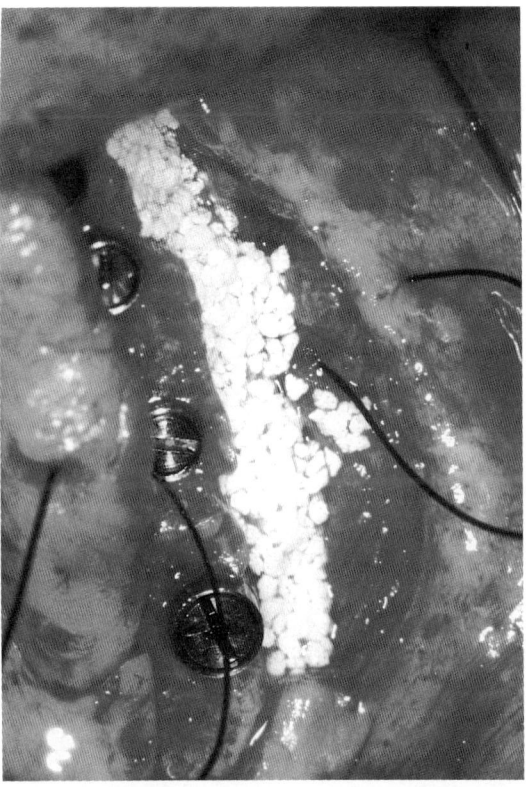

Fig 5b Due to a severe buccal concavity, porous hydroxyapatite granules were used to augment and recontour this area.

Case IV

A 59-year-old woman presented with total asymmetry of the maxilla and mandible (Fig 11a). She had been reviewed by numerous practitioners for potential reconstruction and none of them would develop a treatment plan for her. She was evaluated as a potential candidate for orthognathic surgery involving revision of the asymmetric jaws and ultimately had a bilateral sagittal split osteotomy with repositioning of the chin (Fig 11b). Following these procedures she was evaluated with CT-Dentascan to determine the potential for reconstruction of her totally edentulous maxilla and bilateral posterior mandible (Figs 12a to d). A left antroplasty with augmentation grafting was carried out in the maxilla. Ultimately, her maxilla was reconstructed with two split segment connector bars and an overdenture with internal clip fixation. In

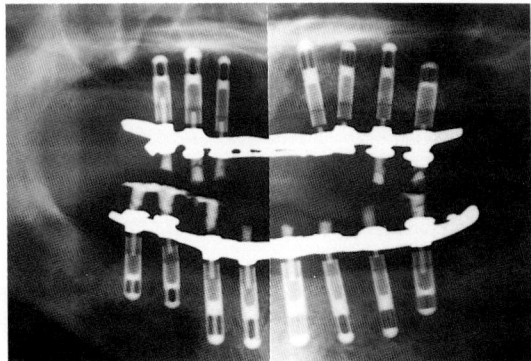

Fig 5c A totally implant-supported screw-retained prosthesis was fabricated for both arches. The postoperative 1-year panoramic radiograph.

the mandible, bilateral placement of two IMZ implants provided support for fixed prostheses (Fig 13).

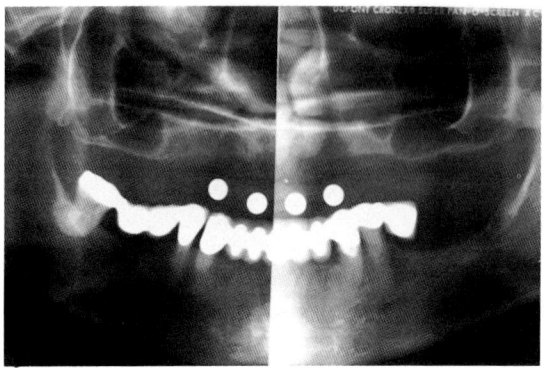

6a

Fig 6a Preoperative panoramic radiograph.

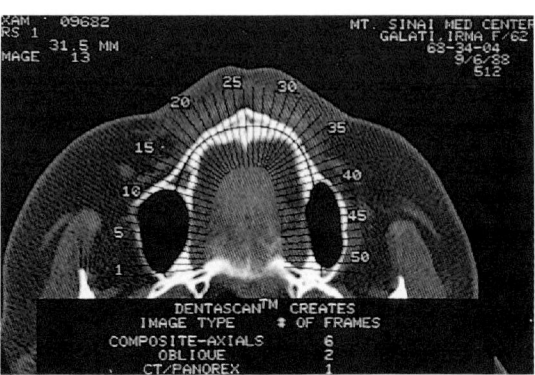

6b

Figs 6b to e CT-Dentascan was carried out in the maxilla.

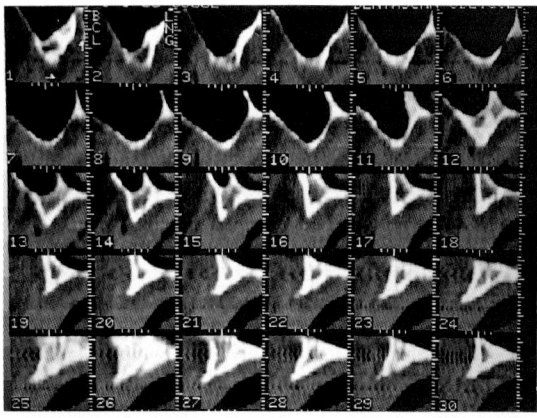

6c

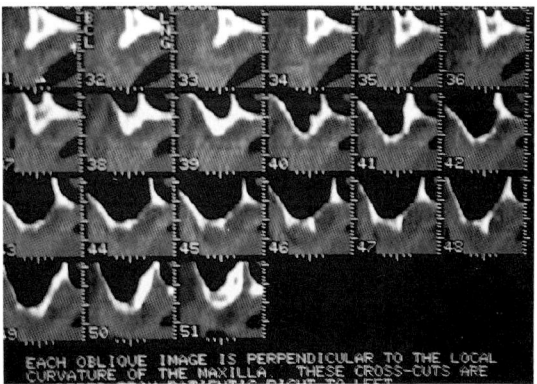

6d

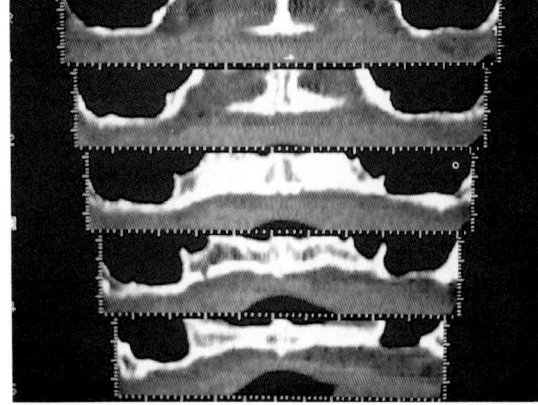

6e

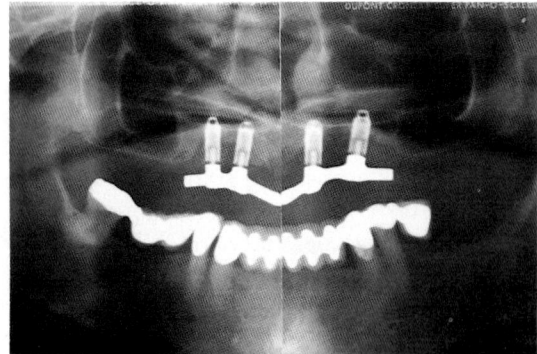

Fig 7 The patient was restored with four 4.0 × 8.0 mm IMZ implants with a connector bar and overdenture with internal fixation. Postoperative panoramic radiograph.

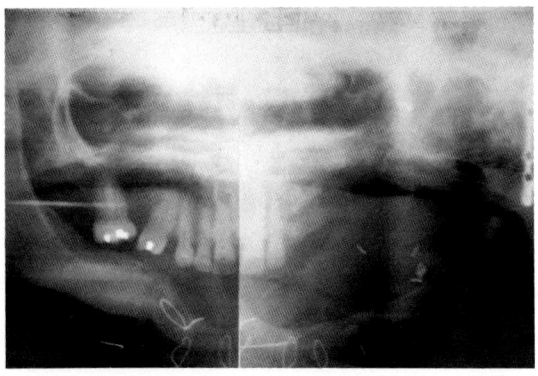

Fig 8 Postreconstruction panoramic radiograph demonstrating mandibular resection with secondary rib graft reconstruction.

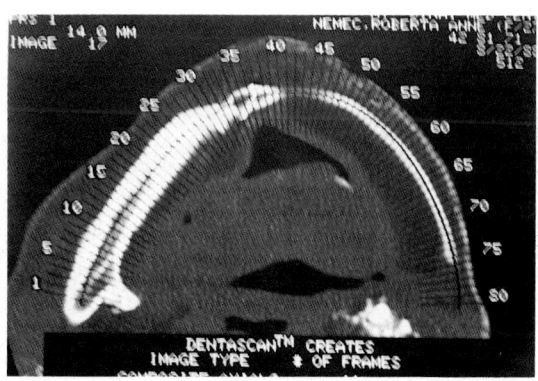

9a

Figs 9a to d CT-Dentascan views of the mandible.

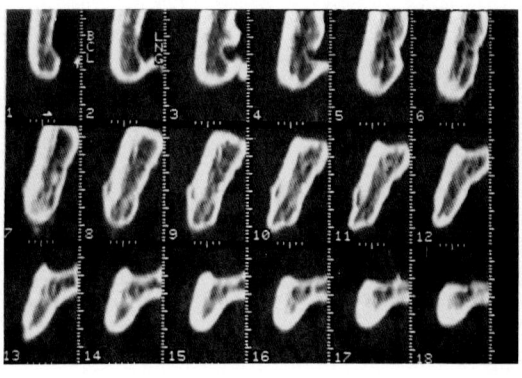

9b

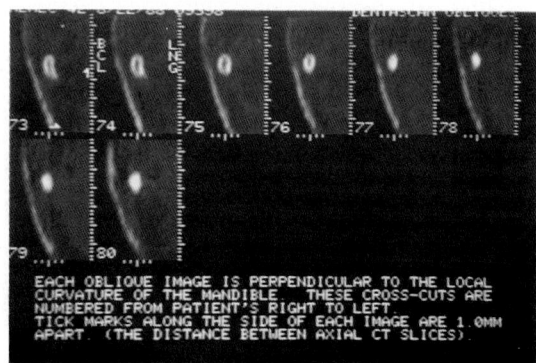

9c

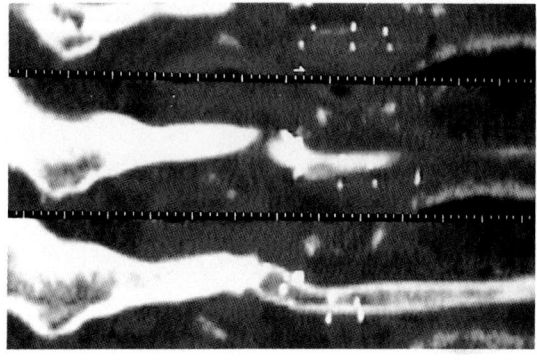

9d

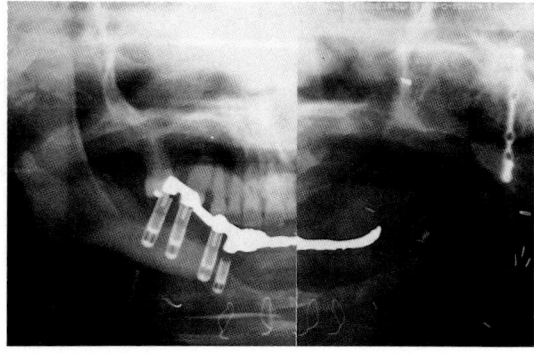

Fig 10 Postoperative panoramic radiograph.

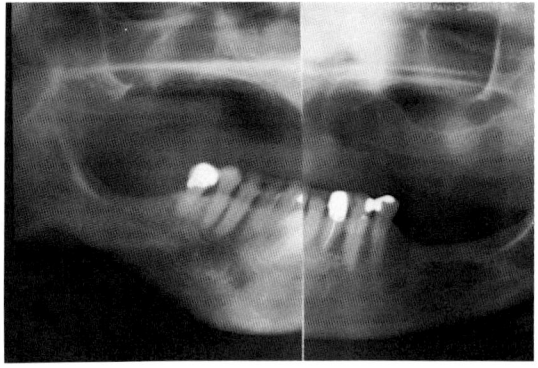

Fig 11a   Presurgical panoramic radiograph.

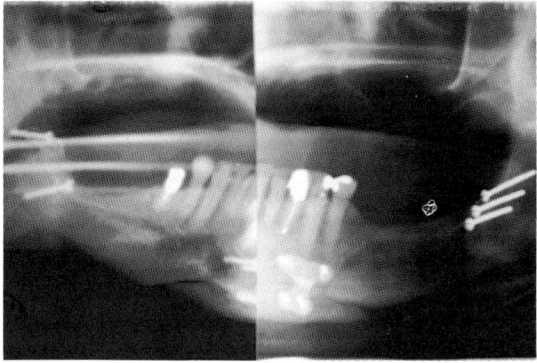

Fig 11b   Postoperative panoramic radiograph demonstrating bilateral sagittal split osteotomy and chin repositioning with accompanying fixation hardware.

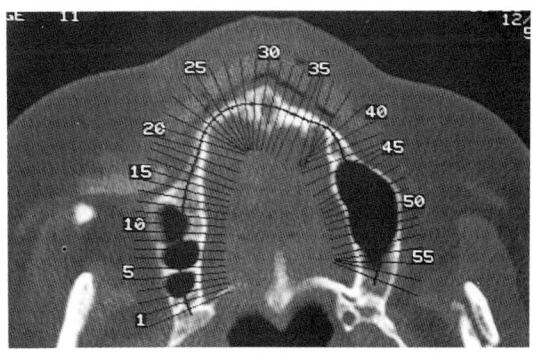

12a

Figs 12a to d   CT-Dentascan demonstrating potential implant receptor sites.

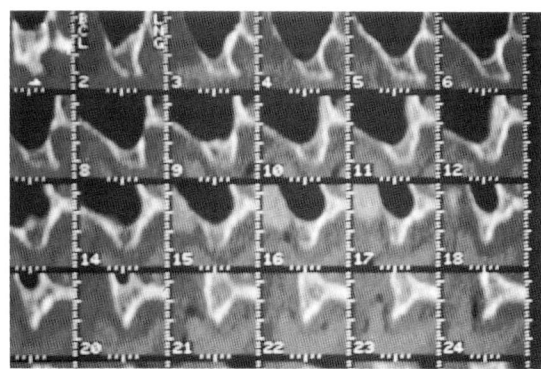

12b

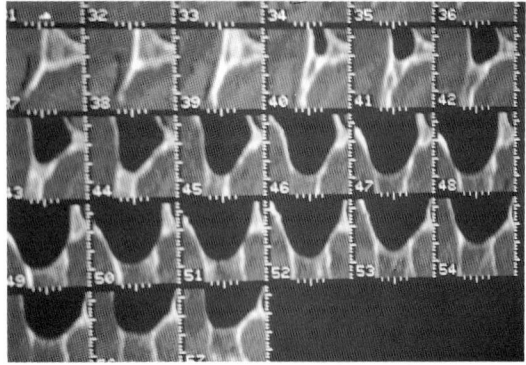

12c

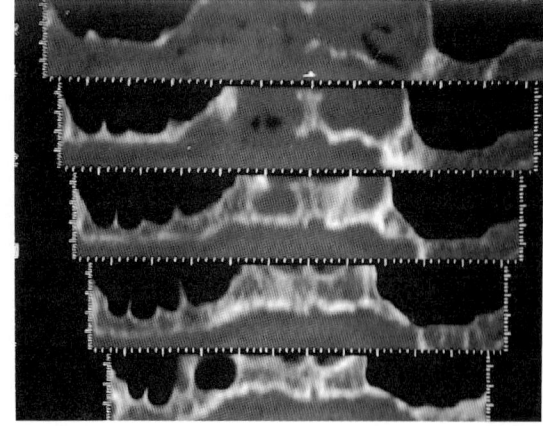

12d

Conclusion

This series of cases demonstrates the potential for defining the three-dimensional configuration of possible implant receptor sites in severely compromised individuals. The use of three-dimensional CT-Dentascan with three-dimensional reformation and two-stage osseointegrated implants has permitted us to treat patients who may not have realized successful results without this advanced technology.

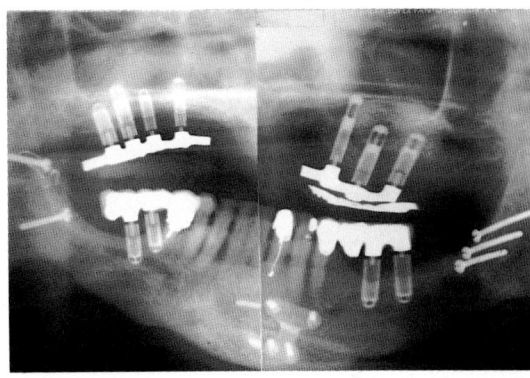

Fig 13 Postreconstruction panoramic radiograph demonstrating completed reconstruction.

References

1. Babbush CA. *Surgical Atlas of Dental Implant Techniques*. Philadelphia: WB Saunders Co, 1980.
2. Berland LL. *Practical CT: Technology and Techniques*. New York: Raven Press, 1987, pp 1–265.
3. Engstrom H, Svendsen, P. Computed tomography of the maxilla in edentulous patients. *Oral Surg Oral Med Oral Pathol* 1981;52:557–560.
4. McGivney GP, Haughton V, Strandt JA, Eichholz JE, Lubar DM. A comparison of computer-assisted tomography and data gathering modalities in prosthodontics. *Int J Oral Maxillofac Implants* 1986;1:55–68.
5. Schwarz MS, Rothman SLG, Rhodes ML, Chafetz N. Computed tomography: Part I. Preoperative assessment of the mandible for endosseous implant surgery. *Int J Oral Maxillofac Implants* 1987;2:137–141.
6. Schwarz MS, Rothman SLG, Rhodes ML, Chafetz N. Computed tomography: Part II. Preoperative assessment of the maxilla for endosseous implant surgery. *Int J Oral Maxillofac Implants* 1987;2:143–148.
7. Shimura MS, Babbush CA, Majima H, Yanagisawa S, Sairenji E. Presurgical evaluation for dental implants using a reformatting program of computed tomography: Maxilla/mandible shape pattern analysis (MSPA). *Int J Oral Maxillofac Implants* 1990;5:175–181.
8. Babbush CA, Kirsch A, Mentag PJ, Hill B. Intermobile cylinder (IMZ) two-stage osteointegrated implant system with the intramobile element (IME) Part I. Its rationale and procedure for use. *Int J Oral Maxillofac Impants* 1987;2:203–216.

Nasal Inlay Bone Graft Technique

K.W. Higuchi

In the past, bone graft augmentation of the resorbed edentulous maxilla has involved various onlay techniques, or has utilized an interpositional graft in conjunction with the Le Fort I osteotomy. A number of authors have addressed this area of reconstruction.[1–6]

Advanced or extreme resorption following long-term edentulism appears to be the most common indication for augmentation procedures. While a number of patients have benefitted from a variety of onlay and interpositional grafts of autogenous bone, clinical results were often disappointing. Significant surgical morbidity, early and progressive graft resorption, compromised prosthesis function and stability, and limited patient satisfaction were frequently associated with these procedures.

Since 1978, Brånemark has pioneered the use of corticocancellous onlay graft augmentation with simultaneous fixture placement for patients having extreme resorption. His long-term results have proven to be very favorable with stable and successful implant-anchored prostheses in 90% of the patients observed (Table 1).

However, this effective method does have some attendant general disadvantages. A relatively high patient morbidity at operation and donor sites occurs primarily because of the generous exposure needed to harvest the horseshoe-shaped graft, and to secure soft tissue closure over it. Necessary inpatient hospitalization with the use of operating room and general anesthesia increases financial costs. The onlay augmentation requires that the patient refrain from using a maxillary prosthesis for at least 4 to 6 weeks after graft and fixture placement. Following that period of time, a new denture intended for cosmetic purposes only can be fabricated, with the patient remaining on a nonchewing diet for the next 6 months. These practical and financial considerations may be unacceptable for certain patients. As a variation of the full onlay graft, bone grafting into the nasal floor was first utilized by this author in 1986. The material for this paper has been adapted from a chapter on the same topic in a forthcoming surgical textbook edited by Worthington and Brånemark (*Advanced Osseointegration Surgery;* Quintessence Publ Co, 1992). My purpose is to focus on surgical rationale and technique.

Nasal inlay bone graft concepts

To add dimensional thickness to a flattened surface, material may theoretically be added to either the superior or inferior aspects. The superior surface of the maxilla or nasal floor provides an enclosed environment within the nasal cavity and is protected from the normal loading forces of a maxillary prosthesis. Surgical access to the region is good, and the necessary amount of graft material is less than that required for onlay augmentation. The limiting anatomic structures of the edentulous anterior maxilla include the location and configuration of the incisive foramen, nasal cavity, and the anterior margins of the maxillary sinuses. The average mediolateral width of each piriform aperture is approximately 10 mm from septum to the lateral extent of the piriform opening. A thin lip of bone several millimeters wide defines each opening, extends above the nasal floor, and shields the lateral extent of aperture. Bell[7] has observed that typically there is between 5 to 9 mm of space between the nasal floor and the level of the inferior turbinates. Years of experience with Le Fort I superior repositioning has indicated that maxillary intrusion has not significantly interfered with clinical airway resistance.

Surgical technique

Surgical exposure to accommodate grafting to the nasal floor is less than that needed for onlay augmentation. To accommodate the resorbed vertical anterior maxilla, a modified Le Fort I incision is used to develop a mucoperiosteal flap to expose the residual maxillary ridge and piriform apertures. The nasal mucosa is reflected intact off the floor of the nose and medial and lateral bony margins. Access to the nasal floor is improved by reducing the lipped rim with Kerrison bone forceps to just above the nasal floor and mediolaterally to accept the width of the graft. At this time, it seems prudent to recommend that a minimum of 4 to 5 mm of residual maxillary bone height be present to serve as anchorage for the securing fixtures.

A corticocancellous bone graft is then harvested from the medial table and crest of the hip, or alternately from the mandibular symphysis. The graft dimensions are approximately 8 × 10 mm, and between 6 to 10 mm in thickness, depending upon the donor site anatomy. If the graft is taken from the hip, a portion of iliac crest is obtained, leaving the lateral table of the crest intact. This will permit a compact bone surface facing anteriorly when the graft is to the nasal floor. While the quality and quantity of bone obtained from the hip may be superior to that from the symphysis, mandibular bone can be harvested and placed on an outpatient basis.

Table 1 Grafted maxillary cases (P-I Brånemark)*

	After 1 year	At present
Bridge	73 (75%)	72 (74%)
Overdenture	15 (15%)	16 (16%)
Denture	9 (9%)	9 (9%)
Total patients	97	97

*Observation time: 1.5 to 11 years, from June 1978 to June 1990.

Table 2 Nasal floor bone grafts (Spokane and Mayo Clinic)

Number of patients	10
Fixtures placed into grafts	20
Fixtures uncovered	18
Fixtures removed	0
Observation time	1.5 to 4.0 years

Using low-speed drilling, two rectangular osteotomies are made through the lateral cortex to, but not including, the inner lingual cortex. The graft segments are removed with thin osteotomes. They are then transferred directly to the prepared nasal floor recipient sites and positioned so that the cancellous surfaces are against the nasal floor and the cortical sides oppose the mucosa. The grafts are then stabilized with firm downward pressure during drilling and fixture placement. Additional conventional fixture placement may be possible in other regions of the maxilla prior to soft tissue closure. Following suture removal in 7 to 10 days, the complete denture prosthesis may be adjusted and temporarily relined to allow for usage and a soft diet. The number and location of osseointegrated fixtures will determine the ultimate design of the prosthesis, either fixed or removable.

Preliminary results

Combined results from the Spokane Center for Tissue Integrated Reconstruction and the Mayo Clinic are presented as preliminary data (Table 2).

The number of patients treated using nasal inlay bone grafting in conjunction with fixture placement have been limited. While early results are encouraging, it must be emphasized that additional long-term assessment is required before nasal floor bone grafting is considered more than investigational.

References

1. MacIntosh RB, Obwegeser HL. Preprosthetic surgery: A scheme for its effective employment. *J Oral Surg* 1967;25:397.

2. Terry BC, Albright JE, Baker RD. Alveolar ridge augmentation in the edentulous maxilla with the use of autogenous ribs. *J Oral Surg* 1974;32:429–434.

3. Farrell CD, Kent JN, Guerra LR. One-stage interpositional bone grafting and vestibuloplasty of the atrophic maxilla. *J Oral Surg* 1976;34:901–906.

4. Male AJ, Gasser J, Fonseca RJ, Nelson J. Comparison of onlay autologous and allogeneic bone grafts to the maxilla in primates. *J Oral Maxillofac Surg* 1983; 42:487–499.

5. Kahnberg KE, Nyström E, Bartholdsson L. Combined use of bone grafts and Brånemark fixtures in the treatment of severely resorbed maxillae. *Int J Oral Maxillofac Implants* 1989;4:297–304.

6. Starshak TJ, Sanders B. *Preprosthetic oral and maxillofacial surgery.* St Louis: CV Mosby Co, 1980.

7. Bell WH, Proffit WR, White RP. *Surgical Corrections of Dentofacial Deformities,* vol 1. Philadelphia: WB Saunders Co, 1980.

Immediate Placement of Osseointegrating Implants Into the Maxillary Sinus Augmented With Mineralized Cancellous Allograft and Gore-Tex: Second-Stage Surgical and Histological Findings

O.T. Jensen and R. Greer

Posterior maxillary placement of dental implants has been complicated by deficiencies in both bone quality and quantity,[1] prominent sinus anatomy or sinus disease,[2] difficult surgical or prosthetic access,[3,4] perforation into the sinus cavity with increased epithelial downgrowth or infection potential,[5] high bite force requirements,[6–8] and difficult oral hygiene maintenance.[9]

Zarb described the posterior maxilla as the most problematic area (zone II) in the jaws for treatment with osseointegrating implants because of morphologically compromised surgical and prosthetic demands.[10] In Adell's 15-year study, the highest proportional incidence of fixture loss occurred in the posterior maxilla.[11]

Sinus or nasal penetration has been reported to reduce success rates about 10%.[5] Because of bone deficiency in the posterior maxilla, endosseous implants have been avoided or the subperiosteal implant has been advocated.[12,13]

To improve posterior maxillary jaw morphology, various augmentation procedures have been advocated and include: iliac, rib, or allograft alveolar augmentation grafting[14–16]; Le Fort I downgraft[17,18]; titanium cribs with iliac graft; collagen tubes with iliac graft; maxillary alveolar split with autograft; or alloplast, composite alloplast autograft combinations.[19] Breine and Brånemark recommended immediate or delayed iliac grafts with rigid fixation by implants that could be used for prosthetic anchors.[20] Most all of these maxillary grafting procedures have focused on the anterior maxilla. Until sinus bone grafting procedures were developed over the past decade, endosseous implants were seldom placed into zone II.[21]

Subsequently, multiple grafting regimens have been used to augment the sinus floor. These include the use of tricalcium phosphate, hydroxyapatite,[22] maxillary osseous autograft and xenograft,[23] resorbable hydroxyapatite, iliac onlay or inlay corticocancellous graft,[24] demineralized freeze-dried bone,[25] composite or combination grafts, and mandibular grafts to the sinus using alveolus, chin, ramus, or coronoid process.[26]

The biological basis for osseous incorporation in the maxillary sinus area has not been well studied, especially in regard to allografting independent of alloplasts, xenografts, or autografts. The use of nonresorbable hydroxyapatite alone is not described in the literature despite clinical reports of success, and has been criticized as being of modest value in participating in implant integration.[22,27]

There appears to be a better biological basis for the maxillary downgraft procedure. Studies have shown autograft or allograft alone to produce significant sinus floor augmentation, ie, increased alveolar height in *Macaca fascicularis*[28,29] and in humans.[15,16]

Histological studies examining sinus augmentation via the Cardwell-Luc sinus membrane lift approach have not been published extensively in the literature. Whittaker recently reported an 8-month postsurgical human autopsy specimen that had combined demineralized allograft and bovine resorbable hydroxyapatite placed in the sinus simultaneously with titanium screw-form implants. The implants were never loaded but appeared to be integrated histologically.[23] Block and Kent used immediate hydroxyapatite-coated implant placement with cancellous iliac autograft.[25]

Despite the greater certainty of iliac autograft incorporation, the sinus graft requirement is not always conducive to harvesting bone from the ilium for various preferential or medical reasons. The purpose of this paper is to discuss clinical experience from the past 4 years with various sinus graft techniques and report recent findings accumulated over the past 18 months using a Gore-Tex (W.L. Gore and Associates, Flagstaff, Ariz) membrane barrier placed laterally over the antroplasty site.

Materials and methods

Patients who presented with atrophic edentulous posterior maxillary ridges were selected for inclusion in the clinical study. Most patients' teeth had been restored with partial or complete dentures. All patients had lost their teeth through periodontal disease and/or dental caries. Patients were screened for medical conditions including chronic sinus disease, diabetes, and tobacco abuse. No medical contraindications were found in any patient included in the study.

Jaw and sinus morphology was analyzed using computed axial tomography (CAT) scans and panoramic and periapical radiographs. Prospective implant sites were selected and classified with respect to available bone mass.[30] Most sites were identified as either Class B (7 to 9 mm) or Class C (3 to 6 mm) based on vertical measurement. Class D sites (>3 mm) were also selected.

Preoperative medications included either amoxicillin 500 mg or cephalexin (Keflex) 500 mg administered orally 1 to 2 hours prior to surgery. Betadine facial and chlorhexidine oral preparations were made. The local anesthetic used was 2% lidocaine with 1:100,000 epinephrine and nerve block, and infiltration procedures were utilized. Most patients were treated with

intravenous sedation using midazolam and nalbuphine. A few patients were operated on under general anesthesia. Two patients received local anesthesia only.

The first-stage surgery consisted of a full-thickness degloving of the residual alveolar process and the lateral posterior maxilla. A palato-crestal incision was made from the canine area posteriorly and extended to vertical-releasing incisions in the tuberosity and canine fossa areas. The entire flap was freed and dissected so that the lateral maxilla could be well visualized, providing access to the maxillary antrum. The antrum was usually translucent through the thin cortical plate of bone.

Access to the sinus membrane was usually made a few millimeters above the inferior extent of the translucency or just above the sinus floor using a high torque rotary drill with a small round bur. At high speed, a sinus window was cut through the bone approximately 8 to 10 mm × 10 to 15 mm in size, starting near the height of contour of the maxillary zygomatic buttress. Care was taken to avoid perforation through the sinus membrane when developing the osteotomies. The osteotomies were generally incompletely cut with the drill and completed with hand instrumentation. After the plate of bone was freed of bony attachment, but still attached to the sinus membrane, the sinus lining was stripped broadly within the sinus to include the inferior, lateral, anterior, nasal, and sometimes posterior walls. The freed plate of lateral bone that remained attached to the sinus membrane was transferred superiorly in the sinus to provide a roof for the graft and implants. Any small perforations were not sutured but instead collapsed in on themselves via dissection of adjacent adherent sinus membrane (Figs 1a and b and 2a and b).

Two to four Brånemark (Nobelpharma USA, Inc, Chicago, Ill) implants 13 to 15 mm in length were placed through the alveolar process according to a previously fabricated guide splint. If monocortical stabilization was achieved, the implant was retained; if not, it was removed. Occasionally bicortical stabilization occurred via the lateral nasal wall, canine fossa, or tuberosity

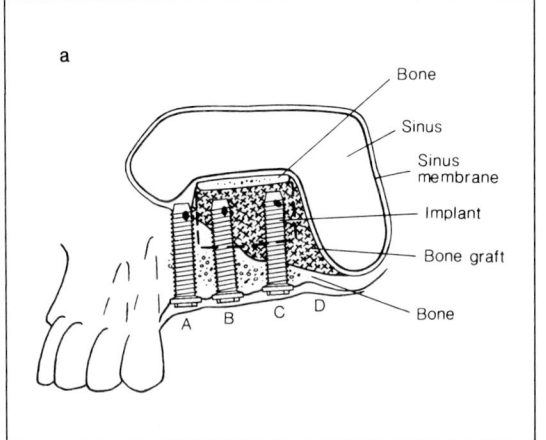

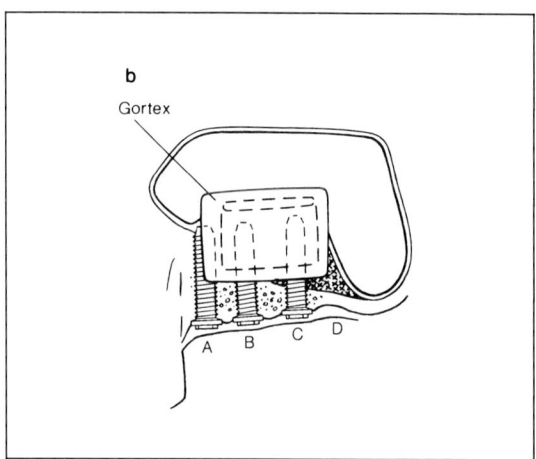

Fig 1a A lateral view of the posterior maxilla showing the sinus window held superiorly by graft material and fixtures. The site class is designated for each implant site based on available residual bone. The Class D site has inadequate bone for implant stabilization.

Fig 1b Following grafting and implantation, a Gore-Tex filter is placed over the osteotomy site.

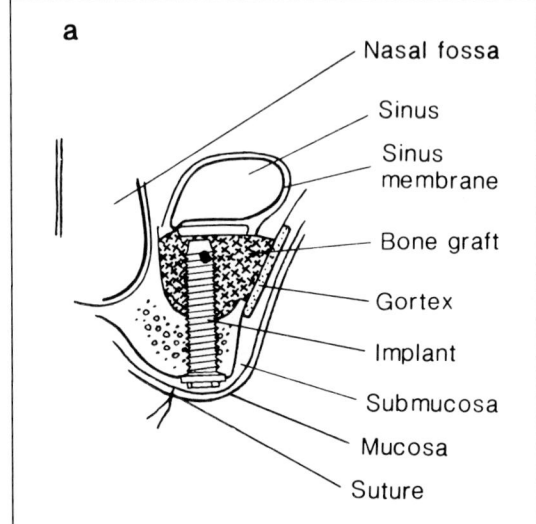

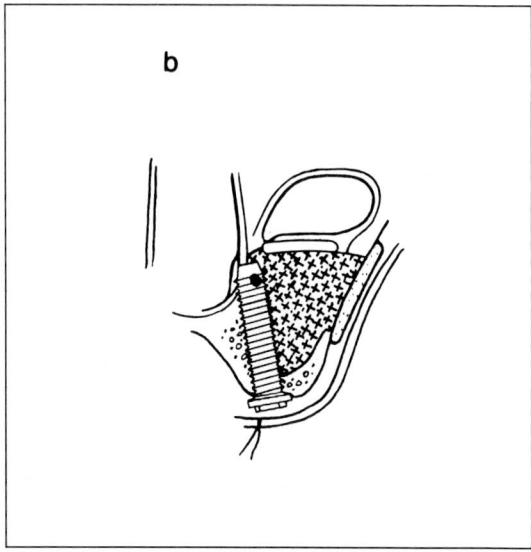

Fig 2a A coronal view through the posterior maxilla in the area of the antrum demonstrating the "lifted" sinus membrane, the subsinus grafting, monocortical implant location, lateral Gore-Tex membrane position, and suture location.

Fig 2b Bicortical stabilization can occur in highly resorbed ridges in the premolar regions with the lateral nasal wall, pyriform rim, or sinus buttress.

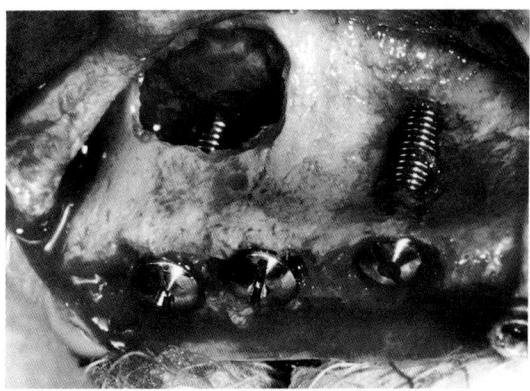

Fig 3a Three implants are placed into the sinus via sinus antrostomy with the lateral plate of bone transposed within the sinus to the superior wall of the defect. The sinus membrane is dissected from the sinus walls, taking care to avoid perforation. Implants are placed as planned prosthetically.

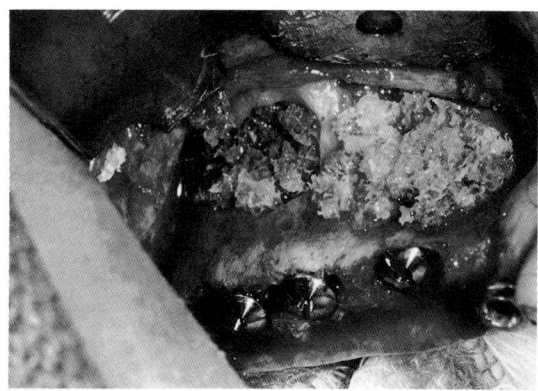

Fig 3b Mineralized allogeneic cancellous bone chips are packed into the sinus around the implants and the cavity is overfilled laterally. The dehisced implant is also grafted.

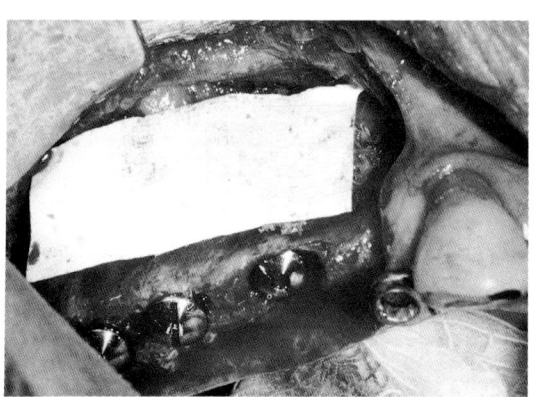

Fig 3c A Gore-Tex membrane is placed over the graft site and the wound is closed primarily.

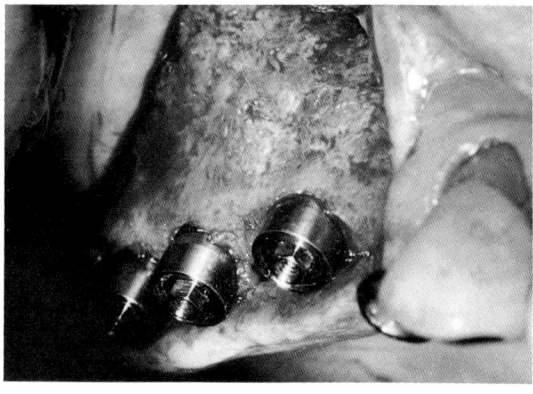

Fig 3d Six months later the Gore-Tex membrane is removed. Marked osseous filling of the defect is observed.

bone (Fig 2). Unusual or abnormal sinus variations including septal and buttress points were infrequently encountered.

The implants were usually not countersunk so as to preserve cortical engagement. In a few instances the alveolus was relatively hypertrophic vertically and required reduction with loss of the cortical crest of the aveolus. All fixtures used were self-tapping. Cover screws were seldom used, depending upon the profile prominence of the fixture.

Following fixture placement, various graft materials were used to fill the newly created subsinus cavity, including iliac autograft, demineralized freeze-dried bone powder or cancellous chips, radiated mineralized cancellous allograft, and maxillary alveolar autograft. No alloplast or xenogeneic materials were used. Cancellous graft material was generally cut into fine pieces or injected and packed into the subsinus cavity around the implants as densely as possible. Cortical graft material was not used.

The subsinus was overpacked a few millimeters laterally and one group of patients then had a Gore-Tex filter placed using augmentation material (GTAM; W.L. Gore, Flagstaff, Ariz) that covered the grafted defect by at least 2 or 3 mm on all sides. Gore-Tex filters were generally cut to sizes of about 10 to 12 mm × 14 to 18 mm. Gore-Tex membranes were placed initially in odd-numbered cases during the early phases of the study and in all patients as determined by clinical impression in the later phase of the study (Figs 3a to d).

Patients were instructed not to wear overdenture prostheses for 1 month or not at all following surgery and to follow a soft diet protocol. All patients were also instructed not to blow their noses for 10 days after surgery. Allograft patients were kept on antibiotics for 3 weeks, and decongestants were used in most situations for a few days postoperatively. The patients were asked to use oral chlorohexidine rinses for 7 to 10 days after surgery. Radiographs were taken immediately following surgery and at the 6-month exposure appointment.

Six months after the first surgery, the implants were exposed and 3-mm abutments were placed. The lateral wall of the maxilla was exposed for removal of the Gore-Tex membrane and/or direct observation of the antroplasty site. A 3-mm trephine drill was used to remove a biopsy core of bone vertically, parallel to the axis of the implants. This was done in the first molar region and sent to the laboratory for decalcification and histological analysis usng hematoxylin and eosin stain.

A provisional loading scheme was used in which the final prosthesis or overdenture restoration was delayed in some patients up to 6 months after exposure of the implants. However, in other patients soft-lined overdentures were used immediately after exposure so that no single early loading protocol was possible.

Results

Fifteen patients with 26 sinus grafts were treated with 74 implants during a 2½-year development period by immediate placement of implants into grafted maxillary sinuses (Table 1).

Of the 26 first-stage surgeries, there were no immediate postoperative infections. Three patients had sinusitis develop within the first 2 months of surgery. All were successfully treated with antibiotics.

Almost all patients had some wound dehiscence at the palatocrestal margin of the wound (Fig 4). The areas of wound breakdown were generally 1 to 3 mm in width and rarely led to healed exposure of the cover screws. In one patient, a 10-mm dehiscence developed and the cover screws became exposed and remained so throughout the healing phase. In three sinus graft sites the dehiscence led to exposure of the Gore-Tex filter at and fistulation of the allograft occurred, requiring removal of the Gore-Tex filter at 3 weeks in two patients and at 4 weeks in an additional patient.

In three patients who wore metal-based partial dentures against natural dentition, late (2 to 3 months postsurgery) dehiscence of the cover screws or implants occurred and implant mobility developed, preventing integration and leading to loss of the implants.

By the 6-month exposure date, no patient had sinus symptoms or oral discomfort; however, five patients had exposed implants or cover screws, two from early wound dehiscence and three from overdenture trauma.

Of the 15 patients, 7 wore no provisional restoration during the healing phase. In the group that wore provisional overdentures of various types, 18 of 42 implants were not integrated at the time of exposure or lost integration within the first few months of exposure.

At the exposure operation, there were differences in the clinical findings of the osteotomy sites depending on the treatment rendered. Those patients treated with Gore-Tex and mineralized allograft showed clinically dense bone laterally. The lateral bony anatomy was found to be outpouched and protruded to the extent of the previous graft overfill and conformed intimately to the Gore-Tex membrane cover (Figs 5a to c). No instance of fibrous tissue clefting or intrabony scarring was evident. In one patient the Gore-Tex was removed

Table 1 Results of 2½-year study of 15 patients treated with 74 implants placed into grafted maxillary sinuses

Pt.	Site class	No. implants	Success	Sinus perforation	Restored	Gore-Tex	Graft material	Biopsy	Provisional denture
1 (WW)	BBB	3	3	Yes	FB	Yes	RMCA	Good	No
2 (RG)	BCC	6	6	No/Yes	FB	Yes	RMCA	Good	No
3 (BK)	BCC	3	3	No	FB	Yes	RMCA	Good	No
4 (FB)	CCC CCC	6	5	No	FB	No	RMCA	Good	Yes
5 (LJ)	BCC CCC	6	6	No	FB	Yes	RMCA	Good	Yes
6 (RG)	BCD	3	2	No	FB	No	RMCA	Poor	No
7 (BC)	BDC	3	2	No	FB	No	RMCA	Fair	No
8 (HH)	CD	2	1	Yes	Prov	Yes(infect)	RMCA	Fair	No
9 (FG)	CCC CCC	6	2	No	Prov	No	RMCA	Fair	Yes
10 (MC)	CCCC	4	4	Yes	OD	No	DCA	N/A	Yes
11 (CT)	CDD CDD	6	2	Yes	Fail	Yes	DCA	Poor	Yes
12 (ML)	CDD CCC	6	2	Yes	Fail	Yes(infect)	DCA	Poor	Yes
13 (FL)	CDC CCD	6	4	No	Fail	No	DCA	Poor	Yes
14 (JHe)	CCD CCC	6	0	No	Fail	No	AA	Poor	Yes
15 (JHa)	DDD DD	5	5	No	OD	No	IA	Good	(At 3 months)

FB = fixed bridge; Prov = provisional prosthesis; OD = overdenture; RMCA = radiated mineralized cancellous allograft; DCA = demineralized cancellous allograft; AA = alveolar autograft; IA = iliac autograft.

at 4 weeks after the initial surgery because of inflammation. Outpouching of bone was not present and scarification had occurred at the osteotomy site. When the Gore-Tex was in place the entire 6-month period, all 21 implants placed had integrated.

In the three patients who experienced infections associated with Gore-Tex filters, which were removed, four of eight implants had integrated: one of two in mineralized graft and three of seven in demineralized graft.

Ten patients treated with irradiated mineralized bone graft (Rocky Mountain Transplant Bank, Denver, Colo) in 15 sinus grafts received 41 implants placed with and without Gore-Tex filters. These patients had nine implant failures, with eight of those failures occurring within the non–Gore-Tex group and the additional failure occurring within the infected Gore-Tex group.

When a mineralized bone graft was used without a Gore-Tex membrane, greater scarring appeared to be present on gross examination of the osteotomy site.

One 41-year-old patient was treated without immediate placement of implants and without Gore-Tex filters. In this patient radiated mineralized allograft was used as a graft, but minimal bone formation was found on biopsy 7 months after surgery.

Patients treated with demineralized bone (Mile High Tissue Bank, Denver, Colo) with or without Gore-Tex filters did poorly. Only 10 of 22 implants were firm at the time of exposure. All bone specimens were clinically soft and appeared poorly mineralized at the time of trephine biopsy.

Two patients were treated with autografts. One patient had six implants placed within the

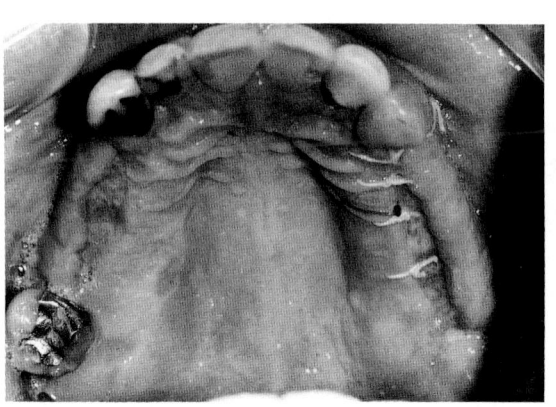

Fig 4 Flap dehiscence in a patient treated with allograft antroplasties.

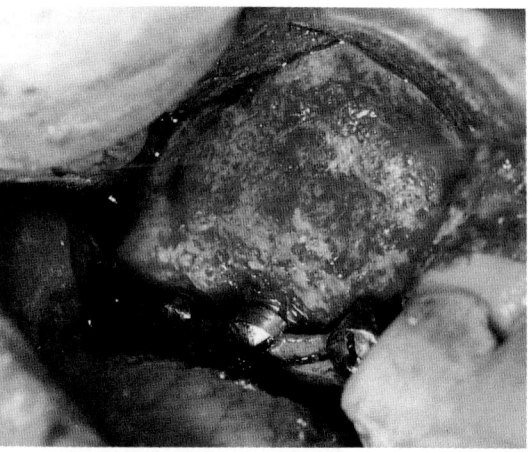

Fig 5a The contrasting finding in another patient treated with immediate implant placement, mineralized allograft, and Gore-Tex. Note the marked evagination of the lateral maxilla and highly vascular clinically firm bone.

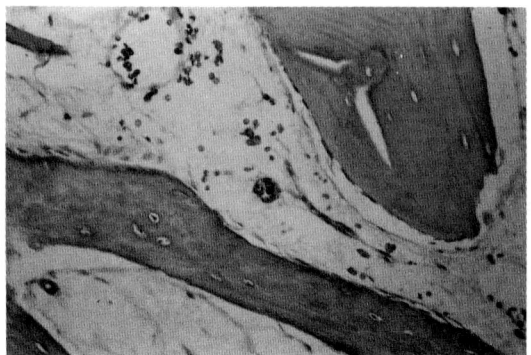

Fig 5b Viable woven bone is set in a loose reticular fibrofatty collagen and marrow. Dilated vascular channels are prominent throughout the supporting stroma.

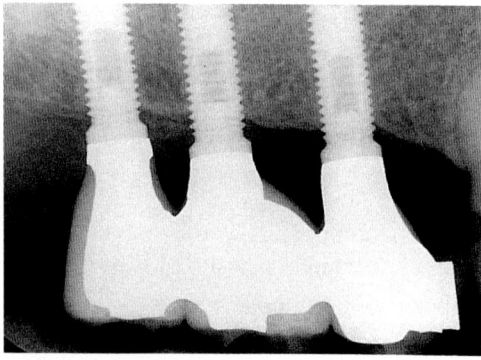

Fig 5c Periapical radiograph taken 14 months after implant placement.

sinus using grafted maxillary alveolar bone that was hypertrophic and had reduced interarch distance significantly. All six implants had compromised integration. One implant was dislodged into the sinus 2 months after exposure by overdenture compression and required surgical retrieval. All six implants eventually failed. The second patient was treated with an autograft (iliac corticocancellous) and five implants, which had all integrated.

Six patients had small perforations of 2 mm or less in the sinus membrane at the time of stage-one surgery. Two patients had blood flow from the nasal fossa following surgery, indicating a probable communication in 8 of 26 sinus grafted cases. Of the eight patients, two were in the group of three patients who had sinusitis 3 weeks beyond surgery.

Of the patients who experienced sinus perforations, there appeared to be no direct corretion to implant success or failure according to position nearest the perforation site. Four of the eight patients had all implants integrate. In the remaining four patients, other contributing reasons for nonintegration were apparent, ie, poor site selection, type of graft material used, or Gore-Tex filters not used.

Discussion

The histological findings for the mineralized bone graft Gore-Tex membrane group showed a fairly consistent bone fill, with the most common feature being immature woven bone with focal areas of lamellar compaction present in a loose trabecular pattern consistent with maxillary alveolar bone (Figs 6a and b). Tetracycline bone markers indicated a viable physiological process with graft incorporation and remodeling occurring.

No biopsy specimen was taken with an implant surface intact. Therefore, integration can only be inferred by the lack of poorly differentiated fibrous reparative tissue. However, in most specimens there were small areas devoid of bone that healed over by fibrous repair.

Radiographic findings for the radiated mineralized group indicated a fairly consistent trabecular bone pattern similar to adjacent maxillary bone (Fig 5c). The demineralized cases appeared highly radiolucent or almost devoid of bone (Figs 7a and b). Many of the implant sites appeared to have lost at least a millimeter of bone at the crest of the ridge probably because of avascular necrosis from periosteal stripping (Fig 5c).

Implants that were placed in Class B sites were most successful. All of these implants were clinically firm at the time of exposure even in the demineralized cases. Of the Class C implant failures, 6 of 15 were in radiated bone graft without Gore-Tex; the rest were in demineralized bone. All of the Class D sites failed except for the iliac graft situation in which all five implants succeeded (Fig 7a).

Grouping all of the implants together regardless of technique, there were 74 implants immediately placed into the sinus using various grafting materials. Ten implants were placed into Class B sites, 47 implants were placed into Class C sites, and 17 implants were placed into Class D sites. There were no failures in the Class B sites. Fifteen of 47 failures occurred in the Class C sites and 12 of 17 failures occurred in Class D sites.

The technique of using immediate implant placement with mineralized allograft and Gore-Tex membrane evolved based on trial and error in an attempt to treat the posterior edentulous maxilla without resorting to iliac graft surgery. The integration of an implant into the grafted area in the sinus is, however, not proven by this study.

There are four questions of theoretical and practical importance based on these clinical and historical results: *(1)* Is immediate implant placement in a sinus graft site favorable for graft incorporation? *(2)* What type of graft material is best for the sinus bone graft? *(3)* Is the Gore-Tex barrier of significance or is its function only a surface phenomenon? *(4)* To what extent does site selection or deferred loading benefit implant survival?

Immediate implant placement

There is no theoretical precedent for immediate placement of an endosseous implant into allograft. Implants placed with iliac cancellous autograft have been successful both immediately and after a period of time.[20] However, reports of procedures incorporating allograft and the immediate placement of implants are lacking in the literature.

Immediate placement of implants into the graft bed may serve as a stimulus or vehicle during the course of graft consolidation. Wolff's law would suggest that the functional state of the sinus graft is proportional to the structure and architectural persistence of the graft.

It has been shown that a sinus inlay graft with immediate implant placement led to incorpora-

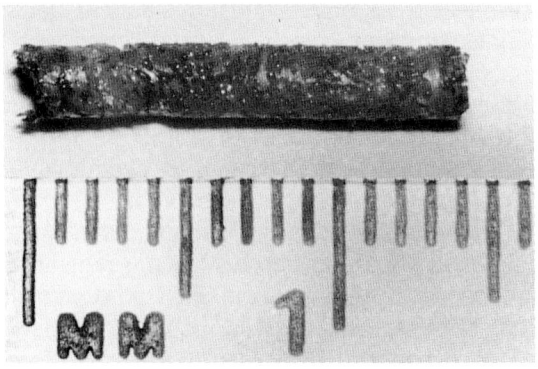

Fig 6a A 3-mm trephine biopsy specimen at the first molar area shows a 15-mm core of clinically firm bone.

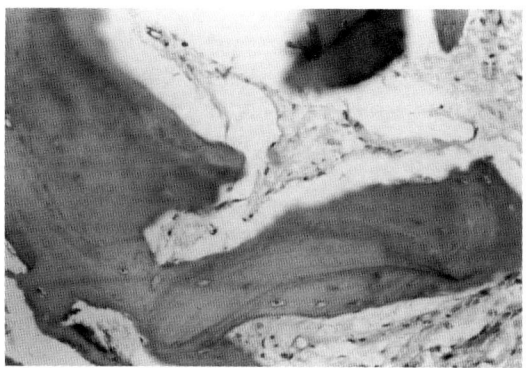

Fig 6b Lamellar bone is surrounded by reticular collagen, endothelial cells, and dilated vascular spaces (hematoxylin-eosin, original magnification ×120).

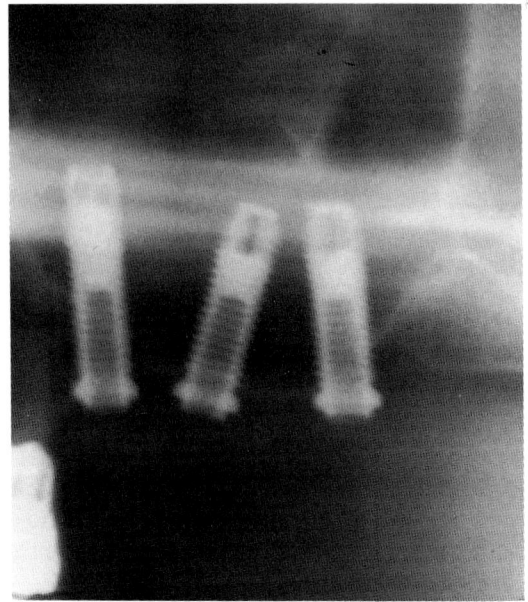

Fig 7a Class C and D sites treated with demineralized graft. Radiographic view is 6 months after grafting. Note loss of stabilization of middle implant. The distal two implants were not integrated.

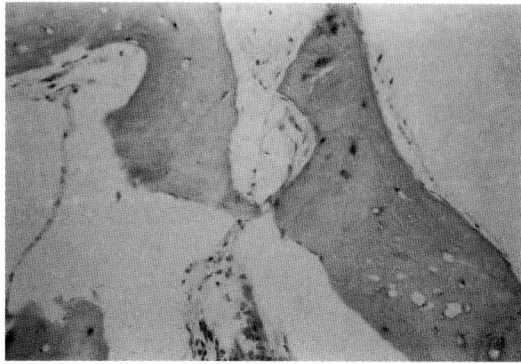

Fig 7b Poor quality bone is seen in woven fragments with thin peripheral supporting strands of fibrillar collagen.

tion and preservation of the graft, whereas onlay or inlay techniques not later treated with fixture placement led to loss of the graft.[20]

Despite leaving the implant submerged and undisturbed for several months, load is transferred to the implants through an elastic flexion of the maxillary bone under occlusal function. Enneking found that in canine fibulae treated with cortical autograft, physiologic stress led to more complete graft incorporation and repair.[31] The union of the graft-host junction appeared to be the trigger for the appositional phase in graft repair and determined the final admixture of necrotic and viable bone. He also observed better graft incorporation in those animals that were more active and placed greater stress on the graft. The question of whether or not small flexion loads within the maxilla are transferred via implants through the sinus graft serving as favorable modeling stimuli following the demineralization phase remains unproven.

In the single patient treated with mineralized allograft without implant placement, ossification of the graft failed to occur sufficiently enough for a drilling procedure to be performed. The failed graft required removal. The presence of implants did not sufficiently affect demineralized allograft induction for mechanical stabilization of an implant to occur (Figs 7a and b).

The basis for immediate placement of implants into the maxillary sinus when the graft is placed needs to be studied further to determine if there is a measurable effect on the ossification process, vis-à-vis a vehicular or stimulus to function.

Graft materials

The type of graft material appeared to be the most important of all the variables tested clinically. The favored graft material for sinus augmentation is the iliac graft with or without immediate implant placement. Unfortunately, use of the iliac graft is proscribed for many reasons, including surgeon and patient preference, insurance or financial reasons, or orthopedic or medical reasons. The need for developing an allograft, alloplast, or xenograft substitute for dental implant reconstruction is widely recognized.

Miller reports that 69% of orthopedic surgeons and 55% of directors of orthopedic surgery programs use allografts.[32] For dental indications, the use of the ileum as a graft site is much more limited if not eschewed.

Many of the various allograft and alloplast materials have been used with some measure of success in the posterior maxilla. Hydroxyapatite has been used as a carrier vehicle to assist in bone conduction.[33] Successful subsinal placement of a hydroxyapatite implant in conjunction with the placement of titanium implants where there is sufficient osseous structure to obtain integration independent of the graft has been accomplished without the addition of allograft. However, implant surgeons frequently use a combination of allograft and hydroxyapatite.

Ripamonti used autolyzed antigen extracted allogeneic (AAA) bone and Interpore (Interpore International, Irvine, Calif) in rat pouches, and showed that the Interpore delayed or inhibited differentiation of bone.[34] He found evidence of giant cells and macrophages with only 26% of the graft in the 63-day specimens showing calcification compared to 84% when AAA bone was used alone over the same time period. These findings do not support the notion that apatite and the allograft complement each other via conducive and inductive synergism.

The combined use of xenogeneic hydroxyapatite and demineralized freeze-dried bone has shown greater promise perhaps based on the resorbability of the hydroxyapatite.[23]

The inadequate osseous response in the sinus to demineralized freeze-dried bone, with or without Gore-Tex, appears to contradict findings reported in the periodontal and orthopedic literature.[35]

The inductive advantage of freeze-dried demineralized allograft is well documented and is thought to be the result of greater inductability provided by ready access to the morphogenetic protein fraction. Next to fresh autograft, demineralized freeze-dried bone was best for treating bone defects in experimental studies done by Oikarien.[36] According to Urist, for any bone defect the best allograft inducer is AAA bone because it has demonstrated the greatest ability to differentiate mesenchymal cells into osteoblasts in the presence of growth cofactors.[37–39]

Sampath and co-workers isolated a purified protein bone inducer derived from demineralized bovine bone, which they termed osteogenin.[40] Osteogenin was the only growth cofactor that produced calcification in vivo when placed in contact with insoluble bone matrix.

Use of a demineralized product would delay the incorporation process by osteoclastic activity so as to get to inducer proteins within the calcified tissue. A mineralized graft would require greater "work" by the host and empirically would be an inherent disadvantage to the host modeling response.

Use of the radiated mineralized allograft was thought to have other disadvantages besides delayed osteogenesis because of radiation denaturation of the bone morphogenetic protein, increased antigenicity, greater potential for viral contamination, and increased incidence of sequestration, infection, or rejection of the graft.

Burchardt showed in two separate studies that segmental mineralized allografts in azanthroprine-immunosuppressed dogs revascularized and incorporated less in 8 months than in 1 month for fresh autograft.[41] He observed weak incorporation, fatigue fractures, and very little internal remodeling with the mineralized allograft. Independent of the immunological consequences, these findings demonstrated a very poor graft performance when used in a segmental or block form.

Hiatt successfully used fresh allograft in cancellous particulate form in treating periodontal osseous defects.[42] The osseous fill was consistent, with only 1 lesion out of 30 not undergoing osseous incorporation with the majority of the defects filling in excess of 80% above controls. Using irradiated (8 megarads) mineralized allograft, Schrad found a 50% greater bone fill in periodontal defects treated with the allograft versus controls.[43]

Schallhorn suggested that radiated allograft has several potential advantages, including adequate grafting material for extensive grafting,

suppressed antigenicity, and accessibility from a bone bank with little fear of disease transfer.[44] The remote possibility of slow virus disease transfer from central nervous system-related tissues such as dura and cornea do not appear to apply to calcified tissues.

The successful use of radiated mineralized allograft in this study is contrary to the anachronistic view that radiation sterilization leads to a loss of inductive capacity and the bone matrix fibrillar network.[45,46]

The success of mineralized allograft in the sinus graft setting may be attributed to carrier (osteoconduction) and residual osteoinduction functions. Since all grafts treated with the mineralized allograft had areas of scarring and poorly differentiated reparative tissue, further investigation is required to determine optimal graft preparation and modem requirements.

Mechanical aspects

The initial mechanical stabilization provided by the threaded titanium implant is paramount. If the implant is not firmly anchored it will not integrate and in these situations there is often only 4 or 5 mm, or less, of bone available to engage.

The use of a screw-form implant provides an advantage over the press fit implants in that it is less likely to be forced into the sinus. A consistent finding in this study was the inability to obtain integration when there less than 3 mm of bone to engage the implant. Implants placed in this setting are particularly vulnerable to prosthetic trauma as well.

The protocol for postexposure loading was based on the suggestion by Roberts that a progressive loading regimen might be helpful to convert less mineralized tissues to better load-bearing bone.[47,48] However, in the orthopedic literature woven bone has been found to be an adequate loading-bearing bone for endosteal implants.

The protocol that evolved in this study for restoration cases was as follows:

1. Exposure of the implants followed by imme-

diate resin or metal prosthesis fabrication with a very narrow occlusal table out of occlusion. This was maintained for 2 to 3 months.

2. The prosthesis was then brought into centric occlusion for an additional 3 months.
3. A final fixed prosthesis was constructed using various restorative materials depending upon the opposing dentition.

When an overdenture was required, the use of a bar-retained resilient liner-based prosthesis was preferred. One of the most important features in successful integration in the posterior maxilla was that the patient wore no provisional overdenture during the incorporation period. The placement of multiple, splinted, relatively long fixtures, carefully loaded and restored postexposure, may all be secondary considerations if the healing period is disturbed mechanically.

Conclusion

Radiated mineralized allograft used in conjunction with maxillary antroplasty, the placement of a screw-form implant, and a Gore-Tex barrier provided the most predictable ossification findings of the sinus graft techniques studied. Demineralized freeze-dried bone alone provided inadequate ossification for the integration of implants, even when Gore-Tex filters were used as a barrier membrane. Both Class B and Class C sites were treated successfully. No Class D sites were treated successfully using allograft.

Patients who wore prostheses during the healing period were much more likely to lose an implant than patients who did not wear a provisional prosthesis. Patients who did not use a progressive loading regimen or splinted implants in the postexposure provisional period were more likely to lose implants.

Overall, preliminary findings indicate that the use of mineralized allograft with a Gore-Tex membrane and immediate implant placement into the sinus may be a viable alternative to iliac autograft treatment in selected cases.

References

1. Lekholm U, Adell R, Brånemark P-I. Possible complications. pp 233–240 In P.-I. Brånemark, G.A. Zarb, T. Albrektsson (eds) *Tissue-Integrated Prostheses: Osseointegration in Clinical Dentistry.* Chicago: Quintessence Publ Co, 1985.
2. Pedersen KN, Huanes HR, Faehn O. Subperiosteal transmucosal porous ceramic titanium implants: Clinical experience from three cases. *Int J Oral Surg* 1979;8:349.
3. Tatum H. Maxillary and sinus implant reconstruction. *Dent Clin North Am* 1986;30:207.
4. Tulasne JF. Implant treatment of missing posterior dentition. pp 103–115 In T. Albrektsson, G.A. Zarb (eds) *The Brånemark Osseointegrated Implant.* Chicago: Quintessence Publ Co, 1989.
5. Brånemark P-I, Adell R, Albrektsson T, Lekholm U, Lindström J, Rockler B. An experimental and clinical study of osseointegrated implants penetrating the nasal cavity and maxillary sinus. *J Oral Maxillofac Surg* 1984;43:497–505.
6. Craig RG. Mechanical properties. pp 60,61 In R.G. Craig (ed) *Restorative Dental Materials.* 6th ed. St Louis: CV Mosby Co, 1980.
7. Haraldson T, Karlsson U, Carlsson GE. Bite force and oral function in complete denture wearers. *J Oral Rehabil* 1979;6:41.
8. Brunski JB. Biomechanics of oral implants: Future research directions. *J Dent Educ* 1988;52:775–787.
9. Meffert RM. The soft tissue interface in dental implantology. *J Dent Educ* 1988;52:811.
10. Zarb GA, Zarb FL, Schmitt A. Osseointegrated implants for partially edentulous patients. *Dent Clin North Am* 1987;31:457–472.
11. Adell R, Lekholm U, Rockler B, et al. Osseointegrated titanium fixtures in the treatment of edentulousness: A 15-year follow-up study. *Int J Oral Surg* 1981;10:387.
12. McKinney RV Jr, Koth DL, Steflik DE. Clinical evaluation standards for dental implants. pp 1–11 In J.F. Hardin (ed) *Clark's Clinical Dentistry.* Philadelphia: JB Lippincott Co, 1984.
13. Golec TS. CAD-CAM Multiple Diagnostic Imaging of Subperiosteal Implants. *Dent Clin North Am* 1986;30:85–89.
14. Terry, BC, Allbright JE, Baker RD. Alveolar ridge augmentation in the edentulous maxilla with the use of autogenous ribs. *J Oral Surg* 1974;32:429.
15. Wolford LM, Epker BN. The use of freeze dried bone as a biologic crib for ridge augmentation: A preliminary report. *Oral Surg* 1977;43:499.
16. Bell WH, Buckles RL. Correction of atrophic alveolar ridge by interpositional bone grafting: A progress report. *J Oral Surg* 1974;32:429.
17. Bell WH, Proffitt WR, White RP. *Surgical Correction of Dentofacial Deformities. vol 1: Maxillary and Midface Deformity.* Philadelphia: WB Saunders Co, 1980, p 493.
18. Bell WH, Fonseca RJ, Kennedy JW, Levey BM. Bone healing and revascularization after total maxillary osteotomy. *J Oral Surg* 1975;33:253.
19. Kent JN, Quinn HH, Zide MF, Guerra LR, Boyne PJ. Alveolar ridge augmentation using nonresorbable hy-

droxylapatite with or without autogenous bone. *J Oral Maxillofac Surg* 1983;41:629–642.

20. Breine U, Brånemark P-I. Reconstruction of alveolar jaw bone. *Scan J Plast Reconstr Surg* 1980;14:23.

21. Boyne PJ, James RA. Grafting of the maxillary sinus floor with autogenous marrow and bone. *J Oral Surg* 1980;38:613.

22. Smiler D, Holmes RE. Sinus lift procedure using porous hydroxyapatite. A preliminary report. *J Oral Implantol* 1987;23:239.

23. Whittaker JM, James RA, Lozada J. Histological response and clinical evaluation of heterograft and allograft materials in the elevation of the maxillary sinus for the preparation of endosteal dental implant sites. Simultaneous sinus elevation and root form implantation: An eight month autopsy report. *J Oral Implantol* 1989;15:141–144.

24. Kahnberg KE, Nystrom E, Bartholdsson L. Combined use of bone grafts and Brånemark fixtures in the treatment of severely resorbed maxillae. *Int J Oral Maxillofac Implants* 1989;4:297–304.

25. Kent J, Block M. Simultaneous maxillary sinus floor bone grafting and placement of hydroxylapatite-coated implants. *J Oral Maxillofac Surg* 1989;47:238–242.

26. Wood RM, Moore DL. Grafting of the maxillary sinus with intraorally harvested autogenous bone prior to implant placement. *Int J Oral Maxillofac Implants* 1988;3:211–214.

27. Jensen O. Allogeneic bone or hydroxylapatite for the sinus lift procedure? *J Oral Maxillofac Surg* 1990;48:771.

28. Stroud SW, Fonseca RJ, Sanders G, Burkes E. Healing of interpositional bone grafts after total maxillary osteotomy. *J Oral Surg* 1980;38:878–885.

29. Frost D, Fonseca RJ, Burkes E. Healing of lypholysed allogeneic bone grafts following total maxillary osteotomies. *J Oral Surg* 1982;40:776–786.

30. Jensen OT. Site classification for the osseointegrated implant. *J Prosthet Dent* 1989;61:228.

31. Enneking WF, Burchardt H, Puhl J, Pioptrowski G. Physical and biological aspects of repair in dog cortical bone transplants. *J Bone Joint Surg* 1975;57A:232.

32. Miller F, Sussman M, Stamp W. The use of bone allograft: A survey of current practice. In *Proceedings of the Scoliosis Research Society. 17th Annual Meeting.* Denver, Colo: University of Colorado Press, 1982.

33. Boyne PJ, Fremming BD, Walsh R, et al. Evaluation of a ceramic hydroxylapatite in femoral defects. *J Dent Res* 1978;57A:108.

34. Ripamonti U, Schnitzler CM, Cleaton-Jones RC. Bone induction in a composite allogeneic bone/alloplastic implant. 1989;47:963.

35. Sepe WW, et al. Clinical evaluation of freeze dried bone allografts in periodontal osseous defects. Part II. *J Periodontol* 1978;49:9.

36. Oikarien J, Kochonen LK. The bone transplant materials used for treatment of experimental bone defects. *Clin Orthop* 1979;140:208.

37. Urist MR. Chemosterilized antigen extracted surface demineralized autolysed allogeneic (AAA) bone for arthrodesis. p 193 In G.E. Friedlander, H.J. Mankin (eds) *Osteochondral Allografts.* Boston: Little, Brown and Co, 1983.

38. Urist MR, DeLange RJ, Fineman GAM. Bone cell differentiation and growth factors. *Science* 1983;220:680.

39. Urist MR, Lietze A, Mitzutani H, Takagi K, Triffitt JT, Amstutte J, et al. A bovine low molecular weight bone morphogenetic protein (BMP) fraction. *Clin Orthop* 1982;162:219.

40. Sampath TK, Mulhullan A, Reddi AH. Isolation of osteogenin, an extracellular matrix-associated bone inductive protein by heparin affinity chromatography. *Proc Natl Acad Sci USA* 1987;84;7109–7113.

41. Burchardt H, Glowczewskie FP, Enneking WF. Allogeneic segmental fibula transplants in azanthroprine immunosuppressed dogs. *J Bone Joint Surg* 1977;59A:881.

42. Hiatt H, Lorato D, Hiatt W, Lindfors K. The induction of new bone and cementum formation. VA comparison of graft and cortical sites in deep infrabony periodontal lesions. *Int J Periodont Rest Dent* 1986;6(5):9–21.

43. Schrad SC, Tussing GJ. Human allografts of iliac bone and marrow in periodontal osseous defects. *J Periodontol* 1986;57:205–210.

44. Schallhorn RG. Present status of osseous grafting procedures. *J Periodontol* 1977;48:574.

45. Urist MR. Surface decalcified allogeneic bone implants. *Clin Orthop* 1968;56:37.

46. DeVries PH, Badgly CE, Hartman JT. Radiation sterilization of homogenous bone transplants utilizing radioactive cobalt. *J Bone Joint Surg* 1958;40A:187.

47. Roberts WE: Bone tissue interface. *J Dent Educ* 1988;52:804–809.

48. Roberts WE, Helm FR, Marshall KJ, Gongloff RF. Rigid endosseous implants for orthopedic and orthodontic anchorage. *Angle Orthod* 1989;59:247–256.

The Role of Insertion Site and Inflammation on the Integration of Pure Titanium Implants

L. Sennerby and P. Thomsen

We have compared the tissue response to screw-shaped titanium implants inserted in the knee joint and tibia of rabbits that were observed for 6 weeks and 3 and 6 months, as quantitated by morphometry on ground sections and measurements of the removal torque. In a separate set of experiments, the effect of a local inflammatory response in the knee joint, induced by repeated injections of bovine serum albumin (BSA) in previously BSA immunized rabbits that were observed for 6 weeks, was evaluated by morphometry.

The removal torque force required to unscrew the intra-articular implants increased with time in contrast to the tibial implants. Less force was needed to remove the intra-articular implants at 6 weeks but not later. More bone was always found around the intra-articular implants. The bone surrounding the intra-articular implants was mostly cancellous except for the part in the subchondral compact bone, whereas cortical bone surrounded the tibial implants. There was a correlation between the amount of bone found in the threads situated in the subchondral and cortical passage.

The titanium implants within the arthritic joints had less degree of bone-to-implant contact and less amount of bone within the threads. In contrast, a higher degree of bone-to-implant contact and amount of bone was found around the tibial implants at the arthritic side compared to the control side.

In conclusion, using light microscopic morphometry, both the insertion site and the state of the implant bed determined the healing of pure titanium implants in bone and joint.

Evaluation of Different Granular Hydroxyapatite (Algipore), Polymeric (HTR), and Ionomeric (V-0$_3$) Bone Substitutes in the Rabbit

H.-J. Schmitz, S.A. Jovanovic, and J. Krauser

The bone substitute properties of the naturally interconnecting, microporous, hydrothermally converted, phycogenic hydroxyapatite-granulate Algipore (Friedrichsfeld Ltd, Mannheim, Germany) were studied in Chinchilla rabbits in periods up to 1 year. Filling of alveoli after extraction of mandibular premolars yielded an exfoliation of most of the hydroxyapatite particles without improvement of regeneration of mandibular bone. In trabecular bone of the distal femur, the phycogenic granulate induced an acceleration of concentric formation of woven bone with concomitant reduction of central soft tissue regenerates.

In simulation of ridge augmentation techniques, the hydroxyapatite granulate within resorbable Vicryl (Ethicon GmbH, Nordstedt, Germany) nets was attached to the petaled ventral aspect of the femur shaft. Osseous incorporation was observed in juxtacortical particle layers only, accompanied by secondary, unwanted, resorptive remodeling of pre-existent cortical bone. Addition of cancellous bone and bone chip increased neither osteoinductive nor osteoconductive properties of the phycogenic hydroxyapatite materials.

Comparative results of polymeric hydroxethylacrylate (HTR) and ionomeric (V-0-Cem) (Ionos Ltd, Seefeld, Germany) granulates for application as bone substitutes in identical experimental procedures is presented.

Session V Discussion

E. Keller (Rochester, Minnesota): Dr Slack, when moving the lower teeth forward, a lot of the movement is tipping. Is it possible to move the teeth bodily forward and in essence move the alveolar process? Could treatment be expanded in those cases that need dental alveolar advancement rather than just dental advancement?

J. Slack (Spokane, Washington): It is possible to tip teeth in the alveolar process. In all of the people treated, the incisors were tipped back and we just tipped them forward. One must work within the limitations of the alveolar process. I would not try to bodily push the teeth forward since they could be pushed right out of the alveolus with stripping, etc. Molars can be moved bodily right through the alveolar process, but basically it is tipping of the anteriors and bodily movement of the molars.

G. Schuetz (Woodstock, Vermont): Dr Slack, how soon after second-stage surgery would you consider using the implant for active orthodontic movement?

J. Slack: We surgically placed the implants, then instituted conventional orthodontic care. Aligning and leveling was done and then when I was ready to protract the teeth, the implants were uncovered. We tried to coordinate treatment so as not to extend treatment time too long. Six months after we started, the implants were engaged.

G. Schuetz: That's 6 months after second-stage surgery, not 6 months after first-stage surgery, is that correct?

J. Slack: No, 6 months after the first-stage surgery.

R. Baier: Professor Lundborg, could you give us more information about the silicone joint, the hinge area; in particular, is there a special way that you are making that by increased cross-linking? Does it have a tendency to take up lipids and subsequently become brittle in the joint? Could that be a possibility for failure?

G. Lundborg (Malmo, Sweden): Silicone material was chosen because we have the greatest experience with this specific material in hand surgery. We know that it is fairly nonreactive, it can take movement, and it is accepted for many clinical uses. I do not have exact information concerning the chemical composition, but it is not different from what has been used in ordinary-occurring silicone implants. We had just a few cases of fracture. In one patient, the proximal interphalangeal (PIP) size joint was used for the metacarpal phalange joint in a tiny hand, which might perhaps explain why it ruptured. We do not think this is the ultimate solution. We are working on a thesis for a specific material. There may be many ways to increase the biocompatibility by treating the surface, for instance, in various ways.

E. Keller: Dr Lundborg, sepsis in the intraoral application of the osseointegrated implant is relatively rare. Could you discuss what were factors in the wrist that led to the infection or made it more probable?

G. Lundborg: These two cases were among the first we did and I think that this could be explained by the long time of surgery. We have not had those kinds of problems since. Infections in elective hand surgery are very uncommon.

E. Keller: Did the infections originate from the bone portion of your surgery or more soft tissue?

G. Lundborg: It was a soft tissue infection that migrated to the joints.

A. Garg (Miami, Florida): Dr Slack, can you briefly elaborate on the fabrication of the crown with the attached bracket that was placed on the implant?

J. Slack: In the laboratory, we waxed the hexagonal end of a fixture for lubrication and then applied some Adaptic restorative material around this area. We placed the bracket on it, polished it, and fixed it in the mouth. Our biggest mistake was making them too thin. The patients actually would try to chew with them if they could.

S. Sachs (Lake Success, New York): Dr Brown, of the patients in whom you placed craniofacial fixtures in the orbit, what percentage had received a full course of therapeutic radiation and how did the fixtures do that were placed in that field?

A. Brown (Birmingham, England): Of our orbital cases, probably only two have received radical radiotherapy, and that one patient I showed you is the only one who has lost a fixture.

S. Sachs: Did this particular patient go on to develop other than a local phenomenon (radionecrosis)?

A. Brown: No, we have not seen any problems like that at all. One should remember that the loss of fixtures in the orbital region is not so extraordinary as it would be in the temporal region. Our current procedure in treating an orbit would be to put in as many fixtures as we could find room for around the orbit because there is a fair chance that a fixture will be lost even in a nonradiated orbit.

S. Sachs: Dr Holt, are you aware of any ongoing clinical trials with jaw lengthening, face lengthening, or cranial expansion with integrated fixtures serving as anchors?

G.R. Holt (San Antonio, Texas): I am not aware of clinical trials. I have read some articles in the literature related to canine snout protrusion with fixtures and I think that has been an exciting area for thought. I have also read some articles about distracty therapy from a discontinuity defect of the mandible, not using our specific integrated fixture techniques, but rather by slowly displacing that defect it grows new bone with it. Maybe Dr Higuchi would like to comment on that.

K. Higuchi: In the area of facial skeletal reorientation using mechanics, to my knowledge there is nothing in the literature about clinical application of this procedure. In 1988, Smalley demonstrated that this is certainly possible using conventional skull bone flange, craniofacial flange fixtures, with extended long-term pressure. He has been able to disarticulate portions of the facial skeleton rather dramatically as reported in the *American Journal of Orthodontics*.

E. Keller: Dr Higuchi, would you share your experience regarding placement of implants in the third molar region?

K. Higuchi: Dr Slack covered some of the surgical access problems in the third molar region. Of the fixtures I placed, all were 10 mm in length; seven patients were treated, six had fixtures in the retromolar or third molar area. None of these fixtures were countersunk because of the presence of the nerve. We also found that because of the soft tissue anatomy, it was more favorable to incline the fixtures toward the lingual side. You may have noticed that the rigid attachment coming from the single-tooth abutment was from the lingual-medial aspect. Initially we used the buccal aspect and, in fact, created some soft tissue problems. We now incline these a bit toward the lingual side. We have not lost fixtures at this point despite the amount of loading we have placed on them. All of the fixtures to date have remained stable. After the course of treatment is completed, the single-tooth attachment is removed, cover screws are placed, and soft tissues are closed. It is necessary to adjust the length of the abutment so that the opposing occlusion is accommodated.

S. Wallach (Greenwood, Illinois): Professor Lundborg, what was the postsurgical protocol for your patients immediately after the replacement of PIP and metacarpophalangeal joints?

G. Lundborg: We applied some of the principles used for other types of hand injuries, especially flexor tendon injuries. The hands were completely immobilized for about 1 week. After that we started on mobilization for the purpose of loading the joints as little as possible. A static splint was used at nighttime and most of the daytime with the exception of 2-minute periods of passive flexion and extension carried out by the occupational therapist for the first 2 or 3 weeks; then continuously increasing the length of these passive motion periods. After some time, a splint with rubber bands helped them to extend the fingers while the patient could flex actively. Periods of so-called active-hold technique, in which the therapist flexed the fingers for the patient and then the patient was asked to keep the fingers in flexion to put on some intermediate load, were also used. This basic protocol was used as we then continuously increased the load until 3 months after surgery; then a full load was allowed.

S. Wallach: In that sense, it is significantly different than intraorally where we rest these im-

plants for 4 to 6 months before loading them. Apparently, you found no significant difficulty.

G. Lundborg: No, I think this is a very important point. If you immobilize the hand for more than 2, 3, or 4 weeks, it would be completely stiff and the whole concept would be completely useless. Therefore, we just have to start mobilizing the things a very short time after surgery and it has proved to be successful.

S. Wallach: Have you done any comparative strength measurements in these joints compared to a normal joint, of the similar type index finger or middle finger?

G. Lundborg: No, we have not.

S. Wallach: How would you extrapolate this to our unhappiness with temporomandibular joints using silicone derivative that have since fragmented and broken down?

G. Lundborg: I am not too familiar with that joint. I would suspect that one would have to consider the various types of forces active on that joint. The hand joints are very different in terms of loading from the joints of the lower extremities, for example. The temporomandibular joint is quite special in that respect too, but I cannot see why the main concept should not be valid for this joint as well as for the joints of the hand.

K. Tidstrom (Minneapolis, Minnesota): Dr Brown, have you used tissue expanders at all in these regions when you had to excise hair-bearing tissue? If you have, do they result in thicker hairless tissue in the temporal region or have you not used expanders and done free grafting?

A. Brown: We have not used tissue expanders at all.

S. Sachs: Dr Higuchi, when you used autologous mandible as the nasal inlay, did you find it necessary to pretap the bone?

K. Higuchi: I have done it both ways and I think it is easier if it can be held in place, not tapped. It seems to react with a little more compression if you thread it conventionally.

S. Sachs: Dr Jensen, how was the sinus health in your patients afterward?

O. Jensen (Denver, Colorado): After sinus augmentation with allograft, the patients were on antibiotics for 3 weeks. The basis for that is if an iliac graft with cancellous bone is used, you may not need to put the patients on antibiotics for more than a few days. But when an allograft is used, the potential exists for sequestration of dead bone. I kept the patients on antibiotics for 3 weeks because the average time when there will be fluid levels in the sinuses is 3 weeks after surgery. So complicationwise, most of the patients had sinus-type headaches, drainage, etc, for about 3 weeks, but I never had a single infection.

S. Sachs: When you treated these patients and you used various approaches and different types of materials, did you discuss with the patients the fact that they were subjects of experimentation?

O. Jensen: Yes, we had special consent forms. Actually I had five pages of consent forms, three different consent forms, one from the Gore-Tex Company, etc.

M. Hall (Lexington, Kentucky): Dr Greer, is it possible that you may not have gotten any osseointegration from any of the materials except possibly the iliac crest bone graft, and that this clinical success of the implants was all due to the natural bone that was present in those conditions?

R. Greer (Denver, Colorado): I totally agree with that. I have not proven that allograft osseointegrates in this setting and you cannot confirm that unless you remove an implant and look at it under a microscope. I did not intend to get a consent form for doing that.

R. Baier: A comment to Dr Schmitz and then a question for Dr Sennerby. Dr Schmitz's paper excellently demonstrated a lack of complete bone incorporation of particulates. We have experienced, not in his setting but in other cases where we have had to use similar particles, better particle incorporation into matrices if the particles are first tumbled in a glow-discharge chamber, where they are rapidly cleaned, energized, and made more wettable. There may be a chance in a future study to get greater and deeper penetration of the bone into such materials, particularly the hydroxyapatite particulates, by cleaning the "junk" off the surface that comes from manufacturing.

Dr Sennerby, in regard to the very interesting and most important conclusion that the torsional back-out strength is due to the cortical bone only in these cases, did you count as cortical bone that bone which grew down from the original cortex by this "cornering" phenomenon, or recorticalization, that we talked about earlier; or did you define it in a more geometric way, that since it was in the marrow space, it was considered marrow and not cortex?

L. Sennerby (Göteborg, Sweden): Yes, we were measuring only the threads within the cortical bone and that means thread numbers 1 and 2 in this case.

R. Baier: I assume, then, that what seems to be an excellent histologic appearance of downgrowth, or recorticalization to the deeper threads, is, in your view, not contributing to any additional mechanical strength?

L. Sennerby: That is my feeling; however, this torque removal technique is not very sophisticated. But, I think the data were very clear.

E. Keller: Dr Jensen, with your allogeneic bone grafts in the sinus, where are you hypothesizing that there is osteogenesis? If you do get osteogenesis with remineralization/revascularization, how long do you think that takes in this particular setting?

O. Jensen: I am not certain how long it takes, but the biopsies I presented were mostly at 6 months. In some cases I waited up to 14 months but never tried anything less than 6 months. However, ossification may occur before that time. As far as the mechanism of action in this technique, when grafting cortical bone, it takes the body more energy to get down to the morphogenetic protein and it is necessary to dissolve or resorb the calcified matrix in order to get down to osteogenic stimulatory factors. That material also acts as a conductive mechanism. Some of the rationale for using hydroxyapatite and demineralized bone combinations comes into play there. I think the mechanism is that it acts as a carrier to allow time for the body's machinery to get going and that delay is reached by using the Gore-Tex membrane.

E. Keller: Are the osteoprogenitor cells coming from the membrane of the sinus?

O. Jensen: They are endosseous. There is no interaction from the periosteum. In peeling off this membrane, it was interesting to note that it was very adherent to the osteotomy site and there was no periosteum growing up underneath it. So I think all of the bone formed was from endosteal osteoprogenitor cells.

E. Keller: From the alveolar bone?

O. Jensen: Yes, from the floor of the sinus.

E. Keller: Dr Babbush, you showed some photographs of sinus lift procedures. It was not clear whether you used just hydroxyapatite grafts or whether you mixed them with bone.

C. Babbush (Beachwood, Ohio): The procedure that we have been using for about 15 to 18 months involves a combination of porous hydroxyapatite and freeze-dried cortical cancellous bone that we get from the Red Cross bone bank at a 1:1 ratio. We are aspirating hemopoietic marrow from the iliac crest and combining it with those two materials.

For ankle fusion, two of the orthopedic surgeons at our institution have been aspirating bone marrow essentially from the iliac crest. Their research and reporting has demonstrated that the quality and quantity of cellular activity from hemopoietic aspirant is the same that one would get from harvesting particulate marrow from the iliac crest. We are doing the procedure under intravenous sedation on an ambulatory outpatient basis in the hospital. In those patients where sufficient bone exists to place the implant—a minimum of 4 to 5 mm of the patient's own residual crest—the implants were placed and the augmentation done simultaneously. When there is less bone, the augmentation is done, and after 9 to 12 months we go back in. Several implants are loaded, but it is too early to draw any definitive conclusions yet.

The Longitudinal Clinical Efficacy of Core-Vent Dental Implants in Partially Edentulous Patients: A 5-Year Report

D. Patrick, J. Zosky, R. Lubar, and A. Buchs

The Core-Vent system (Core-Vent Corp, Encino, Calif) of dental implants has been widely used for rehabilitation of partially edentulous jaws since its introduction by Niznick in 1982.[1] It has a versatile prosthetic protocol that does not require a radical departure from traditional prosthodontic treatment and a simplified surgical technique that promotes predictable osseointegration (Figs 1a and b).

Studies by Lum and others using dogs[2] and primates[3] have shown that Core-Vent implants achieve and maintain osseointegration at the light microscopic level as defined by Brånemark et al.[4] Using this same definition, Niznick[5] and Gores et al[6] have reported osseointegration for Core-Vent dental implants in the edentulous jaws of humans. In light of these reports and the longitudinally documented results of Adell et al[7] and Patrick et al,[8] long-term osseointegration and survival of Core-Vent dental implants are suggested.

Materials and methods

Four hundred twenty male and female partially edentulous patients (173 men and 247 women) were included in this study. Ages ranged from 16 years to 81 years. From November 3, 1982 to March 29, 1988, 826 implants were consecutively placed in these patients by three oral/maxillofacial surgeons (Zosky, Lubar, and Buchs) and a prosthodontist (Patrick).

After routine medical, dental, and radiographic assessment, each patient was evaluated by one of the investigators to determine whether the procedure was feasible for the patient. Each patient was counseled concerning the nature of the treatment, and a properly executed consent form was obtained. Potential patients with a history of drug abuse or those having unrealistic expectations regarding esthetic results were excluded.

All implants were placed by a gentle surgical procedure and aseptic technique. The two-stage surgical procedure consisted first of the placement of the Core-Vent implant; then secondly, attachment of the prosthetic insert (abutment). The surgical placement of the implants included the following basic steps performed under local anesthesia. The patient was prepared and draped for surgery. A mid-crestal, buccal, or labial incision was made at the discretion of the surgeon and a full-thickness flap was elevated so that the underlying bone was exposed. An osteotomy was performed for each implant by the use of trephines internally cooled with either sterile normal saline or sterile distilled water. Retention of a bone core for the basket portion of the implant was determined by the surgeon. The implant was then placed in the site of the osteotomy and hand-ratcheted into place by use of the appropriate hex instrument in the implant's hex-hole. Polysulfone inserts were then placed into the hex-hole of each implant, and the flaps were coapted and sutured over the implants with either black silk or polyglycol sutures.

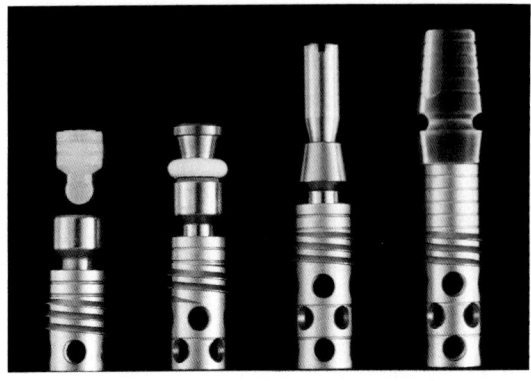 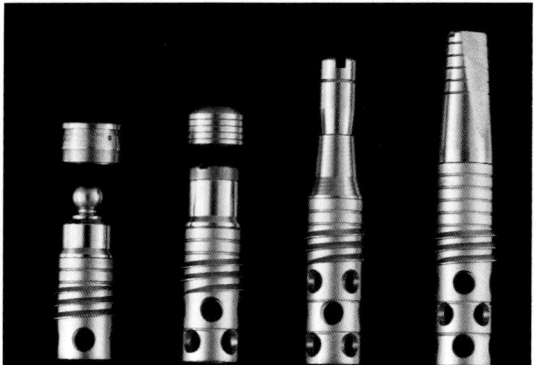

Figs 1a and b Core-Vent implants are available in three diameters—3.5 mm (a), 4.5 mm (b), and 5.5 mm—and four lengths—16 mm, 13 mm, 10.5 mm and 8 mm—with an array of titanium and castable abutments and attachments providing many prosthetic options.

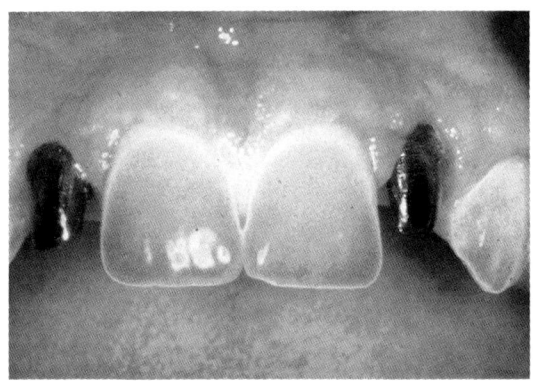

Fig 2 Core-Vent implant-cemented cast abutments prepared for crowns.

Three of the investigators prescribed phenoxymethyl penicillin or erythromycin (if the patient had a penicillin allergy) 1 hour preoperatively and then regularly for the first 7 postoperative days. One investigator prescribed cephalosporin 1 hour preoperatively and for 7 postoperative days.

Occasionally, a transitional prosthesis was relieved over the surgical site and lined with soft temporary lining material and placed immediately after implant placement. However, all patients were requested not to wear a prosthesis over the surgical site for 3 weeks. Liquid or soft diets and saline mouthrinses were prescribed for the first and second postoperative weeks.

Prosthetic treatment began after 3 months of healing in the mandible and after 6 months in the maxilla. Under local anesthesia, the polysulfone inserts were located and exposed with either a scalpel or a diamond bur in a high-speed handpiece with copious irrigation. The surgical inserts were removed and replaced with cemented titanium or custom-cast, high-noble metal inserts (abutments) corresponding to the prosthetic application planned. The titanium or cast inserts were cemented with composite cement. The excess cement was carefully removed before final setting. Prior to cementation of the prosthetic inserts, the implants were evaluated for osseointegration. Any implants that were not osseointegrated were removed.

Most of the osseointegrated implants were restored with single crowns and fixed prostheses either totally implant-supported (Fig 2) or in combination with natural teeth (Fig 3). Seventeen implants held attachments, such as magnetic keepers, for removable partial dentures. The fixed restorations were either retained by dental cement or screws (Figs 4a and b), and all of the single crowns were retained by dental cement.

Within 1 to 3 months after final placement of

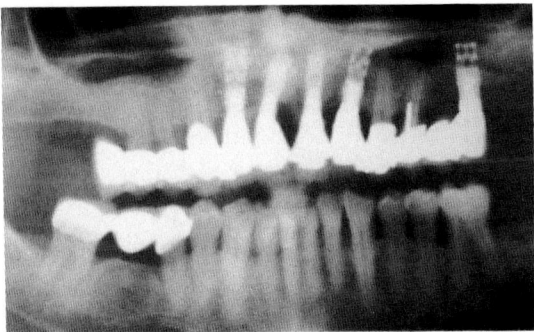

Fig 3 Radiograph of implants and natural teeth supporting restoration.

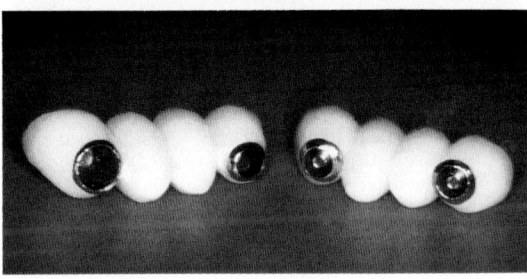

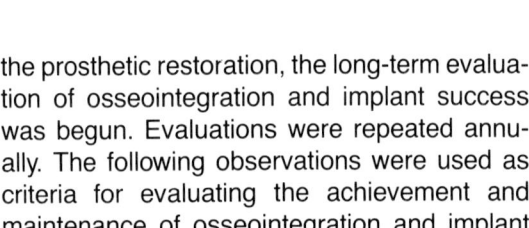

Figs 4a and b Occusal views of two fixed partial dentures: (a) to be cement-retained, (b) to be screw-retained.

the prosthetic restoration, the long-term evaluation of osseointegration and implant success was begun. Evaluations were repeated annually. The following observations were used as criteria for evaluating the achievement and maintenance of osseointegration and implant success.

Mobility

Implant mobility was assessed by placing the prosthetic abutment with or without the definitive prosthesis attached between the metal handles of two dental instruments, such as mirrors or cement spatulas, and subjecting it to a rocking force. If clinical mobility was found, the implant was removed.

Peri-implant radiolucency

Panoramic radiographs were taken annually of all implants, and long cone periapical radiographs of the implants were taken individually beginning 1 to 3 months after placing the prosthetic restoration. These radiographs were viewed without magnification on a standard radiograph viewbox. If a peri-implant radiolucency was present, this was viewed as absence of osseointegration and the implant was removed.

Gingival inflammation

Gingival inflammation was not evaluated by any particular index. However, if the gingiva around an implant appeared red and edematous, pressure was applied to the facial and lingual implant gingiva with gloved index fingers. If purulent exudate was expressed, and if antibiotic therapy and surgical intervention did not correct the pathology, the implant was removed.

The panoramic and periapical radiographs used to determine the presence or absence of peri-implant radiolucency were also used for observation of the mesial and distal vertical bone loss of each implant on a yearly basis. However, this examination was not used as a criterion for implant success because the radiographic technique was not standardized. The

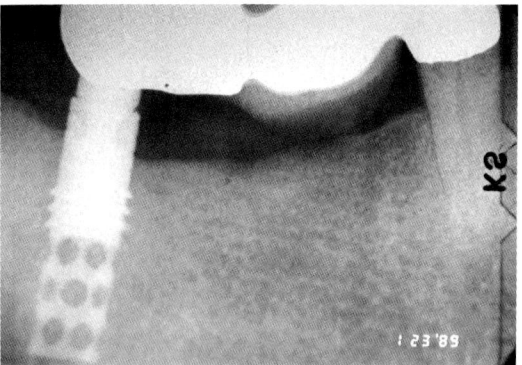

Fig 5 Radiograph of Core-Vent implant after 3 years in function, showing minimal bone loss.

Table 1 Implants in partially edentulous jaws*

Investigators	Maxillary implants				Mandibular implants			
	Inserted	w/Follow-up	Removed	% Success	Inserted	w/Follow-up	Removed	% Success
Lubar	45	43	0	100	95	95	5	94.7
Patrick	72	70	1	98.6	43	40	0	100
Buchs	106	106	3	97.2	239	229	0	100
Zosky	128	121	3	97.7	98	98	5	94.9
Cumulative results	351	340	7	97.9*	475	462	10	97.8†

*Total implants consecutively inserted and checked for osseointegration in partially edentulous jaws were 826.
†Statistically significant as computed by the standard Chi-square test at the 95% confidence level.

radiographs were placed on a standard viewbox and evaluated without magnification. The neck grooves and threads of Core-Vent implants are easily visualized. They are spaced approximately 1 mm apart. Observation of a change in mesial and distal bone height relative to the same groove or thread allows vertical bone loss to be approximated (Fig 5).

Results

By the end of the data collection period (March 30, 1988), all 826 implants were uncovered, checked for osseointegration, loaded, or removed (Table 1). During this investigation, six male and two female patients (representing 24 implants) did not return for annual evaluations and were dropped from the study (Table 2). However, any of these implants that failed while in the study are indicated in the tables as "removed." Thus, of the total 826 placed and uncovered, 802 implants were followed through the 9 to 64 month observation period.

The median observation period for the entire study was 27 months. Each investigator's median observation period was more than 13 months. The longest median observation period was 42 months and the shortest was 14 months. The shortest period of observation was 9 months and the longest was 64 months (Table 3).

Only 7 of the 340 maxillary implants placed and followed up were lost, for an overall maxillary

Table 2 Implant locations in six male and two female patients lost to recall (LTR)

Patient gender	Maxillary implants		Mandibular implants		Cumulative LTR
	Anterior	Posterior	Anterior	Posterior	
Male	10	1	2	3	16
Female	0	0	5	3	8
Total	10	1	7	6	24

Table 3 Observation period

Investigator	Interval (mo)	Patients entering interval	Implants entering interval	Median observation period (mo)
Lubar	11–64	80	140	42
Patrick	9–57	62	115	32
Buchs	15–40	167	345	20
Zosky	9–42	110	226	14

Table 4 Distribution and success of implants supporting single crowns in partially edentulous jaws

	Maxilla	Removed	Success	Mandible	Removed	Success
Anterior	43	0	100%	16	0	100%
Posterior	8	0	100%	28	0	100%
Total	51	0	100%	44	0	100%

success rate of 97.9% (Table 1). These maxillary implants were separated according to anterior or posterior location. Forty-three maxillary anterior implants supported single crowns (Table 4), and 129 supported fixed prostheses (Table 5). Eight maxillary posterior implants supported single crowns and 160 supported fixed prostheses. None of the implants supporting single crowns were lost. However, seven maxillary implants supporting fixed prostheses were removed. Maxillary implant position showed a difference of only 0.6% between anterior and posterior positions (Table 6). Table 6 also demonstrates that only one implant (0.03%) failed after 1 year in function.

Of the 462 mandibular implants placed and subsequently evaluated, 10 were removed because of nonosseointegration, for an overall mandibular implant success rate of 97.8% (Table 1). The mandibular implants were also divided into anterior and posterior implants for evaluation. There was no difference in the success rates between anterior and posterior mandibular implants (Table 7). There were 16 anterior mandibular implants supporting single crowns and 76 supporting fixed restorations (Tables 4 and 5). None of the implants supporting single crowns were lost. However, two anterior mandibular implants supporting fixed prostheses failed (Table 5). In the posterior

Table 5 Distribution and success of implants supporting fixed prostheses in partially edentulous jaws

	Maxilla	Removed	Success	Mandible	Removed	Success
Anterior	129	4	96.9	76	2	97.4
Posterior	160	3	98.1	339	8	97.6
Total	289	7	97.6*	415	10	97.6*

*Statistically significant as computed by the standard Chi-square test at the 95% confidence level.

Table 6 Number failed and % success over time in partially edentulous maxillae*

	Anterior maxilla† 172 Implants with followup				Posterior maxilla† 168 Implants with followup			
Months	Failed to integrate, removed	Failed in function, removed	Osseo-integrated, retained	% Success	Failed to integrate, removed	Failed in function, removed	Osseo-integrated, retained	% Success
3–6	0	0	172	100	1	0	167	99.4
7–12	2	2	168	97.6	0	1	166	98.8
13–24	0	0	168	97.6	0	1	165	98.2
25–64	0	0	168	97.6	0	0	165	98.2

*Total maxillary implants placed: n = 351. Total maxillary implants followed: n = 340. Total maxillary implants removed: n = 7.
†Statistically significant as computed by the standard Chi-square test at the 95% confidence level.

Table 7 Number failed and % success over time in partially edentulous mandibles*

	Anterior mandible† 98 Implants with followup				Posterior mandible† 364 Implants with followup			
Months	Failed to integrate, removed	Failed in function, removed	Osseo-integrated, retained	% Success	Failed to integrate, removed	Failed in function, removed	Osseo-integrated, retained	% Success
3–6	2	0	96	98.0	2	1	361	99.2
7–12	0	0	96	98.0	3	0	358	98.4
13–24	0	0	96	98.0	2	0	356	97.8
25–64	0	0	96	98.0	0	0	356	97.8

*Total mandibular implants placed: n = 475. Total mandibular implants followed: n = 462. Total mandibular implants removed: n = 10.
†Statistically significant as computed by the standard Chi-square test at the 95% confidence level.

mandibular area, 28 implants supported single crowns and none were lost in function. Table 5 also demonstrates that 339 posterior mandibular implants supported fixed prostheses, and 1 of the total 8 removed was lost in function prior to 7 months (Table 7). Three successful mandibular posterior implants supported removable partial denture attachments. The cumulative success rate for the anterior and posterior mandibles supporting single crowns and fixed restorations was 97.8% (Table 1).

The success rate for both maxillary and mandibular implants supporting single crowns was 100% for this observation period (Table 4). The combined anterior and posterior success rates for maxillary and mandibular implants supporting fixed prostheses was 97.6% (Table 5).

The success rate for 340 maxillary implants placed and evaluated was 97.9% and 97.8% for 462 mandibular implants, giving a total success rate of 97.9% (Table 1).

Discussion

The long-term predictability of osseointegrated implants has been described by Albrektsson et al,[9] Cox et al,[10] Patrick et al,[8] and others. Osseointegration has been described at the clinical, radiographic, and microscopic levels, indicating that it is a close intimate contact between living bone and the implant surface, without any intervening fibrous tissue. The Core-Vent implant has been shown to fulfill this criterion for osseointegration in animals and humans. In this study, success was equated with osseointegration. Reported success rates reflect the status of each implant as opposed to the prosthesis it supported.

There have been many definitions of implant success, including the quality of implant survival as part of the success criteria. However, the only standard measure of osseointegrated implant success to be found in the literature is implant survival, absence of implant mobility, and absence of peri-implant radiolucency. In his "17-Year Study on 4,100 Brånemark Implants,"[11]

Adell states: "The anchorage function or the fixture survival rate was defined as the number of stable, prosthesis supporting, osseointegrated fixtures in relation to the total number of fixtures installed."

In the textbook *Tissue-Integrated Prostheses*,[12] "fixture anchorage function" and "fixture survival rate" were the criteria of success. Eleven Swedish teams[13] reported their results, using osseointegrated implants in edentulous jaws, fixture immobility, and absence of peri-implant radiolucency as their criteria for success. They also stated that it was not possible to register marginal bone loss with acceptable accuracy because their radiographic technique was not standardized.

In the textbook, *The Brånemark Osseointegrated Implant*,[14] the clinical results of a 24-team multicenter study using the Brånemark implant in edentulous jaws are reported. It states that the participants agreed to use degrees of crestal bone loss as part of their success criteria. However, the data collection questionnaire provided to the teams did not include bone loss measurements. To allow comparison of results, the above criteria, including survival without chronic infection, absence of implant mobility, and absence of peri-implant radiolucency were used as the criteria for success in this report.

According to Cox and Zarb,[10] "There appears to be growing evidence that conventional soft tissue health indices are not yardsticks to monitor implant efficacy." This suggests that gingival indices are not reliable indicators of implant success. However, gingival infection has been cited as a main etiologic factor of implant failure.[15] All implants included in this report as successful remained free of chronic infection.

The long-term experience with osseointegrated Brånemark fixtures in the treatment of edentulous jaws is described by Adell in the textbook, *Tissue-Integrated Prostheses*.[12] The 5- to 12-year results demonstrated that "the majority of fixture losses did occur during the first year." In this report, surviving implants were considered successful. Maxillary implants were not as successful as mandibular implants. In the maxilla, of 734 fixtures inserted, 88% were considered suc-

Table 8 Four-year life table: Failure analysis of 826 implants followed annually

Year	340 Maxillary implants		462 Mandibular implants	
	Failed	% Success	Failed	% Success
0–1	6	98.2	8	98.3
1–2	1	97.9	2	97.8
2–4	0	97.9	0	97.8
Total	7	97.9	10	97.8

cessful after 1-year, dropping to an 84% "survival rate" by 5 to 12 years. In the mandible, of 721 fixtures inserted, 94% achieved and maintained osseointegration for the first year, dropping to 93% by the 5- to 12-year evaluation period. These results led Albrektsson et al[9] to conclude that "the Brånemark results ... clearly underscore the basic concept of osseointegration as being the major, if not the exclusive reason for successful long-term dental implant attachment." In the same article, Brånemark is referenced as stating, "Any implant losses after the first one to two years of function seem to be unlikely, provided osseointegration has occurred."

In this report of Core-Vent implants in partially edentulous jaws, of 340 maxillary implants inserted and evaluated annually, 334 were successful after 1 year, dropping to 333 by 2 to 4 years (Table 8). In the mandible, of 462 implants inserted and evaluated annually, 454 were successful after 1 year, dropping to 452 after 2 to 4 years (Table 8). No statistically significant difference was observed between the success rates for maxillary implants and mandibular implants in this investigation. This finding is favorable when contrasted with the results reported by both Adell[12] and Mito et al,[16] who observed less success in the maxilla than in the mandible with Brånemark implants.

All implant losses occurred prior to the second year in function (Table 8). This lends support to Brånemark's statement, "Any implant losses after the first one to two years of function

seem to be unlikely, provided osseointegration has occurred."[9] All individual implants supporting single crowns maintained osseointegration throughout the study. Implant position in partially edentulous jaws does not seem to be a factor in determination of success or failure. It was observed that the success rates for both jaws were greater than 97% whether the implants were placed anteriorly or posteriorly.

Summary and conclusions

Core-Vent implants achieve and maintain osseointegration on a highly consistent basis in partially edentulous jaws. Of the implants placed in partially edentulous jaws and evaluated, 97.9% of the maxillary implants and 97.8% of the mandibular implants achieved and maintained osseointegration throughout the 64-month observation period. There was no statistically significant difference in the implants achieving and maintaining osseointegration between the maxillary or mandibular jaws. There was no significant difference in implants achieving and maintaining osseointegration between the anterior and posterior sites of either maxillary or mandibular jaws. Implants supporting single crowns in this study were 100% successful in both the maxilla and mandible. Implants supporting fixed prostheses were 97.6% successful in both the maxilla and the mandible. Most of the implants that failed did so within the first year of placement. The total success rate of 802 implants placed in partially edentulous jaws and followed for the entire observation period was 97.8%.

References

1. Niznick GA. The Core-Vent implant system. *J Oral Implantol* 1982;10:379–418.
2. Lum LB, Beirne OR. Viability of the retained bone core in Core-Vent dental implants. *J Oral Maxillofac Surg* 1986;44:341–345.
3. Lum LB, Beirne OR, Dillings M, Curtis TA. Osseointe-

gration of two types of implants in nonhuman primates. *J Prosthet Dent* 1988;60:700–705.

4. Brånemark P-I, Adell R, Albrektsson T, Lekholm U, Lindström J, et al. An experimental and clinical study of osseointegrated implants penetrating the nasal cavity and maxillary sinus. *J Oral Maxillofac Surg* 1984; 42:497–505.

5. Niznick GA. Osseointegration—An idea whose time has come. *Destinations* 1986;10:44–45,53.

6. Gores RJ, Hayes CK, Unni KK. Postmortem examination of six maxillary Core-Vent implants: Report of a case. *J Oral Maxillofac Surg* 1989;47:302–306.

7. Adell R, Lekholm U, Rockler B, Brånemark P-I. A 15-year study of osseointegrated implants in the treatment of the edentulous jaw. *Int J Oral Surg* 1981; 10:387–416.

8. Patrick D, Zosky J, Lubar R, Buchs A. The longitudinal clinical efficacy of Core-Vent dental implants: A five-year report. *J Oral Implantol* 1989;15:95–103.

9. Albrektsson T, Zarb GA, Worthington P, Eriksson AR. The long-term efficacy of currently used dental implants: A review and proposed criteria of success. *Int J Oral Maxillofac Implants* 1986;1:11–25.

10. Cox J, Zarb GA. The longitudinal clinical efficacy of osseointegrated dental implants: A 3-year report. *Int J Oral Maxillofac Implants* 1987;2:91–100.

11. Adell R. 17-year study on 4,100 Brånemark implants. *J Prosthet Dent* 1983;50(2):252.

12. Adell R. Long-term treatment results. pp 175–186 In P.-I. Brånemark, G.A. Zarb, T. Albrektsson (eds) *Tissue-Integrated Prostheses: Osseointegration in Clinical Dentistry.* Chicago: Quintessence Publ Co, 1985.

13. Engquist B, Bergendal T, Kallus T, Linden U. A retrospective multicenter evaluation of osseointegrated implants supporting overdentures. *Int J Oral Maxillofac Implants* 1988;3:132.

14. Albrektsson T, Zarb GA. Chapter 15: Clinical results of a 24-team multicenter study of the Brånemark implant. pp 229–232 In T. Albrektsson, G.A. Zarb (eds) *The Brånemark Osseointegrated Implant.* Chicago: Quintessence Publ Co, 1989.

15. Newman MG, Flemmig TF. Periodontal consideration of implants and implant associated microbia. *J Dent Educ* 1988;52:737–744.

16. Mito RS, Lewis S, Beumer J III, Perri G, Moy PK. The UCLA implant study—a three-year review of the Brånemark implant system success rate. *J Calif Dent Assoc* 1989;17:12–17.

Diskimplant System: Intraoral Applications in Small Bone Volumes. Patient Selection and Long-Term Results*

G. Scortecci, H. Zattara, P. Meyer, and P. Doms

Cylindrical titanium implants can provide excellent biologic and prosthetic results when bone height of at least 7 to 10 mm is available and the alveolar ridge is at least 6 mm wide. However, when less than 7 mm are available in the vertical dimension, the technical difficulty of submerging cylindrical implants can create serious problems. Bone grafts, sinus elevation, and nerve displacement provide solutions in selected patients, but results are inconsistent.

Osseointegrated pure titanium Diskimplants (Victory Implantoral Production, Nice, France) represent a possible solution for these small bone volumes. The wide range of base diameters and shaft heights allows the surgeon to make optimal use of all available bone in both horizontal and vertical dimensions[1] (Fig 1). Numerous prosthetic components provide the opportunity to achieve excellent functional and cosmetic results. Connection is also possible with other types of osseointegrated fixtures.[2-4] Prevention of bone fracture is a major concern when dealing with direct bone/implant contact subsequent to successful osseointegration. The rigid Antistress System (Victory Implantoral Production) available for prosthetic abutments protects the osseointegrated implant by absorbing forces; if excess stress is applied, the connection collapses, as with a fuse, thus protecting the implant system and bone structure. The Antistress unit can then easily be retrieved and replaced immediately.

*Paper was orally presented by Dr William Hoisington, Seattle, Washington.

Diskimplant system

The Diskimplant features a 0.5-mm-thick disc at the base of a shaft formed by a series of cylinders. Base diameters vary from 5 to 10 mm, increasing in 1-mm increments. The shaft has a constant diameter of 2 mm but is available in several heights. The appropriate base diameter is determined by the distance between the cortical plates; implant height depends on the available bone depth and abutment location selected by the surgeon.

Because it produces minimal operative trauma without thermal bone injury, the lateral osteotomy procedure is compatible with osseointegration even in small bone volumes (Fig 2). After a full-thickness flap is raised, drilling is performed with a high-speed turbine (pressure = 3 bars) accompanied by sprays of sterile water and air. Microchannels along the cutter shaft promote continuous internal irrigation of the bone during the osteotomy (Fig 3). A silicone surgical suction tube is placed against the zone of osteotomy to guard against emphysema. The lateral bone opening permits the exchange of air and water, thereby preventing accumulation in the tissues. Cooling takes place instantly, as demonstrated by in vivo measurement using thermal transducers with an accuracy of 0.1° (with a water spray at 18°C, drilling occurs between 26°C and 28°C).[5]

The Diskimplant itself is slightly larger than the pure titanium cutter so as to achieve primary retention when inserted into the receptor site along the same lateral path, from the buccal to

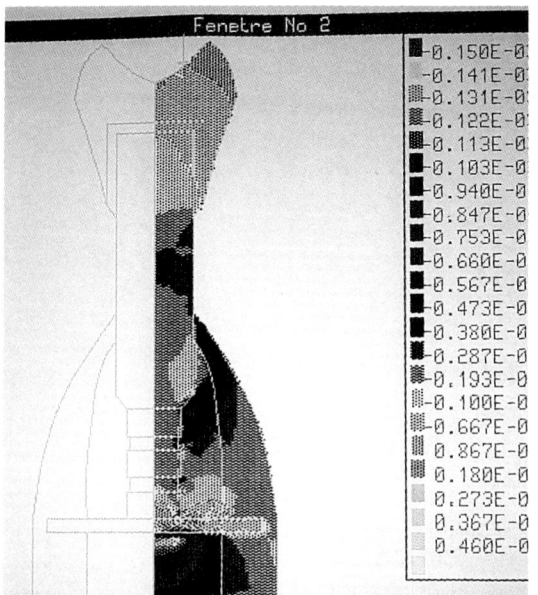

Fig 1 Finite element analysis demonstrating the benefits of cortical support in small bone volumes.

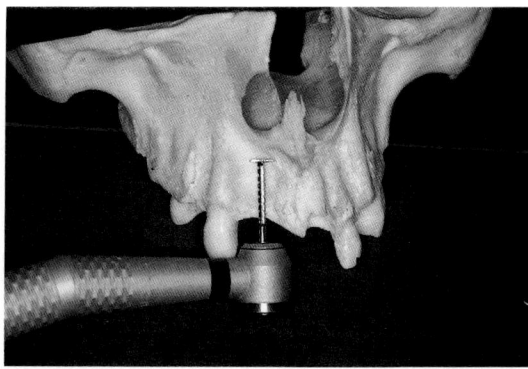

Fig 2 Principle of lateral osteotomy using the pure titanium cutter.

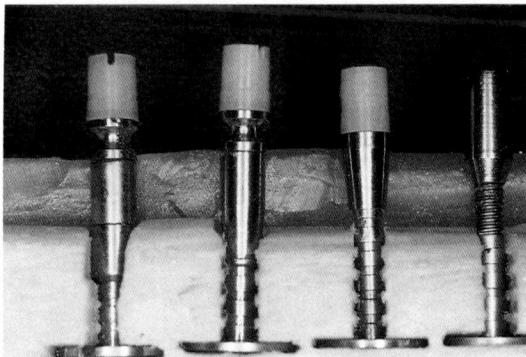

Fig 4 Diskimplants (series I, E, EL) equipped with the Antistress System (bendable or straight pure titanium abutment).

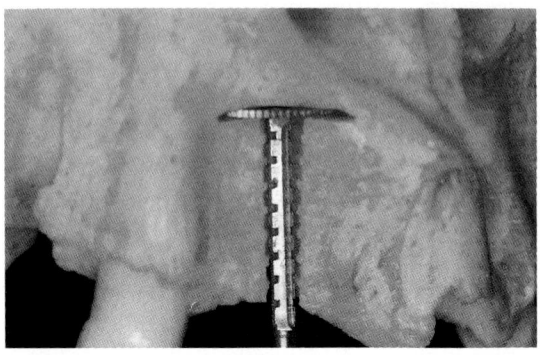

Fig 3 Pure titanium cutter. Note the cutting surfaces on the basal disc and shaft.

the palatal or lingual cortical plate. The lateral flap is then sutured over the implant site. If bone density is sufficient, no additional material is required; coverage of the T-shaped receptor site by the blood clot and periosteum provides enough biological elements for natural bone repair. If the bone is of poor quality and/or the mucoperiosteal flap has been damaged during surgery, a biomaterial such as hydroxyapatite or calcium triphosphate is needed. The implant is left submerged 4 to 8 months for osseointegration. After this healing period, the implant is reexposed for placement of the prosthetic abutment and fabrication of the removable or fixed prosthesis.[6] Fixed prostheses are now connected by means of an Antistress System, which compensates for the lack of a ligament subsequent to direct bone/implant contact (Fig 4).

Double-disc Diskimplants

Introduced some 8 years ago, double-disc Diskimplants are now commonly used in the maxilla in combination with biomaterials for ridge aug-

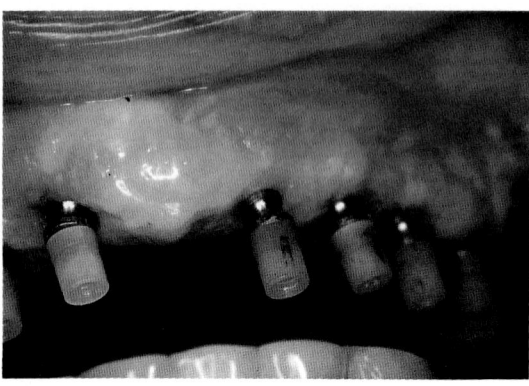

Fig 5a Antistress System with bendable abutments in position in a 71-year-old patient.

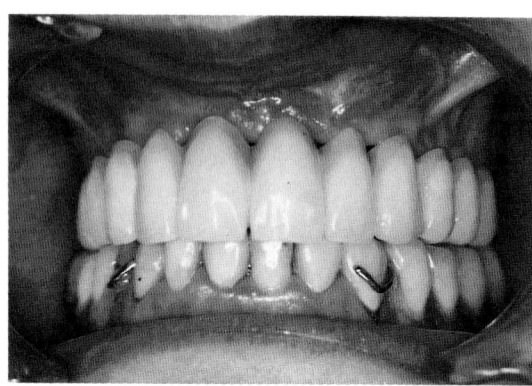

Fig 5b General esthetic appearance (Wiron/cobalt/acrylic) resin fixed partial denture.

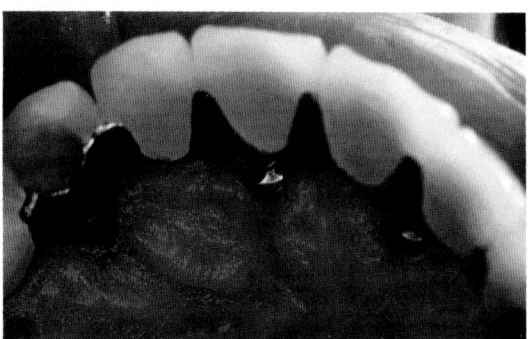

Fig 5c Palatal view.

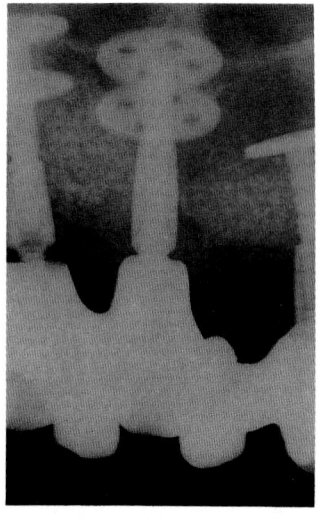

Fig 5d Radiograph at 5 years.

mentation, especially for high and narrow ridges. This is a simple and reliable procedure for achieving support in bone areas where other endosseous implants cannot be used.[7] In very thin ridges, part of the two discs is left protruding beyond the lateral aspect of the ridge to maintain the periosteal flap at a distance from the bone. The space is filled with hydroxyapatite and the blood clot. This procedure for tissue augmentation avoids the need for false gingivae.

Antistress System

Osseointegration has proven to be the best type of biologic bond because it guarantees long-term stability of the implant.[8,9] However, the resultant mechanical rigidity of the bone/implant unit results in direct transmission of forces to the bone tissue, since there is no ligament to absorb stresses.[4,5] From a physiologic standpoint, the main consequence of osseointegration is the absence of proprioception. The exact implications of this situation remain unclear, because the role of proprioception is often assumed by the antagonist teeth, although cases of fracture have been reported in the literature.[6] This could lead to mechanical failures despite successful tissue integration.

To overcome these problems, the Antistress stressbreaker system was introduced in Europe

4 years ago (Figs 5a to d). In the laboratory, the technician constructs a conventional implant-based prosthesis using a screw technique[7]; the dentist substitutes the Antistress unit in the office. A nylon-fiberglass shock absorbing unit screwed onto a titanium support is inserted between the metal framework of the prosthesis and the osseointegrated implant, then it is cemented with a specific surgical resin cement to the prosthesis to achieve rigidity. As soon as the threshold of resistance (predetermined by the manufacturer) is reached, the unit breaks first, like a fuse. The resin cement separates from the nylon-fiberglass component, which itself separates from the titanium support. This chain reaction protects the osseointegrated implant and the surrounding bone as well as the prosthesis.

The Antistress System eliminates several drawbacks encountered with screws: loosening; locking in position, complicating removal; difficulties in controlling the torque applied to individual screws (for example, 15 N on one screw but 17 or 15 N on another). Application of differing torques creates varying internal tensions, thereby increasing the potential for future fractures.

Screws are used only for temporary trials, generally during the first 24 hours after prosthesis positioning, to allow time to check the occlusion and embrasures. The screw is then replaced by surgical cement containing radiodense zirconium (allowing detection of any excess product). As it hardens, the cement takes the place of a screw and the entire Antistress unit becomes a solid and rigid implant-prosthesis connection. Actual screwing of the prosthesis to the Antistress unit remains an option for selected cases.

Along with being easy to use, this cement has the advantage of containing an antibiotic (gentamicin) that combats unpleasant odors. Tested in orthopedic surgery for nearly 20 years, the surgical cement has proven adaptable for use in oral implantology. The Antistress cementing system solves a major problem in implant prosthodontics because the dentist can retrieve the prosthesis at any time if necessary. The nylon-fiberglass component is usually changed every

2 to 4 years, and the prosthesis can be recemented immediately. The possibility for rapid repair and replacement of the shock-absorbing element is a considerable advantage, because it protects subjacent metal components from wear and fracture. This is especially important because of the increasing use of implants in young patients with a life expectancy of over 50 years.

Discussion

Indications and limitations of the Diskimplant System

The system is indicated especially for pyramidal type ridge crests in which lateral insertion is favored by the presence of a more or less vertical bone surface. In nontraumatic and normal occlusal conditions, the number of Diskimplants is calculated by dividing the number of natural roots formerly present in the region by two. In difficult occlusal situations or in patients with bruxism, more abutments and the Antistress System are indicated. For high and thin ridges, a double-disc Diskimplant is indicated, especially in the maxilla. Round, flat crests are best managed with a single-disc Diskimplant or a fixture when ridge height is sufficient. When the amount and quality of bone in the maxilla necessitate use of an autogenous graft, fixtures are indicated and not Diskimplants. The Diskimplant technique provides excellent security provided the indications are respected and the operator has received sufficient training.

Analysis of results for 1,278 Diskimplants placed in the maxilla of partially edentulous patients for 1 to 10 years, with or without an adjunctive biomaterial, revealed a success rate of 85% and excellent functional and cosmetic outcomes in difficult anatomic regions.

Partially edentulous maxilla

Osseointegration provides rigidity of the bone/implant complex and an absence of proprioception provided by the periodontal ligament. The Antistress System overcomes the drawbacks of ligament loss while protecting the bone, implant, and prosthesis from material shear or fractures by reducing stresses at the metal interfaces between the prosthesis and the implant. The Antistress System also makes feasible the use of ceramic occlusal surfaces.

Patient selection criteria

Maxilla

Bone volume requirements: Only those non-smoking patients meeting the following criteria are candidates for Diskimplants in the maxilla:

- 6-mm bone minimum in the vertical dimension
- Alveolar ridge diameters: crest $\geq$ 2.5 mm, base $\geq$ 7 mm
- Bone quality: dense

Smokers are routinely rejected for surgery or requested to stop all smoking for 3 weeks prior to surgery (or longer if the Diskimplant is placed partially within the sinus).

Number of implants: Single-tooth replacement using implants of the IH or IDDH series are possible if occlusal conditions are favorable and if there are a sufficient number of remaining natural abutments to avoid excessive load on the single implant.

A minimum of three implant abutments (series E, EDD, I, or IDD) are required for maxillary freestanding fixed prostheses. Occasionally, if anatomic and occlusal conditions are favorable and the bone is dense, two implants may be sufficient.

The number of implants required for a fixed restoration is determined by dividing the number of natural roots previously present in the anatomic sector by two. Other factors affecting component use are the occlusal conditions of the antagonist elements (teeth or removable denture), dimensions of the dental arch, patient's height and weight, and the possibility of bruxism. Patient sex and age have relatively little importance when there is enough good quality bone. By contrast, menopausal women who already have a small bone volume may not be candidates for dental implants because of the considerable physiologic and pathologic bone loss that can occur over a short period of time.

Mandible

In the mandible, where cortical bone is always present, bone height as small as 5 mm is sufficient, provided a minimum width of 7 mm is available at the base of the alveolar ridge. Diskimplants have also been successfully implanted in elderly patients with bone heights of only 2 to 3 mm whose masticatory force and muscle tone are considerably reduced. For young, much stronger patients, at least 5 mm are needed in height and 7 mm in width at the base. When occlusal conditions are difficult, as can occur with tall and very muscular patients, one or two additional implants are indicated to allow for the anticipated increased functional load.

Conclusion

Long-term clinical results have demonstrated the validity and safety of the Diskimplant system when used by experienced surgeons working as a team with skilled prosthodontists. Furthermore, should failure occur, the Diskimplant is retrieved using the same lateral pathway as for insertion; the small amount of bone used for anchorage (5 to 8 mm) favors subsequent healing and repair, and thus a reduced risk of permanent injury.

References

1. Michel MC, Veyret D, Pantaloni J, Martin R. Analyse comparative par éléments finis d'implants odontologiques avec et sans appui cortical. *Le Chirurgien-Dentiste de France* 1990;510:83–89.

2. Gomez Gonzalez MA. El implante endooséo: Diskim-plant. Alternativa de tratamiento protesico en la odonto-estomatologia. Thèse, Universidad Del Pais Vasco, 1986.

3. Bourbon B, Scortecci G. Prothèse sur Diskimplant. *Revue Française de Prothésistes Dentaires* 1990;13:31–48.

4. Crousillat J, Scortecci G, Foesser P, Bourbon B. La prothèse implantaire au laboratoire. *Les Cahiers de Prothèse* 1989;67:89–103.

5. Scortecci G. Etude comparative de l'échauffement lors du fraisage de l'os. *Industries Dentaires* 1988;22:34–37.

6. Hoisington W. Osseointegrated Diskimplant System: Tissue-integrated prosthesis for small bone volumes. Presented at the UCLA Symposium on implants in the partially edentulous patient, Palm Springs, Calif, April 19–21 1990.

7. Scortecci G. Double Diskimplants in thin maxillary ridges for fixed prosthodontics. Report on seven years' use in Europe. Proc 54th Annual Meeting, Pacific Coast Society of Prosthodontists, Los Angeles, June 1990.

8. Brånemark P-I, Zarb GA, Albrektsson T. *Tissue-Integrated Prostheses: Osseointegration in Clinical Dentistry.* Chicago, Quintessence Publ Co, 1985.

9. Adell R, Lekholm U, Rockler B, Brånemark P '. A 15-year study of osseointegrated implants in the treatment of the edentulous jaw. *Int J Oral Surg* 1981;10:387–416.

Evaluation of Titanium Implants in Alveolar Ridges Reconstructed with Hydroxyapatite

W.B. Donohue and E.A. Stuebner

Hydroxyapatite (HA) has been shown to be of use in the reconstruction of atrophied alveolar ridges.[1] Marshall reported on the simultaneous placement of collagen/HA and endosseous implants in humans.[2] The endosseous implants were first placed in the mandible, and then a solid block of collagen/HA was placed over the implants. Twelve weeks later the implants were exposed, and the transgingival sleeves were placed on the implants and extended through the HA into the mouth. Marshall reported excellent results with this technique. Scattered clinical reports have indicated the successful use of HA in contact with implants.[3–5]

Using rabbits as the experimental animals, we have studied the effects of placing HA around titanium implants.[6,7] In this work the HA was placed in contact with part of the implant body that was purposefully left to project through the cortex into the subcutaneous tissues. The HA was placed at the same time as, or 1 month prior to the time of implant placement. The results indicated that in rabbits the use of collagen/HA did not increase the formation of bone around the implant.

This retrospective cohort study was undertaken to evaluate the feasibility of placing implants though ridges that had previously been reconstructed with various types of HA. This question is important because in some cases preprosthetic HA rehabilitation of the alveolar ridges does not give adequate clinical results. In other instances insufficient bone is present for the placement of endosseous implants. If implants can be placed through HA ridges, these patients might still benefit from the advantages of endosseous implants.

Materials and methods

Sixteen patients were used in this clinical analysis, of which 14 were females. The patients were selected because they were dissatisfied with their denture function despite previous ridge reconstruction with HA. All patients were evaluated clinically and radiographically prior to placing the implants. All patients were white, varying in age from 32 to 67 years with a mean of 47 years. Fifteen of the patients were completely edentulous with various degrees of atrophy. Twelve of the patients previously had preprosthetic surgery involving ridge reconstruction with HA only, two patients received a mixture of HA and freeze-dried bone, and two patients were treated with a particulate bone graft mixed with HA. Seven patients had a lowering of the floor of the mouth procedure with skin grafts several months after the HA had been placed. The time elapsed prior to implant placement varied from 5 months to 7 years (Table 1).

Three different implant systems were the source of 67 implants. In 11 patients, 53 Brånemark implants (Nobelpharma Canada Inc, Willowdale, Ontario, Canada) were placed, four patients received 11 IMZ fixtures (Interpore International, Irvine, Calif) and four Core-Vent implants (Core-Vent Corp, Encino, Calif) were

Table 1 Time elapsed between HA placement and implant insertion

Years	5 mo–1	1–2	2–3	3–4	4–5	5–6	6–7	7–8
No. of patients	3	8	1	1	1	1	—	1
(no. of implants)	(14)	(27)	(4)	(10)	(5)	(4)		(4)

Table 2 Type of HA and implants used in 16 patients

Total no. patients	HA		Implants		
	porous*	nonporous†	Brånemark	IMZ	Core-Vent
16	4	12	11	4	1

* One case with freeze-dried bone + HA.
† Three cases with autogenous bone graft + HA; 1 case with freeze-dried bone + HA.

placed in one patient. Both porous and nonporous HA were used in the ridge reconstructions. The types of implants and HA used are indicated in Table 2.

All of the patients were treated under general anesthesia. Antibiotics were given intramuscularly immediately prior to and after placement of the implants and were continued postoperatively by mouth for 1 week.

The mandibular ridge was exposed by placing a horizontal incision in the vestibular mucosa and then undermining and reflecting the gingiva covering the alveolar crest. The implants were then placed using the standard recognized techniques of low-speed, high-torque drilling, with copious irrigation and a "no touch" technique when handling the titanium implants, the screw-tapping devices, or the trephines.

In five patients, biopsy specimens were taken from the hard HA alveolar ridge using a 5-mm diameter trephine. The specimens were fixed in 10% neutral formalin. After 1 month, they were embedded in methyl methracrylate resin and sectioned with a Reichert-Jung 20-50 supercut microtome (Reichert-Jung Inc, Buffalo, NY). The sections were 5 μm in thickness and stained with hematoxylin-eosin, Gomori trichrome, and silver nitrate counter-stained with toluidine blue.

Camera lucida drawings were made of one section per biopsy specimen using a standard magnification. The whole section was included in the drawing, and areas of fibrous tissue, bone apposition, and HA resorption were traced on the drawing. Using a Zeiss MOP Videoplan Computer System (Karl Zeiss, Oberkochen, Germany), the percentages of the various tissues were computed.

The implants in all patients were exposed after 4 to 6 months and the transgingival sleeves or inserts placed. The prosthetic reconstruction consisted of a fixed prosthesis in seven patients, Dolder bar with clips in the denture in eight patients, and the use of magnets in the remaining patient.

Patients were recalled for clinical examination at 2 weeks, 6 weeks, 6 months, 1 year, and at yearly intervals after placement of the implants. Clinical examination included the evaluation of oral hygiene, measurement of pocket depth around the transgingival sleeves with a periodontal probe, observation of the presence of inflammation or hyperplasia of the gingiva around the posts, the presence of bleeding after pocket probing, and testing for mobility of the implant after removal of the fixed prosthesis or Dolder bar. Orthopantomograms were taken after 3 and 12 months and every 24 months thereafter. The radiographs were examined for

Table 3 Followup period for 16 patients treated with titanium implants and HA

Years in function	0–1	1–2	2–3	3–4
No. of implants	10	11	37	10

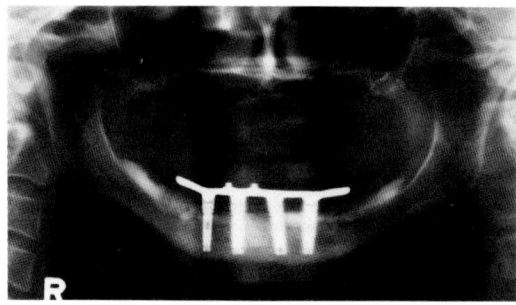

Fig 1 Orthopantomogram showing implants placed through HA.

the presence of pathosis around the implants and sleeves. All pre- and postoperative complications were recorded. Measurements were made on standard orthopantomograms to determine the approximate percentage of the body of the implant in contact with the HA. Only the implants where the fixture and the HA could be clearly seen were used for this measurement (Fig 1). A total of 22 implants were examined in this manner.

Results

The findings in 16 patients who were treated with endosseous implants in two treatment centers are reported here. There were seven patients treated at St. Mary's Hospital, Montreal, and nine at Thorek Hospital and Medical Center, Chicago. The postoperative observation period ranged from 1 to 5 years (Table 3).

The surface consistency of the reconstructed ridge varied. In five patients the HA on the surface of the reconstructed ridge was surrounded by fibrous tissue, while the deeper layers near the cortex were firm and hard, giving the appearance of bone formation around the HA. In 11 patients, the surface of the alveolar ridge had a rough granular structure and was extremely hard (Fig 2). In these situations the ridge was difficult to cut. This made it necessary to change the burs, tapping devices, and trephines frequently as they rapidly lost their cutting edges.

Biopsy specimens taken were from the ridges that were hard and resistant. They showed very dense fibrous tissue formed around the HA granules. In some areas, bone formation was evident. In all of the biopsy specimens, signs of HA resorption were noted. This varied from the

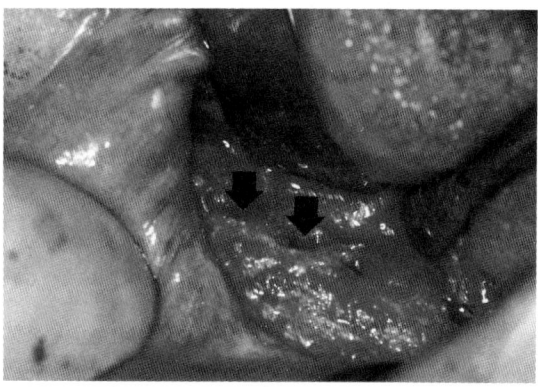

Fig 2 The granular surface of a previously reconstructed ridge. The implant preparations are indicated by the arrows.

presence of Howship's resorption lacunae to active osteoclastic/giant cell resorption (Fig 3). The remaining areas showed accumulations of red blood cells or tissue artifacts.

Histomorphological analysis of the biopsy specimens showed the following tissue distribution (arithmetic mean):

Fibrous tissue	50%
Bone formation	14%
HA resorption	34%

The variation in tissue distribution from one biopsy to the next was large.

In three patients with poor oral hygiene, a gingival sulcus depth of 3 mm or more was

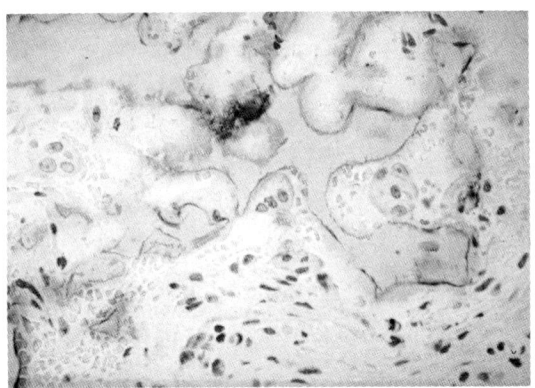

Fig 3 Photomicrograph of an undemineralized section of a biopsy specimen taken from a ridge reconstructed with HA 2 years previously. Note the active osteoclastic resorption of the HA granules (Gomori trichrome, original magnification × 400).

Table 4 Pocket depths, N = 68

Year	0–3 mm	3–8 mm
1	90%	10%
2	96%	4%

Table 5 Bleeding index, N = 68

Year	0 No bleeding on probing	1 Bleeding on probing
1	60%	40%
2	79%	21%

found around three implants after these had been in place for 2 years. These pockets were primarily the result of gingival hyperplasia. In the remaining patients, sulcus depth was 3 mm or less (Table 4). Bleeding was noted on probing around the implants in ten patients (23 implants) at the end of the first year (Table 5). In addition, one patient with scrupulous oral hygiene continued to show pocket formation, bleeding, congested hyperemic gingiva, and occasional purulent exudate from the pockets. This was the only patient using magnets as a retentive device for the prosthesis. Implant mobility was demonstrated in only one of the implants, which was later removed. The fixture, a Core-Vent implant, had been exposed for 13 months. It had been placed through a ridge that had been rebuilt with HA 5 months prior to implant placement and was being used to support a Dolder bar. There were no cases of bone infection. The mean anterior height of the mandible in 15 patients after placement of HA was 6 to 15 mm, with a mean of 11 mm.

Radiographic examination showed no evidence of bone loss around any of the implants. The loss of bone around the neck of the implant, which is commonly observed, was masked by the presence of the HA. Measurements of the HA/implant contact surface indicated that 10% to 70% of the vertical length of the implant body was in contact with HA, with an arithmetic mean of 39.66%. A resume of the patients' treatment schedule is outlined in Table 6.

Discussion

The results indicate that 98.5% of 68 endosseous implants placed through, or partly surrounded by HA, were in function after a postoperative followup period ranging from 12 months to 5 years. One implant was removed because of lack of osseointegration.

Fibrous tissue and bone formation around HA granules has previously been described.[5–8] The tissue reaction to HA placed subperiosteally varies depending on the type of HA used. El Deeb[8] has shown in the rhesus monkey that the use of porous HA leads to a greater proportion of bone being formed, while solid or nonporous HA shows fibrous tissue in and around the HA used to reconstruct infraorbital ridges. In our patients, the hard ridges showed fibrous tissue and bone formation around the HA granules. In some instances, one or other forms of tissue

Table 6 Implants placed after HA reconstruction

HA	Date placed	Time HA → implant placement	Implant	Implant yr function	Prosthesis	Jaw	No. implants
Alvegr*	08/87	5 mo	CV§	3	Dolder	Mandible	4
Alvegr	04/88	5 mo	IMZ¶	2	Fix	Mandible	4
Inter† + freeze-dried bone	12/88	6 mo	B#	1 1/2	Fix	Mandible	6
Alvefr‡	06/87	1 y	B	3	Fix	Mandible	4
Inter	07/87	1 y 1 mo	B	3	Dolder	Mandible	4
Alvefr	07/87	1 y 2 mo	B	3	Dolder	Mandible	4
Inter	10/88	1 y 2 mo	B	2	Dolder	Mandible	4
Autog Bone + Alvegr	10/88	1 y 5 mo	B	2	Dolder	Mandible	4
Inter	10/88	1 y 6 mo	IMZ	2	Fix	Maxilla	2
Autog Bone + Alvegr	06/88	1 y 6 mo	IMZ	2	Fix	Mandible	1
Alvegr	10/88	1 y 7 mo	IMZ	2	Fix	Mandible	4
Alvegr	03/88	2 y	B	2	Dolder	Mandible	4
Freeze-dried bone + Alveogr	08/89	3 y	B	1	Dolder	Mandible	6
				1	Dolder	Maxilla	4
Alvegr	05/88	4 y 7 mo	B	2	Fix	Mandible	5
Alvegr	11/88	5 y 5 mo	B	2	Fix	Mandible	4
Alvegr	03/88	7 y 5 mo	B	2	Fix	Mandible	4

*Alvegr = Alveograf: nonporous HA (Cook-Waite Co)
†Inter = Interpore: porous HA (Interpore International Inc)
‡Alvefr = Alveoform: HA-collagen (Collagen Corp)
§CV = Core-Vent implants (Core-Vent Corp)
¶IMZ = IMZ implants (Interpore International Inc)
#B = Brånemark implants (Nobelpharma Inc)

formation predominated. In all five ridges biopsied there was evidence of HA resorption. The implants placed through this material showed stability and firmness. Kraut et al[5] have shown that implant integration can be achieved when the grafted site contains between 35.9% and 46.2% bone. In our series the bone content varied between 10% and 25%. In five of the nonbiopsied patients, the HA on the crest of the ridges was surrounded by fibrous tissue. Integration of the implants nevertheless occurred despite the lack of complete bone contact with the whole surface of the implant. The lower bone content in this series no doubt stems from the fact that the five biopsied ridges had been reconstructed with HA only; whereas Kraut's case was reconstructed with a mixture of autogenous bone and porous HA. Cobb and his coauthors[9] have shown that the highest percentage of bone integration with HA granules is achieved when the grafted material is a mixture of 50% HA and autogenous bone per volume. The lowest percentage of bone content was noted in grafts consisting of 100% HA, as was the case in 12 of our 16 patients. In our series of clinical cases, implant integration occurred despite the decrease in bone contact with the whole body surface of the implant.

The gingiva in the patient in whom magnets were used as retentive devices showed continued inflammation. The gingival reaction was probably the result of compression of the soft tissues around the implants by the mandibular denture.

Conclusion

Augmentation of the atrophic alveolar process with HA is an accepted method of treatment for edentulous patients. However, there is a limit to the amount of augmentation that can be done in the severely atrophied jaw, and the result may not significantly improve the denture retention area. These clinical results indicate that it is technically feasible to place endosseous implants through HA with minimal complications.

Further evaluation, particularly prospective cohort studies, using standardized HA augmentation and endosseous fixture techniques, will help to assess the benefits and limitations of this combined implant procedure.

References

1. Kent JN, Quinn JH, Zide MF, Guerra LR, Boyne PJ. Alveolar ridge augmentation using non-resorbable hydroxylapatite with or without autogenous cancellous bone. *J Oral Maxillofac Surg* 1983;41:629–642.
2. Marshall SG. The combined use of endosseous dental implants and collagen/hydroxylapatite augmentation procedures for reconstruction/augmentation of the edentulous and atrophic mandible: A preliminary report. *Oral Surg Oral Med Oral Pathol* 1989;68:517–525.
3. Davenport WL, Heldt L, Bump RL. Salvage of the mandibular staple bone plate following bone infection. *J Oral Maxillofac Surg* 1985;43:981–986.
4. Babbush CA. Oral rehabilitation with porous hydroxylapatite granules IMZ implants. *IMZ Update* 1987;1:3.
5. Kraut RA, Kessler HP, Holmes RE. Quantification of bone in dental implant site after composite grafting of the mandible: Report of a case. *Int J Oral Maxillofac Implants* 1989;4:153–158.
6. Donohue WB, Mascrès C. The use of hydroxylapatite (HA) with titanium implants. *J Oral Maxillofac Surg* 1989;47(suppl 1):111–112.
7. Donohue WB, Mascrès C. Effect of hydroxylapatite on bone formation around exposed heads of titanium implants in rabbits. *J Oral Maxillofac Surg* 1990;48:1196–1200.
8. El Deeb M, Holmes RE. Tissue response to facial contour augmentation with dense and porous hydroxylapatite in rhesus monkey. *J Oral Maxillofac Surg* 1989;47:1282–1289.
9. Cobb CM, Eik JD, Barker BF, Mosby EL, Hiatt WR. Restoration of mandibular continuity defects using combinations of hydroxylapatite and autogenous bone: Microscopic observations. *J Oral Maxillofac Surg* 1990;48:268–275.

Tissue Integration of One-Stage ITI Implants

D. Buser, H. Weber, and N.P. Lang

The submerged placement of endosseous implants underneath the soft tissue cover has been required as one of the prerequisites for the achievement of osseointegration. The purpose of the present study was to follow the tissue integration of 100 one-stage ITI (Straumann AG, Waldenburg, Switzerland) implants with a titanium plasma-sprayed surface, which were inserted into 70 partially edentulous patients. During the healing phase of at least 3 months free of functional loading forces, the patients performed careful plaque control. Subsequently, the implants were restored with fixed partial dentures. Following the prosthetic treatment, all patients were enrolled in a recall program with a 3-month interval. In that period, one implant revealed a peri-implant infection, which was successfully treated with antibiotics. The tissue integration of all implants was evaluated 12 months following implantation. Plaque and bleeding indices were obtained. Probing depths, distances between implant shoulder and mucosal margin, and clinical "attachment levels" were assessed. Mobility was measured with the Periotest (Siemens AG, Bensheim, Germany) procedure and standardized periapical radiographs were taken. The peri-implant soft tissues were clinically healthy with a mean bleeding index of 0.26 and a mean plaque index of 0.16, a reflection of excellent oral hygiene.

The mean probing depth was at 2.74 mm and the mean distance between implant shoulder and mucosal margin was at -0.12 mm. The addition of both values gave the mean clinical attachment level of 2.62 mm. All 100 implants revealed clinically no detectable mobility, and no periapical radiographs showed any signs of peri-implant radiolucencies. The obtained Periotest scores ranged from -8 to $+8$, with a mean of -3.78 for 60 mandibular implants. The mean of 40 maxillary implants was at $+0.60$. In summary, out of 100 inserted ITI implants, no early failures occurred and all implants showed a tissue integration with functional ankylosis. The prognosis of 99 implants seems to be good, but the implant with the treated peri-implant infection is questionable. It can be concluded that the one-stage procedure of ITI implants with a titanium plasma-sprayed surface appears to be consistent with the achievement of tissue integration. This research was supported by the ITI-Foundation/Switzerland.

Biomechanical Analysis of IMZ Implants in Goat Mandibles and Maxillae

R.A. Kraut, J. Dootson, and A. McCullen

IMZ (Interpore International, Irvine, Calif) dental implants were placed in the maxillae and mandibles of 17 caprine goats. Biomechanical studies were used to assess the integration at intervals from 2 to 24 weeks. The study[1] indicates that there is a time-dependent progressive increase in pull-out force. The forces were consistently higher for the mandible than the maxilla. Moreover, there was no correlation between the intraoperative stability of the implant and the postoperative pull-out force.

Reference

1. Kraut RA, Dootson J, McCullen A. Biomechanical analysis of osseointegration of IMZ implants in goat mandibles and maxillae. *J Oral Maxillofac Implants* 1991;6:187–194.

Overload Management of Osseointegrated Fixtures to Achieve Optimum Bone Remodeling Through Multistage Prosthodontic Loading

T.J. Balshi

The overload management of osseointegrated fixtures to achieve optimum bone remodeling through multistage prosthodontic loading is a concept that initially evolved out of necessity, rather than pretreatment planning. With increased experience in tissue-integrated prosthesis treatment, some of the overload conditions affecting a bone-anchored prosthesis can be avoided.

Understanding the nature of the attachment between an implant and the host bone is fundamental to the long-range treatment planning process. There are four mechanisms for the interfacial attachment between implants and bone. These include:

1. Highly differentiated fibrous tissue
2. Low differentiated fibrous tissue
3. Use of artificial fixatives (such as bone cements)
4. Direct anchorage of the implant to vital bone—referred to as osseointegration

Brånemark and colleagues have stated that the critical point regarding osseointegration is that living bone and marrow must be made to heal as a highly differentiated tissue and not allowed to develop into low differentiated scar tissue.[1] Implants surrounded by low differentiated scar tissue have been unsuccessful in the past and often have led to a soft tissue inflammatory response and osteitis.

Prosthetic management of patients undergoing implant-supported prosthesis reconstruction begins with the treatment planning process.

Direct management of these patients is critical immediately following fixture placement. It is during this healing period that the hematoma adjacent to the implant screw threads is transformed into new bone through a callous formation. The physiology of healing adjacent to the implant depends on revascularization of the bone followed by demineralization of injured bone and subsequent replacement with remineralized tissue. One highly critical aspect during this phase of the healing process is that no functional loading be applied to the implants.

Using resilient denture base materials provides a cushioned interface between the traditional denture prosthesis and the healing hard and soft tissues.

When cover screws are dehisced following fixture placement, the denture base must be relieved to avoid direct contact, which could transmit loading forces to the fixture. The removable prosthesis should be continually relined and relieved to maintain a soft cushion in the area where contact with the implant might occur under occlusal loading. If prolonged contact with the cover screw occurs at the time of fixture placement, fixtures placed in low-quality bone may be indirectly loaded via the resilient liners. This condition may produce micromovements between the implant and the healing bone, destroying the potential for osseointegration.

Normal loading

Functional loading of the fixtures should only

occur following an initial osseous healing period. Traditionally, the recommended healing period has been 5 to 6 months in the maxilla and 3 to 4 months in the mandible, with bone of suitable quality and quantity. When the quality and quantity of bone is diminished, the initial healing period should be extended.

Excessive loading

For patients known to have parafunctional habits, special prosthetic treatment planning must be undertaken. Before discussing direct implant loading, prosthetic management of these patients following stage 1 surgery should be modified. Strong emphasis should be placed on the complete abstinence from denture use for 3 to 4 weeks immediately following fixture placement. If this is not practical, extra care must be taken in preparing the transitional denture for soft lining over the fixture sites. Patients must be instructed that the denture be removed and left out of the mouth as much as possible and most definitely during sleep, since this is frequently the time when parafunctional loading forces are generated. More frequent change of the soft liners is highly recommended to continuously provide the softest denture surface contact with the healing tissues.

Total initial healing time should also be extended from 3 months to 4 or 5 months in the normal mandible. With good quality and quantity of bone in the maxilla, the initial healing should be extended to 6 or 7 months before stage 2 surgery. If inferior bone quality is noted in either arch, the initial healing period may be extended up to 1 year.

In considering the gradual prosthetic loading concept of osseointegrated implants following stage 1 surgery, five levels of functional loading are suggested. The loading conditions are varied by the prosthesis format and materials used. These loading levels include:

1. Minimal load: The removable tissue-integrated prosthesis with a very soft resilient liner.

2. Light load: A removable tissue-integrated prosthesis with clip-bar retention.[2]
3. Moderate load: An all-acrylic resin fixed conversion prosthesis,[3,4] or rigid metal clip-retained overdenture.
4. Standard load: A fixed tissue-integrated prosthesis constructed of gold framework with acrylic resin veneer.[1]
5. High impact load: A fixed tissue-integrated prosthesis constructed of porcelain-fused-to-gold.

The standard design rules for prosthesis fabrication may require modification for patients exhibiting parafunctional loading. Rather than extending a cantilever two times the abutment width in the molar region, and four times abutment width in the incisal region,[5] one should consider shortening or even eliminating cantilevered extensions, especially in the posterior where loading forces can be magnified.

Through experience, time-frame guidelines have been established to provide optimal opportunity for bone remodeling. These time sequences are as follows:

1. Minimal load: Functional loading with overdentures using very soft tissue conditioner, or soft liner should proceed for 0 to 6 months.
2. Light load: During the next 6 to 12 months, a splinted gold clip-bar may be incorporated to gain additional retention.
3. Moderate load: After a full year of overdenture use with a clip-bar, a fixed conversion prosthesis or rigid clip-bar overdenture may be fabricated and used for 3 to 4 months if the quality of bone has permitted a positive remodeling response.
4. Standard load: Following moderate loading, the traditional gold and acrylic resin tissue-integrated prosthesis should be used for 2 years to produce positive bone modeling. The fabrication of the traditional Brånemark bone-anchored prosthesis, a fixed acrylic resin and gold tissue-integrated prosthesis may then be utilized. It is important to note that this prosthesis should have minimal or no cantilevers. If the patient experiences

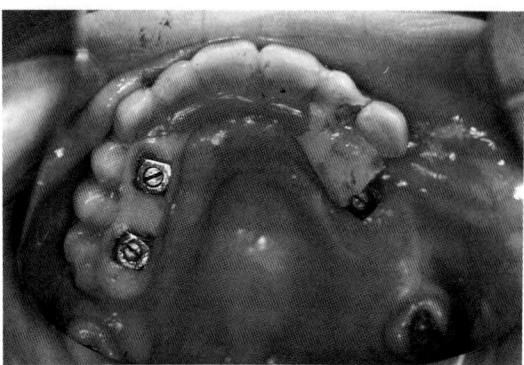

Fig 1a Four-month use of the conversion prosthesis.

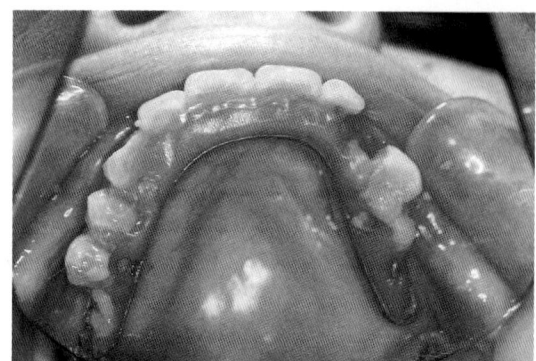

Fig 1b One year postprosthesis. Parafunction produced incisal attrition, fractured teeth, and lost vertical dimension of occlusion.

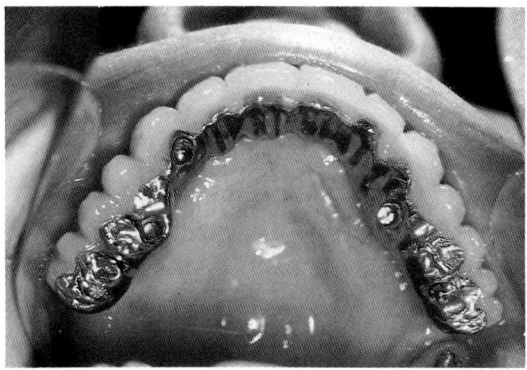

Fig 1c Gold occlusal and lingual surfaces designed to resist rapid wear produced by bruxism.

Clinical applications of the gradual loading concept

Rapid attrition

The first patient presented with oral debilitation, which required prosthetic rehabilitation. Although four long fixtures osseointegrated in relatively dense maxillary bone, it was evident during the 4-month use of the conversion prosthesis that the patient produced intense occlusal loading (Fig 1a).

The traditional Brånemark prosthesis consisting of a cast gold frame veneered with high-impact acrylic resin was placed following a 4-month fixture loading period with the conversion prosthesis.

Parafunctional forces in the form of bruxism produced severe incisal attrition as well as fractured denture teeth 1 year following the placement of this prosthesis (Fig 1b). In addition, severe occlusal wear patterns and deep facets were produced as a result of the bruxing condition. Maintenance and repairs for this prosthesis continued for a 2-year period.

To reduce the continuous maintenance and repair visits, a new tissue-integrated prosthesis was fabricated with a larger cast gold framework designed to deflect occlusal forces and protect incisal edges (Fig 1c) from the rapid attrition experienced with the traditional Brånemark restoration.

severe attrition of the prosthetic materials or is confronted by continuous maintenance problems such as fractured teeth or cracks in the veneering material, use of a more durable porcelain-fused-to-gold tissue-integrated prosthesis should be considered for the future.

5. High impact load: If functional loading remains successful during the previous period, the patient may then proceed with the next level of treatment. Use of a porcelain-fused-to-gold tissue-integrated prosthesis produces high-impact loads on the osseointegrated fixtures.

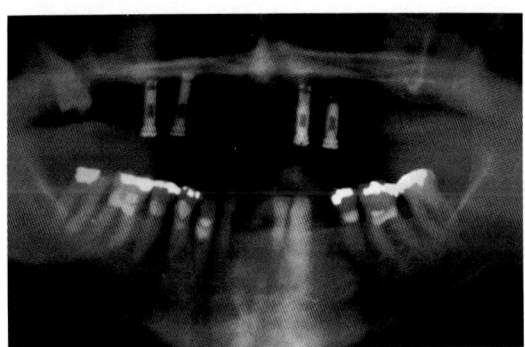

Fig 2a Increase in fixture support ratio illustrated by four additional fixture sites.

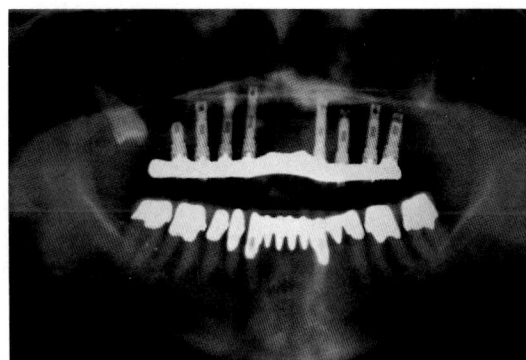

Fig 2b Radiograph of traditional Brånemark acrylic resin/gold tissue-integrated prosthesis.

Diagnostic forecasting

Fixture support ratio

A similar condition was experienced with a 73-year-old patient who presented with a loose maxillary denture and an inability to tolerate this removable prosthesis. During the initial clinical examination, four areas of dehiscence were noted over the cover screws of fixtures previously placed. The existing removable complete denture had been reinforced with a chrome framework. This should have been an indication of the severity of her bruxing and clenching habit as well as potential future problems.

The patient's dental appearance was satisfactory and in harmony with her facial features. Clinical profile view and lateral cephalometric film analysis indicated appropriate lip support provided by the interim removable prosthesis.

Treatment planning provided for a change in the fixture support ratio with additional fixture placement for maximal load distribution to the maxillary bone. The need for the placement of four additional fixtures can be seen in Fig 2a.

A 6-month healing period was permitted before stage 2 surgery. At the abutment connection, the short 7-mm fixture in the maxillary right posterior quadrant was lost.

The traditional Brånemark prosthesis was fraught with maintenance problems over the 2-year period that this prosthesis was in place

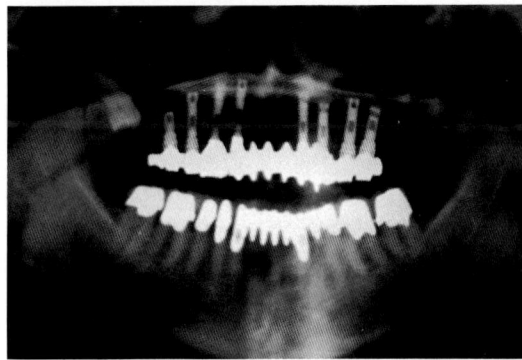

Fig 2c Radiograph of porcelain/gold tissue-integrated prosthesis with heavier framework design.

(Fig 2b). Chronic fracture of the canines and premolars occurred. With continued stability of the osseointegrated fixtures, this prosthesis was then replaced with a porcelain-fused-to-gold bone-anchored restoration. Figure 2c illustrates the framework design for the porcelain-fused-to-gold tissue-integrated prosthesis with heavier framework construction. For patients with heavy occlusal function, the porcelain-fused-to-gold bone-anchored prosthesis provides more durable function.

High stress personality

Periodontally compromised teeth

One month following the placement of the final porcelain-fused-to-gold prosthesis, the patient

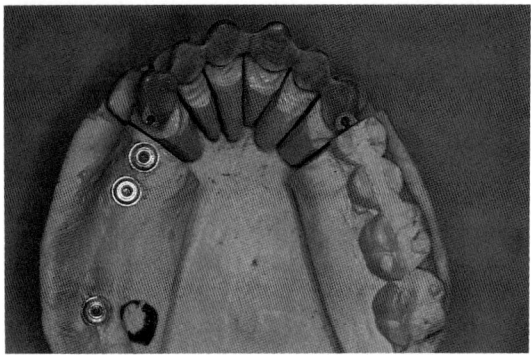

Fig 3a The three fixtures illustrated on the working cast supported a tissue-integrated prosthesis connected to the anterior tooth splint with a precision attachment.

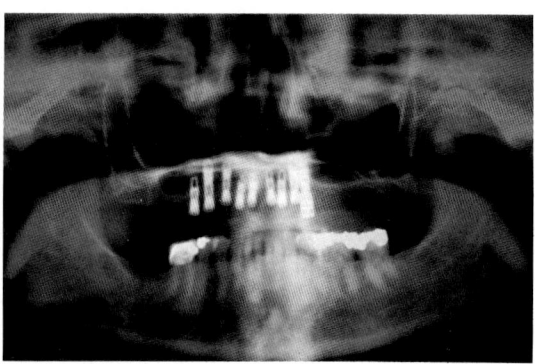

Fig 3b Removal of the maxillary anterior teeth was followed by the placement of Brånemark fixtures.

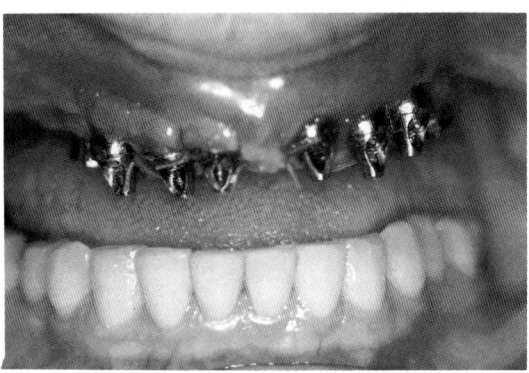

Fig 3c Abutment connection following an 8-month healing period.

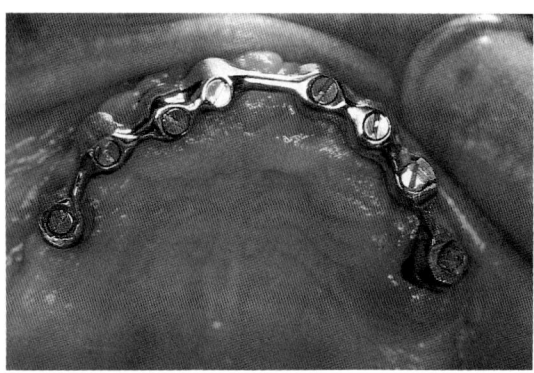

Fig 3d Gold clip-bar splints eight maxillary fixtures.

complained of discomfort in the maxillary posterior area (Fig 3a). Following clinical reevaluation and retrieval of the tissue-integrated prosthesis, the most posterior fixture exhibited clinical mobility and was no longer osseointegrated. The prosthesis was modified by removing the most posterior abutment. During the following 6-month period, a second fixture was lost to functional overload. The decision was then made to use a provisional removable partial denture to replace the missing posterior dentition. The concept of sinus lift grafting procedures was suggested to the patient. The six splinted anterior teeth continued to exhibit anterior-posterior

mobility. The patient rejected the recommendation for bone grafting in the sinus areas and elected instead to have the mobile anterior teeth removed and additional fixtures placed (Fig 3b). Now with eight osseointegrated fixtures, the prosthetic treatment plan called for a gradual loading process to permit additional bone remodeling around these fixtures.

An 8-month healing time was permitted to elapse before the stage 2 surgery was performed. Following the abutment connection (Fig 3c), a non-fixture-retentive overdenture was fabricated to minimize loading of the newly uncovered fixtures. In addition, direct occlusal

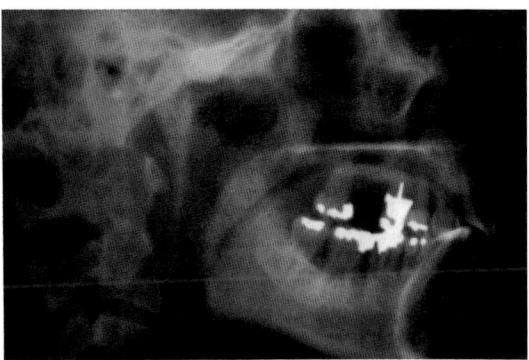

Fig 4a Lateral cephalometric radiograph demonstrates Class II relationship.

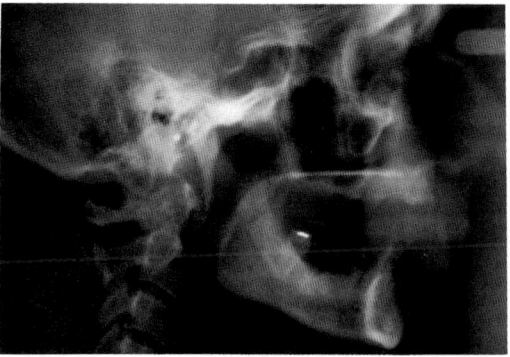

Fig 4b Lateral cephalometric radiograph illustrates maintenance of the patient's profile following removal of all the maxillary teeth.

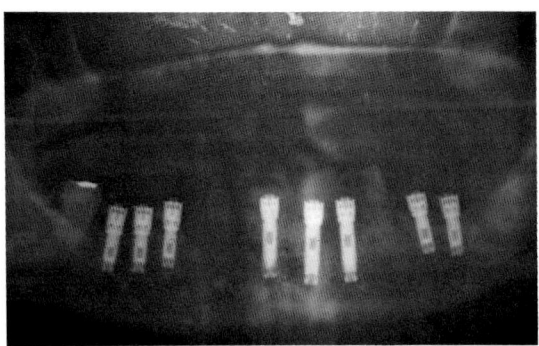

Fig 4c Fixtures placed between periodontally compromised teeth.

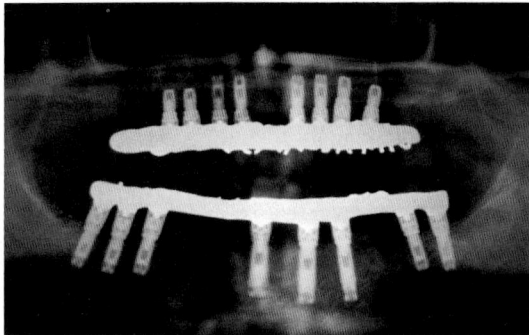

Fig 4d Both maxillary and mandibular arches were restored with traditional Brånemark fixed tissue-integrated prostheses.

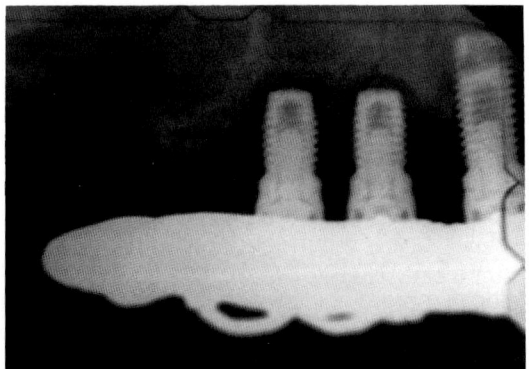

Fig 4e Radiograph of right side illustrating loss of integration around 7-mm fixtures.

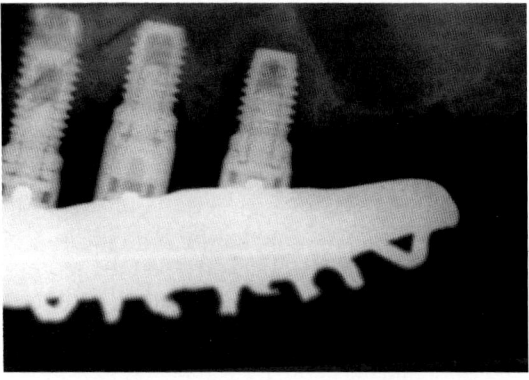

Fig 4f The radiograph from the left side illustrating the loss of integration around the last fixture.

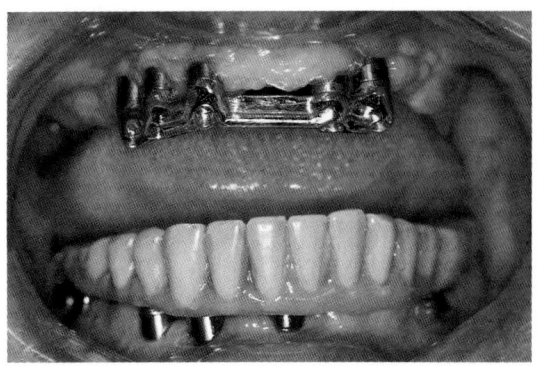

Fig 4g Gold clip-bar supported by five fixtures.

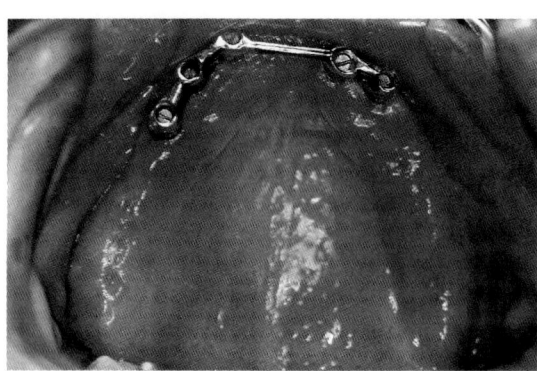

Fig 4h Inflamed residual ridge area resulting from intense occlusal loading.

loading was eliminated. This was accomplished by using dead soft wax placed in the denture to assure contact avoidance between the implants and the hard denture base. A resilient denture base material was then used to reline the overdenture prosthesis.

Six months following the use of the nonretentive overdenture, a gold clip-bar (Fig 3d) was fabricated, splinting the eight fixtures for improved load distribution. The modified overdenture had modest implant-provided retention and transmitted loading forces to the fixture. However, incorporation of the clip itself was postponed for an additional 6 months.

Biologic and mechanical complications attributed to parafunction

A clinical example illustrating biologic and mechanical complications stemming from parafunctional habits was demonstrated by a young woman with severe generalized periodontitis in both the maxilla and mandible, and posterior bite collapse. The cephalometric analysis (Fig 4a), demonstrated a severe Class II skeletal relationship with a deep overbite. Periapical radiographs confirmed the 60% to 70% generalized bone loss around the remaining teeth.

Following removal of all the periodontally involved teeth in the maxilla, the patient was provided with an interim denture to maintain esthetic lip and muscle support.[6,7] This prosthesis provided only limited function. The lateral cephalometric film shows the patient totally edentulous in the maxilla and partially edentulous in the mandible, with maintenance of her soft tissue profile (Fig 4b).

The three remaining mandibular periodontally compromised teeth were used to support a provisional restoration following the Class III modification of the Brånemark method for treatment.[4] Eight Brånemark fixtures were surgically placed between these abutment teeth (Fig 4c).

A new provisional overdenture for the maxillary arch was designed to develop a Class I occlusal scheme. With the fabrication of the final tissue-integrated prosthesis in the mandible and a new maxillary denture, a Class I occlusal relationship was finally established.

The maxillary arch had eight fixtures placed and was reconstructed using the traditional Brånemark bone-anchored prosthesis (Fig 4d). Adequate lip support and dental esthetics were established. Traditional cantilevers, approximately 10 to 13 mm long, extended from the most distal fixtures bilaterally in the maxillary arch.

Mechanical complications related to clenching and bruxism became evident during the first year following delivery of the maxillary fixed prosthesis. The patient presented on several occasions with fractures of the prosthetic materials, most often in the posterior areas.

The occlusal scheme established provided canine guidance in lateral excursion and incisor guidance in protrusion. Biologic complications were noted 1 1/2 years following the delivery of the final prosthesis. The patient then returned with sensitivity bilaterally in the maxillary posterior area. Periapical radiographs indicated that the two most distal 7-mm fixtures on the right side (Fig 4e) and the last 7-mm fixture on the left side were no longer osseointegrated (Fig 4f). This was most likely the result of the patient's intense occlusal loading pattern, which destroyed the bone/implant interface, allowing epithelial migration between the implant and the bone.

The five remaining fixtures were determined to be inadequate to support a fixed prosthesis. A gold clip-bar was then fabricated to splint the remaining fixtures for maximum removable prosthesis (Fig 4g). This overdenture, with a retention clip, was planned for use during the next 6 to 12 months. One month following delivery of this removable implant-supported prosthesis, the inflamed palatal tissues were clinically evident (Fig 4h). Comparing these tissues to the previously healthy mucosal tissues confirmed the intense occlusal loading produced by the patient.

Conclusion

In summary, gradual implant loading and progressive bone remodeling for osseointegrated implant patients is an important consideration when parafunctional habits are recognized. The time sequence suggested in the time-frame guidelines provides a simple guide. Each patient's individual occlusal force patterns must be assessed in relationship to the quality and quantity of bone and the number and distribution of osseointegrated fixtures. Management of patients with parafunctional habits can be accomplished with osseointegrated fixtures. However, their treatment plans must include long time periods producing gradual implant loading. This will enable the adjacent bone to remodel and/or the implant/bone interface to strengthen.

Parafunctional occlusal patterns are not always evident at the diagnostic stage or even early in the prosthetic treatment program. The earlier these patterns are noted, the better the opportunity to modify the tissue-integrated prosthesis to establish a more gradual loading environment.

References

1. Brånemark P-I, Zarb GA, Albrektsson T. *Tissue-Integrated Prostheses: Osseointegration in Clinical Dentistry.* Chicago: Quintessence Publ Co, 1985.
2. Zarb GA. Tissue integrated prostheses: Osseointegration research in Toronto. *Int J Periodont Rest Dent* 1987;7(1):9–35.
3. Balshi T. The Biotes conversion prosthesis: A provisional fixed prosthesis supported by osseointegrated titanium fixtures for restoration of the edentulous jaw. *Quintessence Int* 1985;10:667–677.
4. Balshi T. Tissue Integration in Oral and Maxillofacial Reconstruction, *Proceedings of an International Congress,* Brussels, May 1985. Excerpta Medica, 1986.
5. Rangert B, Jemt T, Jorneus L. Forces and moments on Brånemark implants. *Int J Oral Maxillofac Implants* 1989;4:241–247.
6. Balshi T. Osseointegration for the periodontally compromised patients. *Int J Prosthodont* 1988;1:51–58.
7. Balshi T. Converting patients with periodontally hopeless teeth to osseointegration prostheses. *Int J Periodont Rest Dent* 1988;8(2):9–34.

Session VI Discussion

L. Shulman (Boston, Massachusetts): Dr Patrick, in the data you presented it appears that the implant was just as likely to reach 4 years as it was to reach 1 year. Could you tell us the type of life table analysis that was used?

D. Patrick (Encino, California): Basically the life table analysis that was used involved a determination of the number of implants that were successful over a certain period of time, the number that were removed, and a record of that data.

L. Shulman: You did not keep multiplying the numbers as you went on to show that it is less likely to get to 10 years than 5 years? You just took a raw percentage of each time period and it turned out to be about the same; is that correct?

D. Patrick: Precisely.

T. West: Dr Patrick, were all the cases you showed consecutive? As I understand it, these were all the patients seen over a 6-year period

from some time in 1982 until the end of October 1988 in four offices. Were you able to test mobility, since these were all cemented prostheses?

D. Patrick: Not all of the prostheses were cemented and in those that were, we had to rely on prosthesis mobility and not the individual implant. That could introduce some error. However, we then looked at the peri-implant radiolucency as the second criterion of success. Since the prosthesis was not mobile and there wasn't any peri-implant radiolucency or infection, the assumption, right or wrong, was made that the implant was nonmobile.

T. West: How did the protocol deal with a noncemented prosthesis? Was there a screw-retained implant?

D. Patrick: Yes, and in those patients the prosthesis was removed and the implant was individually checked.

Poster Presentations

Special Applications of Osseointegrated Implants in Prosthodontic Treatment

J.C. Abarno

Tissue-integrated prostheses provide new methods to solve difficult clinical situations. Every case must be studied, balancing the advantages of osseointegrated prostheses against conventional ones. A longitudinal study is presented on clinical cases in which the application of osseointegrated implants improve the prosthodontic treatment.

Ridge Mapping and Alveolar Bone Disjunction

G. Sales

A technique for the preoperative evaluation of alveolar ridge shape is described. In those patients who have narrow buccolingual ridges, the ridges can be expanded to allow future fixture location by the disjunction of buccal and lingual compact plates and the placement of bone graft in between. This easy procedure can also be used for unesthetic bone collapses prior to fixed restorations.

Treatment of Intraosseous Peri-implant Defects

S.A. Jovanovic

The present study was designed to evaluate a technique that arrests progressive peri-implant bone loss and which regenerates intraosseous defects. Eleven patients, ranging in age from 32 to 72 years, presented with intrabony defects around seven TPS (Straumann Ltd, Freiburg-Umkirch, Germany) implants and 13 IMZ (Friedrichsfeld, GmbH, Mannheim, Germany) implants. The implants had an average lifetime of 5 years. Probing depth (PD), plaque index (PI), papilla bleeding index (PBI), gingival index (GI), implant mobility, radiographic bone loss, bone defect dimensions, and occlusal scheme were measured at the beginning of the study.

The therapeutic intervention consisted of occlusal equilibration and/or a surgical approach depending on the etiology of the defect and the topography of the bone defect. The surgical intervention included flap management, implant surface treatment, and resorbable membrane technique. Patients were clinically evaluated at baseline, 3, 6, 9, and 12 months. The topography of bony defects in this group could be divided into four classes based on the measured dimensions. The average initial PD was 7.4 mm; 12 months later it was an average of 3.1; GI, PI, and PBI reduced respectively from 2.8, 1.8, and 2.6 to 0.3, 0.5, and 0.6. Implant mobility and radiographic examination remained stable during the course of the study. Radiographic comparison of baseline and 12-month radiographs in four sites treated with a membrane technique demonstrated bone regenerative capacity.

This clinical study suggests that the use of the presented therapeutic interventions in peri-implantitis sites can arrest progressive bone loss and that the membrane technique holds promise for regeneration of peri-implant bone defects.

Surgical Aspects of Nasal and Nasofacial Prostheses: A Report of Two Cases

O.T. Jensen

Attachment of the nasal prosthesis may be best obtained by using noncraniofacial fixtures placed in areas of available bone. The areas available for placement of fixtures in the nasofacial area are: (1) maxilla through the nasal fossae, (2) the maxillary buttress, (3) the zygomatic bone, (4) the infraorbital rim, and (5) the facial maxillary alveolar process. With the exception of the infraorbital rim, regular dental fixtures can be used.

Two cases are reported using osseointegrated implants that retain nasofacial prostheses. Preferred implant placement locations and angulations are discussed with regard to surgical findings, surgical guide splints, and muscles of facial expression.

In case no. 1, an alar cinch and septoplasty and skin graft were performed to restore about a 60% loss of the nose due to squamous cell carcinoma. In case no. 2, long-term adenocystic carcinoma of the maxilla and nose was treated by total rhinectomy, 90% total maxillectomy, removal of the entire upper lip and right and left cheek areas. Immediate placement of osseointegrating implants was done in the zygoma and zygomatic buttress areas. In both cases, successful prosthetic management was accomplished using the integrated fixtures, which were uncovered and loaded 6 months after initial implant placement.

Resilient Ball and Socket Attachment Design for Implant Overdenture Prostheses

C.L. Brownd

A variety of prosthetic attachments have been used with implant prostheses and overdentures. Different designs distribute masticatory forces to the abutments with varying loads. Most mechanical attachments offer inadequate long-term stress breaking for distal extension situations. They may be technically difficult to fabricate and maintain.

A simple, resilient "ball-and-socket" attachment design is described. It minimizes torque and occlusal loading on abutments. Indications and contraindications, technique, materials, and maintenance are discussed. An ongoing clinical study of up to 4 years on over 40 implant patients is documented.

The "ball" portion of the attachment is cast in gold alloy. It is shaped similar to a Hader bar for multiple abutments, or ball-shaped for freestanding abutments.

The "socket" portion of the attachment consists of a 2- to 4-mm layer of "Molloplast B" (Regneri GmbH & Co KG, Karlsruhe, Germany) resilient denture liner processed into the overdenture base. The resilient liner snaps over the contours of the bar or balls to engage the undercuts.

This technique provides a simple resilient attachment for use with distal extension implant overdentures, weak abutments, unfavorable occlusal situations, and maxillofacial prostheses.

Clinical Study of Hydroxyapatite in Minor Jawbone Defect

R.M. Hebballi

The replacement of diseased, destroyed, or degenerative tissue consumes time and financial resources from a large segment of the surgical community, both in medicine and dentistry. During the last 20 years, specialty science devoted much research to finding a material suitable for the replacement of lost and worn parts. Such materials are called biomaterials. Among them, hydroxyapatite (a ceramic) has come into widespread use for various clinical applications in dentistry.

The purpose of this study was to determine the clinical efficacy of synthetic nonporous hydroxyapatite graft material (Orthomatrix HA, 500 and 1000) in various minor bony defects such as intrabony periodontal defects and alveolar bony defects. It was also used for esthetic contouring of the ridge under a pontic area. Followup of cases is encouraging over 6 months. This clinical study suggested the material was well tolerated by the hard and soft tissues of the mouth and jaws and offers potential for its future use.

Implant Design Selection Based on Cortical Bone Quality and Location

G.A. Niznick

Osseointegration has been demonstrated with a variety of cylindrical implant designs and materials. Its achievement on a highly consistent basis is primarily dependent on three factors:

1. Preparation of the receptor site without overheating the bone
2. Insertion of the implant to achieve initial fixation and congruency
3. Avoidance of load on the implant for an initial 3 to 6 months healing period

The design of the implant dictates the surgical protocol and the surgical protocol determines the ability to achieve immediate fixation of the implant in vital bone.

A "system of systems" approach is based on optimizing the success by selecting the appropriate material, design, diameter, and surgical protocol based on differences in ridge height and width, as well as differences in density of trabecular bone and location of cortical bone.

Two of the variables in achieving osseointegration—avoiding overheating and premature loading—can be well controlled. The third factor, achieving initial fixation, is related directly to the selection of the appropriate design length and diameter of implant to engage cortical bone.

Variations in density of trabecular pattern have been referred to as "bone quality" by Brånemark et al (*Tissue-Integrated Prostheses: Osseointegration in Clinical Denistry*, Chicago: Quintessence Publ Co, 1985) and suggested as a guide to predicting implant success. The location, quality, and thickness of cortical bone is a more significant factor in implant selection. Initial stability (needed to achieve osseointegration) and resistance to functional forces (needed to maintain osseointegration) may be achieved if cortical bone can be engaged by the threads of the implant. Selection of implant design and material for optimum success requires consideration of anatomical location of implant placement since this frequently determines where the cortical bone can be found. Four zones can be clearly delineated using the parameters of location, thickness, and density of cortical bone. Implant designs will be suggested for these zones, which should maximize the opportunity for engagement of cortical bone and increase the potential for more consistent success.

Locations and quality of cortical bone/implant design recommendations are:

Zone 1. Anterior mandible/implant: screw

threaded to apex. Buccal and lingual—thick and dense. Inferior border—thick and dense.

Zone 2. Posterior mandible/implant: basket with lateral threads. Buccal and lingual—thin but dense.

Zone 3. Anterior maxilla/implant: cylinder with apical threads. Buccal and lingual—thin but dense. Floor of nasal cavity—dense, of varied thickness.

Zone 4. Posterior maxilla/implant: cylinder with apical threads. Buccal and lingual—thin and porous. Floor of sinus—thin, dense if palate engaged.

Comparative Study of Hydroxyapatite and Titanium Dental Implants

M. Kohri

This study examined the histological response to hydroxyapatite-coated IMZ (HA-IMZ), Apaceram (AC), Osseodent (OD), and Nobelpharma (NP) mandibular implants in dogs. The HA-IMZ is a pure titanium implant cylinder with a plasma flame-sprayed hydroxyapatite coating. The AC is a clinical implant with its surface consisting of dense hydroxyapatite. The OD and the NP are threaded titanium implants. Four months after implantation, the specimens were fixed and embedded in methyl methacrylate. Light microscopic analysis demonstrated osteogenic ingrowth to the surface of both hydroxyapatite (the HA-IMZ and the AC) and titanium implants (the OD and the NP). For the HA-IMZ and the AC, isolated hydroxyapatite particles were occasionally observed in the bone marrow separated from the implant surface. High magnification scanning electron micrographs of plastic sections revealed that the bone/implant interface showed no gap for the HA-IMZ nor the AC, whereas gaps were observed at the interface with the OD and the NP. Although the histological differences between hydroxyapatite and titanium implants were ob-

served, the results of this study indicate a good biological base for the clinical application of both implants.

Surgical Templates for Placement of Osseointegrated Implants

P.W. Cowan

Since the introduction of osseointegrated implants by Brånemark, much has been learned regarding the importance of optimum positioning of oral fixtures. Not only does this result in improved esthetics, it also allows more axially directed loads to be applied to the fixtures when the superstructure is completed. This will ultimately lead to long-term stability and health of the supporting tissues. Therefore, a great deal of care needs to be taken preoperatively in planning the best sites and angulations for the fixtures. Diagnostic aids including mounted study casts, diagnostic wax-ups, radiographs, and computerized tomography provide information about potential sites. However, this information needs to be translated via some form of guide to the surgeon for use during the surgical template, which in essence is a summary of all the diagnostic procedures previously performed. This presentation deals with the construction of two types of templates—the "same arch" and "opposing arch" templates—and their clinical use in a variety of situations.

Alternative Suturing Technique for Flap Closure

D. Harris

The classical technique for exposing the jawbone when placing Brånemark implants (Nobelpharma AB, Göteborg, Sweden) in fully edentulous patients requires that the incision be made in the labial sulcus anterior to the edentulous ridge. This approach allows a lingually based mucoperiosteal flap to be raised that will give excellent access to the operative site. It also allows clear identification of associated anatomical features and permits good apposition of the periosteum and mucosal tissue layers, thus providing a hermetic seal for the underlying fixtures.

Closure is usually carried out with vertical mattress sutures using a monofilament nonresorbable material inserted through the periosteum and mucous membrane. Such sutures are of necessity tight and can cause considerable discomfort during their subsequent removal. In addition, "bunching" of the tissues in the incision line can leave a hyperplastic scar.

A technique of closing the incision in layers using resorbable sutures for the periosteum and monofilament for the mucosa is described. This technique allows accurate apposition of tissues without tension. It eliminates scarring and greatly reduces patient discomfort postoperatively and on removal of sutures. Results in 80 cases are reported.

PTFE (Polytetrafluoroethylene) Membranes for Guided Bone Regeneration with Brånemark Implants
T.A. Collins

Artificial membranes have been used to guide bone regeneration in crestal and lateral cortical defects and over exposed threads of titanium endosseous implants. Such techniques have been employed with and without demineralized freeze-dried bone or nondemineralized freeze-dried bone.

Use of such membranes is most successful when relaxed primary closure of the overlying tissue is accomplished. Failure of bone regener-ation or risk of infection can occur with immediate or delayed exposure of the membrane.

Potential Referrals for Extraoral Implants
M. Deadman

The introduction of skin-penetrating bone-anchored osseointegrated implants to retain facial prostheses has implications for any service providing craniofacial reconstruction. Our own unit has seen an increase in referrals for prosthetic facial rehabilitation since using this technique.

The Birmingham Unit (Birmingham, England) has had 133 patients referred, over a period of 25 months, with a variety of congenital and acquired facial anomalies. Of these, 121 have now been assessed for possible inclusion in the implant program.

Of the 99 patients requiring facial prostheses, 65 had never before had a prosthesis. Fourteen patients had existing prostheses, while an additional 20 had been offered prostheses previously but had declined them.

Nine patients with Treacher-Collins syndrome were accepted for implant-retained auricular prostheses. Of these, two had had previous orthognathic surgery and seven required orthognathic surgery. However, two of these seven patients declined orthognathic surgery while accepting implantation. An additional three nonsyndromic patients required orthognathic surgery.

When establishing a facial prosthetic service incorporating the use of osseointegrated implants, consideration should be given to the likely increase in patient referrals, many of whom will have had no previous prosthetic rehabilitation. Some of these patients will also require orthognathic surgery and therefore close collaboration must exist with surgeons undertaking this surgery.

The Periotest Method in Osseointegrated Rehabilitation: A Useful Tool for Prosthetic Management

J. Olivé

Previous investigations have shown that the Periotest (Siemens AG, Bensheim, Germany), because of its quantitative and reproducible attributes, permits objective clinical control of bone stability in relation to implant anchorage. The Periotest measurements help the clinician detect early failing implants before building the prosthesis, thus avoiding modifications or unnecessary repetition, and above all, allow the identification of those implants where osseointegration is not completed, reducing the risk of an early load-related failure. This report describes how the Periotest is useful in individualizing the duration of the unloaded period and in deciding the prosthetic design.

Comparative Surface Microanalysis of Failed Brånemark Implants

C. Aparicio

The chemical composition and topography of the implant surface are important in order to understand why the human immunological system responds with different interphases to different materials. This presentation includes a comparative study of the surfaces of 16 Brånemark oral implants (Nobelpharma AB, Göteborg, Sweden), 11 of which came from retrieved samples that did not achieve or that failed osseointegration, and five control samples that were never implanted. The period of implantation in the human maxilla varied between 2 and 22 months. After cleaning and sterilization, the topography, surface chemical composition, and thickness of the oxide layer were studied. The results obtained with scanning electron microscopy did not detect any significant topographical differences among the samples. Radiographs and spectrographic microanalysis showed very similar composition, titanium and amounts smaller than 0.5% of other elements, in the outermost micron layer of the analyzed samples. The Auger spectroscope revealed, in the last monolayers, greater oxide thickness in accordance with the history of the samples and found considerable percentage differences in the amount of carbon and silicon which could be attributed to handling. This places the extracted samples out of the acceptable statistical limits of contamination that were established for the reference surface by long-term clinical studies.

A Comparison of Hydroxyapatite-Coated and Titanium-Sprayed Implants in Fresh Extraction Sites in Dogs

T.L. West

Numerous clinicians and implant manufacturers currently recommend the placement of dental implants into fresh extraction sites. Various bone substitutes are usually packed into the voids around the implant. Clinical observations of good short-term results seem to be encouraging. Although there are extensive human and animal data concerning the placement of dental implants into the healed edentulous maxilla and mandible, little histologic data are available concerning implant placement in the fresh extraction site.

This study attempts to quantify the exact amount of bone and soft tissue present at the tissue/implant interface for 14 hydroxyapatite-coated (HA) and 14 titanium plasma-sprayed (TPS) implants. All 28 implants were placed into the fresh premolar extraction sites of three elderly, periodontally diseased beagle dogs. Porous HA granules were packed into the voids around the implants. Eight maxillary (four HA and four TPS) and 20 mandibular (10 HA and 10 TPS) implants were initially placed and completely covered with soft tissue. All 28 were clinically immobile at the time of sacrifice (6 months). Four of the eight maxillary implants had perforated the nasal cavity but were firm. Two of the 20 mandibular implants showed soft tissue exposure of their cover screws but were also clinically firm. Vascular perfusion with refined India ink was performed at the time of sacrifice.

Histomorphometry was performed by computer on backscatter scanning electron photomicrographs of undemineralized, methyl methacrylate-embedded, cut and ground sections. The sections were cut in both buccolingual and anteroposterior planes. Shallow surface staining with McNeal's stain was performed to examine cell morphology. The stain was then removed and the sections cleared (Spaltheholtz method) to examine the healed vasculature around the implants.

Use of Three-Dimensional Dental Imaging for Treatment Planning of Implant Receptor Sites

R.A. Kraut

Preoperative planning is an essential aspect of any surgical procedure, especially when endosteal implant placement is contemplated. Conventional methods of assessing implant placement sites include clinical examination, mounted diagnostic casts, and periapical, panographic, or cephalometric radiographs. Three-dimensional imaging that has only recently become available allows the surgeon to visualize the implant receptor site in three dimensions, relative to adjacent vital structures. This new modality is particularly useful when planning for the placement of endosteal implants in the maxilla or posterior to the mental foramen in the mandible.

Selected cases illustrating the use of standardized scan protocols that resulted in the ability to plan implant placement in the maxilla and posterior portion of the mandible are presented. Postoperative radiographs are used to demonstrate the accuracy of this treatment planning modality.

A case presentation involving an implant-supported prosthesis in a 30-year-old patient is used to illustrate the importance of being able to visualize structure in three dimensions. The patient was involved in a motor vehicle accident during which he avulsed his maxilla, nasal septum, and vomer. Following autogenous bone grafting to the posterior wall of the antra, three-dimensional imaging allowed for planned placement of endosteal implants. The use of this imaging modality facilitates the safe placement of implants without violation of adjacent vital structures.

Maxillary Denture Retention Utilizing Magnets with IMZ Implants

R.A. Kraut

Twelve patients with existing maxillary dentures participated in a study to determine if denture retention and subsequent patient satisfaction could be improved with the use of IMZ implants (Friedrichsfeld GmbH, Mannheim, Germany) supporting rare earth magnets. A preliminary measurement of the force necessary to break the retentive seal for each patient's denture was obtained using a strain gauge. IMZ plasma-sprayed implants were then placed bilaterally in the maxillary canine area in each patient. Four to 6 months later, following integration of the implants, intramobile and magnet keeper screws were inserted during second-stage surgery. That same day, regular Jackson magnets were inserted in each patient's original dentures and a second measurement of the force necessary to break the retention seal was obtained.

Two months after the magnets had been inserted in each patient's denture, they were asked to complete a survey designed to ascertain whether attitudinal change with regard to denture wear had occurred.

Patient satisfaction with maxillary prostheses can be improved with the use of IMZ implants supporting rare earth magnets.

Proposal for Future Treatment of the Completely Edentulous Patient

W.D. Gates

Rehabilitation of the completely edentulous patient with an implant-supported mandibular prosthesis opposing a conventional denture has become a common treatment modality. The long-term success rates of the Brånemark System (Nobelpharma USA, Chicago, Ill) osseointegrated implant has been well documented.

However, there is a paucity of literature related to the effect of this treatment on the maxillary complete denture and supporting structures. In an ongoing investigation at the University of Iowa of 84 patients treated with the Brånemark System between 1983 and 1988, 48 patients have been restored in this manner. A preliminary survey of 22 of these 48 patients has been made to ascertain any changes in their perception of the success of their prostheses before and after placement of the implants. With increasing time after prosthetic rehabilitation there may be a decrease in the satisfaction with the maxillary denture. Preemptive treatment may be necessary to achieve greater overall long-term patient satisfaction and protect the maxilla from potential detrimental physiologic changes caused by increased masticatory force and stability provided by the mandibular implant-supported prosthesis. Based on the success of natural tooth-supported overdentures, implant-supported overdentures may provide this added stability to the maxillary denture and protect the maxilla without the complications associated with the natural dentition.

Consensus Panel Reports

Basic Science Consensus Panel

John B. Brunski, Chair
Robert E. Baier, Vice-Chair
Robert E. Pilliar, Secretary

The task of the Basic Science Consensus Panel was to address reliably reported and sufficiently verified evidence developed over the last 5 years for implants capable of tissue integration without limitation to any particular system in use today or to any particular part of the human body. Research in oral and craniofacial reconstruction demonstrates the preference for rigidly fixed alloplastic implants. However, tissue integration consisting of sufficiently intimate approximation of the biological components to the synthetic components such that clinical function is fulfilled and retained indefinitely, may also be met by implants of other types in nonosseous sites. Respecting the statutory task of various regulatory agencies to set minimally acceptable standards for any (including tissue-integrated) implants and implant systems, and to define appropriate methods to judge and report evidence of compliance with such standards, the Panel records its agreement with establishment of government standards for oral and craniofacial implants.

Implant materials

All currently accepted implant materials were considered in the previous Consensus Report as a priori candidates for attaining tissue integration. Based on scientific literature concerned with oral and craniofacial implants in humans during the past 5 years, reference has been made to the following specific materials as being most suitable for oral and craniofacial implant applications; commercial purity titanium (cpTi), hydroxyapatite, and aluminum oxide ceramics. This limited list is based on demonstrated acceptance in vivo of these materials. However, it is not intended to exclude other materials such as frequently employed orthopedic alloys that might be demonstrated to be suitable through future studies.

It is important to characterize fully the bulk and surface properties of implant materials. The raw material for a device should meet initial specifications, but it is also necessary to verify the nature of the bulk material and surface properties in the final form of the device. Proper characterization of bulk and surface properties of candidate materials for implant fabrication using state-of-the-art analysis techniques could reveal the introduction of unintended impurities that could adversely affect tissue response and overall implant performance. The equipment for such analyses is currently sufficient to allow the required degree of quality control for material selection by all reputable manufacturers. Greater awareness of the importance of proper and complete material characterization is required by all. In particular, an emphasis on matching the elasticity of implant material and bone has not been demonstrated to be as important as once thought.

Coatings

The area of coatings represents a special case for material selection and use. The increasing use of ceramic coatings onto metal substrata and particularly plasma-sprayed hydroxyapatite or titanium coatings onto titanium, Ti-6Al-4V, or other metal substrata (cast CoCrMo frames for subperiosteal applications) requires that due consideration be given to the characterization of the coating per se and the coating/substratum interface. There is a recognition of the fact that premature failure of the ceramic coating/metal interface can occur; the clinical significance of such failures is not yet known. A need exists to define appropriate test methods for reliably assessing the mechanical characteristics of this interface. In addition, the placement of a coating must not result in unacceptable alteration of the substratum material properties, including mechanical and chemical characteristics (eg, loss in fatigue strength or increased susceptibility to high rates of corrosion).

Implant surface properties

It is generally recognized that surface properties of materials cannot be predicted from their bulk properties, particularly when there will be numerous subsequent treatment steps—including cleaning, sterilization, and packaging—following their initial fabrication into devices. Although the Panel can give no universal definition of what is a "clean" or "optimal" surface state for a specific implant system, it is a basic standard of good biomaterials practice to perform specific measurements to establish the surface properties of materials in their sterile, about-to-be-implanted states prior to any in vitro (eg, cell culture) or in vivo (animal or human implantation) placement. In the absence of secure and documented knowledge of the surface properties of an implant, interpretation of either favorable or unfavorable results will be necessarily ambiguous since even a monolayer of contaminants from any source can completely change the biological reactivity of an implant. At a minimum, final implant surface qualities should be very well defined and reproducible. Conventional means of sterilization, including steam autoclave treatment, are often seen to be processes that add surface contaminants of their own while also leaving behind the sterile residues of microorganisms and other debris. Care should be taken to avoid these residues, where possible, since even sterile organic deposits can change biological responses (diminish adhesion, induce pyrogenicity) to generically inorganic materials.

In this regard, there is an increasing store of reliable evidence that intrinsically low surface energy materials (eg, expanded polytetrafluoroethylene membranes) can be used as minimally adhesive barrier films to separate, during wound healing, cell populations that differ in their potential to differentiate. Those cells capable of forming bone, for example, can be given a selected advantage in repopulating regions of an implant that are to be osseointegrated. Another means of influencing cell behavior is to provide surface textural cues (eg, grooves of various geometries or orientations) to influence cell migration and orientation. This phenomenon, referred to as contact guidance, probably proceeds to some degree on all practical implanted materials with some surface roughness and/or machining marks. Thus, it becomes increasingly critical to better define, specify, and control surface textural features of implants again in their final, sterile states. An important analytical detail is to ascertain how the process utilized for surface textural modification modifies the surface chemical properties of the materials at the same time.

Implant design and biomechanics

A number of factors contribute to the biomechanical performance of oral and craniofacial implants. Progress has been made on a number of fronts since the last International Congress toward a better understanding of these factors.

First, experimental data are now available concerning the general range of vertically directed biting forces in patients having various types of implant-supported prostheses. However, the actual force components transmitted to the implants are not known with certainty. Theoretical models are available to help predict these components, but these models have not yet been verified in vivo.

Second, evidence has been accumulated about those factors that are most important in determining loadings on implants. These include biting loads on the prosthesis, design of the restoration, details of the connections between prosthesis and implant, the number of implants supporting the prosthesis and their angulation. Nevertheless, a completely quantitative understanding of the role of each factor has not yet been provided. Notably, for the case of implants that are meant to support craniofacial prostheses of various types, the loadings on the implants are not yet known.

Third, a growing body of data has been developed on the details of stress transfer at the bone/implant interface. Models for evaluating interfacial stress transfer demonstrate that stress transfer will depend on: loads on the implant, superstructure connections and shape, implant shape, the nature of attachment between implant and bone (or the lack thereof), and the quantity and quality of bone surrounding the implant. Functional bone deformation in either jaw may also cause stresses at the inter-

face. It has been hypothesized that unfavorable stress conditions can develop around some implants, in turn causing bone loss, while in other cases, depending on the stress transfer conditions, there may be bone accretion around implants, or at least a lessening of bone loss, for example, as in the proposed use of implants to preserve height of the edentulous alveolar ridge, or in the use of implants to avoid collapse of tooth alveoli after extractions.

Fourth, there is a consensus that implant stability in the healing wound site (ie, lack of "micromotion") is of paramount importance in permitting bone healing. Also, there is a growing awareness of a need to more fully understand oral and craniofacial bone modeling and remodeling in relation to implants.

Fifth, concerning methods for attaching implants to bone through the use of various surface coatings, there is a need to continue to develop accurate methods for documenting the qualities of such coatings. There is no consensus on a single way to achieve such attachment; indeed a number of macro- and microinterlocking surface textures have been successfully employed as fixation rationales.

Host factors involved in tissue integration

The circumstances prevailing at both sides of the potential implant-host site interface are of utmost importance from the instant of first contact of the biological and synthetic materials and for the remainder of the functional lifetime of the combined system. It is now recognized that the interface is continuously subjected to a dynamic process of remodeling, even at the biomacromolecular scale, with possible reciprocal exchanges of (at least trace) components between the two adjacent phases. During implant placement and thereafter, it remains critical to create and sustain conditions that allow responding cells to maintain tissue building and remodeling capabilities. Although it is now quite clear that implants capable of inducing and sustaining good mammalian cellular approximation are also capable of colonization by oral microflora, such microbial deposits infrequently lead to soft tissue dehiscence, inflammation, or implant loss. It is a tenet of good implant maintenance, however, that routine attention be given to controlling the hygienic qualities of the peri-implant region. This strategy would avoid the possibility of secondary problems associated with the successful restoration of either edentulous or partially edentulous patients. There is clinical followup indicating that skin-penetrating implants in craniofacial applications can be maintained without adverse reactions.

Studies reported during the last 5 years have shown that bone grafts and fresh extraction sites represent acceptable environments for implant placement. It has also been shown that irradiation of bone results in tissue less prone to integration, and therefore placement into irradiated bone should be done cautiously. Given the well-attested use of hyperbaric oxygen for treatment of osteoradionecrosis of the jaw, this might be used as an adjunct to improve the likelihood of osseointegration.

Preliminary research indicates that sensory input changes associated with oral implant abutments appear to influence masticatory cycles, voluntary muscle activity, and occlusal perception. The oral physiological response to implant-supported prostheses deserves extensive study.

Panel Members:
Michael S. Block
Donald M. Brunette
H. David Hall
Bernd d'Hoedt
Magnus Jacobsson
Paul H.J. Krogh
Jukka Lausmaa
Peter K. Moy
Bo Rangert
Heiner Weber
George A. Zarb

Craniofacial Consensus Panel

Patrick J. Henry, Chair
Anders Tjellstrom, Vice-Chair
John Beumer, III, Secretary

Tissue-integrated prostheses provide an important treatment option for individuals suffering from congenital, traumatic, and surgical defects of the craniofacial region. While some defects can be autogenously reconstructed, thus eliminating the need for prosthetic treatment, many defects can only be rehabilitated by conventional prosthetic means. Some are best treated by bone-anchored prostheses.

This modality of treatment should not be undertaken unless essential members of a multidisciplinary team are available including expertise in surgical oncology, oral and maxillofacial reconstructive surgery, prosthetic rehabilitation, and other allied specialties. Success is dependent on proper coordination of all aspects of diagnosis and treatment, and accordingly, it is mandatory that a treatment coordinator fulfill this definitive role, to ensure that all short- and long-term aspects of treatment are met.

Careful planning and coordination between team members needs to be carried out if predictable and effective results are to be achieved in the treatment of these complex defects.

Minimal acceptable standards for clinical use

The use of osseointegrated reconstruction should be based on long-term clinical trials with specific patient selection criteria. The criteria for success rates are complex and have not yet been clearly defined, and they may be site-specific under some circumstances. At the present time there is insufficient data to establish universal guidelines.

The following conditions predisposing to unknown risk factors are evidence of recurrent or residual tumor; history of previous radiation therapy; diabetes, collagen, vascular disease, or AIDS; psychiatric disorders; and unpredictability of patient compliance. Care must be individualized to meet the specific needs of the patient.

Support and load distribution

The loads implants are required to bear in craniofacial defects vary tremendously. In extraoral sites the implants are exposed to minimal loads and generally the load is dependent upon the weight of the prosthesis. Occasionally, however, the implants may be exposed to lateral torquing forces when the prosthesis engages mobile tissue or when used directly or indirectly to retain or support an intraoral prosthesis.

For an auricular prosthesis, two implants are usually sufficient to support the prosthesis. In addition, since the failure rate is so low at this site, extra implants are generally not necessary to ensure against the loss of one fixture. Similarly, in the orbit, two fixtures are usually sufficient to retain a prosthesis used to restore a conventional orbital exenteration defect. Implant success in the orbital region has also proven to be successful in irradiated tissues. The number of implants required may vary according to the defect and regional anatomy.

In most rhinectomy defects, two implants appear to be sufficient to retain a nasal prosthesis. However, insufficient data are available with regard to this site. The rate of loss may be higher than the previous sites described because of the difficulty encountered in gaining access to some of the desirable bone sites with the available instrumentation. In addition, thick tissue in this region may cause difficulty with the long-term maintenance of healthy soft tissue. Consequently, the use of split-thickness skin grafts used to cover raw tissue surfaces at the time of tumor resection (for example, the exposed portion of the floor of the nose) may facilitate the placement of implants at a later date.

In the edentulous radical maxillectomy defect, clinicians are just now beginning to use osseointegrated implants to retain and support maxillary obturator prostheses. The magnitude and nature of the loads brought to bear on the implants in this setting have yet to be determined. The number and positioning of implants necessary to support these restorations will vary according to defect anatomy and the residual skeletal structures. Therefore, maximizing the number of implants placed in these patients will ensure adequate therapeutic reserve.

Likewise in edentulous mandibular continuity defects, little attention has been devoted to determine the required number or positioning of implants necessary to retain and support a mandibular resection prosthesis.

Bone grafting

Bone grafting in the craniofacial region, either simultaneous with implant placement or as a preliminary procedure, may be indicated to restore anatomic continuity, to restore anatomic and cosmetic contour, and to provide sufficient bone for initial implant stability and successful osseointegration. Bone grafting can be carried out at any age. Revascularization and remodeling may take longer in some older patients and in individuals with systemic disease. The younger the age of the patient, the greater may be the healing and osteogenic potential of grafted bone.

Either free or vascularized grafts can be considered in external continuity defects of the craniofacial skeleton. However, no long-term data exist as to success rate, load performance, or treatment requirement.

Long-term concerns

The primary concern has been focused on the risk of potential short- or long-term reaction in bone. There has been no clinical or histological evidence of osteitis even in situations where adverse soft tissue reactions have been noted in more than 10 years of followup.

The possibilities of establishing and maintaining osseointegration in the cortex of the temporal bone are very good. However, in the radiated orbit, implant success rate may be low. With this factor in mind additional implants may need to be placed. No increased frequency of skin reactions is found over time. A limited number of patients are responsible for a majority of the adverse skin reactions. The key factors to avoiding adverse skin reactions include good hygiene, absence of mobility of the skin around the implant, adequate spacing between the implants, and lack of hair follicles at the skin penetration site.

The same low frequency of significant skin reaction is noted in the orbital as in the mastoid region. To date, no difference has been reported concerning the skin reaction in radiated skin as compared to nonradiated skin.

There is still insufficient data available concerning the midfacial region. Currently, there have been no reports of neoplastic change in the tissue around abutments and no signs of allergic reaction to commercially pure titanium implants.

Altered health status

The placement of implants in the craniofacial region is generally a minor surgical operation conducted under local anesthesia as an outpatient procedure. Age is not considered a contraindication. Although systemic conditions such as diabetes or psoriasis are not necessarily a contraindication, placement of implants in such patients should be undertaken with caution. In individuals treated with cytotoxic drugs, wound healing is compromised, and patients with these types of potential risk factors should be followed carefully.

Because personal hygiene around percutaneous implants is extremely important, use of these implants in patients who may be noncompliant can be considered a relative contraindication.

Radiation considerations

Tissue exposed to cancercidal doses of radiation becomes compromised. Osseointegration may therefore be impaired under such circumstances. At extraoral sites the initial data seem to indicate a reduced percentage of implants achieving integration, particularly in the orbital region. There is no evidence of increased skin reactions around implants in irradiated tissues.

The use of implants in heavily irradiated jaws should be considered with caution. The clinical data are short term, with insufficient numbers of patients reported; thus, few conclusions can be drawn from it. The benefit of hyperbaric oxygen in irradiated tissues has yet to be determined, although it is a clinically promising modality.

Financial costs

The cost of the prosthesis and the expense of ongoing replacement usually represent the costly part of treatment. This well-documented problem of long-term costs of care would be greatly reduced if existing techniques for construction and coloration could be improved. However, this will require significant commitments by both research and industrial interests if the problem is to be resolved. Furthermore, health insurance carriers must understand that this area of treatment should receive appropriate insurance coverage to make it possible for more people. Accordingly, to this end, data need to be collected on the efficacy of bone-anchored craniofacial prostheses. These data should include parameters such as retention security, long-term esthetics, ease of patient handling, and comfort and maintenance. The psychosocial effects and cost benefit ramifications must also be considered in the overall assessment of comparative treatment options.

Other considerations

Based on well-documented success in the temporal bone using the two-stage procedure, clinical trials have begun to evaluate whether implant placement and skin penetration procedures can be performed simultaneously. Preliminary data are promising but a longer followup time is needed before this modified procedure can be evaluated.

Lower profile instruments are often needed in patients with orbital and nasal defects. Abutments that could be placed at different angles relative to the direction of the implants are needed, especially in midfacial and orbital midface defects. Sterilizable handpieces would be a useful adjunct. Improved hygiene instrumentation for patient usage and devices for facilitating soft tissue seating would be helpful.

Perfectly placed and osseointegrated implants, by themselves, do not provide facial rehabilitation. The facial prosthesis retained by the anchorage system must be of equally excellent quality, and is dependent upon adequate surgical attention to the preparation of the defect for prosthetic purposes.

A number of specific patient needs in oral and maxillofacial reconstruction have yet to be properly addressed. In patients undergoing resection of portions of the maxilla and mandible for oral and paranasal sinus tumors, defects are created that cause significant functional disability and cosmetic deformity. In edentulous patients particularly, if the prosthesis is not well retained and supported, the quality of speech, mastication, etc, will be compromised.

Although osseointegrated implants may be of significant benefit for these patients, little investigation has been conducted, for example, to determine the feasibility of using onlay grafts in the partially resected maxilla. Furthermore, whether implants can be placed in beds that have been irradiated or are about to be irradiated, or whether it is feasible to place implants at the time of tumor resection is yet to be determined. In addition, the use of implants in mandibular continuity defects restored with either free autogenous bone grafts or free vascularized grafts needs more investigation.

With regard to extraoral defects, significant experiences with a number of defects, particularly using implants in the temporal bone, have been accumulated. However, further work is needed regarding the utilization of implants to restore orbital and rhinectomy defects.

It should be noted that only the osseointegrated implant method ad modum Brånemark has been adapted and tested specifically for tissue-integrated prosthetics in the treatment of craniofacial defects.

Summary

Bone-anchored craniofacial prosthetic techniques replace certain traditional prosthetic as well as autogenous reconstructive procedures. These techniques can be used safely with a high success rate in nonirradiated tissues and with a lower success rate in irradiated tissues. Patient satisfaction rates are very high and a significant effort to generate more data is ongoing.

Bone-anchored hearing devices

As some of the questions regarding implants used in craniofacial prosthetic rehabilitation are not relevant for implants used in hearing rehabilitation, these issues are addressed separately. The considerations for implant and abutment success discussed in the prosthetic section of this document are valid for bone-anchored implants for hearing amplification.

Candidates for this procedure are those patients with conductive or mixed hearing losses who are not candidates for conventional middle ear reconstructive techniques. Additionally, most patients utilizing bone-vibrating hearing aids may receive increased benefit from bone-anchored hearing amplification.

The minimal acceptable standard in hearing rehabilitation is complex and involves a combination of amplification, fidelity, comfort, cosmesis, etc. The total rehabilitative effect should be considered in light of these factors.

Sound amplification through bone conduction has been established by vibrating an implant in the mastoid cortex. This may be accomplished by transcutaneous or percutaneous stimulation. Both techniques appear to be efficacious in patients with a good cochlear reserve, while the percutaneous technique may be better in patients with a reduced cochlear reserve because of the decreased mechanical attenuation from overlying soft tissues.

Clinical experience with skin-penetrating implants utilized for anchoring bone-conducting hearing devices has been similar to the experience with implants utilized for retaining auricular prostheses. Long-term observations have demonstrated high rates of positional stability and low rates of adverse skin reactions.

Recent data indicate that bone-anchored hearing devices also offer enhanced hearing rehabilitation in postsurgical patients who previously used air-conducting hearing aids. Trials are currently under way addressing a one-stage implantation procedure for the temporal bone, a totally implanted hearing device, and direct electrical stimulation of the cochlea. The data will be evaluated after long-term followup of sufficient patient populations has been collected.

Panel Members:
Martin Deadman
Gilian Duncan
Elof Ericksson
Ann Fyler
Matthew B. Hall
Kenji M. Higuchi
G. Richard Holt
Guy Huré
Kerstin Jansson
William W. LaVelle
John K. Niparko
Stephen M. Parel
Thomas A. Taylor
Glen E. Turner

Orthopedic Consensus Panel

Harlan C. Amstutz, Chair
Edmund Y. S. Chao, Vice-Chair
Tomas Albrektsson, Secretary

The Panel agrees that tissue integration for orthopedic implants should achieve sufficiently intimate approximation of the biological components to the synthetic components so that clinical function is fulfilled and retained.

On the light microscopic level, osseointegration is a direct contact between living bone and implant and perhaps is ideal to optimize durability. A functioning biologically fixed prosthesis may or may not show osseointegration. Osseointegration is possible with a number of different biomaterials.

Osseointegration may be achieved in a one-stage surgery but not necessarily in all implant sites or for all applications. One-stage surgery may fail under certain circumstances. Once these circumstances are clearly defined, two-stage surgery might then be considered. Such circumstances include instances where there is inadequate bone stock or substance or where rigid fixation is difficult to achieve, such as the radial head, the ankle, the glenoid, and the proximal tibia and patella, and in limb salvage procedures dealing with segmental graft transplantation on prosthetic replacement.

The magnitude and time of the desired load applied to a system postoperatively is dependent upon the characteristics of the anatomical site, prosthetic design, and initial fixation. There is insufficient experimental or clinical data to predict the desired loads that may be applied to osseointegrated implants in orthopedic procedures. More information on interfacial stresses, however difficult to achieve, is needed in order to correlate with the histomorphometric and histological analyses.

There are insufficient data on the use of permanent skin-penetrating implants to allow conclusions on tissue integration in orthopedic applications.

There is insufficient knowledge at this time regarding the mechanism of osseointegration to say which health factors would adversely affect it. However, it would appear that osseointegration is possible in a wide spectrum of disease states. To determine these effects, we suggest prospective studies of implants in appropriate patient subgroups.

Since osseointegrated devices for orthopedic purposes should be designed to last the lifetime of the patient, it would be unwise to compromise on optimal implant design, technique, and rehabilitation. Any implantation expense will be considerably greater if revision is required. If revision surgery is necessary, reconstruction must be possible.

Irradiation may adversely affect the osseointegration if administered immediately before or after implant insertion. This response is dose and time related. If high energy irradiation is administered to already osseointegrated devices, this does not necessarily affect implant stability. In addition, some drugs, such as anti-inflammatory and immunosuppressive medication, may adversely affect the osseointegration process.

Panel Members:

Björn Albrektsson

Ed Berg

George Van B. Cochran

R. Tass Dueland

David S. Hungerford

Robin Sydney M. Ling

Göran Lundborg

R. Bruce Martin

Greg McNiece

Bernie F. Morrey

Indong Oh

Dale R. Sumner, Jr

Intraoral Consensus Panel

Daniel van Steenberghe, Chair
Eugene E. Keller, Vice-Chair
Leonard B. Shulman, Secretary

Successful implant rehabilitation implies the restoration and maintenance of the health and integrity of the stomatognathic system. It should fulfill patients' needs with respect to function, health, esthetics, and economic considerations.

Success criteria for individual implants include the following:

- Individual implants must be clinically immobile.
- No periimplant radiolucency should appear on intraoral radiographs.
- There should be an absence of persistent or recurrent pain or infection.
- There should be no significant damage to adjacent structures.
- The implant should be loadbearing during function and positioned so as to meet prosthetic needs.

Note: Significant progressive marginal bone loss that fails to stabilize could indicate a future failure.

Endosseous implants that rely on the presence of a direct bone interface that persists during long-term function appear to be more resistant to bone loss, infection, and progressive loosening than those relying on fibrous encapsulation.

The evaluation of an implant system should be related to those implant systems that are well documented. No significant morbidity should result from placement, function, failure, or retrieval. Documented success rates of individual implants in consecutive patients according to the aforementioned criteria are at least 95% after 5 years and 90% after 10 years for fixed reconstruction in the anterior mandible. Results in other locations vary, but are above 85% at 5 years. In assessing implant predictability, the continued use of raw percentage outcomes, unrelated to longevity of the individual implant, is counterproductive. Life table statistical methods must become the standard in the scientific documentation of implant benefit and risk.

Annual examination after the first year is recommended. It should include:

- Assessment of symptoms
- Clinical assessment of soft tissues
- Assessment of prosthesis stability
- Radiographs when clinical indications are present

Note: The prognostic value of periodontal indices around implants remains uncertain. Progressive loss of attachment measured from a fixed reference point is indicative of bone loss. Appropriate radiographs remain the most reliable method of monitoring bone height and status.

Patients' needs in oral and maxillofacial reconstruction that have not been comprehensively addressed include situations where there is insufficient jawbone volume in prosthodontically relevant locations and jawbone discontinuity. These circumstances may indicate the use of autologous bone grafts to facilitate the placement of endosseous implants. As with many augmentation techniques, the long-term results of these procedures are insufficiently documented. No definite answer can be offered to the question of minimal bone dimensions. Implant design, bone quality, the expected loading, and interface strength can all influence these minimal dimensions. Available data indicate that implants as short as 7 mm, completely embedded in favorable bone, can function satisfactorily.

Although documentation is limited, advanced age does not appear to be a contraindication for implant placement. On the other hand, until jaw growth and tooth eruption are completed, implant placement in the young needs a cautious approach and such patients should be treated where appropriate expertise and facilities for proper documentation and followup are available.

Few data are available on the impact of general health factors on the predictability of tissue integration. Uncontrolled endocrine and metabolic diseases affecting bone and soft tissue healing, immunological deficiencies, and radiotherapy can interfere with tissue integration.

Whether to use a resilient or nonresilient layer between the opposing occlusal surface and the implant/bone interface remains an open question.

Whether prostheses on implants should preferably be connected to natural teeth or remain freestanding is uncertain. However, it is recognized that specific clinical conditions may dictate a particular prosthetic protocol. Retrievability of the prosthesis is desirable.

Promising areas for future applications include:

- Anchorage for orthodontic purposes, including tooth movement and possible modification of craniofacial growth
- Inlay grafting techniques in maxillary cavities
- Interpositional grafting
- Composite grafting
- Implant placement in fresh extraction wounds
- Bone augmentation and regeneration by means of membrane techniques

Panel Members:
W. Howard Davis
Ronald P. Desjardins
David S. Harris
Torsten Jemt
Axel Kirsch
Yoshinori Kobayashi
Ulf Lekholm
Guillermo Raspall
Melvyn S. Schwarz
Richard Skalak
Philip Worthington

Concluding Remarks

W.R. Laney

During the course of this Congress, participants heard some 50 scientific paper presentations and viewed 18 poster presentations on various aspects of tissue-integrated prostheses supported by bone-anchored devices in the oral and craniofacial regions, as well as related orthopedic applications. While evidence of considerable progress over the past 2 to 3 decades has been reported, it is obvious that certain questions concerning the efficacy of this treatment modality beg more definitive answers. On behalf of the entire Organizing Committee, I thank all speakers, members of the Consensus Panels, poster clinicians, and back-up speakers for their most significant contributions, cooperation, and willingness to participate in the Congress.

This Second Congress, as did the First, had as its objectives: *(1)* the evaluation of basic scientific and clinical aspects of intra- and extraoral tissue-integrated prostheses, as well as orthopedic applications of the concept, through oral presentations; and *(2)* reporting of state-of-the-art consensus findings determined by expert panels continued from the First Congress.

At first glance, it would appear that the Congress objectives have been satisfied. However, beyond these limited goals and perhaps more importantly, this meeting has provided an opportunity for researchers, scientists, and clinicians from 23 countries and the Republic of Singapore to gather for an exchange of ideas, knowledge, and the results of therapeutic skills focused on the principles of tissue integration, which have survived and grown since their conception by Per-Ingvar Brånemark and colleagues. This and future conferences have already and will continue to contribute to the advancement of science in this field and enhance not only our mutual understanding of progressing treatment modalities and technology, but also the socioeconomic and human relations that so significantly impact our efforts to improve the health and welfare of humankind worldwide.